CLINICAL PEDIATRIC ANESTHESIA

SECOND EDITION

CLINICAL PEDIATRIC ANESTHESIA

A Case-Based Handbook

EDITED BY

ERIN S. WILLIAMS, MD, FAAP

Assistant Professor, Department of Anesthesiology, Perioperative and Pain Medicine
Assistant Director, Hematology-Oncology Sedation Service
Texas Children's Hospital
Baylor College of Medicine
Houston, Texas

OLUTOYIN A. OLUTOYE, MD, MSC

Professor, Department of Anesthesiology, Perioperative and Pain Medicine
Division Chief, General Anesthesiology
Director of Fetal Anesthesia
Vice-Chair for Faculty Development
Texas Children's Hospital
Baylor College of Medicine
Houston, Texas

CATHERINE P. SEIPEL, MD, FAAP

Assistant Professor, Department of Anesthesiology, Perioperative and Pain Medicine
Assistant Director, Procedure Suite Anesthesia
Texas Children's Hospital
Baylor College of Medicine
Houston, Texas

TITILOPEMI A. O. AINA, MD, MPH, FAAP

Assistant Professor, Department of Anesthesiology, Perioperative and Pain Medicine
Clerkship Director, Anesthesiology Medical Student Education
Texas Children's Hospital
Baylor College of Medicine
Houston, Texas

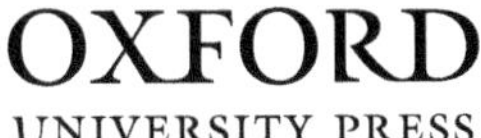

OXFORD
UNIVERSITY PRESS

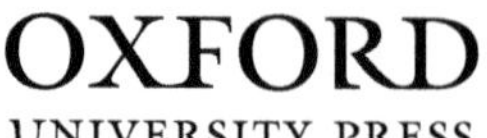

Oxford University Press is a department of the University of Oxford. It furthers the University's objective of excellence in research, scholarship, and education by publishing worldwide. Oxford is a registered trade mark of Oxford University Press in the UK and certain other countries.

Published in the United States of America by Oxford University Press
198 Madison Avenue, New York, NY 10016, United States of America.

CIP data is on file at the Library of Congress
ISBN 978– 0–19–067833–3

EW: To my Saviour, Jesus Christ. Thank you for this opportunity; and to the special people in my life, my husband, George, thank you for your amazing love; my children Eden, Emeri, and Gabriel, thank you for being my sunshine; my mother, Marilyn Barnes-Clay, thank you for teaching me to believe.

OO: To God, I give him ALL the glory, and to my loving husband, Yinka, and our children, Yinka Jr. and Tomi, thank you for your love, patience, and support.

CS: To my husband, Tim, and our son, Andrew, thank you for your steadfast love and the immeasurable joy you bring to life; and to my parents: thank you for your love and commitment to give us every opportunity possible.

TA: I am thankful to God for the opportunity to work on this book with such an amazing group of authors and co-editors. I want to especially thank my family for their tireless support and love, namely: Dr. and Mrs. J.O. Aina, Joke Babalola, Peju Aina, Bola Aina, Bimpe Dada, Paul Babalola, and my wonderful nephews (Dele, Tobi, Nate, Folarin, Dan, and Femi). I would not be here if it wasn't for all of you!

All: This book is dedicated to our patients—you teach, motivate, and inspire us each day.

CONTENTS

ACKNOWLEDGMENTS

Pediatric anesthesiology encompasses the care of the pediatric patient in the perioperative setting as well as in critical care settings; our field is ever changing given the advances in medicine, and though it may be challenging, the encounters with our patients make it most rewarding. Pediatric anesthesiologists have a duty to care for and protect the pediatric patient during perioperative care and beyond. However, it is in the day-to-day interactions with our patients and their families that we gain humility as well as inspiration; it is during these special times that we realize our "calling." Such inspiration also drives us to be the best. In pursuit of excellence we offer *Clinical Pediatric Anesthesia: A Case-Based Handbook*, 2nd edition, for the continued acquisition of knowledge in the field of pediatric anesthesiology.

This book has been an honor for us to complete, and it is with sincere hearts that we thank God for allowing us this opportunity. We could not have done any of this without the support of so many amazing people. It is with the sincerest thanks that we honor and acknowledge all of the previous editors: Dr. Kenneth Goldschneider, Dr. Andrew Davidson, Dr. Eric Wittkugel, and Dr. Adam Skinner. We also acknowledge the contributing authors from both the first edition as well as the second edition of *Clinical Pediatric Anesthesia: A Case-Based Handbook*, for their timely submissions and dedication to this project. To our families, we love you! Your love is patient, your love is kind, your love is what encourages us. We thank our department chair, Dr. Dean B. Andropoulos, for his support of this project. Finally, we thank Oxford University Press for entrusting us with this phenomenal task of continuing the sharing of knowledge in our field of pediatric anesthesiology. It has been our great pleasure to work with Andrea Knobloch and Allison Pratt in creating this book. We are so grateful for this opportunity, and it is our sincere hope that pediatric anesthesiologists everywhere will gain knowledge and provide even better care after reading this book. We hope you enjoy!

CONTRIBUTORS

Adam C. Adler, MD
Assistant Professor
Department of Anesthesiology, Preoperative and Pain Medicine
Baylor College of Medicine
Texas Children's Hospital
Houston, TX

Dean B. Andropoulos, MD, MHCM
Anesthesiologist-in-Chief, Texas Children's Hospital, Department of Anesthesiology, Perioperative and Pain Medicine
Professor, Anesthesiology and Pediatrics
Vice Chair for Clinical Affairs, Department of Anesthesiology Baylor College of Medicine
Houston, TX

Lori A. Aronson, MD
Associate Professor
Clinical Anesthesia & Pediatrics
Director of Liver Transplant Anesthesia
Cincinnati Children's Hospital
Cincinnati, OH

Rahul Baijal, MD
Associate Professor
Department of Anesthesiology, Perioperative, and Pain Medicine
Baylor College of Medicine
Texas Children's Hospital
Houston, TX

Anne C. Boat, MD
Staff Anesthesiologist
Associate Professor
Department of Anesthesia
Cincinnati Children's Hospital
Cincinnati, OH

Carlos J. Campos, MD
Associate Professor
Department of Anesthesiology, Perioperative, and Pain Medicine
Baylor College of Medicine
Texas Children's Hospital
Houston, TX

Lisa Caplan, MD
Assistant Professor
Department of Anesthesiology, Perioperative, and Pain Medicine
Baylor College of Medicine
Texas Children's Hospital
Houston, TX

Arvind Chandrakantan, MD, MBA, FAAP
Assistant Professor of Anesthesiology and Pediatrics
Baylor College of Medicine
Anesthesiologist
Texas Children's Hospital
Houston, TX

Rachel Chapman, MD
Consultant Anesthetist
The Royal Children's Hospital Melbourne
Melbourne, VIC

Kathleen Chen, MD, MS
Assistant Professor of Anesthesiology
Baylor College of Medicine
Anesthesiologist
Texas Children's Hospital
Houston, TX

Vidya Chidambaran, MD
Associate Professor
Department of Anesthesia
Cincinnati Children's Hospital
Cincinnati, OH

Michelle Dalton, MD
Assistant Professor of Anesthesiology
Baylor College of Medicine
Anesthesiologist
Texas Children's Hospital
Houston, TX

Trung Du, MD
Cincinnati Children's Hospital Medical Center
Cincinnati, OH

Mary A. Felberg, MD
Assistant Professor
Department of Anesthesiology, Perioperative, and Pain Medicine
Baylor College of Medicine
Texas Children's Hospital
Houston, TX

Geoff Frawley, BSc, MBBS, FANZCA
Consultant Anesthetist
The Royal Children's Hospital Melbourne
Melbourne, VIC, Australia

Chris D. Glover, MD, MBA
Associate Professor
Medical Director, Perioperative Services Division
Chief, Community Hospital
Department of Anesthesiology, Perioperative, and Pain Medicine
Baylor College of Medicine
Texas Children's Hospital
Houston, TX

Kenneth R. Goldschneider, MD, FAAP
Professor
Director, Pain Management Center
Cincinnati Children's Hospital Medical Center
Cincinnati, OH

Diane Gordon, MD
Assistant Professor
Cincinnati Children's Hospital Medical Center
Cincinnati, OH

Cheryl Gore, MB, MBA, MEd
Assistant Professor
Department of Anesthesiology, Perioperative, and Pain Medicine
Baylor College of Medicine
Texas Children's Hospital
Houston, TX

Erin A. Gottlieb, MD
Associate Professor of Anesthesiology
Baylor College of Medicine
Cardiovascular Anesthesiologist
Texas Children's Hospital
Houston, TX

Kalyani Govindan, MD
Assistant Professor
Department of Anesthesiology, Perioperative, and Pain Medicine
Baylor College of Medicine
Texas Children's Hospital
Houston, TX

Nancy Hagerman, MD
Assistant Professor
Cincinnati Children's Hospital Medical Center
Cincinnati, OH

Melanie Handley, MD
Assistant Professor
Department of Anesthesiology, Perioperative, and Pain Medicine
Baylor College of Medicine
Texas Children's Hospital
Houston, TX

Michele Hendrickson, MD
Anesthesiologist
Pain Management Center
Cincinnati Children's Hospital
Cincinnati, OH

Lisa D. Heyden, MD
Assistant Professor
Department of Anesthesiology, Perioperative, and Pain Medicine
Baylor College of Medicine
Texas Children's Hospital
Houston, TX

Paul Hopkins, MD
Assistant Professor
Department of Anesthesiology, Perioperative, and Pain Medicine
Baylor College of Medicine
Texas Children's Hospital
Houston, TX

Matthew D. James, MD
Assistant Professor of Anesthesiology
Baylor College of Medicine
Texas Children's Hospital
Houston, TX

Aimee G. Kakascik, DO
Assistant Professor
Department of Anesthesiology, Perioperative, and Pain Medicine
Baylor College of Medicine
Texas Children's Hospital
Houston, TX

Megha Kanjia, MD
Assistant Professor
Department of Anesthesiology, Perioperative, and Pain Medicine
Baylor College of Medicine
Texas Children's Hospital
Houston, TX

Helena Karlberg, MD
Associate Professor
Department of Anesthesiology, Perioperative, and Pain Medicine
Baylor College of Medicine
Texas Children's Hospital
Houston, TX

Michael J. Kibelbek, MD
Associate Professor
Department of Anesthesia
Cincinnati Children's Hospital Medical Center
Cincinnati, OH

Matthias W. König, MD
Anesthesiology Specialist
Chapel Hill, NC

Renee Kreeger, MD
Associate Professor of Clinical Anesthesia and Pediatrics
Division of Cardiac Anesthesia
Cincinnati Children's Hospital Medical Center
Cincinnati, OH

C. Dean Kurth, MD
Anesthesiologist-in-Chief
Chair, Department of Anesthesiology and Critical Care Medicine
Children's Hospital of Philadelphia
Philadelphia, PA

Erica P. Lin, MD
Assistant Professor
Department of Anesthesia
Cincinnati Children's Hospital Medical Center
Cincinnati, OH

Michael Lin, MD
Assistant Professor
Department of Anesthesiology
University of Texas Health Science Center at Houston
Houston, TX

Yang Liu, MD
Assistant Professor
Department of Anesthesiology, Perioperative, and Pain Medicine
Baylor College of Medicine
Texas Children's Hospital
Houston, TX

Andreas W. Loepke, MD, PhD, FAAP
Associate Division Chief of Cardiac Anesthesia
Children's Hospital of Philadelphia
Philadelphia, PA

Cheryl Maenpaa, MD
Anesthesiologist
Children's Healthcare of Atlanta
Emory University Hospital
Atlanta, GA

Mohamed A. Mahmoud, MD
Staff Anesthesiologist
Associate Professor
Department of Anesthesia
Cincinnati Children's Hospital Medical Center
Cincinnati, OH

David G. Mann, MD
Associate Professor
Anesthesiology, Perioperative, and Pain Medicine
Texas Children's Hospital
Baylor College of Medicine
Houston, TX

David Martin, MD
Anesthesiologist
Department of Anesthesiology and Pain Medicine
Nationwide Children's Hospital
Washington, DC

Jagroop Mavi, MD
Staff Anesthesiologist
Associate Professor
Department of Anesthesia
Cincinnati Children's Hospital Medical Center
Cincinnati, OH

John J. McAuliffe III, MD, MBA
Research Director
Staff Anesthesiologist
Director, Institute Pediatric Anesthesia
Cincinnati Children's Hospital Medical Center
Cincinnati, OH

Robert McDougall, MBBS, FANZCA
Deputy Director
Anaesthesia and Pain Management
Honorary Clinical Associate Professor
University of Melbourne
Royal Children's Hospital Melbourne
Melbourne, VIC

Rebecca McIntyre, MBBS, FANZCA
Department of Anaesthesia and Pain Management
Royal Children's Hospital
Melbourne, VIC

Caro Monico, MD
Assistant Professor
Department of Anesthesiology, Perioperative, and Pain Medicine
Baylor College of Medicine
Texas Children's Hospital
Houston, TX

David L. Moore, MD
Associate Professor
Clinical Anesthesia and Pediatrics
Cincinnati Children's Hospital Medical Center
University of Cincinnati
College of Medicine
Cincinnati, OH

Emad B. Mossad, MD
Professor
Associate-in-Chief, Clinical Affairs Division Chief, CV Anesthesiology
Department of Anesthesiology, Perioperative, and Pain Medicine
Baylor College of Medicine
Texas Children's Hospital
Houston, TX

Pablo Motta, MD
Associate Professor
Department of Anesthesiology, Perioperative, and Pain Medicine
Pediatric Cardiovascular Anesthesiology
Baylor College of Medicine
Texas Children's Hospital
Houston, TX

Wallis T. Muhly, MD
Assistant Professor
Department of Anesthesiology and Critical Care Medicine
Children's Hospital of Philadelphia
Philadelphia, PA

Ann Ng, MD
Assistant Professor
Department of Anesthesiology, Perioperative, and Pain Medicine
Baylor College of Medicine
Texas Children's Hospital
Houston, TX

Kim-Phuong Nguyen, MD
Associate Professor
Department of Anesthesiology, Perioperative, and Pain Medicine
Baylor College of Medicine
Texas Children's Hospital
Houston, TX

Nihar Patel, MD
Associate Professor
Department of Anesthesiology, Perioperative, and Pain Medicine
Baylor College of Medicine
Texas Children's Hospital
Houston, TX

Mario Patino, MD
Associate Professor
Department of Anesthesiology, Perioperative, and Pain Medicine
Baylor College of Medicine
Texas Children's Hospital
Houston, TX

Miguel Prada, MD
Assistant Professor
Department of Anesthesiology, Perioperative, and Pain Medicine
Baylor College of Medicine
Texas Children's Hospital
Houston, TX

Sharon Redd, MD
Assistant Professor of Anesthesia
Clinical Director, Day Surgical Unit
Senior Associate in Perioperative Anesthesia
Boston Children's Hospital
Harvard Medical School
Boston, MA

Carlos L. Rodriguez, MD
Assistant Professor
Department of Anesthesiology, Perioperative, and Pain Medicine
Baylor College of Medicine
Texas Children's Hospital
Houston, TX

Laura Ryan, MD
Assistant Professor
Department of Anesthesiology, Perioperative, and Pain Medicine
Baylor College of Medicine
Texas Children's Hospital
Houston, TX

Stefano Sabato, MBBS (Hons), FANZCA
Department of Anesthesia and Pain Management
Royal Children's Hospital
Melbourne, VIC

Senthilkumar Sadhasivam, MD, MPH
Associate Professor, Clinical Anesthesia and Pediatrics
Director, Acute and Perioperative Pain Management
Cincinnati Children's Hospital Medical Center
University of Cincinnati
College of Medicine
Cincinnati, OH

Nancy B. Samol, MD
Assistant Professor
Clinical Anesthesia and Pediatrics
Cincinnati Children's Hospital Medical Center
University of Cincinnati, College of Medicine
Cincinnati, OH

Julie Schackman, MD
Assistant Professor
Department of Anesthesiology, Perioperative, and Pain Medicine
Baylor College of Medicine
Texas Children's Hospital
Houston, TX

Brent Schakett, MD
Assistant Professor
Department of Anesthesiology, Perioperative, and Pain Medicine
Baylor College of Medicine
Texas Children's Hospital
Houston, TX

Thomas L. Shaw, MD
Associate Professor
Department of Anesthesiology, Perioperative, and Pain Medicine
Baylor College of Medicine
Texas Children's Hospital
Houston, TX

Jamie W. Sinton, MD
Assistant Professor
Department of Anesthesiology, Perioperative, and Pain Medicine
Baylor College of Medicine
Texas Children's Hospital
Houston, TX

Matthew D. Sjoblom, MD
Department of Anesthesia
Cincinnati Children's Hospital Medical Center
Cincinnati, OH

James P. Spaeth, MD
Director of Cardiac Anesthesia
Department of Anesthesia
Cincinnati Children's Hospital Medical Center
Cincinnati, OH

Caitlin D. Sutton, MD
Assistant Professor
Department of Anesthesiology, Perioperative, and Pain Medicine
Baylor College of Medicine
Texas Children's Hospital
Houston, TX

Brian Tinch, MD
Assistant Professor
Department of Anesthesiology, Perioperative, and Pain Medicine
Baylor College of Medicine
Texas Children's Hospital
Houston, TX

Imelda Tjia, MD
Assistant Professor
Department of Anesthesiology, Perioperative, and Pain Medicine
Baylor College of Medicine
Texas Children's Hospital
Houston, TX

Premal M. Trivedi, MD
Assistant Professor
Department of Anesthesiology, Perioperative, and Pain Medicine
Baylor College of Medicine
Texas Children's Hospital
Houston, TX

Ben Turner, MD, MBBS, FANZCA, FCICM
Department of Anesthesia and Pain Management
Royal Children's Hospital
Melbourne, VIC

Anna M. Varughese, MD, MPH
Anesthesia Divisional Chief
Department of Anesthesia
Cincinnati Children's Hospital Medical Center
Cincinnati, OH

David F. Vener, MD
Associate Professor
Department of Anesthesiology, Perioperative, and Pain Medicine
Baylor College of Medicine
Texas Children's Hospital
Houston, TX

Mehernoor Watcha, MD
Department of Anesthesiology, Perioperative, and Pain Medicine
Baylor College of Medicine
Texas Children's Hospital
Houston, TX

Kenneth Wayman, MD
Assistant Professor
Department of Anesthesiology, Perioperative, and Pain Medicine
Baylor College of Medicine
Texas Children's Hospital
Houston, TX

Eric Wittkugel, MD
Associate Professor
Department of Anesthesia
Cincinnati Children's Hospital Medical Center
Cincinnati, OH

Junzheng Wu, MD, ScD
Department of Anesthesia
Cincinnati Children's Hospital Medical Center
UC Department of Anesthesiology
Cincinnati, OH

Karla E. K. Wyatt, MD, MS
Assistant Professor
Department of Anesthesiology, Perioperative, and Pain Medicine
Baylor College of Medicine
Texas Children's Hospital
Houston, TX

David A. Young, MD, MEd, MBA
Professor of Anesthesiology and Pediatrics
Co-Chair, Medical School Admissions Committee
Baylor College of Medicine
Committee Chair, Pediatric Anesthesiology Simulation, CHSE
Medical Director, Pediatric Advanced Life Support Program
Department of Anesthesiology, Perioperative, and Pain Medicine
Texas Children's Hospital
Houston, TX

Michael Blaine Zelisko, MD
Clinical Director of Anesthesia
Texas Children's Hospital West Campus
Assistant Professor of Anesthesia
Department of Anesthesiology, Perioperative, and Pain Medicine
Texas Children's Hospital
Baylor College of Medicine
Houston, TX

INTRODUCTION

How to Use This Book

ERIN S. WILLIAMS AND TITILOPEMI A. O. AINA

Clinical Pediatric Anesthesia: A Case-Based Handbook, 2nd edition, reviews important clinical considerations and perioperative management of pediatric patients. The chapters are divided into clinical subspecialties and include the most relevant and/or common scenarios, thus making it easy for the reader to find the topic of interest. Additionally, the new electronic or digital version of the book allows the pediatric anesthesiologist to easily obtain this information from any location and utilizes keywords to also facilitate quick navigation of the text. The second edition has also added new chapters that address advances in our field, such as "Anesthesia for Ex Utero Intrapartum Therapy."

The format of the book uses case presentations to help the reader learn about the various practical aspects of pediatric anesthesiology. In contrast to traditional content-based textbooks, case-based learning offers the opportunity to focus on high-yield, clinically relevant topics. Traditional textbooks remain incredibly useful as a resource or reference tool. This book was created to help readers in their discovery of the field of pediatric anesthesiology. We anticipate that the material covered in these pages will be a useful primer for nurses, nurse anesthetists, medical students, junior doctors, residents, fellows, and anesthesiologists, to name a few. Additionally, this book can be used to assist anesthesiologists formulate a well-thought-out plan as they prepare for clinical pediatric anesthesia cases.

Problem-based or case-based learning involves a specific case scenario followed by a series of questions that promote critical thinking and problem solving. Because the student can answer as well as pose questions a more interactive experience is created thus, making the learning environment primarily student directed. Clinical Pediatric Anesthesia 2nd Edition allows such self-directed learning. This active process of thinking through a scenario and analyzing information will allow the learner to have true understanding of the material compared to rote memorization.

Each chapter of this book contains an abstract, keywords, case presentation, introduction, learning objectives, discussion, and summary. The case presentation is relevant to the title of the chapter; and the learning objectives drive the discussion that follows each presentation. The discussion is in the form of answers to questions that will help the learner meet the learning objectives. Each chapter concludes with references. In some chapters a few references have been identified by the author as particularly informative and are annotated. A list of other informative references follows for those wishing to pursue specific subtopics. When specific material is cited in the text, the sources will be so identified. Generally, the references provided, and the suggestions for further reading, will help students to further explore the topics and may help readers achieve objectives that vary from those set out by the authors.

The reader should think of each case as a "simulation" and, after reading the objectives and case presentation, decide how he or she would manage the case. For the solo learner, it is recommended that ideas be written down. If learning in a group of two or more, discussing the case can be productive. Group members can take turns asking the questions of one another, allowing members to think through an answer prior to sharing the explanations in the text.

HOW TO GET THE MOST OUT OF THE DISCUSSION SECTION

Because there are tables, figures along with questions and answers this text provides the reader with multiple resources that promote critical thinking. The clinician can use the discussion section as an opportunity to review various options as well as advantages and disadvantages regarding the perioperative management of the pediatric patient. In summary, the book promotes and strengthens the clinical evaluation and critical thinking skills required of the pediatric anesthesiologist in a variety of thought-provoking clinical scenarios and can be utilized during single or group study.

We hope you enjoy using this book to learn more about pediatric anesthesiology. It has been our pleasure creating this resource for each one of you!

PART 1

Challenges in Preoperative Consultation and Preparation

1

Preoperative Anxiety Management

THOMAS L. SHAW

INTRODUCTION

Anesthesiologists who care for children are faced with a patient population that is more likely to be extremely anxious compared to adults. Additionally, children are less likely to tolerate preoperative intravenous access placement, thereby preventing the possibility of intravenous administration of anxiolytic drugs. Knowledge of the consequences of preoperative emotional distress, combined with knowledge of available pharmacological and behavioral interventions, can help enhance the patient's and the parents' experience, as well as perioperative outcomes.

LEARNING OBJECTIVES

1. Identify children at high risk for anxiety and emotional distress during induction of anesthesia.
2. Describe the negative consequences of preoperative anxiety.
3. List the correct dosing and timing of administration of midazolam.
4. List alternatives to midazolam and indications for their use.
5. Design an anesthetic plan to prevent or treat preoperative anxiety.

CASE PRESENTATION

A 3-year-old healthy boy presents to an outpatient surgery center for circumcision due to phimosis. He had a prior anesthetic for magnetic resonance imaging (MRI) 1 month ago. To facilitate mask induction before the MRI, the father reports that he, the nurse, and the anesthesiologist all had to hold the screaming child down. The father therefore requests to be present for today's mask induction, so he can "help out" the medical team. The smiling, friendly anesthesiologist is unable to get the child to make eye contact. The child also declines to interact with the anesthesiologist or even to give the anesthesiologist a "high five."

DISCUSSION

1. What are the risk factors for preoperative anxiety and distress?

Children between 1 and 5 years of age have a very high risk of preoperative anxiety, as many may not have started school or had the opportunity to socialize with others outside their family members and familiar faces. Children who are shy and inhibited are also at a high risk. If a child has had frequent prior visits to the operating room, previous stressful medical experiences, or repeated hospitalizations, the risk is also increased. Finally, the children of anxious parents and children of separated or divorced parents are also more anxious (Kain et al., 2000).

2. How can you predict which children will have emotional distress upon parental separation?

Behaviors that predict poor separation include poor eye contact with the medical provider, clinging to parents, refusal to speak, and inability of the provider to establish rapport with the child. Feedback from the nurses regarding the child's cooperation while obtaining vital signs and changing of clothes can also provide valuable insight. The anesthesia provider can assess a child's cooperation by trying a quick "practice run" of separation from the parents. This may involve asking the child to come along to look at stickers, toys, pictures, or wagons, leaving parents behind, and proceeding to a different section of the preoperative holding area or toward the operating room. The child is likely to show the same level of cooperation or resistance at this time as well as the actual time of separation from the parents to go to the operating room. This test allows for better prediction of likely emotional distress in a child following separation.

3. What are the different anxiety-provoking moments that children encounter before and during induction of anesthesia?

In a sequence of events, children may be stressed during separation from parents, entry into the operating room, positioning on the operating room table, placement of monitors, and initiation of mask induction. Introduction of the anesthesia mask at the onset of induction of anesthesia has been found to be the time of maximum anxiety (Fortier et al., 2010). Optimal management of preoperative anxiety would result in a calm child during all of these moments, not just during separation from the parents.

4. From our case presentation, is the parent a good candidate for parental presence during induction?

Despite the father's desire to be present and help facilitate mask induction again, the previous mask induction where the father and two health care providers had to hold the child down should be considered a failure. The parent is a good candidate to participate in induction, if he or she is able to calm the child and actually facilitate the child's cooperation. A pharmacological strategy may be indicated to manage this child's anxiety. Midazolam has been shown to be more effective at reducing anxiety in both the child and the parent and is also more effective than parental presence during induction (Kain et al., 1998).

5. As you are writing the order for oral midazolam, the recovery room nurse states that she believes patients who receive midazolam as a preoperative medication seem to wake up delirious or agitated. Is the nurse's anecdotal observation scientifically validated?

Patients with high levels of preoperative anxiety are more likely to experience emergence delirium (Kain et al., 2004). In an institution that selectively administers midazolam to at-risk children, there may be a selection bias that results in an erroneous anecdotal perception. In fact, a randomized study with emergence delirium as an endpoint showed no difference in the rates of emergence delirium in patients who received midazolam compared to placebo (El Batawi, 2015).

6. What are the negative postoperative effects of preoperative anxiety?

Patients with high preoperative anxiety experience more pain and have higher analgesic requirements in the recovery room and also during the first 3 days of recovery from surgery (Kain et al., 2004). After the surgery and anesthesia experience, children may experience negative behavioral changes which include disruption of sleep, separation anxiety, enuresis, temper tantrums, and aggressive behavior. The degree or level of a child's preoperative anxiety determines the incidence of new postoperative maladaptive behaviors that the child may exhibit following surgery (Kain et al., 2006). Recent studies have shown that changes in postoperative sleep patterns are the same in children who received preoperative midazolam and those who did not receive any preoperative anxiolysis (Min et al., 2016).

7. What are the potential benefits of administering preoperative anxiolytics?

Administering a preoperative anxiolytic has the potential to cause anterograde amnesia, smooth parental separation, and facilitate mask acceptance. It also reduces pain scores and postoperative negative behavioral changes. Finally, parents of children who receive midazolam report higher patient satisfaction scores.

8. What are some potential unintended consequences of administering preoperative anxiolytics?

Late identification of a child in need of an anxiolytic will likely delay the operating room start time and decrease operating room efficiency as the team waits for the oral medication to take effect. Also, for very short cases, there may be a delay in recovery room discharge time.

9. What is the dose range and ideal timing of administration of oral midazolam?

Children will rarely willingly accept placement of an intravenous catheter while awake without premedication or sedation. As an alternative, oral administration of an anxiolytic for preoperative

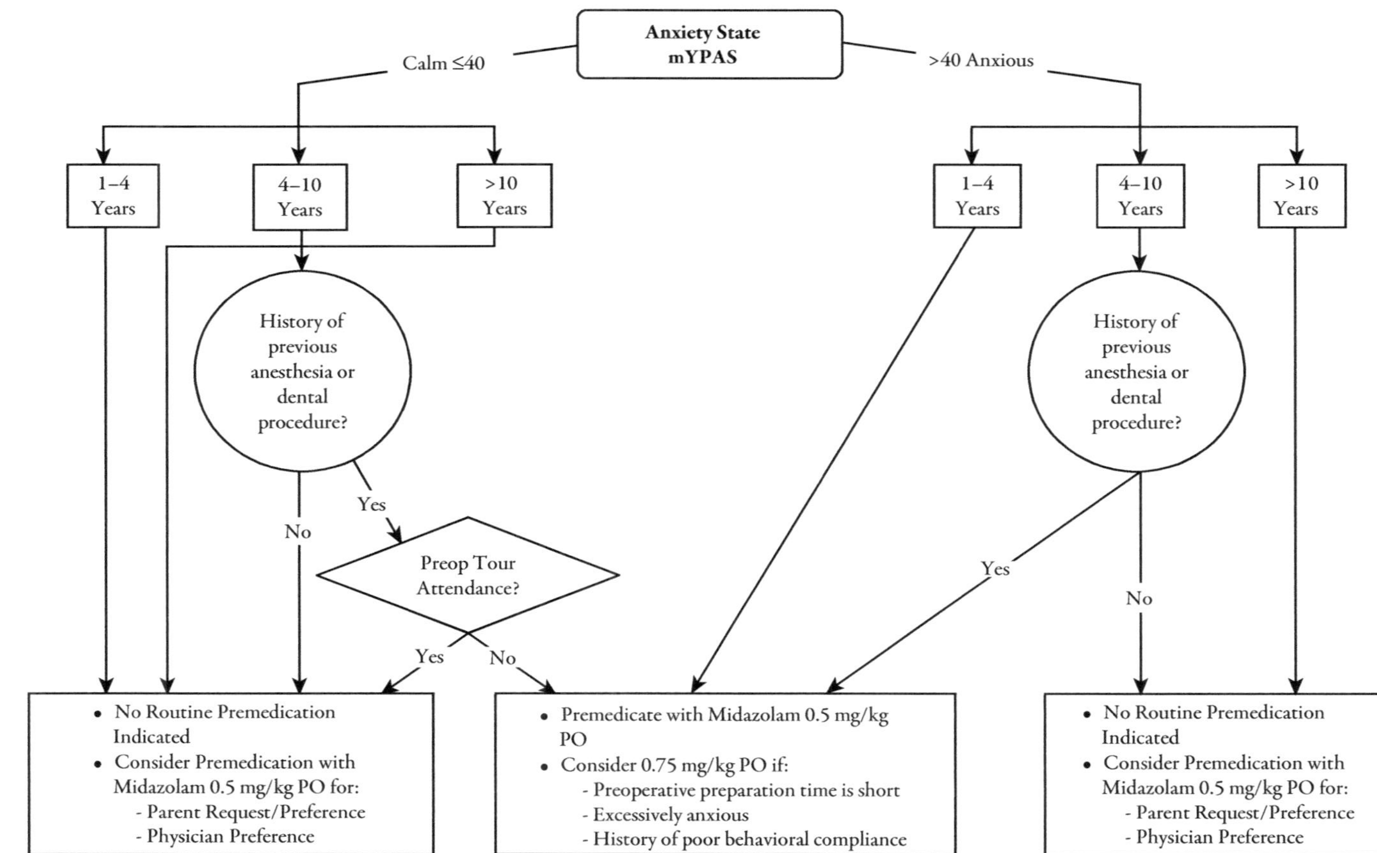

FIGURE 1.1 Premedication clinical algorithm.

sedation is commonly preferred. Midazolam is the most common agent administered via the oral route. The usual dose is 0.5 mg/kg. Anterograde amnesia commences within 10 minutes, and the sedation effect starts after about 15 to 20 minutes. Midazolam can also be administered via the nasal, intravenous, or intramuscular routes at doses of 0.2 mg/kg, 0.1 mg/kg, and 0.1 to 0.2 mg/kg, respectively. Figure 1.1

10. What other alternatives to midazolam are available and when might one choose to use them?

A history of allergy, paradoxical reaction, or refusal to take oral midazolam may preclude its use. Ketamine can be administered per oral (PO) at a dose of 5 mg/kg. Alternatively, intramuscular ketamine at a dose of 2 to 4 mg/kg may be administered for very combative or delayed children. Potent sedation can be achieved by combining oral ketamine 3 mg/kg with oral midazolam 0.5 mg/kg or intramuscular ketamine 2 to 4 mg/kg with intramuscular midazolam 0.1 mg/kg. Ketamine is associated with side effects of sialorrhea and hallucinations and is therefore typically combined with both atropine 0.1mg/kg and midazolam for intramuscular administration to a combative child. Clonidine can be administered PO at a dose of 2 to 4 mcg/kg. Dexmedetomidine is another option and may be administered PO at a dose of 4 mcg/kg (Jannu, 2016) or via the intranasal route at 1 mcg/kg.

11. What behaviors of caregivers can affect a child's preoperative anxiety level?

There are some empathetic behaviors naturally performed by providers that have actually been shown to have unintended consequences. A program called Provider-Tailored Intervention for Perioperative Stress (P-TIPS) teaches provider behaviors that decrease perioperative anxiety (Martin et al., 2011). Anxiety can be reduced with distracting talk, humor, and giving the child actual choices with clear limitations. On the other hand, anxiety is increased by reassuring, apologetic, or empathetic comments that mean well but actually distress children by causing them to focus on their own feelings or stress. Finally, implying a choice when the child actually has none is quite distressing to the child; for example, "Do you want to go back for surgery?" is not a real choice. However, giving the child an actual choice, with limitations, is best; for example, "Do you want to walk back or ride the wagon?"

SUMMARY

The anesthesia provider should be aware that seconds or minutes of terror experienced by a child during induction can have significant negative consequences postoperatively. Children can exhibit detrimental emotional effects for days, weeks, or even months after the anesthetic. Fortunately, there are pharmacological and behavioral interventions that anesthesia providers can employ to allay the fear and stress that surround the surgery experience. Midazolam remains the gold standard for pharmacological therapy and is helpful in preventing or treating preoperative anxiety; however, alternatives do exist, and their use should be explored as the situation dictates.

ACKNOWLEDGMENTS

The author wishes to acknowledge the first edition authors, Anna Varughese and Nancy Hagerman.

ANNOTATED REFERENCE

Zain ZN, Caldwell-Andrews A, Shu-Ming W. Psychological preparation of the parent and pediatric surgical patient. *Anesth Clin North Am.* 2002;20(1):29–44.

This comprehensive review article of behavioral preoperative anxiolytic interventions details the risks of not treating preoperative anxiety and reviews studies on the usefulness of nonpharmacological interventions, including preoperative preparation programs for children, parental preparation programs, parental presence during anesthesia induction, the use of perioperative music and sensory stimuli, and the preoperative interview process.

REFERENCES

El Batawi HY. Effect of preoperative oral midazolam sedation on separation anxiety and emergence delirium among children undergoing dental treatment under general anesthesia. *J Int Soc Prev Community Dent.* 2015;5(2):88–94.

Fortier MA, Del Rosario AM, Martin SR, Kain ZN. Perioperative anxiety in children. *Paediatr Anaesth.* 2010 Apr;20(4):318–322.

Jannu V, Mane R, Dhorigol M, Sanikop C. A comparison of oral midazolam and oral dexmedetomidine as premedication in pediatric anesthesia. *Saudi J Anaesth.* 2016;10(4):390–394.

Kain ZN, Caldwell-Andrews AA, Maranets I, et al. Preoperative anxiety and emergence delirium and postoperative maladaptive behaviors. *Anesth Analg.* 2004;99(6):1648–1654.

Kain ZN, Mayes LC, Caldwell-Andrews AA, Karas DE, McClain BC. Pre-operative anxiety, post-operative pain, and behavioral recovery in young children undergoing surgery. *Pediatrics*. 2006 Aug;118(2):651–658.

Kain ZN, Mayes LC, Wang SM, Caramico LA, Hofstadter MB. Parental presence during induction of anesthesia versus sedative premedication: which intervention is more effective? *Anesthesiology*. 1998;89(5):1147–1156; discussion 9A-10A.

Kain ZN, Mayes LC, Weisman SJ, Hofstadter MB. Social adaptability, cognitive abilities, and other predictors for children's reactions to surgery. *J Clin Anesth*. 2000;12(7):549–554.

Martin SR, Chorney JM, Tan ET, et al. Changing health-care providers' behavior during pediatric inductions with an empirically based intervention. *Anesthesiology*. 2011;115(1):18–27.

Min CB, Kain ZN, Stevenson RS, Jenkins B, Fortier MA. A randomized trial examining preoperative sedative medication and postoperative sleep in children. *J Clin Anesth*. 2016 May;30:15–20.

2

Electrolyte Disturbance in Pyloric Stenosis

BEN TURNER AND IMELDA TJIA

INTRODUCTION

Pyloric stenosis is a common condition that represents a challenge to the pediatric anesthesiologist. Managing these children requires an understanding of fluid, electrolyte, and acid–base abnormalities. The key perioperative message is to realize this is a *medical* rather than a *surgical* emergency. Preoperative correction of the fluid, electrolyte, and acid–base abnormalities is vital in reducing perioperative morbidity. The anesthesiologist needs to be able to accurately assess when a baby's condition is adequately optimized before proceeding to pyloromyotomy. Other anesthetic considerations include induction techniques when patients may have an aspiration risk and perioperative pain management choices for young patients.

LEARNING OBJECTIVES

1. Understand the acid–base and electrolyte disturbances associated with pyloric stenosis and how to correct them.
2. Evaluate the alternative anesthetic techniques.
3. Develop a postanesthetic management plan.

CASE PRESENTATION

A 3.6-kg 5-week-old boy presents to the emergency department with failure to gain weight and ***nonbilious projectile vomiting*** *after feeds in the last week. He was a full-term baby delivered without complications or history suggestive of cardiac, respiratory, or renal disease. The child does not take medications regularly. The child's mother has been instructed by the pediatrician to change formula many times due to a possible formula allergy, and the baby now only consumes soy formula However, he continues to spit up. There is a paternal history of pyloric stenosis. On examination, the baby has a sunken fontanel and a capillary refill time of 3 seconds. He is pale and mildly lethargic, with a pulse of 120 bpm. His mother notes that he has not had a wet diaper for 10 hours. His pre-illness weight is unknown; however, he is estimated to be 5% to 10% dehydrated. A* ***palpable olive-sized mass at the upper right costal margin*** *is noted. His chest is clear and there are no murmurs. There is no jaundice. Laboratory results reveal the following: sodium cation (****Na+****)* ***133 mmol/L****, potassium (K^+) 3.9 mmol/L, chloride (****Cl–****)* ***87 mmol/L****, bicarbonate (****HCO_3^-****)* ***32 mmol/L****, BE + 10.1 mEq/L. The diagnosis of pyloric stenosis is confirmed on ultrasound. He is kept nil by mouth. His* ***volume, Na+, and Cl– deficit is corrected with intravenous (IV) fluid replacement*** *(Table 2.1). After 2 days his laboratory results reveal* ***Na+ 134 mmol/L****, K^+ 4.6 mmol/L,* ***Cl– 97 mmol/L,HCO_3^-28 mmol/L****, BE + 1 mEq/L. The child is assessed as being adequately fluid-resuscitated, and he is scheduled for a laparoscopic pyloromyotomy.*

In a warmed operating room, the patency of his peripheral IV catheter is confirmed. After the monitors are placed, an orogastric tube is inserted and suctioned while he is still awake. During suctioning, the child is turned supine, in left and right lateral and prone positions (four-quadrant suction). The baby is induced using cricoid pressure during intubation. Anesthesia is maintained with sevoflurane with oxygen/nitrous oxide. The patient undergoes a laparoscopic pyloromytomy. The surgeon insufflates using carbon dioxide to create a pneumoperitoneum of 8 mmHg of pressure. When the surgeon has completed the repair, he asks the anesthesiologist to push air through the orogastric tube.

At the end of the operation, the surgeon ***infiltrates the wound with 0.25% bupivacaine.***

The baby is extubated once awake, demonstrating regular spontaneous breathing. He is transferred to recovery with orders to advance oral feeds as tolerated over the next 12 hours.

DISCUSSION

1. What is pyloric stenosis and how is it diagnosed?

Pyloric stenosis (PS) is a condition of pyloric outflow tract obstruction caused by hypertrophy of the circular muscularis layer of the pylorus. PS is the most common surgical cause of vomiting in babies (Table 2.1). The incidence is approximately 0.9 to 5.1 per 1,000 live births and is more common in Caucasian infants compared to African American or Asian ethnic groups (Kamata et al., 2015). It affects males more than females in a ratio of approximately 4:1. It generally presents 3 to 6 weeks after birth. In pyloric stenosis the **vomiting is nonbilious**, which often differentiates the condition from other causes of vomiting. Palpation of an "olive-sized" mass in the upper abdomen occurs in only 48% of examinations (Kamata et al., 2015). Confirmation of the diagnosis with ultrasonography leads to earlier diagnosis as the accuracy "approaches 100% in experienced hands with 99.5% sensitivity and 100% specificity" (Kamata et al., 2015). Infants with PS can be diagnosed early with ultrasound before experiencing severe dehydration and electrolyte derangements (Acker et al., 2015). Recent evidence proposes that infants presenting with PS are diagnosed early before experiencing severe dehydration or electrolyte imbalances likely due to a combination of factors, "including parental pressure, medico-legal concerns and the widespread availability of ultrasound" (Taylor et al., 2013). Due to early diagnosis and minimal metabolic changes, surgical repair may be able to take place on the first day of admission, thereby decreasing overall length of hospital stay (Poon et al., 1996).

2. What is the underlying acid-base disturbance?

The classic metabolic derangements of hypochloremia, hypokalemia, and metabolic alkalosis is seen less frequently, "perhaps related to early diagnosis by ultrasound" (Kamata et al., 2015). Vomiting in the presence of pyloric obstruction causes *unopposed loss of gastric acid (HCl), water, Na^+, and K^+*. The patient therefore develops a metabolic alkalosis. Under physiological conditions, HCl entering the duodenum is neutralized by pancreatic secreted bicarbonate. In pyloric stenosis, pancreatic HCO_3^- is absorbed, contributing to the alkalosis. The net raised bicarbonate concentration overwhelms the resorptive capacity of the proximal convoluted tubule of the kidney, causing an initial alkaline urine pH (Fell & Chelliah, 2001).

The fluid loss and reduced oral intake causes extracellular **fluid volume depletion**. This stimulates the renin-angiotensin-aldosterone system; Na^+ is therefore retained at the expense of K^+ loss in the urine. Total body potassium falls for two other reasons: alkalosis causes a shift of K^+ into the intracellular space and a small amount of K^+ is lost in the

TABLE 2.1 PREOPERATIVE MAINTENANCE FLUID REGIMEN FOR PYLORIC STENOSIS

Assessed Fluid Deficit	*Fluid Regimen (Note: K^+ is added only if baby is passing urine)*
Less than 5% (well, reduced urine output)	No bolus required. 0.45% NaCl and 5% dextrose with 20 mmol/L KCl at 150% of normal. maintenance rate for 12 hours
5%–10% (mildly lethargic, pale, dry mouth, poor urine output)	Bolus 0.9% saline 20 mL/kg in 30 minutes; then 0.45% NaCl and 5% dextrose with 30 mmol/L KCl at 200% of normal maintenance rate for 12 hours
Greater than 10% (lethargic, pale, mottled, anuria, tachycardia)	Bolus 0.9% saline 20 mL/kg in 30 minutes; then 0.45% NaCl and 5% dextrose with 30 mmol/L KCl at 200% of normal maintenance rate for 16 hours or more

Note. NaCl = sodium chloride; KCl = potassium chloride.

Glucose, urea, electrolytes, and creatinine should be monitored q4–6h if >10% dehydrated and q6–12h if <10% dehydrated.

Reproduced and modified with permission from Thompson K, Tey D, Marks M. *Paediatric Handbook*. 8th ed. Malden, MA: Wiley-Blackwell, 2009.

vomitus. Thus the anesthetic implication of the potassium level (which may be low, normal, or high) must be taken in context of the overall acid–base and electrolyte pattern (Schwartz et al., 2003).

The expected renal response to metabolic alkalosis is to reduce H^+ ion secretion; this causes a net loss of bicarbonate. In PS, elevated aldosterone levels prevent this. Aldosterone stimulates sodium reabsorption in exchange for K^+ and H^+. Paradoxically, a more acidic urine and worsening alkalosis will result.

Cl^- is lost with H^+ during vomiting. This results in **hypochloremia.** Normally, the kidneys attempt to reabsorb Cl^- (with Na^+) in exchange for the secretion ofHCO_3^-; however, there is insufficient Cl^- in the glomerular filtrate for this process to occur. Hence there is complete bicarbonate reabsorption, acidic urine, and maintenance of alkalosis. Urine $[Cl^-]$ is thus very low or zero in metabolic alkalosis with a contracted volume state. Correction of the alkalosis therefore cannot occur until the serum (Cl^-) is restored. Therefore, by giving volume, Na^+, and Cl^-, the homeostasis will be restored.

In extreme uncorrected cases, profound hypovolemia may lead to reduced tissue oxygen delivery and a metabolic acidosis; hemoconcentration may result in polycythemia.

3. What are the principles of preoperative fluid and electrolyte management and subsequent timing of surgery?

- **Correction of volume deficit**
- **Replenish sodium and chloride** to enable the kidney to correct the alkalosis by excreting bicarbonate.

One regimen is outlined in Table 2.2. Targets for resuscitation are **a normal volume state, serum** (HCO_3^-) **<30 mmol/L,** and **serum** (Cl^-) **> 105 mmol/L.** Although not commonly measured in practice, a urine (Cl^-) >20 mmol/L provides evidence in PS that volume state has been corrected and the kidney is no longer maximally reabsorbing sodium chloride (NaCl; Goh et al., 1990). In the absence of adequate resuscitation, perioperative risks include *central respiratory depression due to alkalosis, dysrhythmias due to electrolyte imbalance,* and *hypotension due to hypovolemia.*

4. Why is it necessary to correct metabolic derangements prior to surgical correction?

Metabolic alkalosis can affect the respiratory drive placing an infant with metabolic derangements associated with pyloric stenosis at risk of apnea (Kamata et al., 2015). The partial pressure of carbon dioxide ($PaCO_2$) and the partial pressure of PO_2 affect ventilation. The respiratory center is composed of central and peripheral chemoreceptors; with alterations of the $PaCO_2$, the pH in the cerebrospinal fluid (CSF) changes, thereby impacting the respiratory center. PaO_2 influences peripheral chemoreceptors in the aorta and the carotid bodies. As the PaO_2 decrease, minute ventilation will increase; however, in neonates and infants, the "primary stimulus for ventilation remains $PaCO_2$ (the pH of the CSF)" (Kamata et al., 2015).

Abreu et al. (1986) performed a study that demonstrated infants with elevated serum bicarbonate levels experienced central sleep apnea due to

TABLE 2.2 DIFFERENTIAL DIAGNOSIS OF VOMITING IN A 1-MONTH-OLD

Category	*Example*
Sepsis	Septicemia
	Urinary tract infection
	Meningitis
Mechanical	**Pyloric Stenosis**
	Malrotation with volvulus
	Strangulated inguinal hernia
	Gastroesophageal reflux
Others	Overfeeding
	Congenital adrenal hyperplasia

"loss of stimulus to wakefulness and/or a defect in metabolic control affecting central or peripheral chemoreceptor mechanisms". Although serum pH is corrected prior to surgical correction, there is a delay in the correction of alkalosis in the CSF (Kamata et al., 2015).

5. What anesthetic techniques are appropriate?

The principal goals of anesthesia for pyloromyotomy are to safely secure the airway in a patient with a recognized increased risk of aspiration and to discharge the patient to recovery with adequate analgesia but minimal risk of postoperative apnea.

Prior to induction of general anesthesia, aspiration precautions must be observed by inserting a **large-bore orogastric tube** to reduce residual gastric volumes in most patients (Cook-Sather et al., 1997). Preoxygenation is advised before either IV or inhalational induction of general anesthesia. IV induction can be achieved by a rapid sequence induction (RSI) using a sedative-hypnotic agent and succinylcholine or a modified RSI integrating bag-mask ventilation (<10–12 cm H2O), elective use of cricoid pressure, and a nondepolarizing muscle relaxant (Kamata et al., 2015). The use of cricoid pressure could compromise intubating conditions by altering the anatomy: It increases "the incidence of failed intubation by a factor of 8 in adults and this complication might occur even more frequently in infants for anatomical reasons" (Scrimgeour et al., 2015).

Neonates are more inclined to desaturate very quickly despite adequate preoxygenation due to "small airway closure secondary to high closing capacity to functional capacity relationship and higher oxygen consumption" (Kamata et al., 2015), making the modified RSI technique the more ideal choice, and enabling practitioners to use bag-mask ventilation at low pressure (Kamata et al., 2015).

An inhalational induction technique may also be used when patients present without IV access (Kamata et al., 2015) or in patients suspected of having a difficult airway (e.g., Pierre Robin, Treacher Collins, etc.). Scrimgeour et al. (2015) demonstrated that inhalational inductions were safe in children undergoing pyloromyotomy; however, "they cautioned that the aspiration of gastric contents during induction is extremely rare . . . and that further study is needed to demonstrate that inhalation induction is superior to modified RSI". One potential advantage would be the avoidance of succinylcholine. Although succinylcholine poses risks for rhabdomyolysis, hyperkalemia, arrhythmias, and cardiac arrest in situations of undiagnosed skeletal muscle myopathy, these risks are rare in infants (Kamata et al., 2015).

Awake intubation is used by some but is generally not recommended. The use of this method has decreased over the years due to possible "soft-tissue injury, bradycardia, breath-holding, laryngospasm and even aspiration" (Kamata et al., 2015).

Maintenance with shorter-acting volatile agents such as sevoflurane or desflurane is increasingly being used due to a faster wake-up and the theoretical reduced incidence of postoperative apneas. Maintenance using remifentanil and N_2O has also been described (Davis et al., 2001).

Analgesia is frequently provided by a multimodal approach including infiltration of local anesthetic at the surgical site by the surgeon and acetaminophen. The rate and extent of absorption of rectal acetaminophen is variable, so, if available, the IV form is more reliable. Studies revealed the peak plasma concentrations of oral acetaminophen (45–60 minutes), rectal route (4 hours) was much longer than the 15 minutes following IV acetaminophen administration; however, data suggests that a clinical benefit of IV acetaminophen over rectal acetaminophen in terms of pain scores or length of stay is not clear (Yung et al., 2016). Limiting the use of opioids is necessary since "the combination of corrected peripheral venous alkalosis, persistent and slower correction of cerebrospinal fluid alkalosis, intraoperative hyperventilation and opioids can lead to postoperative apnea" (Fell & Chelliah, 2001). Although a low-dose opioid can be used, it may delay emergence and increase the incidence of postoperative apnea.

Currently, laparoscopic pyloromyotomy is the more common approach to treatment which has proven to be equally safe as the open technique (Acker et al., 2015). Advantages of the laparoscopic technique include shorter time to feeding and shorter length of stay as well as better cosmetic results with smaller incision sites (Siddiqui et al., 2011). Moreover, the laparoscopic technique is preferred as it helps to "minimize surgical stress, parietal trauma and postoperative discomfort" (Leclair et al., 2017). Because of the decreased parietal trauma and subsequent postoperative pain, a study by Lemoine et al.

(2011) confirmed that patients undergoing an open pyloromyotomy required increased doses of acetaminophen and morphine compared to patients who underwent laparoscopic pyloromytomy. Although past arguments against the laparoscopic approach included a longer procedure time and increased cost, Siddiqui et al. (2011) demonstrated "dramatically similar procedure times, [with] the total increase [found] in equipment cost alone".

Lemoine and colleagues further demonstrated that both approaches were found to be equally safe without any significant difference in hospital length of stay (Lemoine et al., 2011). Another study did not demonstrate any difference in the incidence of postoperative nausea and vomiting or cosmetic advantage. However, the laparoscopic approach did place patients at a greater risk of incomplete pyloromyotomy (Leclair et al., 2007).

The laparoscopic technique requires instillation of a pneumoperitoneum that can lead to hemodynamic and perfusion changes in the head and neck region. A study has however, disproved these concerns by monitoring brain oxygenation using near-infrared spectroscopy monitoring indicating that "regional brain oxygenation remained unaltered throughout the whole anesthetic period . . . [when] using a pressure of 8mm Hg and flow rate of 5L/minute" (Tytgat et al., 2015).

6. What is an appropriate postoperative management plan?

Postoperative anesthetic issues include analgesia, maintenance fluids, and monitoring for postanesthesia apnea. For analgesia, acetaminophen is usually sufficient. IV 0.45% NaCl with 5% dextrose as maintenance IV fluids should be administered postoperatively as these infants are at risk for hypoglycemia as a result of hepatic glycogen depletion. Oral intake is often re-established between 6 and 12 hours postoperatively. Although the feeding regimen may differ, vomiting increases when feeding is reintroduced early; the timing of feeding does not impact the hospital length of stay. Vomiting occurs due to persistent decreased gastric motility postoperatively. Gastric motility returns to normal activity approximately 1 week after surgery (Ross et al., 2016).

For term babies, postoperative apnea monitoring and line-of-sight nursing is required "in young full- term infants who undergo general anesthesia" (Andropoulos et al., 1994). Ex-premature infants are often managed on the neonatal intensive care unit in some institutions.

SUMMARY

1. The vomiting of pyloric stenosis causes loss of water, HCl, Na^+, and K^+. This causes dehydration and a hypochloremic metabolic alkalosis; these metabolic abnormalities must be corrected before surgery.
2. Laparoscopic pyloromytomy is the common approach for repair.
3. Adequate analgesia is usually achieved without opioids using a combination of local anesthetic infiltration and acetaminophen.
4. The risk of postoperative apneas should be considered.

ANNOTATED REFERENCES

Bissonnette B, Sullivan PJ. Pyloric stenosis. *Can J Anesth* 1991;38(5):668–676.

An excellent overview of the pathophysiology and management of pyloric stenosis.

Eaton DC, Pooler JP. Regulation of hydrogen ion balance. In: Vander AJ, ed. *Renal Physiology*. 6th ed. New York: McGraw Hill; 2004: 174–176.

A clear explanation of renal mechanisms during metabolic alkalosis.

BIBLIOGRAPHY

Abreu F, Silva E, Macfaydens UM, Williams A, Simpson H. Sleep apnoea during upper respiratory infection and metabolic alkalosis in infancy. *Arch Dis Child.* 1986;61(11):1056–1062.

Acker SN, Garcia AJ, Ross JT, Somme S. Current trends in the diagnosis and treatment of pyloric stenosis. *Pediatr Surg Int.* 2015;31(4):363–366.

Andropoulus DB, Heard MB, Johnson KL, Clarke JT, Rowe RW. Postanesthetic apnea in full-term infants after pyloromyotomy. *Anesthesiology.* 1994;80:216–219.

Cook-Sather SD, Tulloch HV, Cnaan A, et al. A comparison of awake vs paralysed tracheal intubation for infants with pyloric stenosis. *Anesth Analg.* 1986;86:945–951.

Cook-Sather SD, Tulloch HV, Liacouras CA, Schreiner MS. Gastric fluid volume in infants for pyloromyotomy. *Can J Anesth.* 1997;44(3):278–283.

Davis PJ, Galinkin J, McGowan F, et al. A randomised multicenter study of remifentanil compared with halothane in neonates and infants undergoing pyloromyotomy. I. Emergence and recovery profiles. *Anesth Analg.* 2001;93:1380–1386.

Fell D, Chelliah S. Infantile pyloric stenosis. *Contin Ed Anesth, Crit Care Pain.* 2001;1:85–88.

Goh D, Hall S, Gornall P, Buick R, Green A, Corkery J. Plasma chloride and alkalaemia in pyloric stenosis. *Br J Surg.* 1990;77:922–923.

Kamata M, Cartabuke RS, Tobias JD. Perioperative care of infants with pyloric stenosis. *Pediatr Anesth.* 2015;25(12):1193–1206.

Leclair M, Plattner V, Mirallie E, et al. Laparoscopic pyloromyotomy for hypertrophic pyloric stenosis: a prospective, randomized controlled trial. *J Pediatr Surg.* 2007;42(4):692–698.

Lemoine C, Paris C, Morris M, et al. Open transumbilical pyloromyotomy: is it more painful than the laparoscopic approach? *J Pediatr Surg.* 2011;46(5):870–873.

MacDonald NJ, Fitzpatrick GJ, Moore KP, Wren WS, Keenan M. Anaesthesia for congenital hypertrophic pyloric stenosis: a review of 350 patients. *Br J Anaesth.* 1987;59:672–677.

Mostafa S, Gaitini LA, Vaida SJ, et al. The effectiveness and safety of spinal anaesthesia in the pyloromyotomy procedure. *Pediatr Anaesth.* 2003;13:32–37.

Pappano D. Alkalosis-induced respiratory depression from infantile hypertrophic pyloric stenosis. *Pediatr Emerg Care.* 2011;27(2):124.

Poon T, Zhang A, Cartmill T, Cass DT. Changing patterns of diagnosis and treatment of infantile hypertrophic pyloric stenosis: a clinical audit of 303 patients. *J Pediatr Surg.* 1996;31(12):1611–1615.

Ross A, Johnson PR. Infantile hypertrophic pyloric stenosis. *Pediatr Surg.* 2016;34(12):609–611.

Schwartz D, Connelly NR, Manikantan P, Nichols JH. Hyperkalemia and pyloric stenosis. *Anesth Analg.* 2003;97:355–357.

Scrimgeour GE, Leather NW, Perry RS, Pappachan VJ, Baldock AJ. Gas induction for pyloromyotomy: a service evaluation. *Pediatr Anesth.* 2015;25:677–680.

Siddiqui S, Heidel RE, Angel CA, Kennedy AP. Pyloromyotomy: randomized control trial of laparoscopic vs open technique. *J Pediatr Surg.* 2012;47(1):93–98.

Taylor ND, Cass DT, Holland AJ. Infantile hypertrophic pyloric stenosis: Has anything changed? *J Paediatr Child Health.* 2012;49(1):33–37.

Tytgat SH, Stolwijk LJ, Keunen K, et al. Brain oxygenation during laparoscopic correction of hypertrophic pyloric stenosis. *J Laparoendosc Adv Surg Tech.* 2015;25(4):352–357.

Yung A, Thung A, Tobias J. Acetaminophen for analgesia following pyloromyotomy: does the route of administration make a difference? *J Pain Res.* 2016;9:123–127.

3

Upper Respiratory Infection

KENNETH WAYMAN, NANCY B. SAMOL, AND ERIC WITTKUGEL

INTRODUCTION

Upper respiratory tract infections (URIs) are common in children, with most children experiencing 6 to 8 episodes per year. Evidence suggests that the airway reactivity associated with these infections persists for several weeks after resolution of clinical symptoms and increases the risk of perioperative adverse events. Thankfully, data also suggests that the majority of these complications are easily managed and are seldom associated with any lasting adverse sequelae. Unfortunately, day of surgery cancellation of patients with URIs is not without economic and emotional implications for the patient, the family, and the health care system as a whole. Understanding the risks associated with anesthetizing a child with a URI is paramount to formulating a well thought out anesthetic plan and minimizing burden to the patient, the family, and the medical system.

LEARNING OBJECTIVES

1. Understand the basic pathophysiology and clinical presentation of the pediatric patient with a URI, particularly as it affects the decision to proceed with elective anesthesia.
2. Define and stratify adverse events during anesthesia.
3. Identify factors evident in the preoperative evaluation that may predict adverse anesthetic events in the perioperative period.
4. Develop evidence-based practice guidelines to optimize perioperative management and reduce risk in the child with a URI who undergoes general anesthesia.

CASE PRESENTATION

A 2-year-old girl with a history of recurrent adenotonsillitis, adenotonsillar hypertrophy, and chronic otitis media presents to the operating room for elective adenotonsillectomy and placement of pressure-equalizing tubes. She is a former full-term baby with a history significant for recurrent ***URIs*** *concurrent with her adenotonsillitis, recurrent otitis media, and* ***reactive airway disease****.*

On review of systems, her mother reports near-constant URIs and a ***chronic cough*** *that is "at baseline" today. Though febrile last week, she has been* ***afebrile*** *for 5 days. The patient* ***snores*** *loudly at night, with 1- to 2-second* ***pauses****, but no witnessed gasping. The mother is quick to remind the staff that this is their third attempt at this surgery. Previously the patient has been cancelled twice due to URI. The mother also relays that the family drove 2 hours to the hospital this morning. The child received a nebulized albuterol treatment this morning as her mother hoped that would "help." The exam room smells of cigarette smoke; both parents smoke but deny smoking in the house.*

On physical exam, the girl is alert but fussy; she weighs 12.2 kg and is in no distress. She is afebrile with normal vital signs and an oxygen saturation of 98% on room air. She is a mouth-breather with large tonsils that are nearly touching and has ***clear rhinorrhea****. Her pulmonary exam demonstrates* ***coarse upper airway sounds*** *and a* ***wet cough*** *but no* ***rales, rhonchi****, or* ***wheezing.*** *The anesthetic plan and risks are discussed with the family, including* ***exacerbation of cough, airway obstruction, postoperative oxygen requirement, prolonged intubation****, and* ***hospital admission****.*

During induction of anesthesia with oxygen, nitrous oxide, and sevoflurane by mask, the child coughs, holds her breath, becomes difficult to ventilate, and begins to ***desaturate****. While an intravenous line is placed, the* ***laryngospasm*** *is broken by positive-pressure mask ventilation. The child is intubated and the remainder of the procedure proceeds uneventfully.*

Upon emergence, the child begins to ***cough*** *and* ***desaturate*** *with audible* ***wheezing*** *bilaterally. The wheezing improves with albuterol administration per endotracheal tube. Moderate thick* ***secretions*** *are suctioned from her nose and endotracheal tube before deep extubation. Following extubation, the child is breathing spontaneously with minimal support; the child remains in the operating room until she opens her eyes and then is taken to the postanesthesia care unit. In recovery, she* ***requires a single nebulized albuterol treatment and supplemental oxygen*** *for 3 hours before transfer to the floor. She is discharged the next day.*

DISCUSSION

1. What constitutes a URI and how common is it?

URIs are common and frequent in children, especially during the winter months and in those attending daycare or school. Data suggest that anywhere from 3% to 33% of children presenting for *any* anesthetic or surgery do so with active URIs and an astonishing 3% to 70% have had a recent URI (defined as within 4 weeks of clinical symptoms; Elwood & Bailey, 2005). In an unselected cohort, 30% to 40% of children presenting for *elective procedures* have an active URI (Levy et al., 1992; Stasic, 2004). The mean annual incidence of URI is highest in infants and preschool-aged children who typically experience 6 to 8 URIs per year (Becke, 2012). Typical symptoms of an uncomplicated URI include some combination of rhinorrhea, sneezing, congestion, nonproductive cough, fever less than 38.5°C, sore or scratchy throat, and laryngitis. Subclinical manifestations include upper and lower airway edema, increased respiratory tract secretions, and bronchial irritability.

Patients with **fever** greater than 38.5°C and constitutional symptoms such as lethargy or signs of lower respiratory tract involvement such as **wheezing**, mucopurulent secretions, **rales**, **rhonchi**, or productive cough should not be treated as a simple URI. These symptoms suggest that infection extends beyond the upper respiratory tract or the infection may be bacterial in nature. Unless the need for surgery is urgent, it is best not to proceed in the face of a lower respiratory tract infection.

2. What is the basic pathophysiology of a URI?

Approximately 95% of these infections are of viral etiology, often reflecting the viral prevalence in the community at any given time, though rhinovirus is most commonly implicated (Tait et al., 2000). Unfortunately, multiple pathogens produce similar URI-like symptoms making the differential diagnosis broad. Infections such as croup, influenza, bronchiolitis, pneumonia, epiglottitis, and strep throat may mimic a URI. Even noninfectious diseases such as allergic or vasomotor rhinitis can masquerade as a URI.

At the tissue level, viral infections damage respiratory mucosa and epithelium leading to sensitization of airways to the irritant effects of anesthetic vapor, increased production and viscosity of secretions, increased ventilation-perfusion (V/Q) mismatch, and increased closing volumes (Dueke et al., 1991; Jacoby & Hirshman, 1991). The mechanism of viral-induced airway hyperreactivity is poorly understood. However, mounting evidence suggests viral sensitization of both chemotactic and neurologically mediated bronchoconstriction reflex arcs (Jacoby & Hirshman, 1991; Tait, 2002; Tait & Malviya, 2005). Furthermore, several studies have proven URI to have adverse effects on pulmonary function studies, including decreases in forced vital capacity, forced expired volume, and peak expiratory flow, as well as decreases in diffusion capacity (Elwood & Bailey, 2005; Tait & Malviya, 2005). Animal studies indicate that URI exacerbates the decrease in functional residual capacity and increases intrapulmonary shunting created by anesthesia (Dueck et al., 1991). Clinical symptoms are usually self-limited, but the associated airway hyperreactivity persists. Anesthetic URI-related adverse respiratory events are high in children with active URI symptoms or those with symptoms in the preceding 4 weeks. The highest rate was in those whose clinical symptoms had resolved for less than 2 to 4 weeks at the time of anesthesia (Rachel Homer et al., 2007; Tait & Malviya, 2005).

3. What adverse perioperative respiratory events may occur in a child with a URI? What are the consequences?

Large-scale studies have identified active or recent URI as a statistically significant risk factor for adverse respiratory events associated with anesthesia (Cohen & Cameron, 1991; Elwood & Bailey, 2005; Parnis et al., 2001). These studies defined adverse events as breath holding, significant arterial oxygen desaturation (<90%), severe coughing, airway obstruction, laryngospasm, bronchospasm, postextubation croup/stridor, reintubation, pneumonia, copious secretions, and unanticipated admission. It should be noted that while URIs are to be associated with a higher incidence of respiratory complications, most are minor and easily managed; there is very little morbidity directly attributable to URI. Indeed, there are no cases in the pediatric or adult anesthesia closed-claims literature implicating URIs with serious adverse events (Tait & Malviya, 2005). In fact, increased mortality has not been demonstrated in any controlled study (Tait & Malviya, 2005). In light of current evidence, it is important that cancellation of surgery is not considered as a blanket policy but instead considered on a case by case basis. The risks of respiratory complications are multifactorial, and, in the modern era, anesthesiologists have a vast armamentarium to predict, diagnose, and treat common URI-related complications of anesthesia (Tait, 2002, 2005; Tait et al., 1995).

4. What factors in the preoperative history and physical exam may predict adverse respiratory events during and after anesthesia?

The window of opportunity for providing anesthesia to a URI-free child is extremely small—nonexistent in some cases. Therefore, it is helpful to assess these children for elective surgery armed with criteria to logically weigh the risks and benefits of proceeding with surgery versus cancellation. To this end, several studies have identified criteria in the history and physical assessment that are useful predictors of adverse respiratory outcomes (Becke, 2012; Elwood & Bailey, 2005; Parnis et al., 2001; Rachel Homer et al., 2007; Tait 2005; Tait & Malviya, 2005). *Active or recent (<4 weeks since diagnosis) URI alone is a statistically significant risk factor for adverse respiratory events. Additional harbingers of perioperative respiratory complications include planned airway surgery, planned intubation, history of prematurity (<37 weeks at birth),* ***reactive airway disease, passive smoking****, copious secretions, nasal congestion, history of* ***snoring****, and parent's statement that the child has a "cold."* Of note, confirmation of URI by a parent was consistently found to be a reliable predictor and, in one study, a better predictor of laryngospasm than symptom criteria alone (Rachel Homer et al., 2007; Tait & Malviya, 2007).

5. Why not cancel the pediatric patient with a URI presenting for elective procedures?

Following McGill et al.'s initial 1979 report of URI related complications (Tait et al., 2000), cancellation or postponement of surgery due to URI became common practice in anesthesia (McGill et al., 1979). However, in today's health care environment, the decision to cancel a surgical procedure is a complicated one. Parents may take time off from work, arrange childcare, travel significant distances, and often go to great lengths preparing a child both mentally and physically for surgery. The economic consequences of cancellation are significant for both the family and the surgical facility, while the emotional consequences are shouldered mainly by the child (Elwood & Bailey, 2005; Tait & Malviya, 2007; Tait et al., 1995). Current evidence suggests that, if anesthetized, most children with URIs will experience mild complications that can be safely managed without the need to postpone surgery. Multiple large-scale studies have suggested this (Parnis et al., 2001; Tait et al., 2000), with one study showing only 3 out of 1,078 children developing sequelae requiring rehospitalization. A survey conducted by Tait et al. in 1995 reported that anesthesiologists appear less likely to cancel cases due to URI than in the past. About 40.4% of anesthesiologists with less than 10 years in practice reported "seldom" (1%–25% of the time) cancelling a case solely due to URI. In contrast, only 27.2% of those with greater than 10 years in practice reported the same (Tait et al., 1995). If the data demonstrate that delaying a procedure will not markedly change the incidence of adverse respiratory events, then cancellation cannot be taken lightly and may gain little except to inconvenience the family, the surgeon, and the surgical schedule.

6. What evidence-based guidelines exist to minimize perioperative risk to the patient with a URI?

Management of the patient with a URI should be directed at minimizing stimulation of a potentially irritable airway (Becke et al., 2012; Flick et al., 2008; Parnis et al., 2001; Tait & Malviya, 2005). Premedication with a bronchodilator such as albuterol or ipratropium showed no decrease in adverse airway events in children with symptoms of URI. Pretreatment with anticholinergic agents such as glycopyrrolate, in hopes of decreasing secretions and attenuating airway hyperreactivity, did not result in fewer complications (Parnis et al., 2001; Tait et al., 2007).

Intraoperatively, the risk for complications increase with intubation (up to 11-fold in some studies) and decreased with laryngeal mask airway or facemask use (Flick et al., 2008; Parnis et al., 2001; Rachel Homer et al., 2007; Tait & Malviya, 2005). Propofol appears to be the safest induction agent likely due to the rapid blunting of airway reflexes and sevoflurane is best for inhalational inductions (Parnis et al., 2001). For intraoperative maintenance of anesthesia, sevoflurane appears to impair airway mechanics less than desflurane or isoflurane in children with susceptible airways. Instrumentation and suctioning of the airway should be undertaken only after a deep plane of anesthesia has been attained. Muscle relaxants are an indirect risk factor for perioperative complication both due to the potential for residual weakness and the need for reversal. Anticholinesterase reversal (e.g., neostigmine) is an independent risk factor for respiratory complications (Parnis et al., 2008). For long procedures, humidification of inhaled agents avoids drying and inspissation of secretions. Figure 3.1

SUMMARY

1. Cancellation of patients harboring URIs has economic and emotional implications for the patient, the family, and the health care system as a whole.
2. The airway hyperreactivity associated with URIs may persist for up to 6 weeks after apparent resolution of clinical symptoms.
3. Although URIs appear to be associated with a higher incidence of respiratory complications, most sequelae are minor and easily managed. To date, there has been very little residual morbidity and no increased mortality demonstrated that is directly attributable to URI.
4. The following factors predict perioperative respiratory complications in children with URI: *active or recent (<4 weeks since diagnosis) URI alone is a statistically significant risk factor for adverse respiratory events. Additional harbingers of perioperative respiratory complications include planned airway surgery, planned intubation, history of prematurity (<37 weeks at birth), reactive airway disease, passive smoking, copious secretions, nasal congestion, history of snoring, and parent's statement that the child has a "cold."*
5. Safe management of a pediatric patient with a URI includes minimizing airway instrumentation, vigilant monitoring, hydration, humidification of gases, consideration of anticholinergics and preoperative bronchodilators if appropriate, and prudent cancellation.

ANNOTATED REFERENCES

Elwood T, Bailey K. The pediatric patient and upper respiratory infections. *Best Pract Res Clin Anaesthesiol.* 2005;19(1):35–46.

A thorough overview of anesthetic management in the child with a URI. It examines patient, anesthetic, and surgical risk factors, with an emphasis on prediction and prevention of complications. It highlights shortcomings in the current data and suggests future areas of research.

Parnis SJ, Barker DS, Van Der Walt JH. Clinical predictors of anaesthetic complications in children with respiratory tract infections. *Pediatr Anesth.* 2001;11(1):29–40.

This Australian study uses statistical analysis to create discrete checklists used in the preoperative and intraoperative setting that may predict adverse respiratory outcomes based on history and physical exam findings. The authors use logistic regression to stratify risk numerically, allowing clinicians to better predict outcomes.

Tait AR, Malviya S. Anesthesia for the child with an upper respiratory tract infection: still a dilemma? *Anesth Analg.* 2005;100(1):59–65.

This concise and generously referenced review is co-written by Alan Tait, a pioneer and prolific author on the subject of anesthesia in the child

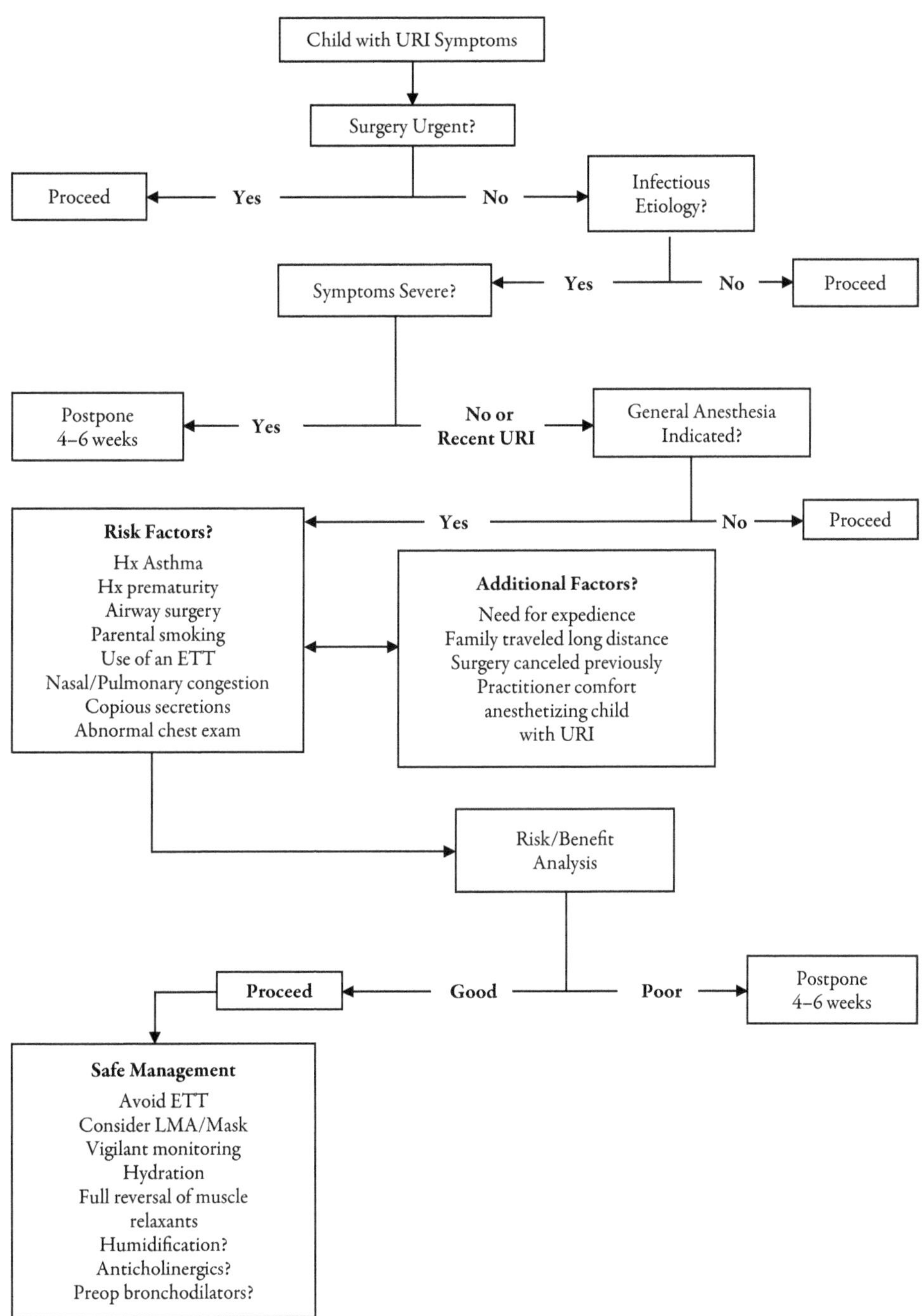

FIGURE 3.1 Suggested algorithm for the assessment and anesthetic management of the child with an upper respiratory tract infection. Reprinted with permission from Tait AR. Anesthetic management of the child with an upper respiratory tract infection. *Curr Opin Anesthesiol.* 2005;18(6):603–607.

with a URI. This article synthesizes over 50 years of observational and clinical research, much of it Tait's, to offer a useful algorithm for the assessment and management of these patients as well as to suggest future research directions to minimize anesthetic risk.

BIBLIOGRAPHY

Becke K. Anesthesia in children with a cold. *Curr Opin Anesthesiol.* 2012;25(3):333–339. doi:10.1097/aco.0b013e3283534e80

Cohen MM, Cameron CB. Should you cancel the operation when a child has an upper respiratory tract infection? *Anesth Analg.* 1991;72(3):282–288. doi:10.1213/00000539-199103000-00002

Drake-Brockman, TF, Ramgolam, A, Zhang, G, et al. The effect of endotracheal tubes versus laryngeal mask airways on perioperative adverse events in infants: a randomsed control trial. *Lancet.* 2017;389:701–708. doi:10.1016/S0140- 6736(16) 31719-6.

Dueck R, Prutow R, Richman D. Effect of parainfluenza infection on gas exchange and FRC response to anesthesia in sheep. *Anesthesiology.* 1991;74(6):1044–1051. doi:10.1097/00000542-199106000-00012

Elwood T, Bailey K. The pediatric patient and upper respiratory infections. *Best Pract Res Clin Anaesthesiol.* 2005;19(1):35–46. doi:10.1016/j.bpa.2004.08.004

Flick RP, Wilder RT, Pieper SF, et al. Risk factors for laryngospasm in children during general anesthesia. *Pediatr Anesth.* 2008;18(4):289–296. doi:10.1111/j.1460-9592.2008.02447.x

Jacoby DB, Hirshman CA. General anesthesia in patients with viral respiratory infections. *Anesthesiology.* 1991;74(6):969–972. doi:10.1097/00000542-199106000-00001

Lee BJ, August DA. COLDS: a heuristic preanesthetic risk score for children with upper respiratory tract infection. *Pediatr Anesth.* 2013;24(3):349–350. doi:10.1111/pan.12337

Levy L, Pandit UA, Randel GI, Lewis IH, Tait AR. Upper respiratory tract infections and general anaesthesia in children. *Anaesthesia.* 1992;47(8):678–682. doi:10.1111/j.1365-2044.1992.tb02389.x

Mamie C, Habre W, Delhumeau C, Argiroffo CB, Morabia A. Incidence and risk factors of perioperative respiratory adverse events in children undergoing elective surgery. *Pediatr Anesth.* 2004;14(3):218–224.

McGill WA, Coveler LA, Epstein BS. Subacute upper respiratory infection in small children. *Anesth Analg.* 1979;58(4):331–333. doi:10.1213/00000539-197907000-00017

Parnis SJ, Barker DS, Van Der Walt JH. Clinical predictors of anaesthetic complications in children with respiratory tract infections. *Pediatr Anesth.* 2001;11(1):29–40. doi:10.1046/j.1460-9592.2001.00607.x

Rachel Homer J, Elwood T, Peterson D, Rampersad S. Risk factors for adverse events in children with colds emerging from anesthesia: a logistic regression. *Pediatr Anesth.* 2007;17(2):154–161. doi:10.1111/j.1460-9592.2006.02059.x

Rolf N, Coté CJ. Frequency and severity of desaturation events during general anesthesia in children with and without upper respiratory infections. *J Clin Anesth.* 1992;4(3):200–203. doi:10.1016/0952-8180(92)90065-9

Schreiner MS, O'Hara I, Markakis DA, Politis GD. Do children who experience laryngospasm have an increased risk of upper respiratory tract infection? *Anesthesiology.* 1996;85:475–480.

Stasic AF. Perioperative implications of common respiratory problems. *Sem Pediatr Surg.* 2004;13(3):174–180. doi:10.1053/j.sempedsurg.2004.04.004

Tait AR. Anesthetic management of the child with an upper respiratory tract infection. *Curr Opin Anesthesiol.* 2005;18(6):603–607.

Tait AR. Upper airway infection and pediatric anesthesia: how is the evidence based? *Curr Opin Anesthesiol.* 2002;15(3):317–322. doi:10.1097/00001503-200206000-00007

Tait AR, Burke C, Voepel-Lewis T, Chiravuri D, Wagner D, Malviya S. Glycopyrrolate does not reduce the incidence of perioperative adverse events in children with upper respiratory tract infections. *Anesth Analg.* 2007;104(2):265–270. doi:10.1213/01.ane.0000243333.96141.40

Tait AR, Malviya S, Voepel-Lewis T, Munro HM, Seiwert M, Pandit UA. Risk factors for perioperative adverse respiratory events in children with upper respiratory tract infections. *Anesthesiology.* 2001;95(2):299–306.

Tait AR, Malviya S. Anesthesia for the child with an upper respiratory tract infection: still a dilemma? *Anesth Analg.* 2005;100(1):59–65. doi:10.1213/01.ane.0000139653.53618.91

Tait AR, Pandit UA, Voepel-Lewis T, Munro HM, Malviya S. Use of the laryngeal mask airway in children with upper respiratory tract infections: a comparison with Endotracheal Intubation. *Surv Anesthesiol.* 1999;43(2):87. doi:10.1097/00132586-199904000-00030

Tait AR, Reynolds PI, Gutstein HB. Factors that influence an anesthesiologist's decision to cancel elective surgery for the child with an upper respiratory tract infection. *J Clin Anesth.* 1995;7(8):725. doi:10.1016/0952-8180(95)90086-1

Tait AR, Voepel-Lewis T, Malviya S. Perioperative considerations for the child with an upper respiratory tract infection. *J Perianesth Nurs.* 2000;15(6):392–396.

Tait AR, Voepel-Lewis T, Malviya S. Perioperative considerations for the child with an upper respiratory tract infection. *J Peri Anesth Nurs.* 2000;15(6):392–396. doi:10.1053/jpan.2000.19503

Tait AR, Voepel-Lewis T, Munro HM, Gutstein HB, Reynolds PI. Cancellation of pediatric outpatient surgery: economic and emotional implications for patients and their families. *J Clin Anesth.* 1997;9(3):213–219.

von Ungern-Sternberg B, Boda K, Chambers N, et al. Risk assessment for respiratory complications in paediatric anaesthesia: a prospective cohort study. *Lancet.* 2010;376:773–783.

von Ungern-Sternberg B, Saudan S, Petak F, Hantos Z, Habre W. Desflurane but not sevoflurane impairs airway and respiratory tissue mechanics in children with susceptible airways. *Anesthesiology.* 2008;108:216–224.

4

Acute Fluid Resuscitation for Intussusception

ERIN S. WILLIAMS

INTRODUCTION

Intussusception is a process that involves a bowel segment invaginating into a distal segment of bowel in an anterograde direction. Peristalsis causes progression of this occurrence. Typically, the ileum goes through the ileocecal valve and invaginated into the cecum; this process also involves the blood vessels (Jiang et al., 2013). It is the most common cause of intestinal obstruction in infants, with an incidence of 1 in 2,000 and if intussusception is left untreated, or not relieved can lead to bowel ischemia due to compromised blood flow, as well as necrosis, perforation, peritonitis and potentially death (Jiang et al., 2013). Early recognition and treatment within 24 hours can prevent the need for surgical intervention and complications. Intussusception can also result in significant dehydration due to vomiting and diarrhea. An essential aspect of the perioperative management is to identify and treat dehydration.

LEARNING OBJECTIVES

1. Identify signs of dehydration in an infant and use them to quantify the degree of dehydration.
2. Know the principles of resuscitation of a dehydrated infant.
3. Understand the principles of fluid management therapy in children in the perioperative period.
4. Identify the key management issues and anesthetic implications of a bowel obstruction in an infant.

CASE PRESENTATION

A 6-month-old, full-term, previously healthy baby boy weighing 7 kg presents to the emergency department with a 2-day history of vomiting, rhinorrhea, and lethargy. His vomiting is becoming increasingly frequent, and he is now unable to tolerate any oral intake. He has not had any breast milk for more than 6 hours. He has had loose bowel movements (the most recent appeared to be red and jelly-like in consistency) and few wet diapers during the past 24 hours. ***He appears pale, mottled, lethargic,*** *and* ***miserable.*** *His* ***heart rate is 182 and blood pressure 85/45, with O_2 saturations of 98%.*** *His* fontanelle is sunken and ***capillary refill time is 4 seconds***. *Of note, he grimaces and cries during abdominal examination but there is no mass appreciated.*

He receives an intravenous (IV) bolus of ***120 mL (20 mL/kg) of 0.9% NaCl (normal saline),*** *then an infusion of Lactated Ringer's with 1% dextrose at 24 mL/hr in the emergency room, and a further bolus of 60 mL 0.9% NaCl is repeated while awaiting surgical review. Morphine is administered for analgesia and he is kept nil orally. His capillary refill improves to 2 seconds, and further investigations are arranged.*

A plain abdominal x-ray shows central air fluid levels but no evidence of perforation. A nasogastric tube (NGT) is placed and free drainage commenced. An ultrasound scan demonstrates an intussusception in the ileocolic region. He is given intravenous cefazolin and metronidazole. An ***air enema*** *is attempted but fails to reduce the intussusception. He is transferred to the operating room for laparotomy and surgical reduction.*

On arrival in the operating room he is again noted to have sluggish capillary refill. A bolus of 120 mL of Lactated Ringer's is administered, followed by an infusion of the same solution at 24 mL/hr. His NGT is aspirated prior to a rapid sequence induction with propofol and succinylcholine (suxamethonium), and he is intubated with a 3.5 cuffed endotracheal tube. Anesthesia is maintained with oxygen, air, and sevoflurane and a caudal anesthetic. Surgical reduction is performed without complication. The surgeon reduces the segment of telescoped bowel and there is no ischemia. Once the surgical site is closed, the baby successfully emerges from anesthesia, is extubated awake in the operating room, and is transported to the postanesthesia care unit for recovery.

Postoperatively, the baby continues on IV maintenance fluids and nasogastric losses are replaced with 0.9% NaCl. These losses gradually reduce over 24 hours and oral intake is reintroduced as bowel sounds return. ***Electrolytes are monitored every day while receiving IV fluids****, which are gradually reduced as oral intake increases. Analgesia is achieved with morphine infusion and regular acetaminophen (paracetamol). He is discharged home on day 5 tolerating a full oral intake, with no signs of recurrence.*

DISCUSSION

1. How is dehydration detected and quantified in an infant?

Preoperative resuscitation of the dehydrated child is imperative, as delayed diagnosis and inadequate resuscitation is a significant cause of death in children. Dehydration in this case occurred due to a combination of diarrhea and vomiting, as well as losses into the interstitium (third-space losses), which are not visible and hence are often underestimated. Fever can also contribute to fluid loss.

Dehydration is categorized as either mild, moderate, or severe. The designation depends upon a multiplicity if clinical findings (Table 4.1). Mild dehydration (3%–5% of body weight) is often not associated with any clinical signs. Signs of moderate dehydration (6%–10% of body weight) include a reduction in capillary refill time (>2 seconds), reduced tissue turgor, and an increased respiratory rate. With more severe degrees of dehydration (>10% of body weight), capillary refill time is further slowed (>3 seconds), skin becomes **mottled**, and breathing becomes deeper with developing acidosis. As the child's volume status worsens, **tachycardia** and hypotension develop, and **consciousness** becomes **impaired**. The most reliable measure of the degree of dehydration is comparison with a recent documented weight, but this is often not available. **Lethargy** and sunken eyes are often referred to, but these are unreliable signs. In this case presentation, the child had significantly **slowed capillary refill** with **tachycardia** and **mottling of the skin**, indicating severe dehydration. Given the many clinical signs and symptoms to consider, bedside ultrasound has also been described as a potential objective tool for determining the degree of dehydration. By calculating the ratio of the inferior vena cava (IVC) diameter to the aorta diameter one can assess the volume status of the patient.

2. What are the principles of resuscitation of a dehydrated child and subsequent fluid management?

Resuscitation of the dehydrated child should be considered in three phases. First, the preexisting deficit should be calculated. This will include losses from the gastrointestinal tract (through vomiting, diarrhea, and interstitial losses), as well as other deficits from the renal tract, bleeding, and preoperative fasting if present. This deficit should be replaced with 0.9% NaCl, usually as a bolus dose of 10 to 20 mL/kg, repeated as needed to correct hypovolemia.

TABLE 4.1 SIGNS OF DEHYDRATION

Degrees of Dehydration		
Mild (<4% body weight)	Moderate (4%–6% body weight)	Severe (>7% body weight)
Often no signs	Slowed capillary refill (>2 sec)	Greatly reduced capillary refill (>3–4 sec)
Perhaps dry tongue	Reduced tissue turgor	Mottling, cold
Thirsty	Dry mucous membranes	Acidosis
	Tachypnea	Tachycardia, hypotension
	Restless, lethargic, irritable	Reduced urine output
		Altered conscious state

The initial bolus of **20 mL/kg of 0.9% NaCl** in the case presentation resulted in some improvement in the boy's clinical status but not full symptom resolution, so it was repeated.

The second component of fluid replacement is the maintenance fluids which contain the correct combination of water and electrolytes to cover, the ongoing losses through respiration, perspiration, gastrointestinal losses, evaporative losses and urine (Gregory et al., 2012). They are usually calculated over a 24-hour period and include fluid, electrolytes, and glucose. Halliday's "4–2–1 rule" (4 mL/kg/hr for the first 10 kg of the child's weight, plus 2 mL/kg/hr for the next 10 kg of weight, plus 1 mL/kg/hr for every kg thereafter) was first proposed in 1957 and has been the mainstay of hourly maintenance fluid calculations for many years (Gregory et al., 2012). However, this has been recently revisited, particularly in sick or perioperative children (Neville et al., 2010). In these cases, *elevated antidiuretic hormone (ADH) levels in response to stress, surgery, and pain, combined with the use of hypotonic solutions, are associated with an increased risk of hyponatremia and cerebral edema*. Children are particularly susceptible to this due to their larger brain: cranium ratio, and an immature Na^{+} K^{+} ATPase at the blood–brain barrier, meaning that they become symptomatic at lesser degrees of hyponatremia than adults. Maintenance fluid rates should be reduced by up to 50% of the regular 4–2–1 rule or intraoperative rehydration with 20 to 30 mL/kg of a balanced salt solution followed by a 2-1-0.5mL/Kg postoperative maintenance rate if the child is at risk of elevated ADH secretion. Further, the 4–2–1 rule presupposes normal renal function, and patients with anuric renal failure may need their maintenance fluid rates reduced by 60% from that calculated.

The final component is the replacement of ongoing losses, such as, in this case, those via an NGT. As this patient's nasogastric losses reduced and oral intake increased, his IV fluid rate was reduced by an equivalent amount.

Given these considerations, a child's ongoing fluid requirement after major surgery must be carefully considered. Hydration status and ongoing losses must be assessed frequently, along with serum electrolytes. The rate will be determined by any deficit that still needs correction, any expected ongoing losses, and the maintenance requirement. Note that while the maintenance component will usually be less than the 4–2–1 rule (due to ADH secretion), the total volume administered is often initially more than the 4–2–1 rule when there are anticipated ongoing losses.

3. What is the best fluid to use in children?

The fluid used to replace an existing deficit should reflect the composition of the fluid being replaced. In most cases, 0.9% NaCl is an appropriate starting solution.

There has been much discussion recently about the optimal fluid for maintenance therapy in children. Once the mainstay, 4% dextrose with 0.18 NaCl ("4% and a fifth") is now no longer recommended in children, other than in very specialized areas (e.g., intensive care unit). It should not be used for routine maintenance therapy. Four percent dextrose with 0.45 NaCl ("4% and half normal saline") is generally safe for most children; however, there are some instances when only isotonic solutions should be given. These include in the perioperative period, in patients with low initial sodium levels, and in children with central nervous system infections or head injuries, bronchiolitis, or salt-wasting conditions.

There are several fluid preparations available that are isotonic, or nearly isotonic, but all have potential problems with their use. Hartmann's and Ringer's lactate solutions contain calcium, making them potentially incompatible with certain medications. The high chloride: sodium ratio in 0.9% NaCl can cause a metabolic acidosis when large volumes are infused. After initial resuscitation with 0.9% NaCl, it may be advisable to avoid such an acidosis by changing to another solution with less chloride relative to sodium. Last, Plasmalyte 148™ contains acetate, which can accumulate and cause hypotension.

Dextrose should be included in maintenance fluids, with solutions of 1% to 2.5% dextrose proving adequate to meet the needs of most children, especially children less than 6 months of age. Higher concentrations are likely to increase blood sugar levels, resulting in deleterious cerebral effects, and an osmotic diuresis, which can worsen hypovolemia. Most importantly, children receiving prolonged periods of IV hydration should be closely monitored and their treatment individualized. Electrolytes should be checked at the start of therapy and daily thereafter. If sodium levels are low (e.g., <130 mmol/L), they should be monitored up to every 6 hours. Blood glucose levels should also be monitored

TABLE 4.2 KEY FEATURES OF INTUSSUSCEPTION

Demographics	Age: most common 2 months to 2 years, peak at 5–9 months Males > females
History	Intermittent, colicky pain, often severe Vomiting, often bilious Blood in bowel movements (classically described as red-currant jelly appearance), Diarrhea common May follow a respiratory viral-like prodrome
Examination	Pallor, lethargy Abdominal mass or distention Dehydration to hypovolemic shock
Investigations	Abdominal x-ray: often normal unless evidence of obstruction Ultrasound: high sensitivity and specificity Air enema: both diagnostic and therapeutic
Differential Diagnosis	Gastroenteritis Appendicitis or other infections Other causes of bowel obstruction
Management	Rehydration Analgesia, antibiotics Nil orally, nasogastric tube Air enema ~80% success rate Ultrasound-guided hydrostatic enema Surgical reduction
Outcome	May recur after air enema (~9%) Low mortality with appropriate management

for the duration of treatment. Children who have alterations in their plasma osmolality (e.g., high blood glucose or hypernatremic dehydration) will be sensitive to rapid correction, and frequent rechecks of electrolytes and osmolality are advisable.

4. What are the anesthetic implications of a bowel obstruction due to intussusception?

Usually there is an initial failed radiographic attempt at reduction, in this case an **air enema,** prior to the patient being scheduled for surgical reduction/repair. Anesthetic management of an infant requiring surgical intervention for intussusception should be performed in a specialist pediatric center. Overall characteristics of intussusception are shown in Table 4.2. Adequate fluid resuscitation is vital *prior* to general anesthesia. This is due to the combined effect of loss of sympathetic tone and direct effects of the anesthetic agents at the time of induction, which result in peripheral vasodilation, hypotension, and even cardiovascular collapse. The child will continue to lose fluid during this procedure, and thus if the procedure is lengthy it is not uncommon for the child to become significantly dehydrated again. The child's hydration state should be assessed prior to induction, even if it was deemed adequate earlier.

Prior to induction, the NGT should be aspirated, and even though its use is controversial in some circumstances, rapid sequence induction is still recognized as the safest form of induction in children with bowel obstruction. Nitrous oxide should be avoided during the procedure as there is potential for further distention of already-threatened bowel. Analgesia may be provided with a caudal injection and a morphine infusion for postoperative analgesia. IV fluids and nasogastric drainage should be continued postoperatively until bowel function returns to normal. In this case an isotonic solution was chosen as the child was deemed to be at risk of hyponatremia. The rate was based on regular assessment of the child's hydration status and **electrolytes were checked regularly**.

SUMMARY

1. Significant dehydration from any cause in an infant warrants immediate attention.
2. The type of fluid used will depend on the type of fluid lost, but hypotonic solutions

(such as 4% dextrose with 0.18 NaCl) should be avoided.
3. Isotonic solutions are recommended for initial resuscitation followed by maintenance using a balanced salt solution with 1% or 2.5% glucose for full-term neonates and infants <6 months or any child with potential for hypoglycemia.
4. Regular monitoring of hydration state, as well as electrolytes and blood glucose levels, is important for the duration of IV fluid therapy.

ACKNOWLEDGMENT

The author wishes to acknowledge the first edition author, Britt Fraser.

ANNOTATED REFERENCES

Jiang, J, Jiang B, Parashar, U et al. Childhood intussusception: a literature review. *PLOSone*. 2013;8.

This article reviews the epidemiology, diagnosis, clinical manifestations and management of intussusception from 2002–2012.

Justice FA, Auldist AW, Bines JE. Intussusception: trends in clinical presentation and management. *J Gastroenterol Hepatol.* 2006;21:842–846.

This article reviews all patients with intussusception at a tertiary children's hospital over a 6.5-year period.

National Patient Safety Agency. *Reducing the Risk of Hyponatraemia When Administering Intravenous Infusions to Children.* Patient Safety Alert 22. 2007. http://www.nrls.npsa.nhs.uk/resources/?entryid45=59809

This paper provides comprehensive recommendations regarding fluid management in children, with background material about hyponatremia and hyponatremic encephalopathy. Compares the most commonly used fluids.

Jauregui J, Nelson D, Choo E, et al. The BUDDY (Bedside Ultrasound to Detect Dehydration in Youth) Study. *Crit Ultrasound J.* 2014;6:2–8.

The authors discusses the use of ultrasound in measuring the IVC/ aorta ratio and then utilizing this as a predictor of degree of dehydration.

Neville, KA, Sandeman, DJ, Rubenstein, A. Prevention of Hyponatremia during maintenance intravenous fluid administration: a prospective randomized study of fluid type versus fluid rate. *Journal of Pediatrics.* 2010;156:313–319.

This prospective, randomized trial looks at 124 hospitalized children undergoing elective or emergent surgery to determine the importance of sodium content versus intravenous fluid rate in the development of hyponatremia.

BIBLIOGRAPHY

Applegate KE. Intussusception in children: imaging choices. *Semin Roentgenol.* 2008;43(1):15–21.

Kaiser AD, Applegate KE, Ladd AP. Current success in the treatment of intussusception in children. *Surgery.* 2007;142(4):469–475.

Brett, C, Charr, D. Fluids, electrolytes, and nutrition. In: Andropoulos, DB, Gregory GA, eds. *Gregory's Pediatric Anesthesia.* Malden, MA: Wiley-Blackwell; 2012:205–223.

Lerman J, Sampathi V, Watt S. Induction, maintenance, and emergence from anesthesia. In: Andropoulos, DB, Gregory GA, eds. *Gregory's Pediatric Anesthesia.* Malden, MA: Wiley-Blackwell; 2012:352–354.

McClain CD, McManus ML. Fluid management. In Cote CJ, Lerman J, Todres ID, eds. *A Practice of Anesthesia for Infants and Children.* Philadelphia: Saunders Elsevier, 2009:159–175.

5

Asthmatic for Adenotonsillectomy

ERIN S. WILLIAMS

INTRODUCTION

Asthma affects up to 20% of children in some countries and affects approximately 7 million in the United States. This number is increasing. Although many children have mild asthma and require only intermittent treatment, there is a potential that the child with significant symptoms may present for elective surgery and experience preoperative respiratory adverse events (PRAEs). Acute exacerbations of asthma usually result from exposure to triggers—commonly pollen, tobacco smoke, dust mites, cold air, or viral upper respiratory tract infections (URIs). General anesthesia is usually uneventful in asthmatic children; however, they are more susceptible to intraoperative bronchospasm. Intraoperative bronchospasm is more common if there has been instrumentation of the airway. In the vast majority of cases, these exacerbations are mild with no major sequelae. However, bronchospasm can on rare occasions be severe and very challenging to manage. In order to prevent PRAEs the anesthesiologist must focus on optimization of anesthesia management with the goal of minimizing bronchial hyperactivity and optimizing lung function (Regli et al., 2014).

LEARNING OBJECTIVES

1. Know how to identify undiagnosed or not well controlled asthma.
2. Know how to identify patients at risk of intraoperative bronchospasm.
3. Employ various strategies for the optimization of respiratory status to prevent intraoperative bronchospasm.
4. Review the acute management of intraoperative bronchospasm.
5. Summarize the ventilatory strategies for patients with severe asthma.

CASE PRESENTATION

An 8-year-old 45-kg girl presents to the day surgery floor for removal of her tonsils and adenoids. Her past medical history is significant for having asthma. She uses an albuterol inhaler weekly as needed and is on scheduled inhaled steroids twice a day. Her last hospitalization was 3 months ago due to an asthma exacerbation. She received a dose if intravenous (IV) steroids and nebulizer albuterol and was discharged to home after approximately 6 hours. Her mother states that she also snores and pauses when she sleeps. She does not have a formal sleep study.

Her vital signs on the morning of surgery are heart rate 98, blood pressure 100/50, respiratory rate RR 24, oxygen saturation 96%, temperature 98.

The anesthesiologist performs a physical exam, which is normal. The child is given 2 puffs of albuterol as well as 2 puffs of her scheduled inhaled steroid. She is then taken to the operating room (OR) for removal of her tonsils and adenoids. An uneventful inhaled induction is performed and a peripheral IV is placed. She receives IV lidocaine, propofol, dexmedetomidine 0.5 mck/Kg, fentanyl 1 mcg/Kg, acetaminophen 15 mg/kg, and dexamethasone 0.5mg/Kg. She is intubated with a 5.0 cuffed oral RAE endotracheal tube (ETT).

After intubation, the anesthesiologist auscultates and hears diffuse wheezing in both lung fields. He decides to give 2 puffs of albuterol via the ETT (Figure 5.1) and deepens the anesthetic by increasing the sevoflurane concentration. He listens again and finds the wheezing has resolved.

The tonsils and adenoids are removed. The patient is given ondansetron and the anesthesiologist decides to extubate deep in the OR. The patient breathes spontaneously, 2 puffs of albuterol are given, and she is suctioned while deeply anesthetized. The

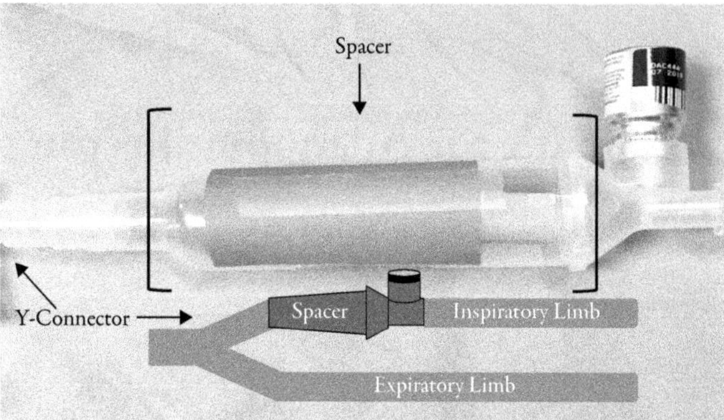

FIGURE 5.1 Albuterol administration via endotracheal tube.

ETT is pulled and the patient is given supplemental oxygen. She is comfortable and transported to the postanesthesia care unit with supplemental oxygen.

DISCUSSION

1. What is asthma?

Asthma is one of the most common chronic respiratory conditions characterized by reversible bronchoconstriction, airway hyperresponsivness, inflammation, and increased mucus production. Such pathophysiology leads to clinical manifestations such as wheezing, coughing, shortness of breath, and chest tightness. Of note, asthma is most prevalent in countries that have a "Western" lifestyle such as the United States, Scotland, Australia, and Brazil.

The incidence of preoperative bronchospasm in children without asthma is 0.2% to 4.1%, and this is increased to 2.2% to 5.7% in asthmatic children.

2. What are the key features of a preanesthetic assessment in an asthmatic patient?

A key aim of preoperative assessment in an asthmatic child is to gauge the severity, control, and "brittleness" of the asthma (Table 5.1). A brittle asthmatic (a patient characterized by intermittent severe asthmatic attacks) is more likely to develop perioperative bronchospasm that is difficult to control. These patients would benefit from a preoperative consultation with their respiratory physician to optimize their asthma control. The major determinant of the severity of asthma is how well symptoms are controlled (Table 5.2). Subsequently this helps guide the clinician in maintaining current therapy or changing it. A short preoperative course of oral steroids may be considered as prophylaxis, although controlled clinical data to substantiate this practice are lacking.

The National Heart, Lung, and Blood Institute and the Global Initiative for Asthma Control have

TABLE 5.1 KEY FACTORS IN DETERMINING SEVERITY OF ASTHMA

Number of acute exacerbations, hospital presentations, and admissions in a year
Recent asthma symptoms, medical interventions, and hospital visits
Usual level of maintenance "preventer" therapy
Usual albuterol frequency, recent use, and especially recent escalation of therapy
Number of episodes of oral corticosteroid use for acute exacerbations within the past year
Previous intensive care admission and invasive ventilation
Any specific triggers for bronchospasm (including previous NSAID exposure)
Presence of a recent cold or coryzal symptoms within the last
2 weeks (this would lower the threshold for delaying surgery more than for a nonasthmatic patient)
Functional exercise tolerance (compared with peers) is a useful marker of severity.

Note. NSAID = nonsteroidal anti-inflammatory drug.

TABLE 5.2 ASTHMA CONTROL

Asthma Control	*Well Controlled*	*Not Well Controlled*	*Poorly Controlled*
Symptoms	≤2 days per week	>2 days per week	Throughout the day
Rescue bronchodilator	≤2 days per week	>2 days per week	Multiple times per day
Early awakening	No		
Nocturnal awakening	No	≥2 times per month	>Once per week
Limitations of work, school, or exercise	No	Yes, some limitation	Yes, extreme limitation
PEF/FEV1	Normal or PB	60% to 80% PB/Predicted	Less than 60% PB/Predicted

Note. PEF = peak flow; FEV1 = forced expiratory volume in 1 second; PB = personal best.

produced a guide to assist the anesthesiologist in determining not only the severity of asthma but also how well its controlled. This provides insight for the appropriate intervention. Severity is determined based on two key features: impairment and future risks. A patient can be assumed to have well-controlled asthma if symptoms present twice a week or less; there is no nocturnal or early awakening and no limitation of work, school, or exercise; and peak flow/forced expiratory volume in 1 second is normal or at the personal best. Thus, when approached with a patient with an asthma diagnosis, the anesthesiologist must determine if the asthma is well controlled, not well controlled, or very poorly controlled.

The absence of the signs of severity and a well-controlled patient is reasonably reassuring; however, some studies have found a poor correlation between assessment of disease severity and the occurrence of perioperative bronchospasm. Asthma is often undertreated, or even undiagnosed, so the absence of intensive control medication should not lead the anesthesiologist to assume the disease is mild or well controlled or not present at all. Many deaths occur in asthmatic patients who have been stratified as having "mild" or "moderate" disease. Perioperative vigilance and preventive measures are required in all children with asthma and other comorbidities to prevent PRAEs (Box 5.1).

A history of prolonged oral prednisolone or high-dose inhaled corticosteroid administration within the previous 12 months is likely to produce some degree of adrenal suppression, and the child will benefit from an intraoperative dose of IV corticosteroid. It is unknown what length and cumulative dose of corticosteroid is required before perioperative corticosteroid supple mentation is required; however, it is commonly thought that the potential benefit obtained from a single intraoperative dose of corticosteroid outweighs the risk of adverse effects.

2. What is the preoperative management of children with undiagnosed asthma?

In general, a short-acting beta 2 (β_2) agonist should be administered, and further investigation is not recommended with resolution of symptoms.

3. What is the preoperative management of the pediatric patient with poorly controlled asthma?

Elective surgery should be rescheduled until the asthma is better controlled.

4. Are objective tests and studies needed preoperatively?

Chest x-rays should not be routinely obtained unless there is a concern for decreased oxygenation or increased work of breathing, volutrauma, or barotrauma. Other tests not recommended include skin tests and simple lung function tests. Because asthma demonstrates reversible bronchoconstriction and inflammation, a normal result does not indicate the absence of disease.

5. What medications should be administered preoperatively?

It is recommended that all asthma medications be given in the preoperative setting. This includes long-term oral corticosteroids. Additionally, inhaled β_2 agonists should be given since they have been shown to improve lung function and reduce PRAEs. In addition to beta 2 agonists, the alpha agonists dexmedetomidine and clonidine may be beneficial given they have been shown to blunt reflex bronchoconstriction after intubation.

BOX 5.1
RISK FACTORS FOR PERIOPERATIVE RESPIRATORY ADVERSE EVENTS

RISKS FOR PRAES

Asthma
Wheezing at exercise
Wheezing more than 3 times in the last 12 months
Nocturnal dry cough
Recent upper respiratory tract infection
Hay fever
Eczema
Family history of asthma, hay fever, eczema
(Passive) smoking
Young age
Higher American Society of Anesthesiologists classification
History of congenital heart disease
Prematurity
Low birth weight
Obesity
Obstructive sleep apnea

6. What are the common triggers for childhood asthma?

The most common trigger for a childhood asthma exacerbation is a **URI**. This is usually viral in nature. Other triggers include inhaled irritant gases (e.g., smoke), pollen, and foreign bodies. Crying or coughing (e.g., during uncooperative inhalational induction) may also trigger acute bronchospasm. During anesthesia, instrumentation of the airway is the most common trigger (e.g., placement of an ETT or tracheal suctioning). Carinal irritation in particular may precipitate bronchospasm. Irritant volatile agents such as desflurane may also predispose to bronchospasm. The differential diagnosis of wheezing always needs to be considered (see Chapter 17).

7. How is bronchospasm prevented?

Delay elective surgery:

Delaying surgery should be considered in the presence of poor asthma control, recent or current URI, or lower respiratory tract infection. Airway hyperreactivity related to a viral URI persists for approximately 4 weeks. The threshold for delaying surgery in an asthmatic child with a URI would be lower than for a child who does not have asthma.

Experienced pediatric anesthesiologist:

Several studies have shown that having an experienced pediatric anesthesiologist during airway management decreases the risk for PRAEs.

Preoperative medications:

The usual inhaled and oral medications should be given on the day of surgery. In addition, it is suggested that giving patients an inhaled bronchodilator 30 to 60 minutes before induction of anesthesia will reduce the incidence and severity of perioperative bronchospasm. Inhaled β_2-agonists are known to attenuate the increased airway resistance associated with tracheal intubation (Scalfaro et al., 2001). In addition, the use of sedative premedication such as midazolam in selected patients can avoid or reduce the child's distress on induction. Crying may in itself induce bronchospasm. Anticholinergic drugs (e.g., glycopyrrolate) have been used to dry secretions but may worsen mucus plugging postoperatively.

ETT versus laryngeal mask airway (LMA) versus bag mask ventilation:

This is a controversial issue; although intubation has been associated with an increased incidence of pulmonary complications, causation is not always clear and there are inadequate outcome data to make definitive recommendations. When considering the risks versus benefits of choice of airway device, the ETT should not be avoided "at all costs"; LMA insertion can also produce bronchospasm, and it would be much more difficult to manage the consequent ventilatory requirements without an ETT. If an ETT is inserted, it is important not to place the tube close to the carina to avoid airway stimulation. It is also recommended to use a cuffed ETT to reduce air leak.

Depth of anesthesia.

A deep plane of anesthesia reduces airway reactivity associated with intubation. Patience is the key: wait until the child is deep enough, and then wait a little more. If possible, deep extubation is recommended for the same reasons. Topical anesthesia of the airway with local anesthetic seems appealing but may increase bronchomotor tone and cause an increased risk of PRAE.

Avoidance of histamine-releasing drugs: This is somewhat controversial because not all histamine-releasing drugs will reliably trigger bronchospasm. However, with alternatives available, it is simple enough to avoid histamine-releasing drugs such as atracurium and morphine.

Avoidance of certain anesthetic agents: Desflurane should be avoided in children with asthma since it is known to be associated with increased risk of bronchospasm. Other agents to avoid include thiopentone, neuromuscular blocking drugs, and neostigmine.

8. What is the risk in children of worsening asthmatic symptoms with nonsteroidal anti-inflammatory drugs (NSAIDs)?

Some asthmatic adults have an aspirin-sensitive condition in which NSAIDs are relatively contraindicated. This seems to be less of a problem in children. Most children with asthma are able to take NSAIDs with no adverse effect. In general, older children (teenagers) with **atopy** and severe brittle asthma are the group most likely to suffer ill effects of NSAIDs (Palmer, 2005). NSAIDs are still only relatively contraindicated in this group, since there is a low risk of causing bronchospasm. Of note, patients with nasal polyps and asthma have shown an increased risk of NSAID-induced asthma and therefore this subgroup of asthmatic patients should not receive NSAIDs. A debate remains as to whether or not IV acetaminophen causes asthma symptoms, thus it is not contraindicated.

9. Should morphine be given to patients with asthma?

Morphine has the potential to cause airway constriction and should be used with caution.

10. What is the acute management of an intraoperative asthma exacerbation and bronchospasm?

Acute management is initially supportive, ensuring adequate oxygen delivery and reasonable carbon dioxide clearance. Mechanical causes should be considered (e.g., blocked/kinked ETT, carinal irritation, defective circuit) as well as other causes of raised airway pressures (pneumothorax, abdominal splinting due to light anesthesia, anaphylaxis). Where possible, ventilatory pressures should be limited to reduce the risk of barotrauma and cardiovascular collapse (from high intrathoracic pressure). Simple measures include **increasing fraction of inspired oxygen, reducing the respiratory rate,** and **reducing the I:E ratio** (prolonging expiratory time) to avoid gas trapping. Permissive hypercarbia is often employed. High positive end-expiratory pressure should be avoided since this can predispose patients to dynamic hyperinflation.

Be aware that patients tend to be hyperventilated (especially during manual ventilation) during an acute respiratory crisis. This runs the risk of increasing **gas trapping**. Placing the patient on a mechanical ventilator reduces this risk. Also consider intermittently reducing the intrathoracic pressure by disconnecting the patient from the breathing circuit and manually compressing the chest to produce a more complete exhalation of trapped gas within the lung.

Concurrent specific treatment of bronchospasm is equally important. This is rapidly achieved by the use of **volatile anesthetic agents**, most appropriately sevoflurane or isoflurane, although this must be balanced against its cardiovascular-depressant effects at higher concentrations. Repeated doses **of inhaled albuterol** (Fig. 5.1) is a simple method of delivering topical bronchodilator quickly. However, it is thought that as little as 3% of the nominal dose if aerosolized drug reaches the airways, though a spacing chamber can increase the delivered dose (Duarte, 2004). Inhaled ipratropium bromide may also be given every 20 to 30 minutes for continued bronchospasm. Terbutaline is available for subcutaneous injection in circumstance in which inhaled β_2 agonists cannot be delivered dependably. Should the wheezing result from anaphylaxis, intravenous epinephrine (adrenaline) is the drug of choice.

Corticosteroids should be given early to those who do not respond promptly to β_2 agonists; although the onset time of the anti-inflammatory effects of corticosteroids take 4 to 6 hours, it does enhance and prolong the effects of β_2 agonists within an hour. It is thought the latter effect occurs due to an increase in the expression of the β adrenoreceptor, restoring G-protein/β_2 receptor coupling and decreasing desensitization (Johnson, 2004).

Status asthmaticus under anesthesia is extremely uncommon. Ventilatory management of these patients is a very complex area, and early involvement of intensive care should be sought. If the patient does not respond to inhaled albuterol and basic ventilation maneuvers (as discussed earlier), more advanced ventilator and pharmacological management is required. A meta-analysis concluded that IV magnesium sulfate has been shown to probably provide additional benefit in moderate to severe acute asthma in children treated with bronchodilators and steroids (Cheuk et al., 2005). IV magnesium sulfate 40 mg/kg over 20 minutes has been shown to be safe in treating asthma exacerbation; it also has the advantage of an apparent paucity of side effects. IV aminophylline has been used in severe asthma, but it is often associated with cardiovascular side effects under anesthesia as well as nausea and vomiting, thus is not advantageous. Studies have failed to show whether IV albuterol or aminophylline is more effective in children with acute severe asthma (Roberts et al., 2003). The most severe cases may potentially require high-frequency oscillation or even extracorporeal membrane oxygenator support.

SUMMARY

1. Assessment is targeted at eliciting the severity and control of the disease.
2. Prevention is the key in *all* patients with asthma: patients should take their usual drugs preoperatively and inhaled β_2 agonists before induction. Avoid bronchospasm triggers.
3. Intraoperative management involves excluding mechanical causes of wheezing, considering alternative diagnoses, and simple ventilator measures. Volatile anesthetic agents and inhaled β_2 agonists can rapidly reverse the bronchospasm in most cases.

ACKNOWLEDGMENT

The author wishes to acknowledge the first edition author, Eugene Neo.

ANNOTATED REFERENCES

Doherty G, Chisakuta A, Crean P, Shields M. Anesthesia and the child with asthma. *Pediatr Anesth.* 2005;15:446–454.

A comprehensive review article covering many aspects of anesthetizing a child with asthma.

Regli A, von Ungern-Sternberg B. Anesthesia and ventilation in children with asthma: part I—preoperative assessment. *Curr Opin Anesthesiol.* 2014;27:288–294.

A comprehensive review of the preoperative assessment and management of the pediatric asthma patient scheduled for surgery.

Regli A, von Ungern-Sternberg B. Anesthesia and ventilation in children with asthma: part II—intraoperative management. *Curr Opin Anesthesiol.* 2014;27:288–294.

A comprehensive review of the intraoperative management of the pediatric asthma patient scheduled for surgery.

BIBLIOGRAPHY

Cheuk DKL, Chau TCH, Lee SL. A meta-analysis on intravenous magnesium sulphate for treating acute asthma. *Arch Dis Child.* 2005;90:74–77.

Dinakar C, Chipps B. Clinical tools to assess asthma control in children. *Pediatrics.* 2017;139:1–11.

Duarte AG. Inhaled bronchodilator administration during mechanical ventilation. *Respir Care.* 2004;49(6):623–34.

Mitra A, Bassler D, Ducharme FM. Intravenous aminophylline for acute severe asthma in children over 2 years using inhaled bronchodilators. *Cochrane Database Syst Rev.* 2001;4:CD001276.

Roberts G, Newsom D, Gomez K, et al. Intravenous salbutamol bolus compared with an aminophylline infusion in children with severe asthma: a randomized controlled trial. *Thorax.* 2003;58:306–310.

Johnson M. Interactions between corticosteroids and β_2-agonists in asthma and chronic obstructive pulmonary disease. *Proc Am Thorac Soc.* 2004;1:200–206.

Palmer GM. A teenager with severe asthma exacerbation following ibuprofen. *Anaesth Inten Care.* 2005;33(2):261–265.

Scalfaro P, Sly P, Sims C, Habre W. Salbutamol prevents the increase of respiratory resistance caused by tracheal intubation during sevoflurane anesthesia in asthmatic children. *Anesth Analg.* 2001;93:898–902.

von Ungern-Sternberg B, Habre W, Erb T, Heaney M. Salbutamol premedication in children with a recent respiratory tract infection. *Pediatr Anesth.* 2009;19:1064–1069.

Tait A, Pandit U, Voepel-Lewis T, Munro H, Malviya S. Use of the laryngeal mask airway in children with upper respiratory tract infections: a comparison with endotracheal intubation. *Anesth Analg.* 1998;86:706–711.

6

Preoperative Fasting in the Pediatric Patient

NANCY HAGERMAN AND ERIC WITTKUGEL

INTRODUCTION

The amount of time without food is the fasting period. Typically, this time is initiated with the nil per os (NPO) order. This period of time has a varies greatly depending on the type of liquid or food ingested. The American Society of Anesthesiologists has updated 2017 preoperative fasting guidelines to aid in patient safety as well as patient satisfaction. The longer a patient is without food and drink the more likely the risk of dehydration, electrolyte abnormalities such as hypoglycemia and difficult peripheral IV placement, thus, it is important that the NPO time be as short as possible.

> **LEARNING OBJECTIVES**
> 1. Know the current preoperative fasting guidelines from the American Society of Anesthesiologists.
> 2. Understand the risk of pulmonary aspiration in the pediatric population, common sequelae, and treatment.
> 3. Understand implications for overweight/obese pediatric patients.
> 4. List advantages associated with a liberalized preoperative fast.
> 5. Name common medical conditions that are associated with an increased risk of pulmonary aspiration.

CASE PRESENTATION

An obese 8-year-old 40-kg girl presents for outpatient ***upper endoscopy*** *to evaluate her chronic abdominal pain. On arrival, the patient is chewing gum which she is instructed to spit out. She has been nil per os (NPO) for solids since the evening before and drank a cup of* ***apple juice*** *just* ***2 hours ago****.*

The gastroenterologist informs you he is ready to take her to the endoscopy suite.

DISCUSSION

1. What are the current American Society of Anesthesiologists (ASA) preoperative fasting guidelines? Who is the intended patient population for these guidelines?

The ASA Task Force on Preoperative Fasting published their most recent guidelines in 2017 (Table 6.1). These guidelines evolve according to medical knowledge and technology and were compiled based on an analysis of current literature, expert opinion, open forum commentary, and clinical feasibility data. The guidelines recommend a fasting interval of **2** or more hours after the consumption of **clear liquids**, **4** or more hours after **breast milk** in both neonates and infants, **6** or more hours after the intake of **infant formula**, and **6** or more hours after a **light meal** (typically toast and clear liquids) or **nonhuman milk**. Additional fasting time (e.g., 8 or more hours) may be needed in cases of patient intake of fried foods, fatty foods, or meat, which prolong gastric emptying. The amount and type of foods ingested must be considered when determining an appropriate fasting period; this understanding will maximize patient and parent satisfaction (Cook-Sather et al., 2006). Clear liquids are defined as water, fat-free and protein-free liquids, pulp-free fruit juice, carbonated drinks, clear tea, and black coffee (Kalinowski et al., 2004). Human breast milk has a higher whey to casein ratio, a faster transit time through the stomach, and a lower potential to form curd compared to cow's milk. Cow's milk has gastric-emptying characteristics similar to those of solids as it separates into liquid and solid (curd)

TABLE 6.1 AMERICAN SOCIETY OF ANESTHESIOLOGISTS FASTING RECOMMENDATIONS (2017)

Ingested Material	*Minimum Fasting Period*
Clear liquids	2 h
Breast milk	4 h
Infant formula	6 h
Nonhuman milk	6 h
Light meal	6 h
Fried, fatty foods or meat	8 h or more may be needed

From Practice guidelines for preoperative fasting and the use of pharmacologic agents to reduce the risk of pulmonary aspiration: application to healthy patients undergoing elective procedures: an updated report by the American Society of Anesthesiologists Task Force on Preoperative Fasting and the Use of Pharmacologic Agents to Reduce the Risk of Pulmonary Aspiration. *Anesthesiology*. 2017;126(3):376–393.

phases in the acid environment of the stomach and can remain undigested for several hours.[3]

These **guidelines** are intended only for **healthy patients of all ages** undergoing **elective procedures.** Following the guidelines does not guarantee complete gastric emptying. The guidelines may not apply to or may need to be modified for patients with coexisting diseases or conditions that can affect gastric emptying time or fluid volume (e.g., pregnancy, obesity, diabetes, hiatal hernia, gastroesophageal reflux disease, ileus or bowel obstruction, emergency care, or enteral tube feeding) and patients in whom airway management might be difficult. Anesthesiologists and other anesthesia providers should recognize that these conditions can increase the likelihood of regurgitation and pulmonary aspiration and that additional or alternative preventive strategies may be appropriate. Of note, the ASA guidelines do not recommend the routine use of gastrointestinal stimulants (e.g., metoclopramide), medications that block gastric acid secretion (e.g., omeprazole, lansoprazole), antacids, and/or antiemetics to decrease the risk of pulmonary aspiration in patients who have no apparent increased risk (Cook-Sather et al., 2006).

Other countries carry similar guidelines regarding the preoperative fast (Table 6.2). Guidelines published by the Royal College of Nursing in 2005 and the Canadian Anesthesiologists' Society in 2008 also follow the ASA "2-4-6 rule." Additionally, the Canadian Anesthesiologists' Society recommends an 8-hour fast after a meal that includes meat, fried, or fatty foods. The Scandinavian Guidelines (2005) are different only in that they include infant formula in the 4-hour rule along with breast milk (Brady et al. 2009).

The determination of what constitutes a safe preoperative fasting duration is difficult as the incidence of pulmonary aspiration is very low and sample sizes in studies are often too small. Because of this, surrogate markers for aspiration, usually gastric fluid volume, are used throughout the anesthesia literature to determine safe practice. Increasingly, gastric fluid volume is being determined by gastric ultrasound and magnetic resonance imaging (Schmitz et al., 2016).

2. What is the risk of pulmonary aspiration in the pediatric population?

Fortunately, the **incidence** of perioperative pulmonary aspiration is rare—it is estimated between 1 in 10,000 and 10 in 10,000, depending upon the methodologies used. The **majority** of these events **occur upon induction** of anesthesia, usually associated with patients who **cough** or **gag** during airway manipulation (Cook-Sather et al., 2006).

In a large prospective study published in 1999, Warner et al. found that there was a greater frequency of aspiration in emergency procedures versus elective procedures and that the majority of infants and children less than 3 years of age who aspirated had ileus or bowel obstruction. They also found that **most children who have mild to moderate aspiration events have no significant medical sequelae**. In fact, based on their experience, Warner and colleagues will discharge a child from the recovery room after 2 hours of observation after an episode of aspiration as long as the child does not present with new symptoms such as coughing and wheezing, new hypoxia while breathing room air, or radiologic abnormalities (Warner et al., 1999).

A more recent 12-month prospective survey performed in the United Kingdom by Walker determined an incidence of pulmonary aspiration within pediatric centers to be 24 out of 118,371 cases, or 2 in 10,000 cases. Of note, of the 12 patients in this

TABLE 6.2 GUIDELINES FOR PEDIATRIC PREOPERATIVE FASTING

Age Group	*Solids*	*Clear Fluids*	*Breast Milk*	*Nonhuman Milk + Formula*
Neonates <6 months	N/A	2 hrs (a,b,c)	4 hrs (a,b,c); (d: milk type not specified	6 hrs (a,b); 4 hrs (d: milk type not specified); 4 hrs formula milk (c)
Infants 6–36 months, <12 months (e)	6 hrs (b,c,d,e)	2 hrs (a,b,c,d,e)	4 hrs (a,b,c,e); 6 hrs (d: milk type not specified)	6 hrs (a,b,e), (d: milk type not specified); 4 hrs formula milk (c)
Children > 36 months, >12 months (e)	6 hrs (a,c,e); 8 hrs (d); 6 hrs for light meal and 8 hrs for meal that includes meat, fried or fatty foods (b)	2 hrs (a,b,c,d,e)	4 hrs (a,b,c,e); 8 hrs (d: milk type not specified)	6 hrs (a,b,e); 8 hrs (d); 4 hrs formula milk (c)

Key:

a = American Society of Anesthesiologists, 1999.
b = Canadian Anesthesiologists' Society, 2008, ages not specified.
c = Scandinavian Guidelines (Task Force), 2005, ages not specified.
d = American Academy of Pediatrics, 1992.
e = Royal College of Nursing, 2005.

From Brady MC, Kinn S, Ness V, et al. Preoperative fasting for preventing perioperative complications in children. *Cochrane Database Syst Rev.* Oct 2009;4:CD005285. Copyright Cochrane Collaboration, reproduced with permission.

survey who aspirated intraoperatively, 10 of them were managed with a laryngeal mask airway, 1 with a face mask, and 1 with a nasal cannula. The author notes that there is a potential case for the use of second-generation supraglottic airway devices in patients with potential risk factors for pulmonary aspiration (Walker, 2013).

Severe aspiration classically presents with bronchospasm, tachypnea, wheezing, cyanosis, and fever. This requires supportive care that may escalate to include tracheal intubation, pulmonary lavage, and admission to intensive care for mechanical ventilation.[3] An infiltrate in the right middle or lower lobe on chest x-ray is consistent with aspiration pneumonia. Radiographic changes usually occur within a few hours and show gradual improvement over the next 48 to 72 hours. With appropriate treatment, **mortality from perioperative pulmonary aspiration is very rare**—estimated at 1 in over 70,000 patients.

3. How do these guidelines apply to children with obesity?

Childhood obesity is considered to be one of the most important public health concerns in the United States. It is estimated that approximately one-third of American children are either overweight or obese. More specifically, 2010 data demonstrates that approximately 18% of school-aged children and 18.4% of adolescents are considered obese in the United States. Overweight children tend to be older, probably related to the fact that obesity is a cumulative disease that begins in early childhood.

The Preoperative Fasting Guidelines published by the ASA specifically note that they are not applicable for obese patients, as obesity could affect gastric emptying and fluid volumes. The anesthesia literature on this topic is inconsistent. Cook-Sather's examination of a pediatric population found that although body mass index (BMI) percentile positively correlates with increased gastric fluid volumes, the correlations are exceedingly small and not helpful to the clinician in assessing the potential risk of aspiration. Additionally, they found no difference in fasting duration between those obese patients who vomited during anesthesia and those who did not, suggesting that **prolonged fasting (>2 hours for clear liquids) does not diminish risk in obese patients**. As such, they advocate extending the 2-hour clear liquid ASA fasting guideline to include overweight and obese children who present for day surgery (Cook-Sather et al., 2009). Similarly, Warner's retrospective review of 172,334 adult patients with a BMI of >35 did not demonstrate obesity to be an independent risk factor for perioperative aspiration (Warner et al., 1993).

In contrast, Mahajan and colleagues prospectively analyzed the gastric fluid volumes and gastric pH values of 20 lean adults compared with 40 morbidly obese (BMI >35) adults. They concluded that unpremedicated morbidly obese adults have significantly higher mean gastric volumes (and thus a higher aspiration risk) than lean adults. However, they also found that morbidly obese adults premedicated with ranitidine and metoclopramide had gastric fluid volumes and gastric pH values similar to that of unpremedicated lean patients. As such, they recommend the routine administration of preoperative ranitidine and metoclopramide in morbidly obese adults (Mahajan et al., 2015).

4. Does chewing gum have any significance during the preoperative fast?

Although adult studies do not demonstrate a change in gastric fluid volumes or pH in patients who chew gum prior to anesthesia, **gum chewed for 30 minutes immediately before surgery in pediatric patients is associated with significantly increased gastric fluid volumes and pH.** Therefore, many practitioners **treat gum that has not been swallowed as a clear liquid**, allowing 2 to 3 hours to pass prior to the start of the anesthetic. Others argue that the use of chewing gum preoperatively could indicate other fasting violations and that the child and parent should be carefully questioned about any other NPO violations (Cook-Sather et al., 2006).

Shanmugam reviewed the WebAIRS, a de-identified anesthesia incident database for Australia and New Zealand, and found only 9 incidents involving chewing gum out of 2600 total incidents in a 5-year time frame. None of the incidents resulted in adverse outcomes including pulmonary aspiration (Shanmugam et al., 2016). In a comprehensive review, Poulton concludes that there is no evidence that gum chewing during preanesthetic fasting increases the volume or acidity of gastric juice in a manner that increases aspiration risk. There is also no evidence that unreported swallowing of gum risks subsequent aspiration. On the contrary, there is evidence that gum chewing promotes gastrointestinal motility and physiologic gastric emptying. However, one must be sure that chewing gum is not in the patient's mouth at the time of induction (Poulton, 2012).

5. What are the advantages associated with a more liberal preoperative fasting policy?

Encouraging healthy patients who present for elective surgery to consume clear liquids up until 2 hours prior to their anesthetic may be associated with several advantages. Specifically, these patients may be **less dehydrated,** have **improved hemodynamic stability upon induction** of anesthesia (particularly with inhalational inductions in small children), have **easier intravenous (IV) access**, have **improved glucose homeostasis**, have **reduced irritability**, may have **improved child and parent satisfaction**, and may have a **decreased risk of postoperative nausea and vomiting** (Kalinowski et al., 2004 and Cook-Sather et al., 2006). Indeed, in an observational study of children under 36 months of age, Dennhardt found that children who were encouraged to drink clear liquids up until 2 hours prior to their surgery had lower ketone body concentrations, a higher mean arterial pressure, and a lower incidence of hypotension after the induction of anesthesia with no occurrence of pulmonary aspiration (Dennhardt et al., 2016).

Some pediatric anesthesiologists suggest reducing fasting times beyond those suggested in the ASA guidelines. Andersson and colleagues describe their 10-year experience of allowing children to drink clear fluids until they are called to the operating room. Anesthesia induction occurs at least 30 minutes after the last intake of clear liquids. Although they call this practice the "6-4-0 regime," they state that they actually encourage strict fasting from solid foods from midnight. They speculate that this less complicated regime may lead to fewer NPO violations. In their practice, they usually perform IV inductions and maintain airways with either an endotracheal tube or laryngeal mask airway and have an incidence of pulmonary aspiration of 3 in 10,000 cases (Andersson et al., 2015). This simplified regime may also aid in the staffing and scheduling of surgical cases in situations in which last-minute changes occur to the operating room schedule (Ragg, 2015).

The practice of allowing children to drink clear fluids up to 1 hour prior to surgery is further supported by Schmidt, who reported no significant difference in gastric pH or residual gastric volumes when comparing children fasted for clears for 1 hour versus 2 hours. This study clearly demonstrates that gastric residual volumes vary substantially in "normal" physiology and an empty stomach cannot always be expected. Therefore, a safe and smooth anesthesia technique to prevent regurgitation by coughing and bucking is just as or even more important in minimizing the risk of pulmonary aspiration (Schmidt et al., 2015).

While the evidence for the safety of preoperative clear liquids is strong, the evidence for guidelines on milk products and solids is less robust. Although human breast milk may clear faster than the recommended 4 hours, it is difficult to consider reducing the fasting interval due to individual variation in gastric emptying and human milk content (Ragg, 2015).

6. What common medical conditions are associated with an increased risk of pulmonary aspiration?

Gastric emptying of liquids and solids is delayed by 40% to 50% in both **type I and type II diabetic patients**. Adult literature has shown that this reduced gastric emptying is most likely secondary to diabetic autonomic neuropathy and not related to hemoglobin A1C, preprandial blood glucose, or age (Kalinowski et al., 2004).

Renal failure has also been shown to be associated with delayed gastric emptying both in patients who are on hemodialysis and peritoneal dialysis (Kalinowski et al., 2004). Patients with *both* diabetes and renal failure have a further delay in gastric emptying.

Infants and toddlers may have an increased risk of pulmonary aspiration **compared to older children**. In Warner et al.'s large prospective study of pulmonary aspiration in children, they found that the majority of children who aspirated had bowel obstruction or ileus. Of this subpopulation, the majority of those children were under the age of 3 years. This was thought to occur because infants and toddlers are known to have lower esophageal sphincter tone compared to older children and adults. The frequency of gastroesophageal reflux decreases to a rate similar to that seen in adulthood by the time a child reaches his or her third birthday. Additionally, young children frequently swallow moderate amounts of air while crying or sucking on a pacifier, which can contribute to higher intragastric pressures (Warner et al., 1999).

A study of children presenting for upper endoscopy to evaluate gastrointestinal symptoms demonstrated that when they had fasted for at least 6 to 8 hours, these children did not have gastric contents with increased volume and acidity compared with previously published groups of children without gastric symptoms who fasted the same length of time. The patients in this study had chronic vomiting, abdominal pain, gastroesophageal reflux, esophageal disease, and other symptoms. This study lends support for, but does not prove, the safety of not automatically intubating these patients coming for upper endoscopy (Schwartz et al., 1998). Patients with severe gastroesophageal pathology, particularly those with obstructive disease, dysmotility syndromes, and achalasia, may benefit from longer NPO times and may require rapid sequence induction and intubation in the head up position. Optimal NPO times for these patients is not known.

7. Should medications be included in the fasting instructions that are given to parents preoperatively?

The determination of which medications to administer or discontinue preoperatively is a complex one. Implications of a medication's impact on surgical and anesthetic risk should be considered. For example, antiplatelet agents, anticoagulants, and herbal remedies are likely to be contraindicated in the perioperative setting. However, a patient's chronic medications should often be continued. These can include antiarrhythmic, antihypertensive, asthma, diabetes, immunosuppressive, anticonvulsant, and psychiatric medications. Specific considerations as to which drugs to continue perioperatively are dependent upon patient, surgical, and pharmacologic factors (Mercado et al., 2003).

SUMMARY

1. ASA Guidelines: 2 hours for clear liquids; 4 hours for breast milk; 6 hours for infant formula, nonhuman milk, or light meal; 8 hours or more may be needed for fried, fatty foods, or meat.
2. Risk of pulmonary aspiration is very low. Most children who do aspirate have no significant medical sequelae. If a patient aspirates, consider discharging from the postanesthesia care unit after 2 hours if they have no new symptoms such as hypoxia, cough, or wheezing.

3. Obesity: Restricting oral intake for a time longer than the ASA guidelines may not be of any benefit.
4. Chewing gum: Treat gum as a clear liquid.
5. At-risk medical conditions: Type I and type II diabetes, renal failure, bowel obstruction, ileus, pregnancy, hiatal hernia, gastroesophageal reflux disease, patients in whom difficult airway management is anticipated.

ANNOTATED REFERENCES

Cook-Sather SD, Litman RS. Modern fasting guidelines in children. *Best Pract Res Clin Anaesthesiol.* 2006;20(3):471–481.

This comprehensive but easy-to-read review of fasting guidelines for children provides a nice discussion of the evidence supporting current guidelines, the management of pulmonary aspiration, how fasting affects the patient intraoperatively, as well as its impact on family-centered care.

Practice guidelines for preoperative fasting and the use of pharmacologic agents to reduce the risk of pulmonary aspiration: application to healthy patients undergoing elective procedures: an updated report by the American Society of Anesthesiologists Task Force on Preoperative Fasting and the Use of Pharmacologic Agents to Reduce the Risk of Pulmonary Aspiration. *Anesthesiology.* 2017;126(3):376–393.

It is useful to read these guidelines and the analysis on which they were created to gain a better understanding of NPO guidelines.

Warner MA, Warner ME, Warner DO, et al. perioperative pulmonary aspiration in infants and children. *Anesthesiology.* 1999;90(1):66–71.

This large prospective study of 56,138 consecutive patients under the age of 18 who underwent 63,180 general anesthetics at the Mayo Clinic identified all 24 cases of pulmonary aspiration in that population. It gives great insight into the incidence and outcomes of this rare complication.

BIBLIOGRAPHY

Andersson H, Zarén B, Frykholm P. Low incidence of pulmonary aspiration in children allowed intake of clear fluids until called to the operating suite. *Pediatr Anesth.* 2015;25(8):770–777.

Brady MC, Kinn S, Ness V, et al. Preoperative Fasting for Preventing Perioperative Complications in Children. *Cochrane Database Syst Rev.* 2009;(4):CD005285.

Cook-Sather SD, Litman RS. Modern Fasting Guidelines in Children. *Best Pract Res Clin Anaesthesiol.* 2006;20(3):471–481.

Cook-Sather SD, Gallagher PR, Kruge LE, et al. Overweight/Obesity and Gastric Fluid Characteristics in Pediatric Day Surgery: Implications for Fasting Guidelines and Pulmonary Aspiration Risk. *Anesth Analg.* 2009;109(3):727–736.

Dennhardt N, Beck C, Huber D, et al. Optimized preoperative fasting times decrease ketone body concentration and stabilize mean arterial blood pressure during induction of anesthesia in children younger than 36 months: a prospective observational cohort study. *Pediatr Anesth.* 2016;26(8):838–843.

Kalinowski CPH, Kirsch JR. Strategies for Prophylaxis and treatment for Aspiration. *Best Pract Res Clin Anaesthesiol.* 2004;18(4):719–737.

Kumar S, Kelly AS. Review of Childhood Obesity: From Epidemiology, Etiology, and Comorbidities to Clinical Assessment and Treatment. *Mayo Clin Proc.* 2017;92(2):251–265.

Mahajan V, Hashmi J, Singh R, Samra T, Aneja S. Comparative evaluation of gastric pH and volume in morbidly obese and lean patients undergoing elective surgery and effect of aspiration prophylaxis. *J Clin Anesth.* 2015;27(5):396–400.

Mercado DL, Petty BG. Perioperative Medication Management. *Med Clin North Am.* 2003;87(1):41–57.

Poulton TJ. Gum chewing during pre-anesthetic fasting. *Pediatr Anesth.* 2012;22(3):288–296.

Practice Guidelines for Preoperative Fasting and the Use of Pharmacologic Agents to Reduce the Risk of Pulmonary Aspiration: Application to Healthy Patients Undergoing Elective Procedures: An Updated Report by the American Society of Anesthesiologists Task Force on Preoperative Fasting and the Use of Pharmacologic Agents to Reduce the Risk of Pulmonary Aspiration. *Anesthesiology.* 2017;126(3):376–393.

Ragg P. Let them drink! *Pediatr Anesth.* 2015; 25(8):762–763.

Schmidt AR, Buehler P, Seglias L, et al. Gastric pH and residual volume after 1 and 2 h fasting time for clear fluids in children. *Br J Anaesth.* 2015;114(3):477–482.

Schmitz A, Kellenberger CJ, Liamlahi R, Studhalter M, Weiss M. Gastric emptying after overnight fasting and clear fluid intake: a prospective investigation using serial magnetic resonance imaging in healthy children. *Br J Anaesth.* 2011;107(3):425–429.

Schmitz A, Schmidt AR, Buehler PK, et al. Gastric ultrasound as a preoperative bedside test for residual gastric contents volume in children. *Pediatr Anesth.* 2016;26(12):1157–1164.

Schwartz DA, Connelly NR, Theroux CA, et al. Gastric Contents in Children Presenting for Upper Endoscopy. *Anesth Analg.* 1998;87(4):757–760.

Shanmugam S, Goulding G, Gibbs NM, Taraporewalla K, Culwick M. Chewing gum in the preoperative fasting period: an analysis of de-identified incidents reported to webAIRS. *Anaesth Intensive Care.* 2016;44(2):281–284.

Walker RW. Pulmonary aspiration in pediatric anesthetic practice in the UK: a prospective survey of specialist pediatric centers over a one-year period. *Pediatr Anesth.* 2013;23(8):702–711.

Warner MA, Warner ME, Weber JG. Clinical Significance of Pulmonary Aspiration During the Perioperative Period. *Anesthesiology.* 1993;78(1):56–62.

Warner MA, Warner ME, Warner DO, et al. Perioperative Pulmonary Aspiration in Infants and Children. *Anesthesiology.* 1999;90(1):66–71.

PART 2

Challenges in Pediatric Pharmacology

7

Malignant Hyperthermia

ERIN S. WILLIAMS

INTRODUCTION

Malignant hyperthermia, or malignant hyperpyrexia (MH), is a rare but frightening condition that occurs with an incidence of between 1:4,000 and 1:60,000 general anesthetics. A very busy pediatric hospital may expect to see one case every 2 to 3 years. Its presentation is nonspecific and the course of MH can be insidious or rapidly progressive. With the majority of MH occurring in the pediatric population, it is imperative that the pediatric anesthesiologist have extensive knowledge regarding diagnosis and treatment of this potentially fatal syndrome.

LEARNING OBJECTIVES

1. Know the clinical features of MH.
2. Understand the pharmacogenetic disturbance of skeletal and cardiac muscle in MH and know how to practically make a diagnosis of MH while considering the differential diagnoses.
3. Know the emergency treatment of MH in a team environment.
4. Know how to follow up a suspected case of MH and evaluate the implications for the patient and family.

CASE PRESENTATION

A 30-kg 6-year-old boy presents for strabismus surgery. He has no past medical history and is taking no medication. This is his first surgery. There is ***no family history*** *of problems with anesthesia. All of his vital signs are stable and his exam is unremarkable. He undergoes a smooth inhaled induction followed by peripheral IV placement. A flexible LMA is inserted after 3 mg/kg of propofol, and 1 mcg/Kg of fentanyl is administered.*

Fifteen minutes into the procedure, the heart rate increases from 90 to 120 then to 150 bpm. He is breathing spontaneously but it is noted that the end-tidal carbon dioxide (ETCO$_2$) has increased from 35 to 55 mmHg. He is placed on pressure control ventilation and however, the ETCO$_2$ continues to rise despite manual hyperventilation. There is no increase in airway pressure. Other observations are SpO$_2$ 97%, BP 90/40, nasopharyngeal temperature is now 39°C. Sevoflurane concentration is increased to 5%. No abnormality is seen in the machine, soda lime, or ventilation circuit. The patient continues to deteriorate: ***ETCO$_2$ 70 mmHg, HR 160*** *(sinus), BP 80/40,* ***temperature 39.2°C****, a stat arterial blood gas reveals pH 7.05, pO$_2$ 300 mmHg,* ***pCO$_2$ 75 mmHg****, base excess–8.6. The diagnosis of MH is made. You turn of the triggering agent, call for help immediately and request the dantrolene. The circulator brings you the MH cart and she is concerned because she says there is no dantrolene but there something called Ryanodex. The* ***local MH protocol*** *is instituted with specific roles for all members of the surgical care team (Table 7.1). A bolus of 2.5 mg/kg* ***dantrolene*** *is given, the patient is intubated, an arterial line and foley catheter is placed, ice is placed on the patient; the patient's heart rate, ETCO$_2$, and temperature rapidly return to normal within 5 minutes. The surgery is quickly completed and the patient is transferred (ventilated) to the pediatric intensive care unit. Over the next 12 hours of ventilation and fluid therapy, the patient develops mild hyperkalemia (K$^+$ 5.9 mmol/L) and a rise in serum creatinine kinase to 500 U/L. His electrocardiogram (ECG) shows a few ventricular ectopic beats. No further dantrolene is required. The patient is extubated the following morning and discharged to the ward after 24 hours. His parents are educated and counseled regarding malignant hyperthermia and the new considerations for the patient and other family members regarding anesthetics and MH.*

TABLE 7.1. PROTOCOL FOR THE ROLES OF OR PERSONNEL IN THE MANAGEMENT OF MH

Anesthesiologist

1. ***Call for help*** and ***stop volatile/triggering agent.*** Designate person to call MHAUS MH Crisis Hotline **1-800-MHHYPER** or **1-800-644-9737**
2. Ask the surgeon to stop ***or rapidly complete the surgery.***
3. Change the anesthetic circuit to a clean one (e.g., a bag-valve mask with oxygen reservoir). If this wastes too much time, increase flows to 15 L/min using the original machine.
4. ***Hyperventilate*** the patient in 100% oxygen (e.g., 3 times/minute ventilation)
5. Administer IV ***dantrolene*** (see Question 6) ***2.5 mg/kg*** as a bolus and repeat every 5 to 10 minutes (up to 10 mg/kg) until $ETCO_2$ and temperature decrease.
6. ***Cool the patient.*** Switch off warming devices and expose the patient. Switch convection blower to ambient temperature. Administer cold IV solutions. Ice packs to vascular plexuses (axilla and groin); consider cold lavage of stomach or bladder.
7. Insert an ***arterial line*** for monitoring and ***arterial blood gases,*** electrolytes (especially potassium and calcium), complete blood count, and coagulation studies.
8. Place urinary catheter; ***consider diuretics*** if urine output is <0.5 mL/kg/hr.
9. Insert ***central venous catheter*** to monitor central venous pressure, and administer inotropes if necessary.
10. When under control, transfer to the ***intensive care unit.*** Potassium, lactate, and myoglobin abnormalities can occur for a number of hours or days. Further dantrolene may need to be given several hours later if symptoms or signs of increased metabolic activity recur.

Care must be appropriate, timely, and organized.

Other OR Personnel

Surgeon: Cease surgery temporarily until some control is obtained, then complete surgery ASAP; following this, assist the anesthesiologist.

Anesthetic Assistant: Send for MH trolley; mix dantrolene in the vial or pour into a burette or sterile container. Organize blood gases, monitoring, and ice packs.

OR Nurse: Call for assistance and help mix dantrolene. Notify PICU and help prepare additional monitoring.

Surgical Technician: Collect ice, cool fluids, drugs, and blood specimens.

Note: OR = operating room; MH = malignant hyperthermia; MHAUS = Malignant Hyperthermia Association of the United States; $ETCO_2$ = end-tidal carbon dioxide; IV = intravenous; PICU = pediatric intensive care unit.

DISCUSSION

1. What is the pathophysiology of MH? What are the clinical features?

MH is a pharmacogenetic disease or syndrome characterized by a potentially life-threatening hypermetabolic state in susceptible individuals. It was first described by Denborough et al. (1962). In most cases, the abnormality is a mutation in the *ryanodine receptor*. This receptor is located on the sarcoplasmic reticulum within skeletal muscle cells and, if abnormal, opens and releases calcium into the cell in response to certain anesthetic *triggers*, namely the **volatile anesthetic agents** and the depolarizing muscle relaxant **succinylcholine**. Early suggestions that nitrous oxide, phenothiazines, tubocurarine, amide local anesthetics (lidocaine and bupivacaine), and anticholinergics may be triggers in susceptible patients have been disproven (Hopkins, 2000). In susceptible individuals, these triggers result in *an increase in the intramyoplasmic calcium* levels either from the sarcoplasmic reticulum stores or from the extracellular milieu. This causes a sustained contracture of the muscle and stimulation of the enzyme calcium-ATPase, which leads to a *hypermetabolic state* involving increased aerobic (oxygen consumptive) and anaerobic (glycogen breakdown) metabolic pathways. Heat is generated, carbon dioxide production is increased, and oxygen is consumed. The clinical signs are **tachycardia**, hyperventilation, **rising arterial and $ETCO_2$, hyperthermia**, and muscle rigidity. If undiagnosed this may progress to renal failure, disseminated intravascular coagulopathy, progressive acidosis, and death. If unrecognized and untreated, MH has a mortality rate up to 90%. Early detection and treatment can *decrease this mortality risk to <5%.*

2. What are the molecular genetics of MH?

MH is usually inherited as autosomal dominant with variable penetrance; however, the genetics are not simple and because more than one genetic locus has recently been identified, it appears that both hetero- and homozygote forms exist. The abnormality in more than 50% to 80% of cases is a mutation of the ryanodine receptor subtype RYR1. This receptor subtype is encoded by a gene on the 19th chromosomes (Zhou et al., 2015). Five other loci associated with MH have been identified on chromosomes 17, 1, 3, 7, and 5, but the only other known causative gene for MH is CACNA1S, which encodes a voltage-gated calcium channel on the α subunit of the cell membrane (Zhou et al., 2015).

3. What are the conditions associated with MH?

Although there has been a suggested association with various myopathies, dystonias, exertional stress, and enzymopathies, clear linkage with other pathologies exists for only a few. The conditions for which there is an association with MH are *King Denborough syndrome, central core disease,* and possibly *hypokalemic periodic paralysis.*

4. How is MH diagnosed?

There is no single clinical sign, monitored variable, or biochemical finding specific to MH, and the course can be insidious or rapidly progressive. There may not be a family history. The most frequent early signs are related to increased oxygen consumption and **increased carbon dioxide** and lactate production. This is usually followed by signs of autonomic sympathetic stimulation. The key early features of increased muscle metabolism are **unexpected tachycardia,** increased respiratory rate, **increased $ETCO_2$** (despite adequate ventilation), and **raised temperature** (which may increase by up to 2°C per hour or be delayed for several hours).

Muscle rigidity commonly occurs and is prolonged and nonpropagated. In the unparalyzed patient rigidity may help differentiate the diagnosis from septicemia. Muscle rigidity of the jaw (spasm of the masseter and lateral pterygoid muscles) is commonly seen after **succinylcholine** administration. If this is severe or prolonged ("jaws of steel") and is associated with contracture of skeletal muscle elsewhere, there is a very high likelihood of MH.

If any of these signs develop, MH should be considered, but they should also prompt further investigation to exclude other causes (Table 7.2).

Other features that may develop in an MH event include *cardiovascular collapse* with decreased cardiac output, *arrhythmias* including *hyperkalemic cardiac arrest* (peaked T-waves and ventricular ectopy may be seen on ECG preceding this), *neurological collapse, coma and fixed dilated pupils* (hyperthermia, acidosis, and fluid shifts can cause acute cerebral edema), *disseminated intravascular coagulopathy* (may occur with thromboembolism due to release of tissue thromboplastin), *rhabdomyolysis and myoglobinuria* (this may cause renal failure), and *desaturation or cyanosis, sweating, and being hot to the touch.*

In classic MH, the arterial blood gas analysis will confirm a *mixed respiratory and metabolic acidosis,* an increased serum lactate, and possible hyperkalemia. Later tests may show an *increased creatinine kinase level, continued hyperkalemia, and abnormal renal function.*

TABLE 7.2. DIFFERENTIAL DIAGNOSIS OF MH

- Inadequate depth of anesthesia
- Ventilation delivery problem: defective or inappropriate breathing circuit, inadequate gas flow, inadequate ventilation settings (low minute volume), ventilator mechanical fault, exhausted soda lime, blocked ETT/LMA
- Anaphylaxis
- Tourniquet ischemia
- Endocrine causes: pheochromocytoma, thyroid storm
- Neuroleptic malignant syndrome (e.g., if on neuroleptic medication, antidopaminergic drugs)
- Drugs (e.g., Ecstasy)
- Cerebral ischemia
- Other muscular diseases (e.g., isolated masseter spasm in patients with Duchenne's)
- Other (e.g., overzealous active heating where the patient has reduced ability to lose heat, such as bilateral leg tourniquets)

Note: MH = malignant hyperthermia; ETT = endotracheal tube; LMA = laryngeal mask airway.

In some clinical situations, patients are treated for MH empirically without definite diagnosis.

5. What is the practical treatment of MH?

Early diagnosis of MH is arguably the most important step. Any delay in treatment increases the risk of morbidity and mortality. Even if subsequent follow-up demonstrates another diagnosis, there are few disadvantages in treating a patient with possible signs of MH early; it is better to overtreat than delay treatment. A **local protocol** should allocate tasks to individual members of the operating room (OR) staff (see Table 7.1). The Malignant Hyperthermia Association of the United States (MHAUS) is the central source that all anesthesiologists should utilize in the event of a suspected or definite MH event. The MHAUS website provides a hotline for immediate assistance both within the domestic United States and outside of the United States. This allows physicians to communicate with experts regarding the most up-to-date and complete management of an MH crisis. Other entities such as the Society for Pediatric Anesthesia have also developed a Critical Events Checklist that aids successful management of MH. The Malignant Hyperthermia Australia and New Zealand group has developed a MH Resource Kit (MHANZ, 2007). This kit contains information and aids in the management of patients suspected of an MH diagnosis, including "task cards" for members of the team and OR education posters.

6. What is dantrolene?

Dantrolene is the most important agent in the management of MH. The dose is 2.5 *mg/kg* as a bolus, which is repeated at 1 mg/kg every 15 minutes (up to 10 mg/kg) until $ETCO_2$ and temperature decrease. Dantrolene sodium is a hydantoin derivative that acts as a muscle relaxant but not a paralyzing agent. It appears to work directly on the ryanodine receptor to prevent the release of calcium from the sarcoplasmic reticulum. Each ampoule provides 20 mg of dantrolene. This drug should be kept in every hospital providing general anesthesia along with an MH treatment box. Due to the rarity of this condition, the cost of dantrolene, and its short shelf life, most hospitals have an arrangement with a sister hospital to provide backup supplies of the drug in the event of an MH crisis. Traditionally, dantrolene has been extremely difficult to administer to a patient in MH crisis due to the labor-intensive mixing process that was required. This dantrolene comes as a lyophilized powder with 3 g of mannitol and sodium hydroxide to maintain the alkaline pH of 9 to 10, requiring 60 mL of sterile water and warming to dissolve just 20 mg of dantrolene. Given the recommended 2.5 mg/kg loading dose then 1 mg/kg dose until resolution of symptoms or 10 mg/kg maximum, a minimum of 9 vials or a maximum of 35 vials is used in a 70-kg adult. Effective and quick administration of this only true treatment necessitates many people just to assist with mixing and dissolving dantrolene. Such manpower is problematic especially if the MH crisis occurs during off peak hours when there is limited personnel. In 2014, a new formulation of dantrolene known as Ryanodex was produced. This form of the drug comes in 250 mg vials rather than the original 20 mg vials and only requires 5 mL of sterile water without warming. Because of the high concentration of the dantrolene, one can expect high serum levels of the drug quicker, with less volume, and hopefully a quicker response.

7. How are patients and families managed after the event?

The history should be rereviewed in detail; information regarding triggering agents, previous anesthesia, and family history of incidents during anesthesia should be documented. Some centers measure serum creatinine kinase levels at rest and fasting in the patient and family members. If these are elevated, there is a good correlation with MH susceptibility and biopsy may be unnecessary. However, this is controversial, and many centers will still require a biopsy for diagnosis. Normal levels of creatine kinase are not predictive. Muscle (quadriceps) biopsy contracture studies are the definitive test for MH susceptibility; they are offered to the family but cannot be performed on the patient until several months after the event. These are performed at many designated centers around the world.

Many of these centers will not perform biopsies on prepubertal children, and Australian centers have a minimum age of 12 years. North American centers require children to have a lean body mass of at least 20 kg. The reason for age and weight limitation is to ensure standardization of the test, which requires a relatively large piece of vastus lateralis muscle. The muscle sample is calculated for cross-sectional area using a formula of weight and length and usually measures 3 to 5 cm long and up to 1 cm wide. If a child is too young or small for biopsy, the parents should be offered testing. Only one parent need be biopsied; if the first parent is found to be positive, the child would then be considered MH sensitive. If both parents are found to be MH negative, the child should be considered MH susceptible until old enough for a definitive diagnosis with biopsy.

Two biopsy protocols exist: European and North American. The European Protocol (in vitro contracture test [IVCT]) uses incremental concentrations of caffeine (0.5–32 mM) and halothane (0.5%–3%). The result yields three potential diagnoses: *MH sensitive* if halothane and caffeine are abnormal, *MH negative* if halothane and caffeine are normal, and *MH equivocal* (and therefore considered "sensitive") if one result is abnormal. The North American Protocol (caffeine halothane contracture test) uses graded caffeine (0.5–32 mM) and a halothane bolus of 3%. This yields only two possible diagnoses: normal or sensitive.

If the result is sensitive or equivocal, the patient and family are usually DNA tested for mutation of the ryanodine gene. Family members found to have 1 of 15 known RYR1 mutations are considered sensitive. The patient/family should be supplied with written information of their MH susceptibility, which they should carry with them at all times. This might also include the wearing of a Medic-Alert bracelet.

8. Who are the patients at risk for MH and how should they be approached?

Patients should be considered susceptible if

(a) *Previous MH reaction or*
(b) *A relative* has had either *positive IVCT, positive DNA, or previous MH reaction.*

The key is to identify these patients and avoid the triggering agents. The anesthesia machine should be "cleansed" of volatile agent by removing vaporizers, previous circuits, and soda lime and flushing at 10 L/min with 100% oxygen for 20 minutes. Informed consent should include discussion of risks with the patient. Core temperature should be measured in addition to standard monitoring. Dantrolene should be available but not given prophylactically.

SUMMARY

1. MH is an uncommon, potentially fatal pharmacogenetic condition that results in a hypermetabolic state after exposure to volatile anesthetic agents or depolarizing muscle relaxants.
2. It is usually related to the ryanodine receptor RYR1 gene mutation on skeletal muscle endoplasmic reticulum.
3. There is no single feature that is pathognomonic for MH.
4. The important step in management is to first consider the diagnosis; treatment can reduce mortality from 90% to 5%.

ACKNOWLEDGMENT

The author wishes to acknowledge the first edition author, Philip Ragg.

ANNOTATED REFERENCES

Davis PJ, Brandom BW. The association of malignant hyperthermia and unusual disease: when you're hot you're hot or maybe not. *Anesth Analg.* 2009;109(4):1001–1069.

A thought-provoking editorial discussing various MH issues, including the limitations of our knowledge concerning its pathophysiology, the difficulty in testing for the disease, and the risk stratification of MH with various myopathies.

Hopkins PM. Malignant hyperthermia: advances in clinical management and diagnosis. *Br J Anaesth.* 2000;85(1):118–128.

Good overview of the topic.

Malignant Hyperthermia Australia and New Zealand. ANZCA Publication 2007. http://www.anaesthesia.mh.org.au/mh-resource-kit/w1/i1002692/%3E

An excellent website containing a "kit" with advice on the contents of a MH emergency box, OR posters, and task cards for individual members of the team in the event of a MH crisis.

Zhou J, Bose D, Allen PD, Pessah IN. Malignant hyperthermia and muscle-related disorders. In: RD Miller, LI Eriksson, LA Fleisher, JP Wiener-Kronish, WL Young, eds. *Miller's Anesthesia.* 8th Ed. Philadelphia: Elsevier; 2015:1287–1314.

An extremely well-written, thorough chapter about MH. It covers the biochemical mechanism to the clinical treatment of this rare yet deadly condition.

BIBLIOGRAPHY

Denborough MA, Forster JF, Lovell RR, Maplestone PA, Villiers JD. Anaesthetic deaths in a family. *Br J Anaesth.* 1962;34:395–396.

Larach MG for the North American Malignant Hyperthermia Group. Standardization of the caffeine halothane muscle contracture test. *Anesth Analg.* 1989;69:511–515.

Malignant Hyperthermia Association of the United States of America. http://www.mhaus.org/.

Pollock N, Langton E, Macdonell N, Tiemessen J, Stowell K. Malignant hyperthermia and day stay anaesthesia. *Anaesth Intens Care.* 2006;34:40–45.

Xiao B, Masumiya H, Jiang D, et al. Isoform dependent formation of heteromeric calcium release channels (ryanodine receptors). *J Biol Chem.* 2002;277(44)41778–41785.

8

Anaphylaxis

DIANE GORDON, MATTHEW D. SJOBLOM, AND LORI A. ARONSON

INTRODUCTION

Anaphylaxis is an immediate hypersensitivity reaction that can involve the cardiac, pulmonary, integumentary, and gastrointestinal systems. It can be triggered through allergic or nonallergic mechanisms and can be quite severe, especially if not recognized and treated promptly with epinephrine. During anesthesia, recognition may be delayed due to inability to assess the patient, nonspecific presenting signs, and considerable overlap in clinical presentation with other acute processes.

LEARNING OBJECTIVES

1. Describe the pathophysiology of anaphylaxis.
2. Review the most common triggers and risk factors for anaphylaxis.
3. Recognize perioperative anaphylaxis.
4. Discuss treatment and prevention of perioperative anaphylaxis.

CASE PRESENTATION

A 10-year-old boy is scheduled for surgical repair of a dislocated hip. His past medical history is significant for meningomyelocele that was repaired at 2 days of age. Associated hydrocephalus required a ventriculoperitoneal shunt at 1 month of age followed by three subsequent revisions. At age 5, he had release of his tethered spinal cord. He has a neurogenic bladder requiring scheduled catheterization and is wheelchair-bound. He has no known drug allergies but is on latex precautions due to his diagnosis of meningomyelocele and neurogenic bladder. There is no prior history of anesthetic complications.

The boy has an unremarkable inhalational induction with intubation aided by propofol, fentanyl, and cisatracurium. A dose of cefazolin is administered before incision. Twenty minutes after incision there is profound hypotension, desaturation, increased peak airway pressures, and decreased end-tidal carbon dioxide. Anesthetics are discontinued and the patient is aggressively resuscitated with 100% oxygen, epinephrine, albuterol, bolus crystalloid fluids, diphenhydramine, and hydrocortisone. Blood is taken for tryptase and histamine levels. After cardiopulmonary stabilization, the patient is transferred to the intensive care unit on an epinephrine infusion. Before his discharge, an allergy consultation is obtained to investigate the cause of his intraoperative anaphylaxis and to make recommendations for future anesthetics.

DISCUSSION

1. What is the pathophysiology of anaphylaxis?

Anaphylaxis is an acute, potentially lethal multisystem process resulting from the sudden release of mediators from mast cells and basophils into the circulation. The World Allergy Organization categorizes anaphylaxis as either allergic or nonallergic (Johansson et al., 2004). Allergic anaphylaxis is the result of a cascade of reactions triggered by specific immunoglobulin E (IgE), IgG, and immune complex/complement binding to and initiating degranulation of mast cells and basophils. Nonallergic anaphylaxis (formerly called anaphylactoid reaction) is caused by agents that induce sudden, massive mast cell or basophil degranulation in the absence of immunoglobulins. Regardless of type, the immediate treatment is identical, but subsequent evaluation, testing, and recommendations may vary.

TABLE 8.1. CLINICAL SEVERITY SCALE OF IMMEDIATE HYPERSENSITIVITY REACTIONS

Grades	Clinical Signs
I	Cutaneous-mucous signs: Erythema Urticaria with or without angioedema
II	Moderate multivisceral signs: cutaneous-mucous signs + /– hypotension + /– tachycardia + /– dyspnea + /– gastrointestinal disturbances
III	Life-threatening mono- or multivisceral signs: Cardiovascular collapse: Tachycardia or bradycardia, + /– cardiac arrhythmia + /– bronchospasm + /– cutaneous–mucosal signs + /– gastrointestinal disturbances
IV	Cardiac arrest

Reprinted with permission from Dewachter P, Mouton-Faivre C, Emala C. Anaphylaxis and anesthesia: controversies and new insights. *Anesthesiology.* 2009;111:1141–1150.

The predominantly affected organs are the skin, mucous membranes, gastrointestinal tract, and cardiovascular and respiratory systems. Fatalities are divided between circulatory collapse and respiratory arrest. Anaphylaxis has characteristics of both distributive shock (profound reduction in venous tone) and hypovolemic shock (increased vascular permeability causing massive fluid shifts and reduced venous return). Up to 35% of intravascular volume can shift to the extravascular space within 10 minutes during anaphylaxis. In addition, myocardial function is depressed. Severity of anaphylaxis is commonly graded by the Ring and Messmer criteria (Table 8.1) (Ring, 1977).

Multiple substances and mediators are released, with histamine and tryptase being the most readily measurable. Histamine H_1 receptor stimulation initiates nitric oxide synthesis and has been implicated in the hypotension of anaphylaxis. Blood analysis for histamine level should be drawn within 15 minutes of Grade 1 or 2 reactions and within the first 2 hours for Grade 3 or 4 to have the best positive- and negative-predictive value (Mertes et al., 2011). Tryptase is only released from mast cells and elevation >25 microgram/L is suggestive of an IgE-mediated reaction. Serum tryptase levels may be normal or slightly elevated for Grade 1 and 2 reactions even if drawn at the appropriate time (15–60 minutes after onset of the reaction). Optimal sampling for Grade 3 and 4 reactions is 30 minutes to 2 hours after onset (Mertes et al., 2011). Other inflammatory mediators that may rise during anaphylaxis include platelet-activating factor, prostaglandin D2, and leukotriene 4 (Simons et al., 2015).

Biphasic anaphylaxis (recrudescence) is rare. Most data are from emergency departments after food ingestion or insect sting–mediated reactions. These data suggest an incidence of biphasic reactions in 1.5% to 3% of anaphylaxis cases, with delayed epinephrine treatment being the only reliable risk factor (Lee et al., 2013). Biphasic reactions are of unclear etiology and usually occur within 8 hours of the initial reaction, though later presentations have been reported (Farbman & Michelson, 2016).

2. What are the most common triggers and risk factors for anaphylaxis?

Perioperative anaphylaxis in the United States is estimated to occur in roughly 1 in 34,000 general anesthetics in adults (Gurrieri et al., 2011), and mortality in adults is estimated as high as 9% in surveys from several countries (Gomez et al., 2015). In adults, neuromuscular blocking agents (NMBAs) are the most common cause of intraoperative anaphylaxis, responsible for 50% to 70% of cases, followed by latex and antibiotics. However, the causative agent varies by country, with antibiotics recently being the more frequent cause in the United States (Mertes et al., 2014; Volcheck et al., 2014). All NMBAs can elicit hypersensitivity reactions. Many over-the-counter drugs, cosmetics, and food products contain quaternary or tertiary ammonium ions (also part of the structure of NMBAs) which may cause sensitization and which would explain first-exposure reactions (Mertes et al., 2012) as well as cross-reactivity between NMBAs (approximately 60%–70%). To date, succinylcholine remains the most common NMBA to cause anaphylaxis (Michalska-Krzanowska, 2012). Anaphylaxis usually manifests shortly after induction with NMBAs or antibiotics but may occur at any time with all potentially allergenic agents.

In children, latex is the most common cause of anaphylaxis, followed by NMBAs and antibiotics. Latex-induced anaphylaxis usually occurs 30 to 60 minutes after the beginning of the surgery but may be immediate or considerably delayed. Children at increased risk include those with myelomeningocele, congenital urogenital malformations, and multiple operations (especially in the first year of life) and patients who require daily urinary catheterization. While there may be a genetic component to latex allergy in patients with myelomeningocele, environmental exposure to latex from repeated operations and urinary catheterization appears more likely. Latex anaphylaxis is most likely with parenteral or mucous membrane exposure. The only effective treatment is complete avoidance of latex in the health care setting, including the use of latex-free gloves. Latex has been removed from many operating rooms (and indeed entire hospitals), which has decreased the incidence of anaphylaxis to this agent (Mertes et al., 2011).

Antibiotics, primarily penicillin and cephalosporins, are another frequent cause of anaphylaxis. Cross-reactivity between penicillins and cephalosporins seems to be low (10%) and is attributed to the common beta-lactam ring. Intravenous anesthesia induction agents are a less common cause of perioperative anaphylaxis. Anaphylaxis to propofol is rare, even in patients with anaphylaxis to eggs, and even less likely with etomidate and ketamine. Opiates, especially morphine, commonly cause flushing and urticaria via direct histamine release following intravenous (IV), intramuscular (IM), and intrathecal administration; however, the risk of anaphylaxis remains low.

General risk factors for anaphylaxis are atopic conditions (eczema, asthma, allergic rhinitis) and mastocytosis. Prior to puberty, males and females are at equal risk for anaphylaxis, but with the onset of the influence of sex hormones, anaphylaxis becomes more common in women (Karila et al., 2005; Mertes et al., 2010).

3. What is perioperative anaphylaxis?

The initial diagnosis of perioperative anaphylaxis is clinical, based on history and physical examination, and the retrospective diagnosis relies on serology and skin tests. A survey of anaphylaxis during anesthesia demonstrated that cardiovascular symptoms (74%), cutaneous symptoms (70%), and bronchospasm (44%) are the most common clinical features (Laxenaire et al., 2001). Anaphylaxis may be mild and resolve spontaneously due to endogenous production of compensatory mediators, or it may be severe and progress within minutes to respiratory or cardiovascular compromise and death. During anesthesia the initial symptoms often go unnoticed because the patient is unconscious and the skin is not visible due to surgical drapes. As a result, the reaction may be detected only when dramatic respiratory and cardiovascular changes develop, at which point the differential diagnosis remains broad. This explains why cardiovascular collapse is the first detected manifestation in up to 50% of cases.

The differential diagnosis of an anaphylactic reaction during general anesthesia includes (a) other causes of respiratory symptoms: asthma, postextubation stridor, pulmonary edema, pulmonary embolus, tension pneumothorax; (b) other causes of hypotension: arrhythmia, cardiogenic shock, hemorrhage, hypoglycemia, overdosage of vasoactive drug, pericardial tamponade, sepsis, vasovagal reaction, venous air embolism; and (c) other causes of angioedema: hereditary or acquired angioedema, treatment with angiotensin-converting enzyme inhibitors.

The clinical diagnosis can be supported by documentation of elevated concentrations of plasma histamine and total tryptase. Skin testing based on the likely offending causes remains the gold standard for the detection of IgE-mediated reactions. Skin testing is typically performed 3 to 4 weeks after an anaphylactic reaction to avoid false-negative results because of mast cell depletion but earlier testing (0–4 days after reaction) has been studied and may be useful in addition to later testing (Lafuente et al., 2013). Skin tests are reliable for identifying allergic reactions due to NMBAs, latex, antibiotics, and chlorhexidine but are poor for opiates and benzodiazepines (Gomez, 2015). Comprehensive allergy evaluation may not identify the offending agent but has nevertheless been shown to be useful in planning future anesthetics for a patient who has experienced an intraoperative hypersensitivity reaction (Guyer et al., 2014).

4. What are appropriate treatment and prevention methods for perioperative anaphylaxis?

The management of anaphylaxis consists of immediately removing the offending drug or latex gloves, reduction or discontinuation of anesthetic drugs, early administration of epinephrine, intubation if not already performed, ventilation with 100% oxygen, expansion of the intravascular volume, placing the patient in the Trendelenburg position, and abbreviating the surgical procedure if possible. Epinephrine is the mainstay of treatment of anaphylaxis because of its vasoconstrictor (alpha-1), inotropic and chronotropic (beta-1) and bronchodilation, mast cell- and basophil-stabilization effects (beta-2). Anaphylactic reactions outside the operating room are treated with IM epinephrine, and this route can be considered for treating reactions that occur during anesthesia as well (Gomez, 2015; Society for Pediatric Anesthesia Quality and Safety Committee, n.d.). Grade 4 anaphylactic reactions require code doses of IV epinephrine as per pediatric advanced life support/ adult cardiac life support (PALS/ACLS) guidelines.

All other medications used for treatment of anaphylaxis should be deferred until epinephrine has been given. For additional treatment of bronchospasm, inhaled beta-2 agonists (albuterol) should be administered as needed. Corticosteroids are given on an empiric basis in the treatment of anaphylaxis but efficacy data is lacking, including evidence that steroids decrease the risk of biphasic reactions (Lee, 2013). Similarly, H_1 and H_2 receptor antagonists are often recommended, but there is minimal evidence to support their use. Therefore, they should not be given in place of, or delay the administration of, epinephrine. The treatment of anaphylaxis is summarized in Table 8.2.

Patients receiving beta-blockers may be resistant to treatment with epinephrine and can develop hypotension and bradycardia requiring glucagon for its inotropic and chronotropic effects as they are not mediated through beta-receptors.

TABLE 8.2. CHECKLIST FOR SUSPECTED INTRAOPERATIVE ANAPHYLAXIS

Oxygen FIO_2 1.0 and adequate ventilation
Remove suspected trigger(s)
Turn off anesthetic agents if hypotensive
Crystalloid fluid bolus: 10–30 ml/kg IV/IO
Epinephrine: 1–10 mcg/kg **IV/IO** *or*
10 mcg/kg **IM** for depo effect
If infusion needed: 0.02–0.2 mcg/kg/min IV
Albuterol: 4–10 puffs inhaled as needed
Methylprednisolone: 2 mg/kg IV/IO (max 100 mg)
Diphenhydramine: 1 mg/kg IV/IO (max 50 mg)
Famotidine 0.25 mg/kg *or* **Ranitidine** 0.25 mg/kg IV
Send **histamine** and **tryptase** blood levels immediately to within 2 hours of event
Critical care disposition
Obtain **allergy consult**

Note: IV = intravenous; IO = intraosseous infusion; IM = intramuscular.

Epinephrine-resistant anaphylaxis may require norepinephrine, metaraminol, or arginine vasopressin (AVP). AVP may be preferred because it does not rely on adrenergic receptors.

A careful history regarding adverse drug reactions and allergies, including latex allergy or latex precautions, should be obtained before every anesthetic. Cross-reactivity between several food allergies (banana, avocado, kiwi, mango, pineapple, passionfruit) and latex have been reported. Premedication with steroids and/ or antihistamines is controversial. This practice has been shown to reduce the severity (but not the incidence) of some reactions and has not been shown to prevent immune-type reactions (Gomez, 2015). Additionally, premedication may blunt the early signs of anaphylaxis and therefore delay recognition and treatment. The safest approach for managing future anesthetics in a patient who suffered perioperative anaphylaxis is identification of the offending agent via allergy testing and complete avoidance thereafter, keeping in mind cross-reactivity within the classes of NMBAs and the beta-lactam antibiotics.

SUMMARY

1. Anaphylaxis, immune- or nonimmune mediated, has a similar clinical presentation which can vary from mild cutaneous signs to cardiopulmonary collapse. Maintaining a high index of suspicion along with prompt recognition and treatment with epinephrine is crucial. Steroids and antihistamines may also be beneficial, but should not be given in place of epinephrine. An intensive care unit stay may be necessary for continued monitoring or resuscitation. Biphasic reactions are rare. Environmental sensitization is likely responsible for anaphylaxis in patients without prior exposure to the offending agent.
2. Blood histamine and tryptase levels should be obtained during the event. Allergy consultation and testing can help determine the causative agent and guide future anesthetic care.
3. The three most common causes of intraoperative anaphylaxis in children are latex, neuromuscular blockers, and antibiotics. Latex reactions may be delayed and difficult to recognize. A high index of suspicion is required.

BIBLIOGRAPHY

Farbman KS, Michelson KA. Anaphylaxis in children. *Curr Opin Pediatr*. 2016;28:294–297.

Gurrieri C, Weingarten TN, Martin DP, et al. Allergic reactions during anesthesia at a large United States referral center. *Anesth Analg*. 2011;113:1202–1212.

Guyer AC, Saff RR, Conroy M, et al. Comprehensive allergy evaluation is useful in the subsequent care of patients with drug hypersensitivity reactions during anesthesia. *J Allergy Clin Immune Pract*. 2015;3:94–100.

Johansson SGO, Bieber T, Dahl R, et al. Revised nomenclature for allergy for global use: report of the nomenclature Review Committee of the World Allergy Organization, October 2003. *J Allergy Clin Immuno*. 2004;113(5):832–836.

Karila C, Brunet-Langot D, Labbez F, et al. Anaphylaxis during anesthesia: results of a 12-year survey at a French pediatric center. *Allergy*. 2005;60(6):828–834.

Lafuente A, Javaloyes G, Berroa F, et al. Early skin testing is effective for diagnosis of hypersensitivity reactions occurring during anesthesia. *Allergy*. 2013;68:820–822.

Laxenaire MC, Mertes PM, Groupe d'Etudes des Reactions Anaphylactoides Peranesthesiques. Anaphylaxis during anesthesia: results of a two-year survey in France. *Br J Anaesth*. 2001;87:549–558.

Lee J, Garrett JPD, Brown-Whitehorn T, Spergel JM. Biphasic reactions in children undergoing oral food challenges. *Allergy Asthma Proc*. 2013;34(3):220–226.

Mertes PM, Demoly P, Malinovksy JM. Hypersensitivity reactions in the anesthesia setting/allergic reactions to anesthetics. *Curr Opin Allergy Clin Immunol*. 2012;12:361–368.

Mertes PM, Malinovsky JM, Jouffroy L, et al. Reducing the risk of anaphylaxis during anesthesia: 2011 updated guidelines for clinical practice. *J Investing Allergol Clin Immunol*. 2011;21(6):442–453.

Mertes PM, Tajima K, Regnier-Kimmoun MA, et al. Perioperative anaphylaxis. *Med Clin N Am*. 2010;94:761–789.

Michalska-Krzanowska G. Anaphylactic reactions during anesthesia and the perioperative period. *Anesthesiol Inten Ther*. 2012;44(2):104–111.

Michavila Gomez AV, Belver Gonzales MT, Cortes Alvarez N, et al. Perioperative anaphylactic reactions: review and procedure protocol in paediatrics. *Allegro Immunopathol*. 2015;43(2):203–214.

Ring J, Messmer K. Incidence and severity of anaphylactoid reactions to colloid volume substitutes. *Lancet*. 1977;309(8009):466–469.

Simons FER, Ebisawa M, Sanchez-Borges M, et al. 2015 update of the evidence base: World Allergy Organization anaphylaxis guidelines. *WAO J*. 2015;8:1–16.

Society for Pediatric Anesthesia Quality and Safety Committee. Critical Events Checklists. n.d. http://www.pedsanesthesia.org/critical-events-checklists/.

Volcheck GW, Mertes PM. Local and general anesthetics immediate hypersensitivity reactions. *Immunol Allergy Clin N Am*. 2014;34:525–546.

9

Anesthesia for MRI

TRUNG DU AND MOHAMED A. MAHMOUD

INTRODUCTION

Choosing an appropriate anesthetic or sedative technique for children undergoing diagnostic procedures can be a challenge. Children presenting for magnetic resonance imaging (MRI) may have significant coexisting medical problems including airway obstruction, a difficult airway, and sleep apnea. The MRI suite also poses a unique set of environmental constraints and associated risks. Therefore, a thoughtful plan which is carefully implemented is essential to ensure patient safety and to facilitate high-quality imaging.

LEARNING OBJECTIVES

1. Understand the underlying principles of maintaining patient and staff safety in the MRI environment.
2. Discuss the recognition and management of the difficult airway in the MRI environment.
3. Recognize the risks and challenges of using general anesthesia versus sedation for MRI.
4. Identify suitable sedative and anesthetic choices for children with obstructive sleep apnea presenting for MRI.

CASE PRESENTATION

A 3-year-old, 21-kg boy born at 32 weeks gestation is scheduled for an MRI of the brain. The MRI is being done as part of the workup for recurrent seizures. ***On preimaging evaluation****, the child's exam reveals* ***micrognathia*** *and a* ***cleft palate****. His mother reports that he "snores a lot" and seems to obstruct at night. A look through the medical records shows that the patient recently underwent an* ***overnight sleep study (polysomnography)*** *which demonstrated a moderate degree of* ***obstructive sleep apnea*** *with a minimum oxygen saturation of 86%. Upon inhalation induction with sevoflurane/nitrous oxide in oxygen, mask ventilation is difficult despite placement of an oral airway, and the patient's oxygen saturation drops to 83%. Direct laryngoscopy is performed but no laryngeal structures are seen and the boy desaturates rapidly. A laryngeal mask airway (LMA) is placed successfully and the boy is now adequately ventilated. Anesthesia is then maintained with oxygen/air/sevoflurane. At the end of the MRI scan, the LMA is removed in the MRI suite when the patient is* ***awake****. The patient recovers uneventfully and is discharged home.*

He returns 6 months later for a follow-up MRI evaluation. This time, sedation is planned using ***dexmedetomidine****. An intravenous catheter is inserted after inhalation of 70% nitrous oxide in oxygen. A* ***loading dose*** *of dexmedetomidine (2 mcg/kg over 10 minutes) is given. A significant increase in blood pressure and decrease in heart rate is noticed after the loading dose. A dose of atropine (0.01 mg/kg) corrects the* ***bradycardia.*** *Sedation is maintained with* ***dexmedetomidine infusion*** *(2 mcg/kg/hour). The patient breathes spontaneously throughout the scan,* ***upper airway patency*** *is aided by the placement of a* ***shoulder roll,*** *and supplemental oxygen is administered via nasal cannula. The minimum oxygen saturation recorded during imaging is 94%. At the completion of imaging, the dexmedetomidine infusion is discontinued and the patient recovers uneventfully.*

DISCUSSION

Safety considerations in the MRI environment are vital. First and foremost, it is it is important to remember that the magnet is always on, and the

TABLE 9.1. OUTLINE OF MRI ZONES AND SAFETY CONSIDERATIONS

Zone	Location	Safety Considerations
I	Outside the MRI suite, up to the outpatient entrance.	General public access without restriction.
II	Patient waiting, registration, screening, and changing area	Prescreened individuals Interface between public area and strictly controlled zones
III	Patient holding, preparation, and induction area. MRI control room	Strictly controlled zones begin Entry controlled by MRI staff Electromagnetic fields strength strong enough to present a physical hazard Postscreened individuals only Equipment restrictions and labeling in effect
IV	Magnet room with MRI scanner	Strongest electromagnetic field—most hazardous location Movement of patients, staff, equipment in and out of zone under direct supervision and instruction of MRI staff

Note: MRI = magnetic resonance imaging.

dangers of the electromagnetic field are ever present. The American College of Radiologist recommends that the MRI suite be divided into four zones with increasing safety and access requirements as patients, staff, and equipment move closer to the scanner. This zoned safety approach was acknowledged by the MRI Task Force of the American Society of Anesthesiologists in its updated practice advisory in 2015. (See Table 9.1.)

Portable equipment to be brought into the magnet room (Zone IV) that is wholly nonferrous should be identified with a green square "MRI safe" label. A yellow triangle "MRI conditional" label should be affixed to equipment that requires strict precautions to be observed when used inside the magnet room. For example, the anesthesia machine is a MRI conditional device and needs to be placed at a minimum distance from the magnet to remain safe and functional.

Portable equipment that is required for use in the controlled zones but has ferrous components will have a red circle "MRI unsafe" label and must not be brought into the magnet room. The safety of any unlabeled devices to be brought in the controlled area should be discussed with MRI staff.

The powerful magnetic field also constrains the type of anesthesia and monitoring equipment that can be used. Minimum monitoring requirements for sedation and anesthesia should be instituted with MRI-compatible devices. Standard side-stream capnography and pneumatic blood pressure measurement with nonferrous connectors are unaffected by the MRI environment, and fiber-optic systems are available for pulse oximetry, temperature, and electrocardiogram telemetry.

Anesthesia providers should plan in advance how to respond with an emergency situation that arises in the MRI scanner, keeping in mind additional staff and equipment may be less readily available than in the operating room environment. In most instances, in the event of an emergency, removing the patient from the magnet room to a less hostile environment is the preferred initial course of action.

1. What is the role of preimaging evaluation and why is it important?

Evaluation of children presenting for imaging studies is very similar to the evaluation of children requiring surgery. As in this case, it is especially important to carefully evaluate the airway prior to beginning anesthesia or sedation in the MRI environment. It may be prudent in some cases to start the anesthetic in the more controlled environment of the operating room, secure the airway with an endotracheal tube, and then transport the patient to radiology. The operating room provides a safe, secure, and familiar environment in which the anesthesiologist has access to emergency airway equipment and assistance from colleagues who can help with airway management.

Most imaging studies only require immobilization and are not stimulating. Intubation is frequently not necessary. In a child with a difficult airway, avoiding instrumentation of the airway is a prudent course as long as emergency measures to secure the airway are immediately available. The child in this case did not have a prior procedure requiring intubation; his micrognathia was first recognized on the day of his MRI.

Evaluation of the pediatric airway can be challenging as the patient may be uncooperative and the history given by parents may be misleading. The **overnight polysomnography** provides clues as to the type (obstructive, central, or mixed) and frequency of the airway obstruction during sleep. The lowest documented oxygen saturation may also predict the severity of the obstruction and the likely nadir in oxygenation that may be encountered under anesthesia.

While a supplemental airway was not necessary for the second MRI scan, in all cases, it is critical to have MRI-compatible oral pharyngeal airways, nasal trumpets, and LMAs immediately available to address a deterioration in airway patency.

2. General anesthesia versus sedation? The dilemma still exists

Pediatric sedation can be defined as the use of sedative, analgesic, or dissociative drugs in order to provide anxiolysis, analgesia, and sedation during painful or unpleasant procedures. The Joint Commission and the American Society of Anesthesiologists (ASA) have recently revised their definitions of the levels of pediatric sedation. The four levels of sedation are now minimal, moderate, deep, and general anesthesia. Minimal sedation equates to anxiolysis and has no appreciable effect on vital reflexes. In a state of moderate sedation (previously known as "conscious sedation"), the patient is able to breathe adequately without assistance and responds purposefully to verbal commands/light touch. During deep sedation, the patient cannot be roused easily but will respond purposefully to repeated or painful stimuli and may require assistance with his or her airway or breathing. The sedation level can change rapidly from minimal sedation to general anesthesia; therefore, the expectation of the Joint Commission is that a deeply sedated patient should be able to be rescued from a depth of general anesthesia.

One commonly used general anesthetic technique is an inhalation induction for placement of an intravenous line which is then followed by a propofol infusion. Supplemental oxygen is provided with a nasal cannula. Placement of a shoulder roll and/or an oral airway is helpful in maintaining patency of the airway. If the airway remains obstructed, a LMA or endotracheal tube can then be placed.

The literature suggests that **sedation** may be unpredictable, has a relatively high failure rate (15%), and can be associated with morbidity and, rarely, mortality. That said, sedation can be practiced safely and successfully by appropriately trained practitioners in well-prepared centers that have robust mechanisms to identify and exclude high-risk patients.

For some complex patients, especially those with a difficult airway, an anesthesiologist may provide the safest and most effective sedation or anesthesia and airway management necessary for the imaging studies.

A further consideration in determining whether general anesthesia or sedation is preferred is that it is critical to have an understanding of the requirements for successful completion of the imaging study planned. MRI airway imaging studies may be undertaken specifically to investigate patients with known airway obstruction to examine airway dynamics while asleep and to determine the site and severity of the airway obstruction.

In these cases, in order to obtain effective imaging studies, the patient's airway is ideally not altered with airway adjuncts. Airway obstruction and subsequent desaturation may well occur during the anesthesia and sedation for these children. There is no consensus among anesthesiologists on when to interrupt airway imaging studies. Absolute lower limits of oxygen saturation below which artificial airway adjuncts are required will differ from patient to patient. Some of the factors to take into consideration are the known nadir in oxygen saturations with natural sleep observed on polysomnography, the benefits to be gained from an undisturbed imaging study, and the severity of the patient's other coexistent conditions.

3. What are the challenges associated with safely anesthetizing or sedating a child with a difficult airway and obstructive sleep apnea (OSA)?

Micrognathia in this child most likely contributed to his OSA. Maintaining the **patency of the upper airway** during spontaneous ventilation in sedated or anesthetized children with preexisting sleep-disordered breathing or airway obstruction is a major challenge for anesthesiologists. Anesthetic agents impair the ability of the upper airway muscles to overcome the negative pressures generated during inspiration, resulting in increased upper airway resistance and predisposing the patient to obstructive events, particularly in the retropalatal region. Children with significant OSA are sensitive to all sedative and anesthetic drugs. Upper airway obstruction and/or respiratory depression can occur even with minimal levels of sedation. Pharyngeal airway muscle tone is decreased during sleep; this reduction is even more pronounced during anesthesia or sedation, increasing the likelihood of upper airway obstruction leading to the development of hypoxia and hypercapnia. The genioglossus muscle is sensitive to sedatives and anesthetics, and reduced tone allows the tongue to fall back into an already unfavorable anatomic situation, worsening obstruction. These changes are accentuated in children with OSA, particularly with anesthetic or sedative drugs which exhibit strong respiratory depressant or airway relaxant effects.

Hypoventilation and the resultant hypercapnia may contribute to morbidity in patients with raised intracranial pressure, pulmonary hypertension, and end-stage renal failure. Increased ventilatory control would be indicated in patients with these conditions.

4. What are the suitable sedative and anesthetic choices for children with a difficult airway and OSA presenting for MRI airway imaging?

Sedatives and anesthetics commonly used in children for MRI imaging studies include barbiturates, propofol, benzodiazepines, ketamine, and dexmedetomidine.

Propofol administration has been shown to achieve adequate conditions for imaging in 95% to 99% of cases. It has been reported that minor adverse events are seen in up to 6% of patients, and 1.5% required some form of airway intervention. Independent predictors for these events were the very young age of the patient, a higher ASA status, and the use of supplementary opiates.

Where imaging of the airways in concerned, it must be kept in mind that propofol and barbiturates can exacerbate upper airway obstruction and increase the risk of respiratory depression and apnea. Similarly, benzodiazepines have relaxant effects on the pharyngeal musculature, causing a reduction of the pharyngeal space. In contrast, ketamine has been shown to preserve hypopharyngeal caliber in adults.

A combination of ketamine and dexmedetomidine followed by a dexmedetomidine infusion has also been found to be effective in providing anesthesia without exacerbating respiratory problems during MRI in three children with Down syndrome and OSA (Luscri & Tobias, 2006). **Dexmedetomidine** is an alpha-2 adrenergic agonist with sedative, analgesic, and anxiolytic properties similar to clonidine. Because of its sedative and anxiolytic properties, dexmedetomidine has been shown to be a useful agent for pediatric procedural sedation. In contrast to other sedative agents, dexmedetomidine has been shown to have sedative properties that mimic natural sleep without significant respiratory depression. These advantages make dexmedetomidine an attractive agent for noninvasive procedural sedation in children. A recent retrospective study (Mahmoud et al., 2009) showed that children with OSA anesthetized with dexmedetomidine for MRI sleep studies experienced **fewer episodes of oxygen desaturation** and airway obstruction requiring **airway interventions** than those anesthetized with propofol. The advantages of dexmedetomidine appear particularly dramatic in children with more **severe OSA**.

5. What side effects should be expected when using dexmedetomidine as a sole sedative agent?

In order to use dexmedetomidine as a sole sedative agent for MRI sedation, higher doses are required, as shown in this case. Dexmedetomidine typically causes a decrease in the heart rate and an increase in blood pressure during the loading phase followed by a decrease in blood pressure during the infusion phase due to a reduction in plasma catecholamine levels. Hemodynamic parameters return to baseline within 1 hour of stopping the infusion. Therefore, careful attention to hemodynamics is essential during administration of the **loading dose** Dexmedetomidine causes peripheral alpha-2 receptor stimulation, leading to paradoxical vasoconstriction, **transient hypertension**, and profound **bradycardia**. Other reported side effects include sinus arrest and cardiac arrhythmias. Current understanding of the complete hemodynamic profile of dexmedetomidine, including its effects on pulmonary vascular resistance, remains incomplete. Dexmedetomidine has a half-life of about 2.5 hours, thus full recovery may be delayed in some patients. As a result of its low potential for respiratory depression, dexmedetomidine is seeing widespread, off-label use for pediatric sedation, even in children with congenital heart defects in whom dexmedetomidine administration has been reported during imaging studies, cardiac surgery, and postoperative intensive care unit recovery.

SUMMARY

1. Be aware of the environmental consideration in the MRI environment and the limitations it places on availability of equipment and assistance and access and monitoring of the patient. Have a preplanned emergency response.
2. Children scheduled for MRI imaging may have complex medical problems including airway obstruction; thorough preoperative assessment is essential.
3. Sedation and general anesthesia can be safely used in the MRI suite, but both must be tailored to the individual patient.
4. In the case of a difficult airway, it may be wise to secure the airway in the operating room before proceeding to the MRI suite.
5. Sedation with dexmedetomidine for MRI sleep studies provides sedation that mimics natural sleep without significant respiratory depression. Dexmedetomidine may be a better choice than propofol for children with significant OSA.
6. Dexmedetomidine can cause hypertension and bradycardia with the loading dose, following by a decrease in blood pressure during the infusion phase. Because of its low potential for respiratory depression, it is being used more commonly for pediatric sedation.

ANNOTATED REFERENCES

Mahmoud M, Gunter J, Donnelly LF, Wang Y, Nick TG, Sadhasivam S. A comparison of dexmedetomidine with propofol for magnetic resonance imaging sleep studies in children. *Anesth Analg.* 2009;109(3):745–753.

This article concludes that, compared with propofol, dexmedetomidine has less effect on upper airway tone and airway collapsibility, provides more favorable conditions during dynamic MRI airway imaging in children with OSA, and requires fewer scan interruptions and less aggressive airway interventions.

Coté C, Wilson S. Guideline for monitoring management of pediatric patients during and after sedation for diagnostic and therapeutic procedures: an update. *Pediatrics.* 2006;118 (6):2587–2602.

A structured guideline for the planning and administration of safe sedation and general anesthesia. It provides a clear definition if the various levels of sedation and outlines reasonable expectation as to the personnel, skills, and equipment that must be available in each instance.

Malviya S, Voepel-Lewis T, Eldevik OP, Rockwell DT, Wong JH, Tait AR. Sedation and general anaesthesia in children undergoing MRI and CT: adverse events and outcomes. *Br J Anaesth.* 2000;84(6):743–748.

Quality assurance data were collected prospectively in this study for children who were sedated ($n = 922$) or given general anesthesia ($n = 140$) for MRI or computerized tomography. For preselected children high-risk children, MRI scanning was more successful with general anesthesia than with sedation.

BIBLIOGRAPHY

Cravero JP, Beach ML, Blike GT, Gallagher SM, Hertzog JH. The incidence and nature of adverse events during pediatric sedation/anesthesia with propofol for procedures outside the operating room: a report from the Pediatric Sedation Research Consortium. *Anesth Analg.* 2009;108(3):795–804.

Kanal E, Barkovich AJ, Bell C, et al. ACR guidance document on MR safe practices: 2013. *Magn Reson Imag.* 2013;37:501–530.

Koroglu A, Demirbilek S, Teksan H, Sagir O, But AK, Ersoy MO. Sedative, haemodynamic and respiratory effects of dexmedetomidine in children undergoing magnetic resonance imaging examination: preliminary results. *Br J Anaesth.* 2005;94(6):821–824.

Luscri L, Tobias J. Monitored anesthesia care with a combination of ketamine and dexmedetomidine during magnetic resonance imaging in three children with trisomy 21 and obstructive sleep apnea. *Ped Anesth.* 2006;16:782–786.

Mahmoud M, Mason K. Dexmedetomidine: a review, update and future considerations of the paediatric perioperative and periprocedural applications and limitations. *Br J Anaesth.* 2015;115(2):171–182.

Mason KP, Zurakowski D, Zgleszewski SE, et al. High dose dexmedetomidine as the sole sedative for pediatric MRI. *Ped Anesth.* 2008;18(5):403–411.

Practice Advisory on Anesthetic Care for Magnetic Resonance Imaging: an updated report by the American Society of Anesthesiologists Task Force on Anesthetic Care for Magnetic Resonance Imaging. *Anesthesiology.* 2015;122(3):495–520.

10

Egg and Soy Allergies and Propofol Use

MICHAEL J. KIBELBEK, LORI A. ARONSON, AND LISA D. HEYDEN

LEARNING OBJECTIVES

1. Understand the significance of gastroesophageal reflux (GERD) in this population relative to anesthetic management.
2. Appreciate the significance of egg and soy allergy with propofol usage.
3. Know the options for airway management during endoscopy.

CASE PRESENTATION

A 4-year-old, 14-kg girl presents for repeat surveillance upper endoscopy of her eosinophilic esophagitis (EoE) and GERD. She has a history of reactive airway disease and wheezing, treated with an albuterol (salbutamol) inhaler twice daily. Her last asthma exacerbation was 4 weeks ago, associated with an upper respiratory infection, and it was managed at home with frequent treatments of nebulized albuterol. She has had a previous uneventful anesthetic for endoscopy at another institution, but the records are not available. Since then, radioallergosorbent testing (RAST) has revealed allergies to penicillin, wheat, soy, and eggs. There is no significant family history. Her physical exam is unremarkable. She has fasted 10 hours after solids and 2 hours after apple juice.

The patient receives nebulized albuterol before coming to the operating room, where she undergoes an uneventful inhalational induction with her parents present. A peripheral intravenous line is established, and pharyngeal ***topical anesthesia*** *is provided with* ***2 mL of 1% lidocaine****. The inhalation agent is discontinued and her anesthetic is deepened with 20 mg propofol while maintaining spontaneous respirations.* ***Propofol*** *is provided in* ***intermittent boluses*** *for maintenance anesthesia. During the procedure, supplemental oxygen is delivered at 2 L/min via nasal prongs. The procedure is completed without evidence of gastric reflux or wheezing. After removal of the endoscope and verification of spontaneous respirations and a patent airway, the patient proceeds to the recovery room.*

DISCUSSION

1. What is the significance of GERD to this anesthetic?

Although many pediatric gastrointestinal (GI) patients are being evaluated for **GERD** or are already carrying this diagnosis, regurgitation during induction is a relatively rare event. In general, fasted children presenting for upper endoscopy have gastric volumes and pHs similar to those found in fasted children presenting for other surgeries. The standard pediatric nil per os guidelines (8 hours fatty food or meat, 6 hours light solids, nonhuman milk or formula, 4 hours breast milk, 2 hours clears) appear to be effective in reducing passive regurgitation. It should be noted, however, that children with esophageal dysmotility conditions, such as achalasia, may have very large volumes of food in their esophagus even with prolonged fasting.

2. Does the history of egg and soy allergy preclude the use of propofol?

GI patients frequently present with a history of multiple food intolerance and allergies. They may have been experiencing abdominal pain, vomiting, malabsorption, loose stools, or **EoE**. Adverse immune reactions to various foods are thought to cause EoE through *delayed cell-mediated immunity*. Some children with EoE will also have a history of food allergy capable of producing histamine-mediated systemic reactions, including rash, urticaria, wheezing, and even anaphylaxis. EoE is associated with atopy in 75% of patients. The most common clinical manifestation of EoE in the pediatric population is food refusal and failure to thrive in infants and nausea, vomiting, and abdominal pain in older children. Many patients have food sensitivities, and these patients often have improvement of symptoms after elimination of certain foods from their diet. Food allergens play a particularly important role in the pediatric population. Treatment includes pharmacologic and dietetic approaches. One common dietetic approach in children is the Six Food Elimination Diet (SFED) in which patients exclude the six more probable food allergens: milk and dairy products, **egg, soy**, tree nut/peanut, sea food (fish/shellfish). The efficacy of SFED was about 70% according to a meta-analysis. Parents often report their child to be "allergic" to all foods on the elimination diet and all foods identified by RAST or skin prick tests (SPTs). Oftentimes, confirmation of sensitization to certain food with SPT is challenging. For example, in one study, SPT was able to identify the actual trigger food in only 13% of cases. Although foods associated with oral adverse immune reactions have the potential to re-produce esophageal disease, allergic reaction to **propofol** is rare in EoE patients, even among patients who report being **egg-** and **soy-allergic.**

The anesthetic induction agent **propofol** is poorly soluble in water and must be formulated in an oil–water emulsion. Propofol's active ingredient, 2, 6-diisopropylphenol, is dissolved in an emulsion of highly purified soy oil identical to parenteral lipid infusion. Lecithin, a mixture of phosphatidylcholine and phosphatidylethanolamine, helps prevent the oil emulsion from separating into oil and water layers after manufacturing. The lecithin used is a highly purified extract of egg yolk. The lipid emulsion used in propofol contains 10% soy oil, 2.25% glycerol, and 1.2% egg yolk lecithin.

Patients who report allergy or intolerance to either egg or soy are almost always intolerant to the *egg* or *soy protein*, not egg yolk or soy oil. The manufacturing and purification processes remove all but trace amounts of soy protein and ovalbumin, the strongest allergens. Patients who develop anaphylaxis to soy protein may cross-react with other allergens in the legume family, especially peanuts; this is the genesis of the warnings in the various package inserts. The Diprovan® insert reads, "Diprovan Injectable Emulsion is contraindicated in patients with a known hypersensitivity to Diprovan Injectable Emulsion or its components." In late 2009 and early 2010, the United States experienced a critical shortage of domestically produced propofol, necessitating importation of an alternate preparation, Propoven®. The package insert for Fresenius Propoven 1%®, manufactured in Italy, contains the following warning: "Fresenius Propoven 1% (propofol 1%) is contraindicated in patients who are allergic to soy or peanut." Personal communication with AAP Pharmaceuticals, LLC, the supplier of Propoven®, explains that this warns against the possibility of residual soy allergen in the soy oil. It is also theoretically possible for cross-contamination of the soy oil with residual peanut allergen to occur at the pressing plants, where processing equipment may have been used to press both soy and peanut oils, before it is purified. Reaction to soy allergen as a result of exposure to soy oil is rare. Both the US Food Labeling and Consumer Protection Act of 2004 and the European Food Safety Authority exempt highly refined vegetable oils, including soy oil, from being explicitly listed as ingredients in food products. Instead, the manufacturers are permitted to include a listing of the different oils the product *may* contain.

The incidence of propofol anaphylaxis has been reported as 1 in 60,000, and it accounts for 1.2% to 2.1% of perioperative anaphylaxis cases in France, but the specific allergen in the propofol emulsion was not identified (Hepner & Castells, 2003). Propofol injectable emulsion has also been tested by SPT and intradermal injection with negative results in adult, egg-allergic patients.

The literature has only very rare reports of allergic reactions to parenteral infusion of oil emulsion (Intralipid®). Our gastroenterology colleagues do not consider a history of egg or soy allergy to be a contraindication to the use of Intralipid® parenteral alimentation. Yet, propofol and parenteral Intralipid® differ only in the addition of the active ingredient. It seems that the recommendation for contraindication of soy lipid emulsion in egg- and soy-allergic patients occurs most strongly within the anesthesia community. In general, propofol hypersensitivity reactions are rare and published cases, as well as several retrospective case reviews, do not show a connection between allergy to propofol and allergy to egg or soy. Propofol should *not* be considered to be contraindicated in pediatric or adult patients with ingestible **egg or soy intolerance**.

3. Is intubation required for most upper endoscopy patients?

Endoscopies in adults are commonly performed under conscious sedation, relying upon **topical local anesthesia** of the esophagus and anxiolysis with benzodiazepine or propofol infusion. Pediatric endoscopies are often thought to require general anesthesia with endotracheal intubation for airway control. In a randomized controlled study of children ages 1 to 12 years, insufflation with sevoflurane during upper endoscopy was associated with a higher incidence of adverse airway events, including desaturation and laryngospasm, than patients who received sevoflurane via endotracheal tube (ETT) (Hoffman et al., 2010). Intubation was associated with more frequent complaints of sore throat. Therefore, they recommended endotracheal intubation over insufflation during upper endoscopy, especially in patients who are younger or obese or who have received midazolam premedication. However, the minimum alveolar concentration level required for intubation of the trachea and tolerance of the ETT likely exceeds the stimulation produced by the endoscope in the esophagus, with biopsies being essentially painless.

To improve patient comfort and facilitate turnover, many anesthesiologists choose not to intubate uncomplicated pediatric endoscopy patients aged 4 and older. In addition, tracheal instrumentation of patients with **reactive airways** may precipitate bronchospasm. The oropharynx of these patients is ordinarily large enough to accommodate the endoscope and still allow sufficient room for air exchange. An oral airway or a bite block will protect the scope from the patient's teeth and vice versa, given that many children are in the process of losing deciduous teeth. Several specifically designed products are available that allow the scope to pass through the center of the bite block rather than alongside it.

If necessary to improve the airway with a bite apparatus in place, a jaw lift will usually relieve a partial obstruction. Supplemental oxygen can be provided by **nasal prongs** directed into the nares or the mouth, with blow-by oxygen from a circuit directed toward the nose and mouth or via a nasal trumpet with an ETT adapter inserted. Practically, airway patency often improves once the scope is inserted beyond the oropharynx. Anesthetic maintenance can then be maintained with volatile anesthetic insufflation (with caution, as noted) or with total intravenous anesthesia. When a longer or more involved endoscopic procedure is planned, it is preferable to secure the airway with an ETT. Some institutions use laryngeal mask airways (LMAs) to maintain the airway during upper endoscopy. This works very well, though the endoscopist has to become accustomed to the slightly greater resistance to passing the scope and the anesthesiologist must remain vigilant that the LMA is not dislodged.

Effective **topical anesthesia** of the oropharynx and the esophagus is beneficial to reduce the stimulation of scope insertion and to reduce the amount of anesthesia necessary to produce patient compliance. Patients old enough to be cooperative can gargle and swallow several milliliters of lidocaine (lignocaine) slurry (2% lidocaine mixed with a sweetener to reduce the bitter taste) or permit their oropharyx to be sprayed with topical anesthetic. Asking older patients to suck on two sodium benzonatate vesicles (Tessalon Perles®) 10 minutes before the procedure produces extremely effective anesthesia of the esophagus and oropharynx. Unfortunately, all effective topical oral anesthetic agents have a noxious, bitter, metallic taste, even the flavored ones. Younger patients may not be willing to cooperate with awake application of local anesthetic, due to the taste. The sticky, glutinous consistency of lidocaine jelly will cause many patients to gag when asked to swallow it and is best avoided. Remember that flavored topical oral spray Hurricane® (prilocaine) can cause methemoglobinemia in infants and other susceptible patients.

Younger, noncooperative patients can be given a conventional inhalation induction. After intravenous access is achieved, 2 to 3 mL of **1% or 2% lidocaine** (both work equally well) is trickled into the oropharynx. Following a jaw thrust, the topical agent can be instilled behind the tongue. Next, the inhalation agent is discontinued and 20 seconds of spontaneous or controlled ventilation distributes the topical agent and usually permits the return of spontaneous ventilation. Before allowing the endoscopist to insert the scope, a 1- to 1.5-mg/kg **bolus of propofol** will keep the patient still while usually preserving spontaneous respirations. Additional similar **bolus** doses of

propofol are given **intermittently** as necessary for the remainder of the procedure.

Upper endoscopy can be performed with the patient either supine or in the lateral decubitus position without compromising the airway, according to the preference of the endoscopist. Most diagnostic upper endoscopies take about 15 minutes or less. Ask the endoscopist to suction liquid stomach contents through the scope upon entering the stomach and before withdrawing the scope to remove insufflated air, if this is not his or her routine practice. These steps will aid patient comfort during recovery. Emergence is generally smooth and rapid, with discomfort limited to a sore throat from friction of the endoscope against the mucosa.

SUMMARY

1. Children who present with GI symptoms for GI endoscopy have gastric contents with similar volumes and pHs compared to other children who fasted for similar times. Special precautions are rarely indicated for these patients with GERD.
2. Reports of egg and soy allergy are not contraindications to receiving propofol. Propofol may be used in patients with nonsystemic allergic reactions such as GI symptoms of food intolerance and positive skin and RAST tests.
3. Monitored anesthesia care/sedation with pharyngeal local anesthesia is an appropriate alternate technique to endotracheal intubation for routine diagnostic pediatric upper endoscopy. Endotracheal intubation for upper endoscopy is associated with fewer adverse respiratory events in young children and obese children and may be better for longer endoscopies.

ANNOTATED REFERENCES

Furuta GT, Liacouras CA, Collins MH, et al. Eosinophilic esophagitis in children and adults: a systemic review and consensus recommendations for diagnosis and treatment. *Gastroenterology.* 2007;133:1342–1363.

An excellent review of the symptoms, pathophysiology, and treatment of EoE.

Hepner DL, Castells MC. Anaphylaxis during the perioperative period. *Anesth Analg.* 2003;97:1381–1395.

This extensive review summarizes the literature experience with anaphylaxis from anesthetic and nonanesthetic drugs commonly given in the perioperative period.

BIBLIOGRAPHY

Alalami AA, Ayoub CM, Baraka AW. Laryngospasm: review of different prevention and treatment modalities. *Pediatr Anesth.* 2008;18:281–288.

Asserhoj LL, Mosbech H, Kroigaard M, Garvey LH. No evidence for contraindications to the use of propofol in adults allergic to egg, soy or peanut. *Br J Anaesth.* 2015;116(1):77–82.

Hefle S, Taylor S. Refined soybean oil not an allergen, say food scientists. http://www.foodnavigator-usa.com/Science-Nutrition/Refined-soybean-oil-not-an-allergen-say-food-scientists.

Hoffmann CO, Samuels PJ, Beckman E, et al. Insufflation versus intubation during esophagogastroduodenoscopy in children. *Pediatr Anesth.* 2010;20(9):821–830.

Molina-Infante J, Arias A, Vara-Brenes D, et al. Propofol administration is safe in adult eosiophilic esophagitis patients sensitized to egg, soy, or peanut. *Allergy.* 2014;69:388–394.

Murphy A, Campbell DE, Baines D, Mehr S. Allergic reactions in egg-allergic children. *Anesth Analg.* 2011;113(1):140–144.

Putnam PE, Rothenberg ME. Eosinophilic esophagitis: concepts, controversies, and evidence. *Curr Gastroenterol Rep.* 2009;11:220–225.

Ridolo E, Melli V, De'Angelis G, Martignago I. Eosinophilic disorders of the gastro-intestinal tract: an update. *Clin Mol Allergy.* 2016;14(17).

PART 3

Challenges in Airway Management

11

Obstructive Sleep Apnea

LAURA RYAN AND PAUL HOPKINS

INTRODUCTION

Adenotonsillectomy is first-line treatment for obstructive sleep apnea (OSA), and it is increasingly performed as a day-surgery procedure. A diagnosis of OSA results in a five-fold increased risk of perioperative respiratory complications after andenotonsillectomy (De Luca Canto et al., 2015). Children with OSA have a respiratory drive and airway tone that may be exquisitely sensitive to anesthetic and analgesic agents. The gold standard for diagnosing OSA is overnight polysomnography (PSG), but this is a scarce and expensive resource considering the number of procedures performed. Recognition of OSA in children is largely dependent on clinical examination and parental history. Accordingly, the anesthesiologist needs to identify which patients are at highest risk of complications, what is an appropriate anesthetic regimen, and how best to monitor these patients postoperatively.

LEARNING OBJECTIVES

1. Know how to assess the severity of OSA and decide if ambulatory surgery is appropriate.
2. Recognize the anesthetic considerations for a patient with OSA.
3. Know the anesthetic principles for and complications of adenotonsillectomy.

CASE PRESENTATION

A 2-year-old boy is scheduled for adenotonsillectomy. His parents report labored breathing with ***snoring, pauses*** *in breathing, and* ***gasping*** *at night. He is also noted to be very restless and occasionally sweaty. He is "slow to get going" in the morning,* ***struggles to keep up with his siblings*** *on the playground, and* ***routinely falls asleep*** *as a car passenger. His past medical history is otherwise unremarkable.*

On examination he weighs only 12 kg and exhibits mouth breathing with hyponasal speech, and his resting SaO_2 is 96% on room air. He has clear breath sounds with no added cardiac sounds on auscultation. Results of the ***polysomnogram (PSG)*** *demonstrate an SaO_2 nadir of 64%, an obstructive apnea hypopnea index of 35.4/hr, an rapid eye movement (REM) respiratory disturbance index of 80.5/hr, and an average transcutaneous CO_2 in total sleep time of 46.1 mmHg (with increase in average $TcCO_2$ in REM sleep of 11 mmHg).*

An inhalational induction is performed with 50% nitrous oxide with oxygen and sevoflurane. Significant airway obstruction is noted on induction, though it is easily overcome with jaw thrust and positive pressure. Intravenous (IV) access is established once asleep, and he receives propofol 30 mg and fentanyl 7.5 mcg to optimize intubating conditions. He is intubated with a size 4.5 RAE endotracheal tube (ETT) without muscle relaxants. 200 mL Lactated Ringer's is administered along with dexmedetomidine 6 mcg, dexamethasone 4 mg, and ondansetron 1.2 mg. Anesthesia is maintained with sevoflurane/oxygen/air. After proper positioning, the surgeon inserts a ***Boyle-Davis gag,*** *which is checked to ensure no* ***ETT kinking****, and the child is allowed to breathe spontaneously with pressure support of 10 cmH_2O. Aliquots of* ***fentanyl*** *are* ***titrated*** *to keep the respiratory rate approximately 15 to 20 breaths min^{-1} and the end-tidal carbon dioxide ($ETCO_2$) 40 to 50 mmHg. At the end of the procedure, an oropharyngeal airway is inserted after careful suctioning of residual secretions, and the patient is* ***extubated "deep."*** *The child is turned to the left lateral position and taken to the postanesthesia care unit (PACU) with oxygen and continuous positive airway pressure applied via mask and* *portable SpO_2 monitor. Arrangements are made for an overnight stay on the ward with pulse oximetry, "line-of-sight" nursing, and instructions regarding oxygen application, managing airway, and medical emergency team criteria.* ***Analgesia*** *is provided with regular acetaminophen every 6 hours and oxycodone syrup 0.1 mg/kg every 4 hours as needed. The first dose of oxycodone is given 1 hour prior to discharge from the PACU to observe for any effects on respiration. IV fluids (0.45% saline with 5% dextrose) are run at half-maintenance rate until adequate oral fluid intake. Ondansetron serves as* ***anti-emetic*** *coverage when needed. Overnight, two desaturations to 90% are noted during sleep, which are easily relieved by turning the boy to the left lateral position, applying oxygen, and mouth opening. The patient is discharged on postoperative day 1.*

DISCUSSION

1. What is obstructive sleep apnea?

OSA is a disorder of breathing during sleep characterized by **snoring** (with **pauses** and **gasping**) with continuous partial airway obstruction resulting in ineffective ventilation and hypercarbia and/or hypoxemia. Sleep is restless and sometimes associated with night terrors, sleep-walking, or enuresis. As a result, children may be difficult to awaken in the morning and experience daytime somnolence, poor school performance, or irritability. OSA may lead to a spectrum of symptoms including neurocognitive and behavioral disturbances, cardiovascular dysfunction, and pulmonary diseases. Severe cases of OSA associated with hypoxemia and hypercarbia can lead to respiratory acidosis, constriction of the pulmonary vasculature and right ventricular hypertrophy, and ultimately death from cor pulmonale or arrhythmia.

OSA is at the end of a spectrum of sleep-disordered breathing, which includes snoring, upper airway resistance syndrome, obstructive hypopnea, and OSA. The peak in incidence in children between 2 and 6 years of age relates to when a physiological enlargement of tonsils and adenoids has occurred relative to the midfacial skeleton (which significantly expands after 6 years of age). A susceptibility to OSA relates to the propensity for upper airway collapse, and in any given person this is determined by anatomic and neuromuscular factors influencing upper airway size and function. There is an increased incidence among children with syndromes affecting their upper airway (mandibular hypoplasia in Treacher-Collins or Pierre-Robin; maxillary hypoplasia in Crouzon's, Apert's, or Pfeiffer's syndromes; relative macroglossia in Down syndrome) and among children of Asian or African origin. Neuromuscular conditions can also predispose to OSA due to reduced pharyngeal tone.

2. Which OSA patients need to be monitored in the hospital postoperatively and where?

Children with OSA have a higher incidence of perioperative respiratory complications, which can occur during induction or emergence of anesthesia or postoperatively. Complications include need for supplemental oxygen or oral or nasal airway insertion, assisted ventilation, postobstructive pulmonary edema, pneumonia, and respiratory failure.[1,2] Furthermore, increased *severity* of OSA correlates with increased probability of complications.[1] It follows that patients with more severe OSA should be scheduled admissions to monitor oxygenation postoperatively. Unfortunately, diagnosis of OSA and stratification of severity is not always straightforward. The gold standard for diagnosis is overnight PSG because it provides an objective, quantitative evaluation of respiratory disturbance during sleep. Children with an apnea-hypopnea index (AHI) >10 events per hour, profound recurrent hypoxemia below 80%, or elevated $ETCO_2$ have an increased risk of major medical interventions after adenotonsillectomy (Brown 2011). Unfortunately PSG is a scarce resource considering the high volume of patients with sleep-disordered breathing requiring adenotonsillectomy. The McGill Oximetry Score determined by nocturnal oximetry provides an estimate of the severity of OSA; however, this test is not widely available. When no PSG has been performed, then other clinical factors need to be taken into consideration before deciding on an appropriate place for surgery. Table 11.1 is by no means exhaustive but provides an outline of which patients are at higher risk of respiratory complications and should be monitored overnight.

The perioperative team should be flexible in disposition of patients, as unanticipated admissions may occur based on a patient's intraoperative and PACU course. Adenotonsillectomy patients should be observed for a prolonged period of time in the PACU, and those who experience recurrent desaturations,

TABLE 11.1. CLINICAL INDICATIONS FOR HOSPITAL ADMISSION AFTER ADENOTONSILLECTOMY

- Age <3 years
- Severe OSA based on PSG
  - o AHI >10 events per hour
  - o SaO2 nadir <80%
  - o Peak $ETCO_2$ > 50 mmHg
- Weight <3rd percentile or BMI >95th percentile for age
- Any significant neuromuscular disease (e.g., muscular dystrophies, myasthenia, myopathies, spinal cord disorders, mitochondrial and glycogen storage diseases, severe cerebral palsy—may have associated central apnea)
- Genetic or chromosomal syndromes prone to airway obstruction (e.g., Down syndrome, Pierre-Robin sequence, Treacher-Collins, mucopolysaccharoidoses, craniofacial syndromes, achondroplasia)
- Complex or cyanotic congenital heart disease
- Cor pulmonale/right ventricular hypertrophy/pulmonary hypertension (especially if requiring oxygen therapy)
- Significant hematologic disorders/coagulopathies/factor deficiencies (risk of primary hemorrhage)
- Sickle cell disease

Note: OSA = obstructive sleep apnea; PSG = polysomnography; AHI = apnea-hypopnea index; BMI = body mass index.

oxygen requirement, or frequent airway suctioning may need to be admitted for overnight observation.

It is reasonable to expect that a pediatric surgical ward should be equipped to monitor SaO_2 effectively, deliver supplemental oxygen, and reposition the patient and summon assistance if necessary. If a ward cannot do this, then young OSA patients should be monitored in a high-dependency or intensive care facility.

Patients with mild or moderate OSA who have their surgery in smaller hospitals should be monitored with caution and should preferably have surgery scheduled in the morning. The rationale for this is that the onset of respiratory compromise may be delayed for several hours until a sleep pattern is achieved, and a morning procedure allows a greater period of postoperative observation in the presence of more medical staff.

3. What are the anesthetic principles and management of adenotonsillectomy?

The airway: Anesthesia for adenotonsillectomy involves a ***shared airway*** with the surgeon. Intubation without muscle relaxants is straightforward up to the age of 8 to 9 years or a weight of approximately 35 kg. Older children may require muscle relaxants to facilitate intubation. In older children some anesthetists will choose to use a laryngeal mask airway (LMA) and throat pack rather than a tracheal tube; this practice requires a cooperative surgeon and close vigilance to look for airway dislodgement. One benefit of using an LMA is that a less deep plane of anesthesia is needed for insertion allowing rapid return of spontaneous ventilation; however, there is likely a greater risk of leak of anesthesia gases into the oropharynx. Always check airways for compliance after the **Boyle-Davis gag** has been applied as the ETT or LMA may be compressed. The RAE or "south-facing" ETT is ideally suited as it sits within the gag neatly.

Positioning for surgery usually necessitates a significant degree of ***neck extension*** by the surgeon. This needs to be considered in the preoperative assessment of the child, especially in conditions such as achondroplasia, Morquio's syndrome, Klippel-Feil, Down syndrome, or any disease process involving fused cervical vertebrae, atlanto-axial instability, or surrounding soft tissue deposition. In these cases, it is appropriate to use less neck extension.

Sedation and analgesia: Premedication with midazolam may be useful in separation from parents but should be used with caution in children with OSA as it can be associated with respiratory depression. Typically adenotonsillectomy is a 15- to 30-minute procedure, so premedication with acetaminophen, oxycodone, or hydrocodone may be helpful in establishing a plane of analgesia. Adenotonsillectomy is a painful procedure, and provision of adequate **analgesia** is essential. Excessive doses of opiates may precipitate postoperative hypoventilation and airway obstruction in OSA patients, especially in young toddlers. Children with profound hypoxemia (i.e., nadir saturation <80% on PSG) demonstrate a heightened respiratory and analgesic sensitivity to opioids,[2] so a standard dose of opioid may actually be an overdose in a child with OSA. One approach to administering opiates is to carefully titrate fentanyl to respiratory rate intraoperatively. In patients without severe OSA, morphine or hydromorphone may be more suitable but harder to titrate given longer time to peak effect. A dose of oral oxycodone or hydrocodone can be given in the PACU and a period of observation allowed prior to discharge to ward or home.

The Food and Drug Administration issued a black box warning against the use of codeine to manage postoperative pain in children following tonsillectomy after reports of several codeine-related deaths (Crews et al., 2014). Codeine is bioactivated to morphine by cytochrome P450 2D6 (CYP2D6). Polymorphisms of CYP2D6 have been identified resulting in highly variable metabolism of codeine among the general population. Ultrarapid metabolizers experience increased formation of morphine following codeine administration leading to higher risk of toxicity, while poor metabolizers have greatly reduced morphine formation and insufficient pain relief. Tramadol, hydrocodone, and oxycodone are also partially metabolized by CYP2D6 and should be used with caution. Careful titration of opiates is key, and if airway problems postoperatively are thought to be due to the opiate, then naloxone should be considered.

Acetaminophen (paracetamol) (15 mg/kg) should be used regularly if not contraindicated. Nonsteroidal anti-inflammatory drugs are excellent adjunctive analgesics, but their use after adenotonsillectomy is controversial due to a possible increased risk for secondary bleeding. Dexmedetomidine is a useful adjunct in adenotonsillectomy as it provides mild analgesia and sedation without respiratory depression and may also prevent emergence delirium. A low dose (0.1–0.2 mg/kg) of ketamine provides added intraoperative analgesia but is not sufficient by itself. Ketamine's respiratory-sparing effect makes it attractive; however, accumulated dosing may still cause some hypoventilation, sedation, and possibly nausea. Intraoperative dexamethasone is commonly used to prevent pain and edema as well as to reduce postoperative nausea and vomiting. Administration of high doses (>0.5 mg/kg) of dexamethasone have been linked in some studies to increased risk of post-tonsillectomy hemorrhage, although subsequent studies have not demonstrated this correlation (Shargorodsky et al., 2012). There is no consensus as to ideal dosage of dexamethasone at this point.

Bupivacaine or ropivacaine injection into the tonsillar fossae may be performed by the surgeon and has variable effectiveness in reducing pain and enabling early oral intake of fluids. Great care must be taken to avoid intravascular injection.

Antiemetics: Emesis is a major cause of morbidity after adenotonsillectomy. A single dose of dexamethasone given intraoperatively significantly reduces emesis events in the first 24 hours after surgery and hastens return to soft/solid diet (Thimmasettaiah et al., 2012). Antiserotonergic drugs (e.g., ondansetron) also effectively reduce postoperative vomiting after adenotonsillectomy and are often used in conjunction with dexamethasone. Blood in the stomach is a potent cause of vomiting, so the stomach should be suctioned prior to emergence from anesthesia. Ongoing nausea and vomiting warrants the use of another agent such as metoclopramide or promethazine. IV fluids should be continued until there is an adequate oral intake.

Preventing airway complications: Overall, safe management of the airway is the most important principle of adenotonsillectomy. An estimate of mortality after adenotonsillectomy is 0.6/10,000 cases, with less than one-third of these outcomes attributed to lethal hemorrhage (Brown, 2011). Respiratory events have been implicated in 36% of cases of death or permanent neurological injury after tonsillectomy (Schwengel et al., 2014), highlighting the importance of vigilant respiratory monitoring after adenotonsillectomy, especially in children with confirmed or suspected OSA and those receiving opioid analgesia.

Airway fire is a rare but devastating complication of adenotonsillectomy. Adenotonsillectomy is considered a "high-risk" procedure for the development of an airway fire since the triad of an ignition source (electrocautery), combustible tissue, and an oxidizer-enriched environment (presence of oxygen in a concentration above that of room air and/or the presence of nitrous oxide) exists. Cuffed ETTs should be used whenever possible, as they prevent leakage of oxygen from the breathing circuit into the oropharynx. If an LMA or an uncuffed ETT is used, a moist throat pack should be inserted to minimize leakage of gases into the oropharynx. Whenever possible, FiO_2 should be reduced to 0.21 to 0.30 and nitrous oxide should be avoided to minimize the risk of airway fire once the airway is secured. Spontaneous respirations or low peak inspiratory pressures can also reduce air leak around the ETT/LMA and minimize the risk of airway fire.

Many patients presenting for adenotonsillectomy have frequent and recurrent upper respiratory tract infections. Often parents report nasal congestion, coughing, and secretions at baseline, making it unreasonable to postpone elective surgery for these symptoms. After surgery children may have persistent oozing from the surgical site along with hypersalivation, putting them at risk for laryngospasm or aspiration. Because of this risk, along with lingering effects of inhaled anesthetic on airway muscle tone and subsequent airway obstruction, many anesthesiologists prefer an "awake" extubation. On the other hand, an awake extubation is more likely to be accompanied by coughing and bleeding. A deep extubation can be safely performed in children after adenotonsillectomy but relies on an experienced PACU and readily available equipment to recognize and manage airway problems. If the decision is made to extubate deep, the airway should be cleared of any blood or secretions and the patient positioned such that the airway is patent. An oropharyngeal or nasopharyngeal airway may be helpful to bypass upper airway obstruction. Positioning the patient laterally will allow for secretions to pool on the side of the mouth and reduce stimulation of vocal cords and risk of laryngospasm.

Postoperative care: The postoperative environment must be well equipped and staffed to manage the airway in children. Ongoing upper airway obstruction after adenotonsillectomy is common in the initial postoperative period. This may be due to copious nasal secretions or reactive postsurgical edema in the adenoid and tonsillar beds. Children should be monitored for a prolonged period of time in the PACU after tonsillectomy to assess oxygenation and airway obstruction. It is reassuring to observe a patient maintain normal room air SpO_2 values during sleep in the recovery room. The perioperative team must remain flexible in the disposition of patients, because there may be unexpected hospital admissions, especially in children with suspected OSA. Patients with prolonged oxygen requirement, recurrent desaturations, or inadequate oral intake may need to be admitted for observation.

Mode of analgesia should consider the risk of respiratory depression versus desirability of a relaxed, comfortable patient who is able to tolerate swallowing liquid. Appropriate prescription of analgesics prior to discharge is vital as these patients often have significant discomfort for up to 2 weeks postoperatively. Bleeding after tonsillectomy ranges from minimal to torrential and is often delayed; further discussion can be found in Chapter 15.

ANNOTATED REFERENCES

Schwengel DA, Sterni LM, Tunkel DE, Heitmiller ES. Perioperative management of children with obstructive sleep apnea. *Anesth Analg.* 2009;109:60–75.

Excellent review article on diagnosis of OSA, components of polysomnography, and strategies for postoperative care.

BIBLIOGRAPHY

Brown KA. Outcome, risk, and error and the child with obstructive sleep apnea. *Pediatr Anesth.* 2011;21:771–780.

Coté CJ, Posner KL, Domino KB. Death or neurologic injury after tonsillectomy in children with a focus on obstructive sleep apnea: Houston we have a problem! *Anesth Analg.* 2013;118(6):1276–1283.

Crews KR, Gaedigk A, Dunnenberger HM, et al. Clinical pharmacogenetics implementation consortium guidelines for cytochrome P450 2D6 genotype and codeine therapy: 2104 update. *Clin Pharmacol Ther.* 2014;95(4):376–382.

De Luca Canto G, Pacheco-Pereira C, Aydinoz S, et al. Adenotonsillectomy complications: a meta-analysis. *Pediatrics.* 2015;136(4):702–718.

Schwengel DA, Dalesio NM, Stierer TL. Pediatric obstructive sleep apnea. *Anesthesiol Clin.* 2014 Mar; 32(1):237–261.

Shargorodsky J, Hartnick CJ, Lee GS. Dexamethsone and postoperative bleeding after tonsillectomy and adenoidectomy in children: a metaanalysis of propective studies. *Laryngoscope.* 2012 May;122(5):1158–1164.

Steward DL, Grisel J, Meinzen-Derr J. Steroids for improving recovery following tonsillectomy in children (Review). *Cochrane Database Sys Rev.* 2011;8:CD003997. doi:10.1002/14651858.CD003997.pub2

Thimmasettaiah NB, Chandrappa RG. A prospective study to compare the effects of pre, intra, and postoperative steroid dexamethasone sodium phosphate on post tonsillectomy morbidity. *J Pharmacol Pharmacother.* 2012;3:254–258.

12

Foreign Body in the Airway

VIDYA CHIDAMBARAN AND SENTHILKUMAR SADHASIVAM

INTRODUCTION

Airway foreign body aspiration is associated with significant airway distress that can lead to morbidity and mortality, especially in young children. Children who inhale a foreign body into the airway and require bronchoscopy under general anesthesia present the anesthetist with some of the most difficult and demanding cases in pediatric anesthesia. A literature review by Fidowski et al. (2010) found a total of 12,979 cases of tracheobronchial aspiration of foreign bodies reported between 2000 and 2009. In fact, it is a leading cause of accidental death in children less than 4 years of age. A majority of aspirated foreign bodies are noted to be organic materials (77%–86%), mostly nuts and seeds. Among airway foreign bodies, 83%–91% lodge in the bronchial tree, with a higher inclination for the right versus the left bronchial tree.

LEARNING OBJECTIVES

1. Understand how to recognize and evaluate a foreign body in the airway.
2. Describe the anesthetic management for rigid bronchoscopy, including pros and cons of controlled versus spontaneous ventilation, and likely perioperative airway complications.
3. Explain the postoperative management of children after airway body removal and what problems to anticipate.

CASE PRESENTATION

A healthy, 11-kg 2-year-old girl with ***suspected foreign body aspiration*** *presents for diagnostic and therapeutic rigid bronchoscopy. She was playing with her doll yesterday and suddenly started choking and had transient cyanosis. This morning, the child develops a* ***fever*** *and a* ***croupy cough*** *and has intermittent* ***stridor****. Although a chest x-ray shows no foreign body, the patient has inspiratory stridor, suprasternal and intercostal retractions, and an oxygen requirement. Otolaryngology is consulted and schedules her for urgent rigid bronchoscopy. On arrival in the operating room, an intravenous (IV) line is placed,* ***glycopyrrolate*** *is given, and inhalation induction with sevoflurane begins, maintaining* ***spontaneous ventilation****. During the prolonged inhalation induction, the airway becomes more obstructed and the oxygen saturation falls into the 80s. As soon as the surgeon inserts the bronchoscope to see if the larynx is obstructed, the child coughs, her partial obstruction becomes complete, and the saturation falls to the 50s. The surgeon sees something yellow in the airway beyond the vocal cords but is not able to intubate the trachea. With the rigid bronchoscope, he pushes the object deeper into the right main bronchus. The patient is bradycardic with a heart rate of 65 due to hypoxia, which is treated immediately with atropine 0.2 mg IV. With the foreign body pushed into the right main bronchus, a 3.5 endotracheal tube (ETT) is passed through the cords. Chest movement and breath sounds are heard on the left side only. With positive-pressure ventilation and deepening of anesthesia with propofol, her saturations improve to 91% and her heart rate increases to 120. The surgeon then removes the ETT, sprays her vocal cords and trachea with 1 mL of 4% lidocaine and inserts a rigid ventilating bronchoscope. The patient is ventilated by connecting the anesthesia circuit to the side port of the ventilating bronchoscope and a propofol infusion is started. The surgeon is now able to remove the foreign body, a bead, from the right bronchus. Another look with the rigid bronchoscope reveals modest* ***airway edema****, which is treated with dexamethasone 0.5 mg/kg IV. On awakening, with a mask airway in the operating room, the patient has* *mild stridor. In the postanesthesia care unit, she is given nebulized* ***racemic epinephrine*** *(adrenaline) with good effect before being transferred to the ward for overnight observation.*

DISCUSSION

1. How does one recognize and evaluate a foreign body in the airway?

The presenting symptoms of **foreign body aspiration** vary depending on the location of the foreign body, the degree of obstruction, and the duration of the aspiration. The most common symptoms are **non-productive cough** (48.6%), **wheezing** (44.3%), and **respiratory distress** (18.6%). The most common physical examination findings are unilateral decreased pulmonary sound (62.3%), generalized wheezing (26.1%), and crackles (17.4%). The severity of symptoms may vary from a mild cough to severe respiratory distress. A high degree of suspicion is warranted, especially in young children from 1 to 3 years of age. A history of witnessed choking is especially suggestive of an acute aspiration. Findings on physical examination may also vary considerably, from a normal chest exam to decreased breath sounds, wheezing, and rales in the case of pneumonia. Inspiratory and expiratory chest radiographs, as well as antero-posterior and lateral airway films, are usually performed. Since the majority of aspirated foreign bodies are radiolucent (e.g., organic materials, such as food), a third of children will have a *normal radiograph*. Lateral decubitus chest films are helpful in the diagnosis of foreign bodies in the lower airway in young children who cannot cooperate for expiratory films. With a lateral decubitus film in a normal child, the mediastinum shifts to the down side. In the case of a foreign body in the right main bronchus, for example, a right lateral decubitus film would show no shift of the mediastinum to the right and would show persistent hyperinflation of the right lung. The history and physical examination cannot exclude the suspicion of an aspirated foreign body, and because radiographic findings may be normal, the diagnosis relies on bronchoscopy. A positive history and clinical symptoms are sufficient to justify bronchoscopy for the diagnosis and retrieval of an airway foreign body.

Peanuts are especially hazardous because they cause *profound inflammation* and *edema* of the airway, necessitating urgent removal. Vegetable matter expands with moisture and may fragment into multiple pieces, making its removal more difficult.

Esophageal foreign bodies, often associated with drooling and dysphagia, may mimic airway foreign bodies by compressing the posterior membranous trachea. Of note, irregularly shaped or sharp esophageal foreign bodies pose a risk for puncturing the posterior trachea and represent a contraindication to cricoid pressure. Ingested disc batteries must be removed promptly to avoid tissue necrosis from sodium hydroxide produced by a local current generated by the battery.

Thoracic computed tomography (CT) and virtual bronchoscopy—a reformatted three-dimensional CT image that generates intraluminal views of the airway to the sixth and seventh generation bronchi—are new modalities to diagnose tracheobronchial foreign bodies in children, with the caveat of higher costs, limited availability, and excessive radiation exposure.

2. What are the principles of anesthetic management for a child with an airway foreign body?

Preoperative assessment of the child's condition, including a review of the radiographs, is important. Discussion with the surgeon about the approach and backup plans cannot be overemphasized. Other preoperative considerations are (a) cautious premedication to avoid worsening airway obstruction, (b) IV **anticholinergic** administration (such as the **glycopyrrolate** given here) to decrease secretions and prevent reflex bradycardia during airway instrumentation, and (c) assessment of the risk for aspiration of gastric contents (Fig. 12.1).

Unless the child is moribund, general anesthesia is usually necessary for removal of an airway foreign body. Important factors to consider are (a) the patient's condition (airway, respiratory, and fasting status); (b) size, location, and effects of the foreign body on the airway; and (c) surgical technique. Removal of a foreign body may necessitate laryngoscopy, bronchoscopy, thoracoscopy, thoracotomy, or even a tracheotomy. Use of extracorporeal membrane oxygenation has also been reported. The following discussion focuses on rigid bronchoscopy, which is the most commonly employed technique.

A peripheral IV catheter should be placed prior to bringing the child to the operating room. The surgeon should be present for the induction of

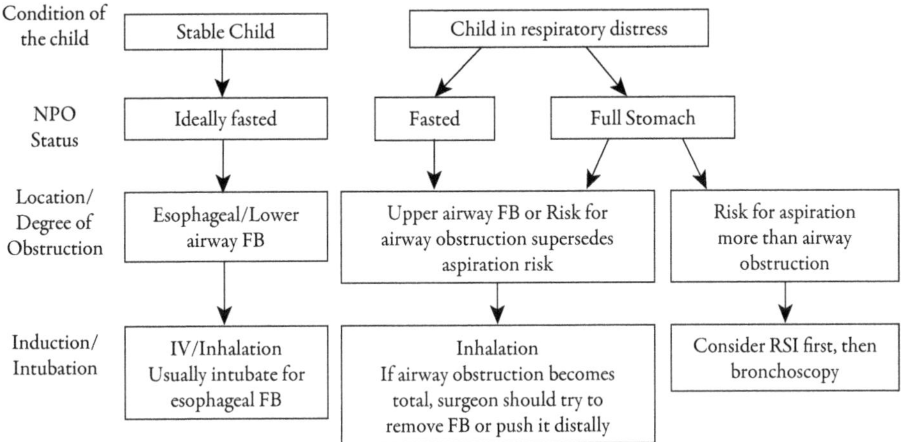

FIGURE 12.1: Anesthetic management options for bronchoscopy for foreign body removal. FB, foreign body; RSI, rapid sequence induction.

anesthesia and should be prepared to address acute airway obstruction. Anesthetic priorities include

1. Safe sharing of the airway with the surgeon/endoscopist, while maintaining the airway and the ability to ventilate, and administering 100% oxygen.
2. The choice of induction is dominated by the consideration of converting a proximal partial obstruction into a complete obstruction. Either inhalation induction, or a judicious IV induction, with maintenance of spontaneous ventilation are acceptable.
3. Adequate depth of anesthesia, use of topical lidocaine on the airway, and judicious doses of opioids, such as fentanyl, during the procedure to blunt airway reflexes.
4. Use of steroids to prevent airway **edema**.
5. Prevention of pulmonary aspiration. If the patient has a full stomach and immediate bronchoscopy is indicated, consider rapid sequence induction, immediate intubation, and gastric suctioning. The rigid bronchoscope is then inserted as the endotracheal tube is withdrawn.
6. Meticulous monitoring of the electrocardiogram (ECG), oxygen saturation, end-tidal carbon dioxide, and blood pressure

Ventilation can be effectively provided through the side port of the ventilating bronchoscope. Maintenance of anesthesia can be accomplished with an inhalation technique, with supplemental boluses of propofol as needed, or a total IV anesthesia (TIVA) technique. TIVA provides an uninterrupted anesthetic even in cases of severe airway obstruction and inadequate ventilation and also decreases operating room pollution which occurs through the open proximal port of the bronchoscope. It was shown that the propofol-dexmedetomidine technique provided more stable respiratory and haemodynamic profiles but required a longer recovery time, compared with remifentanil-propofol TIVA.

3. Is spontaneous or controlled ventilation preferred for maintenance of anesthesia?

It is controversial whether **spontaneous** or controlled ventilation is superior for the maintenance of anesthesia (Table 12.1). While **spontaneous ventilation** has definite theoretical advantages, assisted ventilation often becomes necessary to prevent hypoxia and hypercarbia.

4. What postoperative complications can occur? How should they be treated?

The postoperative course can be associated with various complications related to the procedure, the anesthesia, and the effects of the foreign body having been in the airway. Manipulation of the airway can cause airway bleeding and swelling, resulting in postoperative stridor. **Steroids** are beneficial in preventing postextubation stridor, due to anti-inflammatory actions that inhibit the release of inflammatory mediators and decrease capillary permeability. Doses vary from 4 to 6 doses of dexamethasone (0.25–0.5 mg/kg) given every 6 to 8 hours.

TABLE 12.1. CONTROLLED VERSUS SPONTANEOUS VENTILATION FOR FOREIGN BODY REMOVAL

Spontaneous Ventilation	Controlled Ventilation
Advantages	*Advantages*
1. More effective ventilation as there is less pressure drop across obstruction 2. Ability to ventilate sustained even when proximal port of scope open 3. Less air trapping 4. Less risk for pushing foreign body distally	1. Patient immobility ensured, especially if using muscle relaxants 2. Quicker emergence with use of short-acting muscle relaxants as less need for anesthetic agents 3. Less risk for laryngospasm
PATIENT ALWAYS BREATHING!	
Disadvantages	*Disadvantages*
1. Prolonged emergence due to high concentrations of inhalation agent needed for depth of anesthesia 2. Hypercarbia due to low minute ventilation	1. Air trapping due to stacking of breaths 2. Increased risk of pushing foreign body distally 3. Inability to ventilate with the proximal port of the bronchoscope open 4. Risk of converting a compromised airway to "no airway"

Source: Holzman RS, Mancuso TJ. Point counterpoint: spontaneous vs. controlled ventilation for suspected airway foreign body. *Soc Pediatr Anesth Newslett.* 2001;14(3).

The risk of harm from steroid therapy for 24 hours is negligible. **Racemic epinephrine**, a mixture of the D and L isomers of epinephrine, is also used to treat **airway edema**. The alpha-adrenergic effects of racemic epinephrine mediate mucosal vasoconstriction and its beta effects produce smooth muscle relaxation as well as inhibition of mast cell-mediated inflammation. **Racemic epinephrine** 2.25% in 2 mL normal saline can be used in a dose of 0.25, 0.5, and 0.75 mL for a child weighing 0 to 20, 20 to 40, and >40 kg, respectively. It has a peak effect in 30 minutes and lasts for 2 hours. ECG monitoring should be used as arrhythmias and myocardial infarction have been reported in children after repeated doses of **racemic epinephrine.** Treatment may cause rebound upper **airway edema**, which usually occurs within 2 hours, and therefore close monitoring is essential for 2 hours after the administration of racemic epinephrine. The child can be discharged if free of resting stridor and otherwise stable at the end of the observation period. Sometimes, postoperative intubation may be required to rest the airway and allow the swelling to subside before extubation.

Other possible complications include pulmonary aspiration, pulmonary edema due to sudden relief of airway obstruction, pneumothorax due to barotrauma from ventilation or mechanical trauma from the procedure, and postobstructive pneumonia. A chest x-ray is usually taken postoperatively as a routine to rule out these problems.

SUMMARY

1. Recognize the degree, site, type, and duration of airway obstruction preoperatively. Develop a coordinated plan with the surgeon.
2. Expect a slow and prolonged inhalation induction and maintain spontaneous ventilation until confirmation of the ability to ventilate.
3. Maintain deep planes of anesthesia with minimal airway reflexes via inhalation or IV anesthetic technique. Topical lidocaine is important.
4. In case of total airway obstruction due to a tracheal foreign body, and difficult removal, or when the foreign body is lost during retrieval, a life-saving technique could be to push the object deeper into one of the main bronchi and ventilate the other lung for temporary relief.
5. Postoperative steroids, racemic epinephrine, and intubation/ventilation may be necessary. Obtain a chest x-ray postoperatively.

ANNOTATED REFERENCES

Holzman RS, Mancuso TJ. Point counterpoint: spontaneous vs. controlled ventilation for suspected airway foreign body. *Soc Pediatr Anesth Newslett.* 2001;14(3).

Detailed review of pros and cons of spontaneous versus controlled ventilation for maintenance of anesthesia during bronchoscopic removal of airway foreign body in children.

Kain ZN, O'Connor TZ, Berde CB. Management of tracheobronchial and esophageal foreign bodies in children: a survey study. *J Clin Anesth.* 1994;6(1):28–32.

A survey of anesthetic management of airway foreign bodies that showed that practice type, greater percentage of time spent in pediatric anesthesia, and greater experience are related to a higher likelihood of inhalation induction.

Zur KB, Litman RS. Pediatric airway foreign body retrieval: surgical and anesthetic perspectives. *Pediatr Anesth.* 2009;19(Suppl 1):109–117.

A comprehensive review of the practical aspects of anesthetic management of foreign bodies in the airway in children.

FURTHER READING

Chatterji S, Chatterji P. The management of foreign bodies in air passages. *Anaesthesia.* 1972;27(4):390–395.

Chen KZ, Ye M, Hu CB, Shen X. Dexmedetomidine vs remifentanil intravenous anaesthesia and spontaneous ventilation for airway foreign body removal in children. *Br J Anaesth.* 2014 May;112(5):892–897.

Eren S, Balci AE, Dikici B, Doblan M, Eren MN. Foreign body aspiration in children: experience of 1160 cases. *Ann Trop Paediatr.* 2003;23(1):31–37.

Fidowski CW, Zheng H, Firth PG. The anesthetic considerations of tracheobronchial foreign bodies in children: a literature review of 12,979 cases. *Anesth Analg.* 2010;111:1016–1025.

Haddadi S, Marzban S, Nemati S, Ranjbar Kiakelayeh S, Parvizi A, Heidarzadeh A. Tracheobronchial foreign-bodies in children; a 7 year retrospective study. *Iran J Otorhinolaryngol.* 2015 Sep;27(82):377–385.

Holzman R. Prevention and treatment of life-threatening pediatric emergencies requiring anesthesia. *Semin Anesthesia Periop Med Pain.* 1998;17:154–163.

Liu Y, Chen L, Li S. Controlled ventilation or spontaneous respiration in anesthesia for tracheobronchial foreign body removal: a meta-analysis. *Paediatr Anaesth.* 2014 Oct;24(10):1023–1030.

Markovitz BP, Randolph AG. Corticosteroids for the prevention of reintubation and postextubation stridor in pediatric patients: a meta-analysis. *Pediatr Crit Care Med.* 2002;3(3):223–226.

Matsuse H, Shimoda T, Kawano T, et al. Airway foreign body with clinical features mimicking bronchial asthma. *Respiration.* 2001;68(1):103–105.

Pahade A, Green KM, de Carpentier JP. Non-cardiogenic pulmonary oedema due to foreign body aspiration. *J Laryngol Otol.* 1999;113(12):1119–1121.

13

Laryngospasm

BRENT SCHAKETT AND KATHLEEN CHEN

INTRODUCTION

Laryngospasm is one of the most common complications experienced by the pediatric population when undergoing anesthesia. The incidence is 0.4 to 1 out of every 1,000 children who are at risk (Burgoyne & Anghelescu, 2008). Laryngospasm is a protective reflex of the glottic and supraglottic laryngeal adductor muscles that prevents aspiration. It can be self-limiting; the patient's respiratory drive can override the obstruction by subsequent hypoxia and hypercarbia abolishing the reflex. However, if it is severe with complete airway obstruction, providers that anesthetize children must be able to both recognize and treat this complication quickly. If not managed quickly and correctly, the patient's persistent airway obstruction can lead to hypoxia, hypercarbia, cardiac arrhythmias, pulmonary edema, and even cardiac collapse.

LEARNING OBJECTIVES

1. Understand the pathophysiology of laryngospasm and its clinical significance.
2. Identify the risk factors for laryngospasm.
3. Distinguish the symptomology difference between partial or complete airway obstruction.
4. Understand the measures taken to prevent and treat both partial and complete obstruction.
5. Identify clinical sequelae of laryngospasm.

CASE PRESENTATION

A 4-year-old male presents for a tonsillectomy and adenoidectomy (T&A) due to a diagnosis of mild obstructive sleep apnea. The parents report that their child snores loudly every night with occasional gasps throughout the night. During your preoperative assessment, you learn that the child has had a recent runny nose and a mild nonproductive cough that started a week ago but has improved since then. Parents deny fever, a decreased appetite, or any changes in his normal behavior. On examination, you observe dried mucus in and around the nares. He otherwise presents with a normal exam. The patient is very anxious and cries hysterically upon arrival to the operating room. Inhalational induction is performed with oxygen, nitrous oxide, and sevoflurane. You place your standard American Society of Anesthesiologists monitors on the patient as he slowly falls asleep. As the nurse attempts to place an intravenous (IV) line, the patient begins to exhibit suprasternal notch retractions with no anesthesia bag movement or fogging observed in the mask. You turn off the nitrous oxide and continue with 100% oxygen and 5% sevoflurane. With a chin lift, jaw thrust, and the application of continuous positive airway pressure (CPAP), the obstruction slightly improves after placing an oral airway. The anesthesia breathing bag begins to fill and the end-tidal carbon dioxide returns on the anesthesia machine. The IV is secured and the patient is given an intubating dose of propofol. Clear mucus is suctioned from the back of the pharynx prior to intubation and an endotracheal tube is easily placed. Anesthesia is maintained with oxygen/air/sevoflurane and supplemented with morphine, dexmedetomidine, dexamethasone, and ondansetron.

The surgeon completes the T&A, removes the throat pack, and suctions any remaining blood in the posterior oropharynx. At this point, the patient is spontaneously breathing with a sevoflurane minimum alveolar concentration of 1.2. You suction out secretions in his posterior pharynx and extubate him asleep (deep extubation) without any events. During transport to the recovery room, the patient begins to exhibit suprasternal notch retractions and rocking chest movements. CPAP is given with a Jackson-Rees circuit; with no apparent chest rise and minimal breath sounds on bilateral auscultation upon arrival to the postanesthesia care unit (PACU) bed slot, the patient's oxygen saturation is 92%, and an oral airway is placed. Even with the oral airway, the patient is still unable to be ventilated and his oxygen saturations continue to fall. Propofol 1 mg/kg is given and you hear stridor with a slight increase in his oxygen saturations. As you reach for another dose of propofol, the patient's IV gets dislodged. The stridor ceases and the rocking chest movements return. The patient's lips start to turn blue and his oxygen saturations drop precipitately. Succinylcholine 3 mg/kg is drawn and given intramuscularly. As oxygen saturations continue to drop, the patient's heart rate begins to slow down. A new IV is quickly placed and atropine 0.01 mg/kg is given intravenously. His heart rate improves with a return of his oxygen saturations to 100%. A small amount of blood in the oropharynx is suctioned from the patient and he continues to maintain his oxygen saturations.

As the patient awakens gradually, he becomes agitated and is very restless. Your PACU nurse transfers him to his parent's arms and asks them to comfort him by rocking him and by speaking to him. Nothing seems to calm him down. The nurse decides to administer morphine 0.05 mg/kg because she thinks he is in pain. The morphine dose seems to calm him down. Twenty minutes later, he continues to cry and thrashes in his parent's arms. The PACU nurse calls you to the bedside and you administer dexmedetomidine 0.5 mcg/kg. After this bolus, your patient calms down and falls asleep. Your patient eventually meets PACU discharge criteria and is admitted overnight for observation.

DISCUSSION

1. What are the risk factors for laryngospasm?

Laryngospasm is a serious risk in the pediatric patient with a much higher incidence than in the adult population. The incidence ranges from 1/1,000 up to 20/100 for higher risk surgeries (Burgoyne & Anghelescu, 2008). Risk factors can be divided into patient, procedural, and anesthetic related. Patient-related risk factors include younger children, especially those in the preschool age groups. Patients who have an upper respiratory infection (URI) have a two- to five-fold increased risk of laryngospasm. The highest risk occurs when a URI has ensued in the previous 2 weeks with persistent airway hyperactivity for 4 to 6 weeks and sometimes up to 8 weeks. Conservative recommendations to postpone surgery can be up to 6 to 8 weeks because of this risk (Burgoyne & Anghelescu, 2008). Other personal risk factors include wheezing during exercise, nocturnal dry cough, eczema in the past 12 months, family history of atopy or asthma, and parental or patient smoking (Orliaguet et al., 2012; von Ungern-Sternberg et al., 2010). Chronic smokers have increased airway sensitivity that can trigger laryngospasm more frequently than those with no exposure to smoke. For patients who smoke, those who are abstinent for greater than 48 hours may help reduce the risk of laryngospasm. There are also procedural-related factors that increase the risk of laryngospasm secondary to manipulation of pharynx and larynx. Procedures in the airway with high incidence of blood and secretions include tonsillectomy, adenoidectomy, and nasal and palate procedures (Burgoyne & Anghelescu, 2008; von Ungern-Sternberg et al., 2010). T&A have been shown to have an incidence of laryngospasm ranging from 21% to 26%. Surgeries involving the neck can cause injury to the recurrent laryngeal nerve damage from unopposed cricothyroid muscle contraction. Laryngospasm can also be iatrogenic in nature as with hypocalcemia after parathyroid resection. It has also been shown that urgent procedures carry a higher risk of laryngospasm than elective procedures (Burgoyne & Anghelescu, 2008). Anesthesia-related risk factors normally coincide with insufficient depth of anesthesia especially when the airway is not protected with an endotracheal tube. Triggers of laryngospasm during surgery include blood, secretions, pharyngeal suctioning, oropharyngeal airway placement, and laryngoscopy. It has also been shown that less experienced anesthesia providers have higher incidences of laryngospasm (see Table 13.1).

2. What is the pathophysiology of laryngospasm?

Laryngospasm is a protective mechanism for the upper airway to prevent aspiration of foreign substances into the lungs. In addition to protection of the airway, the upper airway has multiple functions

TABLE 13.1. RISK FACTORS ASSOCIATED WITH LARYNGOSPASM

Patient Related	Procedure Related	Anesthesia Related
Recent upper respiratory infection	Airway surgery	Light anesthesia
Asthma	T&A	LMA
Nocturnal dry cough	Nasal surgery	Inhalational induction
Preschool-age child	Palate surgery	Deep intubation without NMB
Eczema in the past 12 months	Esophageal procedures	Deep extubation
Parental or patient smoking history		Ketamine, presence of secretions
Family history of asthma or atopy		Personnel
GERD		
Elongated uvula		
Obstructive sleep apnea		

Note: T&A = tonsillectomy and adenoidectomy; LMA = laryngeal mask airway; NMB = neuromuscular blockade; GERD = gastroesophageal reflux disease.

including phonation, swallowing, and breathing. To protect the airway, there is a coordination of a network of different neuronal pathways. The afferent pathway involves receptors for different upper airway reflexes. These receptors are located in the pharyngeal mucosa for swallowing, supraglottic larynx for laryngeal closure, and in the larynx and trachea for cough. For the laryngeal reflex, afferent fibers are contained in the internal branch of the superior laryngeal nerve. The efferent pathway stimulates respiratory muscles such as the diaphragm, intercostals, abdominals, and the intrinsic muscles of the larynx. The efferent fibers in laryngospasm run via the superior laryngeal nerve, which upon excitation leads to laryngeal closure. This efferent fiber activation is actually a loss of inhibition of the vocal cord's closing reflex. When blood or secretions contact the vocal cords, laryngospasm can occur.

3. How do you diagnosis laryngospasm?

Laryngospasm can be defined as either complete or partial. Complete laryngospasm involves the false vocal cords closing over the laryngeal surface of the epiglottis and interarytenoids. When complete laryngospasm occurs, there is an absence of air movement with the cessation of noisy respirations (Flick et al., 2008). Partial (or incomplete) laryngospasm, however, occurs when there is a residual gap of the vocal cords posteriorly allowing limited air movement with increasing respiratory effort. When laryngospasm occurs, clinical signs include inspiratory stridor, tracheal tug, paradoxical chest movement, and increased diaphragmatic excursions (Coté et al., 2013; Flick et al., 2008). As greater effort is needed, the volume and severity of stridor increases, resulting in a rocking back and forth chest wall movement resembling that of a rocking horse (Flick et al., 2008). Air movement ceases and inspiratory effort becomes silent as the condition progresses. Late signs include oxygen desaturation, followed by bradycardia and central cyanosis (Coté et al., 2013). The differential diagnosis of laryngospasm includes both supraglottic obstruction and bronchospasm. The clinical presentation of partial laryngospasm and supraglottic obstruction includes inspiratory stridor and intercostal retractions (Coté et al., 2013). Application of jaw thrust and positive pressure with or without an oropharyngeal airway should relieve both partial laryngospasm and supraglottic obstruction. If these maneuvers do not relieve the symptoms, complete laryngospasm should be considered (Coté et al., 2013). The application of the "laryngospasm notch" maneuver can alleviate complete obstruction if maneuvers to relieve partial laryngospasm are refractory to your efforts. The laryngospasm notch maneuver refers to intense pressure against the bilateral styloid processes while applying a jaw thrust. This promotes forward displacement of the mandible and minimizes tongue obstruction. In addition, the intense periosteal pain of this maneuver causes activation of the sympathetic autonomic nervous system and causes relaxation of the vocal cords in response. In the case presentation here, the patient arrives to the PACU with partial laryngospasm as he has inspiratory stridor and difficulty breathing. Despite the use of propofol, the patient's condition progresses to complete laryngospasm. This is shown by cessation of inspiratory stridor. With complete laryngospasm, no air can pass, and cyanosis ensues.

4. What measures can be taken to prevent laryngospasm?

The best way to treat laryngospasm is by preventing it in the first place. Prevention in the preoperative phase relies on identifying risk factors. This includes eliciting patient history from the parents: is there second-hand smoking in the house, does the patient smoke, or has the patient had a recent URI (Alalami et al., 2008)? If an adolescent smokes, abstinence should be at least 48 hours prior to anesthesia, although others say 10 days are needed to decrease the risk of laryngospasm (Alalami et al., 2008). If the patient has had a recent URI, maneuvers to reduce airway irritation should be used. Although postponing surgery 6 to 8 weeks following symptom resolution is ideal, this is likely not feasible as most children will have another URI during this time period. During the induction of anesthesia, inhalational agents like sevoflurane or halothane should be used as they are less irritating to the airway than desflurane and isoflurane. Anticholinergic use is controversial but may decrease the incidence of laryngospasm by limiting secretions (Alalami et al., 2008). Placement of an IV line or manipulation of the airway should only happen after child is deepened with anesthesia and is breathing regularly to prevent being in stage 2. The use of muscle relaxants can reduce the incidence of laryngospasm with tracheal intubation. For placement of a laryngeal mask airway, the application of lidocaine gel may help in decrease the incidence (Alalami et al., 2008). During the procedure, it is important to provide adequate depth of anesthesia and analgesia to prevent the patient from becoming anesthetically light, thus increasing the risk of laryngospasm. Although a patient can have an episode of laryngospasm at any time during anesthesia, the emergence phase seems to be the time of highest incidence. There is controversial data on whether performing an awake versus deep tracheal extubation has difference in the occurrence of laryngospasm. Multiple studies have shown no difference, while other studies have shown a decreased incidence with deep extubations (Lee et al., 2007). Before removal of a patient's endotracheal tube, oropharyngeal and tracheal suctioning should be performed to remove blood and secretions. The artificial cough, which provides positive pressure inflation to the lungs to expel secretions, and decreasing adductor muscles response have been shown to prevent laryngospasm (Alalami et al., 2008). If using a laryngeal mask airway, studies have shown a deep extubation yields lower results of laryngospasm than an awake extubation.

5. What are the treatment options for laryngospasm?

The most appropriate way to treat laryngospasm is to make the diagnosis. The first intervention is to removal of the irritant stimulus by suctioning any excess blood or secretions from the patient's pharynx or trachea. If obstruction persists, airway manipulations should include chin lift and jaw thrust with the application of CPAP with 100% FiO2. As discussed previously, the intense jaw thrust applied to the laryngospasm notch can relieve complete laryngospasm by promoting forward displacement of the mandible and minimizing tongue obstruction (Larson, 1998). Pressure against the bilateral styloid processes while applying jaw thrust can cause periosteal pain, which can activate the sympathetic autonomic nervous system and relax vocal cords (Johnstone, 1999). Interestingly, new studies have shown that gentle chest compressions may have better results with standard airway manipulations (Burgoyne & Anghelescu, 2008). The next decision is to diagnosis if the laryngospasm is partial or complete. If complete laryngospasm is present with no air movement, IV agents need to be considered after airway maneuvers have been attempted. If intravenous access is available, subhypnotic doses of propofol 0.25 to 1.0 mg/kg has been shown to improve the symptoms of laryngospasm. If the initial actions do not relieve the complete airway obstruction, muscle relaxation should be used. The most commonly used muscle relaxant is succinylcholine at 0.1 to 3 mg/kg IV, or 1.5 to 4 mg/kg IM if there is no IV access. The IV route provides immediate relaxation, whereas the intramuscular route takes about 4 minutes for maximal twitch depression. With succinylcholine, atropine at 0.02 mg/kg may need to be supplemented to prevent bradycardia. Succinylcholine may need to be followed by mask ventilation or tracheal intubation. If long-acting muscle relaxants (e.g., rocuronium) are utilized to treat laryngospasm, tracheal intubation may be required. The data on lidocaine, magnesium, diazepam, and nitroglycerin to treat laryngospasm have been studied and controversial. The small sample size of patients has made it difficult for conclusions to be drawn (Burgoyne & Anghelescu, 2008).

Cardiopulmonary resuscitation may need to be implemented if the patient becomes hemodynamically unstable and no improvements are observed with attempted interventions.

6. What is the differential diagnosis if the patient has had prolonged delirium after a laryngospasm episode?

Children 2 to 5 years of age, who are in a high-risk age group for being anxious preoperatively, can be afflicted with emergence delirium. Emergence delirium manifests as a state of confusion, hyperexcitability, agitation, and restlessness upon the end of anesthesia. When patients are young or are not able to verbalize their discomfort, it is difficult to discern the cause of their agitation and delirium. If emergence delirium is suspected, there are several treatment modalities. Dexmedetomidine 0.3 to 0.5 mg/kg can successfully treat emergence delirium. Other pharmacologic treatments include propofol 1 mg/kg, fentanyl 1 mcg/kg, and ketamine (Currie, 2015). Pain, is another diagnosis that must be considered in this young population with delirium and agitation. Pain can be treated with narcotics (morphine, fentanyl, hydromorphone) or other multimodal agents (nonsteroidal anti-inflammatory drugs, acetaminophen, alpha-2 adrenergic receptor agonists, etc.).

However, after partial or complete laryngospasm, delirium secondary to impending hypercapnic respiratory failure must be on the differential as well. As the vocal cords are closed, decreased ventilation and worsening gas exchange can cause carbon dioxide to rise, even if appropriate oxygen saturations are maintained. If the practitioner continues to treat the laryngospasm with propofol or succinylcholine without adequate ventilation to dispel carbon dioxide retention, delirium due to a rising carbon dioxide may be observed. As a result, the patient may not continue to have laryngospasm but hypercarbic-associated delirium might be misdiagnosed as emergence delirium. The use of succinylcholine 0.1 mg/kg to treat laryngospasm may need to involve bag mask ventilation or securing an airway with mechanical ventilation until the administered medications wears off, in order to expel hypercarbia. Both options can adequately reduce carbon dioxide sufficiently enough to improve the patient's condition. Other differential diagnoses that should be considered for delirium include hypoxemia, hypotension, and hypoglycemia.

SUMMARY

1. Laryngospasm is a common emergency in pediatric anesthesia.
2. Secretions and oral airways can trigger laryngospasm.
3. Treatment must be quick and includes continuous positive pressure, as well as pharmacologic intervention if needed.

ACKNOLWEDGMENTS

The authors wish to acknowledge the first edition authors, Kenneth R. Goldschneider and Eric P. Wittkugel.

BIBLIOGRAPHY

Alalami AA, Ayoub CM, Baraka AS. Laryngospasm: review of different prevention and treatment modalities. *Pediatr Anesth.* 2008 Apr;18(4):281–288.

Alalami AA, Zestos MM, Baraka AS. Pediatric laryngospasm: prevention and treatment. *Curr Opin Anaesthesiol.* 2009 Jun;22(3):388–395.

Burgoyne LL, Anghelescu DL. Intervention steps for treating laryngospasm in pediatric patients. *Pediatr Anesth.* 2008;18:297–302.

Coté C, Lerman J, Anderson B. *A Practice of Anesthesia for Infants and Children.* 5th ed. Philadelphia: Elsevier; 2013

Currie P. Understanding and treating emergence delirium. Nurse Anesthesia Capstones Paper 4. Biddeford, ME: University of New England; 2015.

Flick RP, Wilder RT, Pieper SF, et al. Risk factors for laryngospasm in children during general anesthesia. *Pediatr Anesth.* 2008 Apr;18(4):289–296.

Johnstone RE. Laryngospasm treatment—an explanation. *Anesthesiology.* 1999 Aug;91(2):581–582.

Larson CP Jr. Laryngospasm—the best treatment. *Anesthesiology.* 1998 Nov;89(5):1293–1294.

Lee J, Kim J, Kim S, Kim C, Yoon T, Kim H. Removal of the laryngeal tube in children: anaesthetized compared with awake. *Br J Anaesth.* 2007 Jun;98(6):802–805.

Orliaguet GA, Gall O, Savoldelli GL, Couloigner V. Case scenario: perianesthetic management of laryngospasm in children. *Anesthesiology.* 2012 Feb;116(2):458–471.

von Ungern-Sternberg BS, Boda K, Chambers NA, et al. Risk assessment for respiratory complications in paediatric anaesthesia: a prospective cohort study. *Lancet.* 2010 Sep 4;376(9743):773–783.

14

Tonsillar Bleed

TITILOPEMI A. O. AINA AND SHARON REDD

INTRODUCTION

Tonsillectomy (with or without adenoidectomy) is one of the most frequently performed surgical procedures in children in the United States, with over 500,000 tonsillectomies performed annually. **Tonsillar bleed**, or **post-tonsillectomy hemorrhage** (PTH), is a rare but potentially serious complication following tonsillectomy.

> **LEARNING OBJECTIVES**
> 1. Identify the risk factors for PTH.
> 2. Develop a safe anesthetic plan for a patient presenting with PTH.
> 3. Recognize the limitations of airway management in remote locations.
> 4. Describe postoperative complications following control of PTH.

CASE PRESENTATION

*A 20-month-old girl presents to the operating room for control of a PTH. Her past medical history is significant for adenotonsillar hypertrophy status post-**tonsillectomy and adenoidectomy (T&A)** and neurofibromatosis-1, with a laryngeal neurofibroma status post-subtotal resection. About **10 days** after her T&A, she presented emergently, via an air ambulance (MedFlight), with a tonsillar bleed. She had decreased appetite over the last couple of days, and today she presents with blood-tinged secretions, that have progressed to gross blood. Due to concern for acute airway compromise, the MedFlight team attempts to secure the airway en route but is unsuccessful.*

The pediatric anesthesiology team is called to meet the transport team on the helipad to provide urgent airway assistance. It was anticipated that there would be difficulty with managing the airway due to the known laryngeal mass and the multiple laryngoscopy attempts en route. Upon arrival to the helipad, several challenges to airway management in this remote site become apparent: lack of adequate lighting, environmental noise, and limited availability of backup equipment.

The patient is assessed and found to be stable enough to be transported to the operating room for airway management and surgical control of the tonsillar bleed.

*On arrival to the operating room, her **vital signs** were heart rate 130, blood pressure 70/40, respiratory rate 35. A 24G intravenous (IV) line was present in the right forearm. Her **hemoglobin level** was 9 g/dL.*

*After preoxygenation with 100% oxygen via mask, a **modified rapid sequence induction** using a reduced dose of propofol and succinylcholine is performed. Direct laryngoscopy is undertaken, and a laryngeal mass is noted to be blocking the laryngeal inlet. The mass easily moves out of the way by the endotracheal tube and a 4.0 cuffed **oral RAE endotracheal tube** is secured. The surgeon cauterizes the bleeding tonsillar fossa, and the stomach is lavaged and suctioned. The patient is extubated fully awake with return of airway reflexes and placed in the recovery position. She is then transferred to the recovery room for observation, prior to **overnight admission** in the intensive care unit.*

DISCUSSION

1. When does post-tonsillectomy bleeding occur?

Post-tonsillectomy hemorrhage (PTH) is a very serious complication that can occur after a tonsillectomy and is a surgical emergency. There are two broad categories of PTH, based on onset of bleeding: **primary** (less than 24 hours) or **secondary** (greater than 24 hours). *Primary bleeding* occurs 75% of the time and is generally more serious because it is more brisk and profuse. It is often attributed to surgical technique. However, when primary bleeding occurs, one must also investigate the possibility of an undiagnosed bleeding disorder in the patient. Coagulation profile along with consultation with the hematology team may be warranted. *Secondary bleeding* occurs most commonly between **5 and 10 days postoperatively**. Secondary bleeding is traditionally attributed to disruption of the healing clot.

The postoperative bleeding rate after adenotonsillectomy is estimated to be less than 5%. Bleeding is predominantly seen from the tonsillar fossa but can also be from the adenoid bed in the nasopharynx. Obtaining a **hemoglobin** level is crucial, as it will help guide the need for blood transfusion.

2. What are the risk factors for post-tonsillectomy bleeding?

While many studies have been undertaken to identify patient attributes that predispose children to post-adenotonsillectomy bleeding, the studies have conflicting conclusions. In a recent study (Spektor et al., 2016), three significant predictors of postoperative bleeding were identified. A history of recurrent tonsillitis increased bleeding risk by 4.5 times. Children with attention deficit hyperactivity disorder had 8.7 times greater risk, and for every increase in age by 1 year, the risk of postoperative bleeding increased 1.1 times.

According to another study (Windfuhr et al., 2005), the risk factors for PTH include male gender, age greater than 70 years, infectious mononucleosis, and a history of recurrent tonsillitis. Also contributing were known risk factors for hemorrhage, in general, such as hypertension, hyperthyroidism, and intake of oral anticoagulants. Additionally, Collison et al. (2000) found male gender, surgery in the spring and summer when patients are active, and use of vasoconstrictors and steroids as risk factors for tonsillar bleed. Yet another article (Fields et al., 2010) cited prior work recognizing age >5 years and preoperative use of nonsteroidal anti-inflammatory drugs or aspirin as other risk factors for post-tonsillectomy bleeding.

Ketorolac has also been implicated in increasing bleeding. Gunter et al. (1995) compared ketorolac and morphine in terms of analgesic efficacy and side effects, specifically drowsiness, respiratory depression, and emesis. Although both groups needed the same rescue dose of opioid in the recovery room, the ketorolac group had fewer episodes of emesis in both the recovery room and at home after discharge. While the overall incidence of bleeding was not significantly different, patients in the ketorolac group had significantly more episodes of major bleeding. The study was terminated prematurely due to the bleeding finding. Therefore, ketorolac is contraindicated in the perioperative period for children undergoing tonsillectomy.

Dexamethasone, which is commonly used to control postoperative nausea and vomiting (PONV), generated some debate when a study (Czarnetzki et al., 2008) examining PONV incidentally found an increase in postoperative bleeding. However, the authors stated that the data was preliminary. Other studies found no compelling evidence that the perioperative administration of dexamethasone increases the risk of bleeding after tonsillectomy (Brigger et al., 2010; Gunter et al., 2006). However, Mahant et al. (2014), in a retrospective cohort study looking at risk of revisits for bleeding when dexamethasone was given as an antiemetic, revealed a small absolute increase in risk. Dexamethasone administration for the prevention of PONV after tonsillectomy remains an evidence-based intervention commonly practiced internationally.

The otolaryngology literature also focuses on surgical technique as a contributing cause of post-tonsillectomy bleeding. The general comparison is made between cold steel technique and techniques employing electrocautery, either monopolar, bipolar, or coblation. The cold steel technique uses nonthermal instruments such as a scalpel or snare to remove tonsillar tissue and uses suture and packing to control bleeding. Electrocautery, either monopolar or bipolar, is used for both dissection and hemostasis. Coblation is a newer technology that is touted as having less postoperative bleeding with the added benefit of less pain for patients. Electrocautery techniques provide better operative hemostasis and therefore less primary bleeding. However, electrocautery causes more thermal tissue injury and eschar development and thus increases the potential for secondary bleeding. Overall PTH rates are not significantly different.

3. What are the signs and symptoms of hypovolemia due to blood loss?

The cause of hypovolemia in the context of PTH is two-fold. First, acute blood loss and then poor oral intake, due to pain and vomiting, contribute to hypovolemia. Hypovolemia in children usually presents with **tachycardia**, **tachypnea**, and, when severe, **hypotension**. Children will typically maintain their blood pressure despite loss of blood volume for a longer period than adults but will deteriorate rapidly and severely once they do begin to decompensate.

Signs and symptoms of hypovolemia in patients with PTH include **dry mucous membranes**, **pale skin,** prolonged **capillary refill**, and decreased **hemoglobin** levels (however, if the patient is very **dehydrated**, the hemoglobin may be normal or even elevated due to hemoconcentration). If the child has swallowed blood, he or she may present with **nausea** and bloody emesis, though these symptoms may be masked if the patient received ondansetron during or after surgery. A young child will often complain of a "stomach ache," as opposed to nausea, before emesis begins. Evaluation for **orthostatic hypotension** can help quantify blood loss that is hidden in the gastrointestinal system.

4. What are the anesthetic considerations in this case?

All patients with PTH should be considered as having **a full stomach,** regardless of nil per os status, and are at increased risk for pulmonary aspiration and gastric regurgitation due to the swallowing of blood. A **rapid sequence induction (RSI)** and intubation is recommended. In patients with a difficult airway, such as the patient in the case in this chapter, a modification of the RSI technique may be warranted. A modified RSI allows for gentle ventilation after induction and may provide a balance between risk of hypoxemia and risk of pulmonary aspiration. At least one large-bore IV line is needed to **replace intravascular volume loss** and possibly transfuse blood. Resuscitation should begin with an IV bolus of crystalloids. Packed red blood cells may be necessary based on clinical signs and the hematocrit.

Once the diagnosis of tonsillar bleeding that requires surgical hemostasis is made, appropriate fluid resuscitation should begin immediately, prior to the beginning the surgery. While brisk bleeding is more common after early hemorrhage, significant hypovolemia may still occur in children with secondary hemorrhage as well.

Two laryngoscopes, 2 working suctions, and 2 styletted endotracheal tubes should be available and ready for use. The otolaryngologist should be present for the induction of anesthesia since this can be a hazardous time with a high risk of aspiration and hypoxemia secondary to difficult intubation and loss of the airway. If an arterial bleed has been identified, the otolaryngologist may be able to apply compression at the site prior to or during intubation. In this particular case, the known presence of the neurofibroma, which was partially resected, warranted having the otolaryngologist poised to perform a rigid bronchoscopy should that have become necessary to recover the airway. Traditional induction choices are etomidate or ketamine, as their noted hemodynamic stability may be useful in the context of severe hypovolemia. If hypovolemia is not a concern, propofol may be used judiciously. Muscle relaxant choices include succinylcholine or rocuronium.

If the patient is actively bleeding, an assistant may need to place a Yankauer suction into the oropharynx during intubation to allow visualization of the glottis for intubation as blood in the oral cavity can prevent visualization of identifiable structures and inhibit insertion of the endotracheal tube. Placement of a **cuffed oral RAE tube** (named after the inventors: Ring, Adair, and Elwyn) helps to protect the airway from aspiration and facilitates surgical access. Pain medication is used judiciously, noting that this surgery is not very painful. With use of an orogastric tube, the stomach should be lavaged with normal saline and suctioned at the end of the case, though suctioning does not guarantee an empty stomach. Suction should be readily available as a blood clot can be dislodged from the stomach and obstruct the airway.

Awake extubation in the operating room is the safest conclusion of the anesthetic as hypoxemia continues to be a major concern during emergence and extubation. Pain control, vigilance for rebleeding, and reevaluation of hydration status should continue in the recovery period.

5. What are your concerns for airway management in a remote site, such as the helipad in this case?

One of the first steps in the American Society of Anesthesiologists difficult airway algorithm for failed ventilation or intubation is to call for assistance.

Often in remote locations, there is **limited availability of personnel and equipment** to assist with airway management. It is paramount to have available assistance from other anesthesiologists as well as the otolaryngologist. Communicating to colleages regarding the potential difficulties prior to patient arrival is always recommended.

There are several airway management devices currently available, ranging from rigid laryngoscopy blades to modified optical laryngoscopes. However, each device has its limitations. For example, while video laryngoscopes have been noted to improve visualization of the glottis, this view does not always correlate with success of intubation. Furthermore, glottis visualization will be severely limited in the presence of blood.

6. Would you delay the case for a type and cross?

Emergency control of the bleeding tonsil is paramount. A hemoglobin level should have been sent upon presentation, and the result will help determine the need for perioperative transfusion. Delaying the case would only extend the duration and extent of blood loss. A type and crossmatch should be sent, and there should be ongoing communication between the surgeon and anesthesiologist. If blood is required urgently, uncrossmatched blood (O−) should be administered until type and cross is achieved.

7. How should one proceed with an anesthetic if no IV line is in place?

A patient presenting with PTH is considered a full stomach and is at increased risk of aspiration with an inhaled induction. An IV line should be placed to facilitate RSI. A skilled hand is needed to successfully place an IV in a dehydrated child who is cooperative but even more so when the patient is crying and uncooperative. The parents can help calm the child and increase cooperation for placement of an IV catheter.

If multiple attempts at an IV line placement are unsuccessful and the patient is hemodynamically stable, an inhalational induction, although not ideal, can be undertaken if steps are taken to help limit aspiration risk. These steps include keeping the patient breathing spontaneously, having large-bore suction readily available, keeping the head of the bed elevated, and having equipment and personnel ready to gain vascular access and to intubate quickly.

If a peripheral IV catheter cannot be placed in a patient who is severely dehydrated and/or displays symptoms of shock, then timely establishment of IV access is crucial. An intraosseous line should be placed and resuscitation should be undertaken prior to induction to avoid cardiovascular collapse. Central venous catheterization is an alternative, but placement may be more time consuming and can be considered once the patient is stable.

8. What issues should be anticipated in the postoperative period?

Patients with *primary bleeding* continue to be at risk for **rebleeding** in the recovery period. Coagulation studies, including prothrombin time, partial prothrombin time, and platelet count should be drawn to rule out a bleeding disorder. The hemoglobin and hematocrit trend should be followed to guide the need for ongoing blood transfusion. If a coagulopathy is suggested by history or laboratory studies, consultation with a hematologist is indicated.

Wheezing may indicate aspiration, and a **chest radiograph** may be helpful. In patients who may have been intubated following multiple attempts, the risk of **airway edema** and **obstruction** is increased. Postintubation croup should be treated with racemic epinephrine. Also, IV dexamethasone can be given to prevent and treat airway edema. The patient should be **admitted overnight for observation**.

For patients with *secondary bleeding* requiring cauterization in the operating room, hydration status and replacing blood loss are the main issues in the recovery room. Laboratory analysis of the hemoglobin level guides the need for transfusion. Because patients may continue to vomit blood or blood clots, vigilance for aspiration is necessary. Stridor, wheezing, or retractions should be evaluated and treated. Overnight hospital admission for further observation may be indicated.

SUMMARY

1. PTH is a rare but serious complication of T&A.
2. PTH occurs most commonly within the first 24 hours and then again at 5 to 10 days postoperatively.

3. Major anesthetic risks include hypovolemia (due to blood loss and poor oral intake), pulmonary aspiration, and potential difficult intubation or loss of the airway due to bleeding.
4. Volume resuscitation, appropriate choice of anesthetic drugs, RIS with the surgeon at the bedside, and an awake extubation are key steps to safe anesthetic management.

ACKNOLWEDGMENTS

The authors wish to acknowledge the first edition authors, Elizabeth A. Hein and Judith O. Margolis.

ANNOTATED REFERENCES

Fields R, Gencorelli F, Litman R. Anesthetic management of the pediatric bleeding tonsil. *Pediatr Anesth.* 2010;20(11):982–986.

This study describes the incidence rates of difficult intubation, hypoxemia, hypotension, and pulmonary aspiration of patients presenting for surgery for tonsillar bleed.

Windfuhr JP, Chen YS, Remmert S. Hemorrhage following tonsillectomy and adenoidectomy in 15, 218 patients. *Otolaryngol Head Neck Surg.* 2005;132:281–286.

This study identifies patient risk factors that predict post-tonsillectomy bleeding.

Zorik Spektor, Saint-Victor S, Kay D, Mandell D. Risk factors for pediatric post-tonsillectomy hemorrhage. *Int J Pediatr Otorhinolaryngol.* 2016;84:151–155.

This study identified and quantified three significant predictors of postoperative bleeding after tonsillectomy.

BIBLIOGRAPHY

Baugh RF, Archer SM, Mitchel RB, et al. Clinical practice guideline: tonsillectomy in children. *Otolaryngol Head Neck Surg.* 2010;144 (Suppl):S1–S30.

Brigger MT, Cunningham MJ, Hartnick CJ. Dexamethasone administration and postoperative bleeding risk in children undergoing tonsillectomy. *Arch Otolaryngol Head Neck Surg.* 2010;136:766–772.

Collison PJ, Mettler B. Factors associated with post-tonsillectomy hemorrhage. *Ear Nose Throat J.* 2000;79(8):640–646.

Czarnetzki C, Elia N, Lysakowski C, et al. Dexamethasone and risk of nausea and vomiting and postoperative bleeding after tonsillectomy in children: a randomized trial. *JAMA.* 2008;300(22):2621–2630.

Gunter JB, McAuliffe JJ, Beckman EC, Wittkugel EP, Spaeth JP, Varughese AM. A factorial study of ondansetron, metoclopramide, and dexamethasone for emesis prophylaxis after adenotonsillectomy in children. *Pediatr Anesth.* 2006;16(11):1153–1165.

Gunter J, Varughese A, Harrington J, et al. Recovery and complications after tonsillectomy in children: a comparison of ketorolac and morphine. *Anesth Analg.* 1995;81:1136–1141.

Hamid S, Selby I, Sikich N, Lerman J. Vomiting after adenotonsillectomy in children: a comparison of ondansetron, dimenhydrinate, and placebo. *Anesth Analg.* 1998;86:496–500.

Mahant S, Keren R, Localio R, et al. Dexamethasone and risk of bleeding in children undergoing tonsillectomy. *Otolaryngol Head Neck Surg.* 2014;150(5):872–879.

Neuhaus D, Schmitz A, Gerber A, Weiss M. Controlled rapid sequence induction and intubation—an analysis of 1001 children. *Pediatr Anesth.* 2013;23:734–740.

Schmidt R, Herzog A, Cook S, O'Reilly R, Deutsch E, Reilly J. Complications of tonsillectomy: a comparison of techniques. *Arch Otolaryngol Head Neck Surg.* 2007;133(9):925–928.

Windfuhr JP, Schloendorff G, Baburi D, Kremer B. Serious post-tonsillectomy hemorrhage with and without lethal outcome in children and adolescents. *Int J Pediatr Otorhinolaryngol.* 2008;72(7):1029–1040.

Windfuhr JP, Verspho l BC, Chen YS, et al. Post-tonsillectomy hemorrhage—some facts will never change. *Eur Arch Otorhinolaryngol.* 2015;272:1211–1218.

15

Difficult Airway

PAUL HOPKINS AND LAURA RYAN

INTRODUCTION

The management of a difficult airway in a pediatric patient presents a unique set of challenges not frequently encountered in adults. This chapter explores the management of these challenges and the approach to a difficult airway in the pediatric patient.

LEARNING OBJECTIVES

1. Describe and evaluate the differences between the pediatric and adult difficult airway.
2. Develop an approach to managing both the anticipated and unanticipated difficult airway in pediatric patients.
3. Recognize the risk factors associated with difficult intubation in children.

CASE PRESENTATION

A 5-year-old boy with Klippel-Feil syndrome presents to the operating room for incision and drainage and exploration of right hip and knee. He has had 2 days of fever with decreased ambulation over the last 24 hours. His past medical history is significant for cleft palate (status/post repair), inguinal hernia (status/post repair), and asthma. On physical exam his neck has severely limited range of motion. His previous anesthetics were at an outside hospital but the mother reports she was told "it took a long time to secure the breathing tube and a small camera was used to facilitate placement."

He complains of severe pain in right leg and does not want to be touched. Intravenous (IV) midazolam is administered and titrated to anxiolysis in the presence of the parents. Glycopyrrolate is also administered to dry any secretions. He is subsequently less anxious and is calmly transported to the operating room for induction. He was induced using 100% oxygen, sevoflurane, and 1 mg/kg of ketamine IV. After confirmation of easy mask ventilation 1 mg/kg of rocuronium is administered. A direct laryngoscopy with a miller 1.5 blade, with downward pressure applied to the larynx reveals a grade 3 view but the endotracheal tube cannot be inserted. A nasal cannula is placed to passively oxygenate the patient for the second attempt. Using a video laryngoscope to obtain a indirect Grade 1 view of the glottis, the fiber optic scope is inserted orally and the ETT is easily advanced using the Seldinger technique. The second attempt using both a video laryngoscope and fiberoptic scope resulted in the larynx being visualized with the video laryngoscope and the fiberoptic scope was directed into the trachea and facilitated advancement of the endotracheal tube into the trachea. Positive end-tidal carbon dioxide and bilateral auscultation confirm the placement of the endotracheal tube. The case proceeds uneventfully and the patient is extubated awake at the end of the procedure without complication.

DISCUSSION

1. How does airway management of children differ from that of adults?

Head positioning is extremely important in neonates and young children. The optimal position for mask ventilation is obtained when the head is in a neutral or slightly extended position; but the relatively large size of a child's head tends to place the neck in flexion, making airway management more difficult. A small gel pad under the shoulders may improve positioning, especially in neonates. As airway tone decreases during induction of anesthesia, some degree of airway obstruction frequently occurs, especially if the patient has a history of snoring or obstructive sleep apnea. The application of continuous positive airway pressure will help stent the airway open and decrease the severity of obstruction in most cases. The anesthesiologist should pay attention to the **head position** and ensure that the mouth is open and the tongue is not pressed against the palate. Wide mouth opening in combination with a jaw thrust is often useful.

Gastric air insufflation is common during mask ventilation of small children, especially when ventilation has been difficult. This may impair excursion of the diaphragm, and decompression of the stomach with an orogastric tube will alleviate this problem.

It may be occasionally challenging to visualize the laryngeal inlet in small children by conventional laryngoscopy. The larynx is more cephalad, and the epiglottis is long, narrow, omega-shaped, and angled into the lumen of the airway covering the laryngeal inlet. Fortunately, these difficulties are offset by the relative ease with which the larynx can be manipulated by external pressure, either by the little finger of the laryngoscope hand or by the operator's free hand; in the latter case, a colleague may pass the tube under direct vision. It is important to note that extension of the neck of an infant can compress the glottis against the cervical spine and worsen the laryngoscopic view, in contrast to the effect of this maneuver in older children and adults.

The relatively cephalad location of the larynx also means that the "sniffing position" is of little benefit in small children, and a pillow under the large head only makes airway management more difficult by flexing the neck. During the first years of life, the larynx moves distally until the age of 4, when it is located at the adult level of C5–C6, and the sniffing position becomes increasingly useful.

The laryngeal mask airway (LMA) is usually easy to insert in children, but in infants the long epiglottis may get caught and down-folded by the tip of the LMA. Therefore, an alternate method to easily place an LMA in children is to insert it in a reverse fashion, with the opening against the palate, and then rotate it into place when fully inserted.

2. Why do small children tend to become hypoxic on induction more quickly than adults?

Preoxygenation in an upset child is often difficult and ineffective. The oxygen reserve is much smaller, due to a lower functional residual lung capacity and higher oxygen consumption. Desaturation therefore occurs much more rapidly.

3. How should fiberoptic devices be used in children?

Awake fiberoptic intubation is impractical in an uncooperative child, and most published methods are designed to accompany a spontaneously breathing patient under anesthesia. A common method is to use an in situ nasopharyngeal airway attached to an anesthetic circuit via an endotracheal tube connector, while intubation is performed through the mouth or opposite nostril. Fiberoptic video laryngoscopes are available in small sizes but require practice in elective situations.

The LMA has been shown to provide reasonable airway access in a large proportion of patients with a difficult airway, and the fiberoptic view obtained through the LMA provides a good view of the larynx in most cases. A well-known method is to load an endotracheal tube (ETT) over the scope and intubate through the LMA. The problem then becomes how to remove the LMA. It is possible to pass an ETT exchanger over the scope, intubate through the LMA under vision, and railroad an ETT over the exchanger once the scope and LMA have been removed, as described in detail by Thomas (Thomas et al., 2001). Walker and Elwood (2009) also described a similar method, where a guide wire is passed through the scope's suction port and the catheter is advanced blindly over the wire (Walker et al., 2009). Although costly, these methods are a practical choice for even the relatively inexperienced bronchoscopist and will minimize the incidence of a "can't intubate, can't ventilate" scenario. Ellis et al. (1999) have published a useful table showing the uncuffed ETT size that can easily be passed through LMAs of different sizes, enabling the LMA to be removed without an exchanger.

4. What is the risk and benefit of applying topical local anesthetic to a child's airway? What is the best way to apply it?

The aim is to provide an anesthetized airway, which allows the passage of an airway device without coughing or laryngospasm. To avoid toxicity, the required dose of local anesthetic should be carefully calculated. Preoperative administration is ideal, allowing emergency placement of an LMA in a relatively light plane of anesthesia, but most techniques used in an adult are unacceptable to an anxious child. Nebulized local anesthesia is often successful, especially if the child has received nebulized medication before and is familiar with the nebulization mask. Spraying the larynx directly is the most efficient method but requires a deep plane of anesthesia and an adequate view of the larynx, both of which may be challenging to achieve in a child with a difficult airway. Blind administration of local anesthesia into the back of the mouth without laryngoscopy works reasonably well to cover key laryngeal structures (Beringer et al., 2010).

5. Can the ASA Difficult Airway Algorithm be applied to children?

The principles can be directly applied, but many of the advanced techniques are impractical in an uncooperative child. In practice, this usually means that once one has decided to start the case, one proceeds directly to the "Preservation of Spontaneous Ventilation" step. Given that the practical airway management algorithm is truncated, it is important to consider some basic steps in a mental checklist before starting a potentially difficult airway case, as shown in Table 15.1.

6. How many attempts at direct laryngoscopy are appropriate?

Repeated attempts at laryngoscopy lead to trauma to the larynx and are associated with a worse outcome. In general, if the first laryngoscopy has been unsuccessful, one should ventilate while changing the position or equipment in preparation for the second laryngoscopy attempt. If this second attempt is also unsuccessful, it is prudent to ask an experienced colleague to try. After more than two attempts at intubation, the rate of failure and rate of complications are increased (Fiadjoe et al., 2016). Beyond three laryngoscopy attempts, a fiberoptic or other alternative approach to intubation is warranted. For an anticipated difficult intubation, it is important to have a clear plan and have experienced assistance available. It is important for the practitioner to know what equipment the institution has and what he or she is most comfortable using. Knowledge of one's personal "go to" airway device, and how to operate it, is vitally important when an unanticipated difficult airway occurs.

TABLE 15.1. OPTIONS TO CONSIDER IN PLANNING AN ANTICIPATED DIFFICULT INTUBATION IN A CHILD

1. Preparation
   - Are the right people and equipment available in this facility?
   - Is the necessary equipment prepared and on hand?
2. Mode of anesthesia
   - Could the procedure be performed under local anesthetic only?
3. Awake intubation
   - Is awake fiberoptic intubation or awake tracheostomy an option?
4. Intubation under anesthesia
   - Maintain spontaneous ventilation. Consider ketamine in addition to, or in place of, inhalational agents.
   - Positive-pressure ventilation is a last resort. Be mindful of removing the patient's ability to breathe.

7. Should anxious children with an anticipated difficult airway receive sedative premedication?

Many anesthesia providers feel that the use of sedative premedication in a child with an obstructed or potentially obstructed airway is contraindicated. Anything that reduces the child's ability to breathe adequately is potentially counterproductive. On the other hand, it is difficult to approach a terrified child, let alone attach monitoring devices, apply a face mask, or insert an IV cannula. A crying child will produce copious airway secretions which can become an airway irritant, and the crying also increases the anxiety of parents and staff alike. The ability to induce anesthesia in a smooth and calm atmosphere, with full cardiorespiratory monitoring, intuitively adds safety to the process.

8. How should the position of an ETT tube be confirmed in a child?

As in adults, placement should be confirmed by **capnography** and by direct visualization of insertion through the cords, when possible.

9. What are the risk factors for difficult airway in children?

Many of the difficult airways in the pediatric population are associated with syndromes, such as Pierre-Robin, Klippel-Feil, and Goldenhar syndrome, to name a few. The physical features that should be looked for, regardless of syndromic diagnosis, are midface hypoplasia, facial asymmetry, mandibular hypoplasia, retrognathia, large protruding tongue, limited range of motion of the neck, and limited mouth opening.

10. Should neuromuscular blockade be administered to a child with a difficult airway?

There has been much debate and controversy on the use of neuromuscular blockade in difficult airways, and most would agree that the use of muscle relaxation can help optimize ventilation and intubation conditions but should be used judiciously. The literature has shown different outcomes on ventilation and neuromuscular blocking agents, but a recent large study showed improved ability to ventilate with neuromuscular blockade (Sachdeva et al., 2014).

SUMMARY

1. Unexpected difficult intubation in pediatric practice is rare. Potential identifiers include mandibular hypoplasia, facial asymmetry, limited mouth opening, and a history of stridor or sleep apnea.
2. Before starting the case, ensure that adequate assistance and necessary airway devices such as appropriately sized LMAs and a fiberoptic device are available. Consider delaying the case if proper equipment is not available.
3. Maintain spontaneous ventilation if possible, but muscle relaxation can be helpful if adequate mask ventilation has been established.
4. Greater than two laryngoscopy attempts places the patient at increased risk for laryngeal trauma and increased complications.

ACKNOWLEDGMENT

The authors wish to acknowledge the first edition author, Peter Howe.

ANNOTATED REFERENCES

Fiadjoe JE, Nishisaki A, Jagannathan N, et al. Airway management complications in children with difficult tracheal intubation from the Pediatric Difficult Intubation (PeDI) registry: a prospective cohort analysis. *Lancet Resp Med.* 2016;4(1):37–48.

Discusses complications observed in children with difficult tracheal intubation

Holm-Knudsen RJ, Rasmussen LS. Pediatric airway management: basic aspects. *Acta Anaesth Scand.* 2009;53(1):1–9.

An excellent introduction to airway management in children with normal airways.

Practice guidelines for the difficult airway: a report by the American Society of Anesthesiologists Task Force on Management of the Difficult Airway. *Anesthesiology.* 1993;78:597–602.

An overview of the recommended management of the pediatric difficult airway.

Holm-Knudsen RJ, Rasmussen LS. Pediatric airway management: basic aspects. *Acta Anaesth Scand.* 2009;53(1):1–9.

An excellent introduction to airway management in children with normal airways.

Walker RW, Ellwood J. The management of difficult intubation in children. *Pediatr Anesth.* 2009;19(Suppl. 1):77–87.

A well-referenced summary of difficult airway management, which focuses on principles and practical suggestions rather than a rigid protocol.

REFERENCES

Beringer R, Skeahan N, Sheppard S, Ragg P, Martin N, McKenzie I, Davidson A. Study to assess the laryngeal and pharyngeal spread of topical local anesthetic administered orally during general anesthesia in children. *Pediatr Anesth.* 2010;20:757–762.

Caplan RA, Posner KL, Ward RJ, Cheney, FW. Adverse respiratory events in anesthesia: a closed claims analysis. *Anesthesiology.* 1990;72(5):828–833.

Ellis DS, Potluri PK, O'Flaherty JE, Baum VC. Difficult airway management in the neonate: a simple method of intubating through a laryngeal mask airway. *Pediatr Anesth.* 1999;9(5):460–462.

Holm-Knudsen RJ, Eriksen K, Rasmussen LS. Using a nasopharyngeal airway during fiberoptic intubation in small children with a difficult airway. *Pediatr Anesth.* 2005;15(10):839–845.

Holm-Knudsen RJ. The difficult pediatric airway—a review of new devices for indirect laryngoscopy in children younger than two years of age. *Pediatr Anesth.* 2010;21(2):98–103.

Sachdeva R, Kannan TR, Mendonca C, Patteril M. Evaluation of changes in tidal volume during mask ventilation following administration of neuromuscular blocking drugs. *Anaesthesia.* 2014;69:826–831.

Thomas LB, Barry MG. The difficult pediatric airway; a new method of intubation using the laryngeal mask airway, Cook airway exchange catheter and tracheal intubation fiberscope. *Pediatric Anesth.* 2001;11(5):618–621.

Walker RW. The laryngeal mask airway in the difficult pediatric airway: an assessment of positioning and use in fibreoptic intubation. *Pediatr Anesth.* 2008;10(1):53–58.

Wiess M, Engelhardt T. Proposal for the management of the unexpected difficult pediatric airway. *Pediatr Anesth.* 2010;20(5):454–464.

16

Laryngeal Papillomatosis

CARLOS L. RODRIGUEZ

INTRODUCTION

Recurrent papillomatosis is a disease process in which benign tumors arise in the airway due to human papilloma virus (HPV) infection. Lesions may not only be found in the larynx and upper respiratory tract, but the spread of disease can also occur to the trachea and lungs (Soldatski et al., 2005). Papillomas in the airway lead to the narrowing of airway structures and can also lead to laryngeal obstruction when untreated. (Figure 16.1) Patients may present with varying degrees of dysphonia, hoarseness, stridor, and, less commonly, cough, pneumonia, and dyspnea (Derkay & Darrow, 2006). Treatment of these airway tumors primarily involves surgical resection using laser therapy. Those with complete airway obstruction may require tracheostomy. The anesthetic management of patients undergoing surgical removal of laryngeal papillomas can prove to be challenging as the anesthesiologist and surgeon share the airway; therefore, communication between members of the surgical and anesthesia teams is vital.

LEARNING OBJECTIVES

1. Review the possible clinical manifestations of a patient with laryngeal papillomatosis.
2. Develop an appropriate anesthetic plan for the management of a patient undergoing laryngeal airway surgery.
3. List the options for airway management and ventilation for laryngeal surgery.
4. Review laser safety in the context of CO_2 laser microlaryngoscopy.
5. List the required steps when treating an airway fire.

CASE PRESENTATION

A 12-kg, 2-year-old male patient with a history of ***laryngeal papillomatosis*** *presents to the operating room suite for an elective direct laryngoscopy and bronchoscopy with microlaryngeal carbon dioxide* ***laser surgery****. The child presents with hoarseness and* ***stridor*** *that has progressively worsened since his last procedure 6 weeks ago. The patient occasionally becomes short of breath with activity but not significantly worse than before previous surgical procedures and anesthetics. The patient seems extremely anxious and has been tearful since he entered the preoperative area for the surgical suite. Parents state that the patient has been experiencing increasing anxiety related to his multiple doctors' appointments and would like for him to be "calm" before going to the operating room. The parents note that his breathing is "always squeaky" and that he tends to drool "a lot."*

On exam, the patient appears to be tearful and frightened by his surroundings. He is uncooperative upon examination; auscultation of lungs is difficult due to his crying. You hear transmitted sounds from the upper airway. The patient is afebrile. Blood pressure and heart rate are elevated. Pulse oximetry is 97%. The rest of the physical exam is unremarkable.

Inspection of previous anesthetic records show that the patient has undergone both intravenous (IV) and inhalational induction without incident. ***Propofol infusion*** *has been the main mode of anesthesia for his cases. The last anesthetic record showed that the patient experienced laryngospasm during induction and required intermittent intubation during the procedure in order to increase oxygenation. There is no mention of obstruction during mask ventilation. A previous x-ray from a year before does show a soft tissue mass within the larynx (Ugarte & Munoz-San Julian, 2014), but no current radiographs are available.*

Following consultation with the otolaryngologist and parents, the decision is made to premedicate the patient with 0.5 mg/kg of oral midazolam for anxiolysis. This improves the patient's mood, and he is taken to the operating room where an inhalational induction proceeds with sevoflurane in 100% oxygen. Induction is smooth without incident. A 22 gauge IV is placed in the left saphenous vein once the patient is fully asleep. The airway is then handed over to the surgeon after moving the head of the bed 90 degrees to your right. The surgeon performs a direct laryngoscopy with a parson's blade and sprays the vocal cords with 4% lidocaine. At this point, the patient starts to cough and stops breathing. Gentle ventilation is instituted but adequate ventilation is impossible and loss of end-tidal carbon dioxide ($ETCO_2$) occurs with a subsequent decreases in oxygen saturation to the low 60s. Suspicion of laryngospasm leads the anesthesiologist to administer .01 mg/kg of atropine and 2 mg/kg of succinylcholine. This allows resumption of gentle ventilation. Chest rise is now possible and fogging of face mask is noted. The patient recovers to normal saturations and starts to breathe spontaneously again.

*At this point a **propofol infusion** is started at 200 mcg/kg/min and oxygen with 2% sevoflurane is provided via an endotracheal that was passed into the left nostril. The patient is now ready for surgery. A rigid bronchoscope is inserted into the airway and blunt dissection of the papilloma is performed. Five minutes into the procedure, the patient is intubated with a size 3.5 endotracheal tube (ETT) due to desaturations. The patient easily recovers and **laser surgery** continues with the patient continuing to **breath spontaneously** on **21% FiO2. Intermittent endotracheal intubation** occurs 2 more times during the procedure. Once surgery is complete, the patient is reintubated at the request of the anesthesiologist in order to be extubated awake. The patient is extubated awake without complication and is taken to the recovery area with improved breathing.*

DISCUSSION

1. Which signs and symptoms should an anesthesiologist look for when determining severity of disease in a patient with recurrent laryngeal papillomas?

Patients with laryngeal papillomatosis present with varying signs and symptoms (Ugarte et al. 2014). Knowing the features of severe disease will be useful for the anesthesiologist when planning perioperative management. Worsening **stridor** may indicate progression of disease and **retractions of the suprasternal notch** warrant suspicion that laryngeal obstruction is severe. Severe dyspnea or cyanosis indicate most severe form of obstruction (Li et al., 2010). If an anesthesiologist is suspicious of severe disease, it is prudent to be prepared for the patient to have complete obstruction of the airway during induction. This may include having the surgeon present during induction, having various-sized ETTs available, and being prepared for a surgical airway.

2. What is the most appropriate type of anesthetic to be used in this patient? How can anesthesia be maintained?

Maintaining adequate ventilation is key in performing a successful anesthetic in this type of procedure, especially if using the **spontaneous respiration** technique. Because the surgeon may have to perform debridement within the trachea and the larynx, it may not be possible to maintain a protected airway with an ETT throughout the entirety of the surgery. For this reason, maintaining spontaneous respirations is important. Because the goal is to keep the patient breathing spontaneously, the anesthesiologist should be wary of using agents that will induce apnea. Inhalational induction with sevoflurane is appropriate in many patients, as it more likely to allow the patient to maintain spontaneous respirations while he or she is falling asleep. It is also important to note that the laryngologist should be present at the time of induction with appropriate instruments in case of airway obstruction from a papilloma. Once the patient is asleep, maintenance of anesthesia can be performed via **infusions** with medications such as propofol, ketamine, dexmedetomidine, and/or remifentanil. These drugs may be used alone or in combination to provide adequate anesthesia. Of note, some practitioners prefer to administer inhalational agents via a small ETT fitted into the nose or via a naso-tracheal airway once the procedure has begun. These agents are passively administered to a spontaneously breathing patient as ventilation with the anesthesia machine is not possible.

3. Which airway management options are available for patients undergoing suspension laryngoscopic surgery?

The primary goal of an anesthesiologist during laryngoscopic surgery is to maintain a patent airway while the otolaryngologist performs surgery in the area (Li et al., 2010). In this instance both the surgeon and the anesthesiologist share the airway, which can be challenging at times, and constant **communication** between both is vital to the success of the procedure. Current airway management techniques include ventilation via ETT, jet ventilation, apneic anesthesia, and spontaneous respiration under deep anesthesia.

Endotracheal intubation

Management of an airway via endotracheal intubation is the most common airway management technique known to anesthesia providers. This technique is best utilized during laryngoscopic surgery when removal of the papilloma is over the glottis vera. Extubation of the patient during suspension may be required when papillomas are found beyond the glottic opening.

Jet ventilation

Jet ventilation catheters may be placed passed the vocal cords (subglottic) in order to provide ventilation during laryngeal surgery. High pressure is used to channel air into the lungs, providing small tidal volumes to the patient. Anecdotally this tends to be a less favorite mode of ventilation as patients are at risk for barotrauma, pneumothorax, CO_2 accumulation and tracheobronchial injuries (Barakate et al., 2010). In the pediatric population, jet ventilation catheters may still impair the surgical field and obstruct air outflow.

Apneic anesthesia

Apneic anesthesia involves periods of apnea in which the surgeon is able to perform debridement. Oxygenation is optimized by hyperoxygenation via endotracheal ventilation. At this point, administration of a sedative-hypnotic or muscle relaxant agent, can be administered to prevent the patient from achieving spontaneous respirations (Stern et al., 2000). Once apnea is achieved, the surgeon is able to work in the airway until oxygenation is required via intubation. This technique may be repeated multiple times as needed throughout the procedure.

Spontaneous respirations

This technique is previously discussed during the explanation of discussion point #2. It is important to note that the anesthesiologist can accomplish maintenance of anesthesia with inhalational agents, IV agents or a combination of both. Once an adequate depth of anesthesia has been achieved, the surgeon can perform the suspension laryngoscopy while the patient continues to breath spontaneously (Figure 16.2). With this technique, it is difficult to monitor $ETCO_2$. Ventilation is confirmed by monitoring the patient's chest wall movement and assuring that vocal cords are patent during the procedure. Of note, this technique precludes the ability to

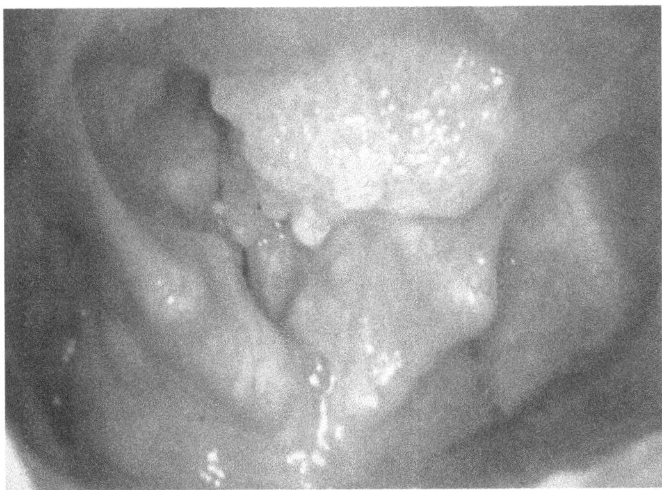

FIGURE 16.1: Laryngeal papillomas obstructing the glottis

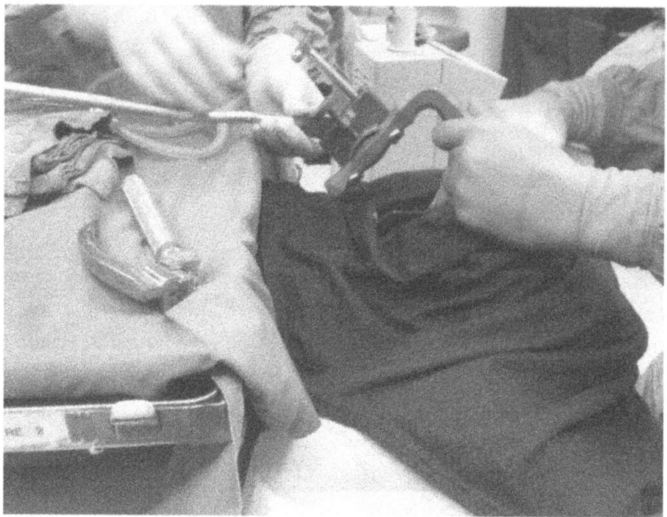

FIGURE 16.2: Suspension laryngoscopy for papilloma excision

scavenge inhalational agents and environmental pollution does occur.

4. What are the risks associated with laser surgery in this scenario?

Laser surgery of the larynx is high risk for the occurrence of an **airway fire**. Lasers are excellent ignition sources, and in the presence of oxygen can create a fire. The Anesthesia Patient Safety Foundation recommends that utilization of oxygen concentrations higher than 30% FiO_2 should be with the use of an ETT or a laryngeal mask airway (Roy & Smith, 2015). Ideally FiO2 of 21% would be best for laser surgery in the patient breathing spontaneously without an ETT. Operating room personnel should be cognizant of wearing protective eyewear while the laser is in use in order to protect their eyes from laser damage. Personnel may also be required to wear protective face masks in order to prevent cross-infection from papillomas during surgical resection.

5. What are the steps needed to manage an airway fire?

Laser surgery is high risk for **airway fire**. The appropriate steps to prevent an airway fire include using a cuffed ETT, laser-safe ETTs, decreasing FiO_2 to less than 29%, and having the surgeon place wet pledgets over the ETT cuff. While appropriate steps may be taken to prevent an airway fire, all personnel should be ready to react in case one develops. Team members should be able to work together in order to eliminate the fire. In case of a fire, the anesthesiologist should eliminate any **flammable gases (oxygen)** contributing to the fire. It is important for flammable materials to be removed from the field as well. This includes pledgets, towels, and ETT. The area should be flushed with saline as soon as possible as well (Roy & Smith, 2015).

SUMMARY

1. HPV infection can lead to recurrent papillomatosis of the airway. Patients have varying degrees of presentation. Poorly controlled disease can lead to complete obstruction of the airway.
2. A variety of anesthetics may be administered for suspension laryngoscopy. Both inhalational agents and IV anesthetics have been used successfully to maintain adequate depth of anesthesia. It is key to ensure adequate ventilation for the procedure and that both anesthesiologist and surgeon keep in close communication.
3. A variety of methods may be used to ventilate a patient undergoing laryngeal surgery. All methods have their own risks and benefits.
4. Laser surgery is high risk for an airway fire. Practitioners should prepare accordingly and be able to control an airway fire if one were to occur.

ACKNOWLEDGMENT

The author wishes to acknowledge the first edition author, Elizabeth Prentice.

ANNOTATED REFERENCES

Derkay CS, Darrow DH. Recurrent respiratory papillomatosis. *Ann Otol Rhinol Laryngol.* 2006;115(1):1–11.

This is a great review article with specific information detailing the etiology, epidemiology, presentation, and management of recurrent papillomatosis.

Li S, Chen J, Fu H, Xu J, Chen L. Airway management in pediatric patients undergoing suspension laryngoscopic surgery for severe laryngeal obstruction caused by papillomatosis. *Pediatr Anesth.* 2010;20(12):1084–1091.

This study reviews techniques of perioperative airway management in pediatric patients undergoing treatment for recurrent papillomatosis.

Soldatski IL, Onufrieva EK, Steklov AM, Schepin NV. Tracheal, bronchial, and pulmonary papillomatosis in children. *Laryngoscope.* 2005;115(10):1848–1854.

This study examines and reviews the disease progression between different patients. The objective of the study was to compare clinical progression of the disease.

Ugarte LK, Munoz-San Julian C. Laryngeal papillomatosis. *Anesthesiology.* 2014;121(5):1092.

This is a journal article showing radiographic evidence of papillomas in the airway with a brief description of the clinical scenario.

BIBLIOGRAPHY

Barakate M, Maver E, Wotherspoon G, Havas T. Anaesthesia for mircolaryngeal and laser laryngeal surgery: impact of subglottic jet ventilation. *J Laryngol ANO Otol.*2010;124(6):641–645.

Roy S, Smith LP. Surgical fires in laser laryngeal surgery: are we safe enough? *Otolaryngol Head Neck Surg.* 2015;152(1):67–72.

Stern Y, McCall JE, Mueller KL, Willging JP, Cotton RT. Spontaneous respiration anesthesia for respiratory papillomatosis. *Ann Otol Rhinol Laryngol.* 2000;109(1):72–76.

Venkatesan NN, Pine HS, Underbrink MP. Recurrent respiratory papillomatosis. *Otolaryngol Clin North Am.* 2012;45(3):671–694.

PART 4

Challenges in Patients with Pulmonary Disease

17

Intraoperative Wheezing

JULIE SCHACKMAN AND ERIN S. WILLIAMS

INTRODUCTION

Intraoperative wheezing is caused by a number of factors, including but not limited to asthma, mucus plugging, airway foreign body, pneumonia, or congestive heart failure. The prevalence of asthma has increased, making asthma a likely cause of intraoperative wheezing. Of note, many patients will present to the operating room with no diagnosis of asthma or reactive airway but may exhibit wheezing. Wheezing occurs when there is an obstruction or blockage of airflow. In order for wheezing to be heard, some air has to pass through the lumen. Thus, with complete airway obstruction, there is no wheezing. The clinician must have a high index of suspicion when considering the likely cause of intraoperative wheezing. It is imperative to consider the age of the patient as well as the preoperative physical exam and medical history. All of these components will assist the pediatric anesthesiologist in the accurate diagnosis and treatment of intraoperative wheezing in the pediatric patient.

LEARNING OBJECTIVES

1. List the causes of wheezing.
2. Recognize the risk factors for perioperative bronchospasm.
3. Know how to manage the child with intraoperative wheezing.

CASE PRESENTATION

A 3-year-old boy with no significant past medical history, except for recurrent ear infections and loud snoring, presents to the ambulatory surgery center for bilateral ear tube insertion and adenoidectomy. He is a former full-term infant and has never had surgery. His parents are in good health, and they deny any anesthetic-related problems in the family. The child has no known drug allergies and has been without food since 8 PM and drink since 10 PM the night prior. The patient is playful and interactive and wants to hurry back with you to the operating room because he was told he can have treats once he is done with surgery.

His vital signs are all stable, and his oxygen saturation is 99% on room air. His physical exam is unremarkable except for some minimal dried mucus under each nare. When you question the parents about the dried secretions, they state that the patient has seasonal allergies and has been sneezing every morning since the weather changed.

Since there are no other concerns, you proceed to the operating room with the patient and begin a smooth inhaled induction with nitrous oxide, oxygen, and sevoflurane. The peripheral intravenous (IV) line is placed uneventfully. A bolus of propofol 3 mg/kg and fentanyl 2 mcg/kg is administered and the patient is intubated atraumatically.

Bilateral breath sounds are confirmed, and the oral Ring-Adair-Elwyn (RAE) endotracheal tube (ETT) is taped in place. The patient is placed on the ventilator with a maintenance anesthetic comprised of sevoflurane, oxygen, and air. Once the surgeon has placed the ear tubes, the bed is turned 90 degrees and the surgeon begins the adenoidectomy. Two minutes later, you note the patient has desaturated to 96% on 30% FiO2. You notify the surgeon of the change and listen to both lung fields while also increasing the FiO2. You appreciate wheezing in seemingly both lung fields. You notify the surgeon and ask that she temporarily pause while you find the cause and treat the wheezing. You deepen your anesthetic by increasing the sevoflurane from 3% to 4% and you administer 2 puffs of albuterol. After 1 minute, there is minimal resolution of the wheezing. You listen again and notice there are no breath sounds on the left and wheezing can be heard on the right. You quickly pull back the ETT and give another 2 puffs of albuterol. Subsequently, you are able to here bilateral breath sounds equally and the wheezing has resolved.

The surgeon and you discuss that the ETT likely moved during the repositioning of the head for ear tube placement. The right mainstem position irritated the airway and led to reactivity. The patient remains stable throughout the surgery and is extubated deep in the operating room. He breathes spontaneously without increased retractions or wheezing. He awakens uneventfully in the postanesthesia care unit and is discharged home.

DISCUSSION

1. What is wheezing?

Wheezing is a high-pitched, musical whistle heard in expiration. In the healthy child, the velocity of airflow is too low to produce sound and breathing is inaudible without a stethoscope. Wheezing occurs from increased speed of airflow and turbulence in narrowed airways. In asthma, bronchospasm, and bronchiolitis, the small airways are affected, but in fact the wheezing comes from the trachea and major bronchi, which are narrowed from secondary compression during expiration. Small airway obstruction leads to forced expiration with positive (rather than the usual negative) intrapleural pressure. This positive intrapleural pressure exceeds the intraluminal pressure in the trachea and major bronchi and results in compression and dynamic expiratory narrowing of these airways.

While obstruction of the small airways is the most common reason for wheezing, obstructive lesions in the trachea or main bronchi may also generate an increase in velocity of airflow causing wheezing. Foreign bodies in the large airways or compression from lymph nodes may also manifest as wheezing.

Extrathoracic obstructive causes of wheezing usually have an inspiratory noise. This distinguishes them from bronchospasm, which usually just has the expiratory wheeze. "Stridor" is the term used to describe the inspiratory noises.

2. What causes wheezing?

There are many potential causes. A useful classification of possible causes is based on age (Table 17.1). Wheezing is common, and 40% to 50% of children less than 6 years of age will wheeze at some time. The majority of these have a condition known as transient infant wheeze, as did the child in this scenario. This is a benign condition that appears to be related to the relatively small caliber and floppiness of the airways. Most children outgrow the condition by age 6 years, but 5% to 7% of all children (30%–40% of those who wheeze) continue to wheeze and are diagnosed with persistent wheezing or asthma (Henry, 2007).

TABLE 17.1. ETIOLOGY OF WHEEZING BY AGE GROUP

Infants, Toddlers, and Preschoolers (0–4 years)	
Obstruction of small airways	Acute viral bronchiolitis (RSV) Aspiration Asthma/bronchospasm Bronchiectasis Chronic lung disease of prematurity Transient infant wheeze
Obstruction of large airways	Airway and vascular malformations Inhaled foreign body Mediastinal cysts/masses
School-Age Children/Adolescents (5–15 years)	
Obstruction of small airways	Asthma Mycoplasma pneumoniae infection Bronchiectasis
Obstruction of large airways	Bronchial adenoma Alpha 1-antitrypsin deficiency Inhaled/ingested foreign body Mediastinal tumors/masses Hysterical wheezing

3. What is the management of the child who is wheezing at the preoperative consult?

First, the cause of wheeze should be determined. The age of the child, a history of prematurity, respiratory tract infection, or reactive airways disease will give clues as to the likely cause. In a child with transient wheeze or asthma, further history is required to determine how well controlled the symptoms are. A history of chronic cough and diurnal or nocturnal symptoms are typical of poorly controlled asthma. Factors that trigger bronchospasm should be recorded. A history of recent viral infection or an exacerbation of asthma requiring hospitalization is associated with an increased risk of perioperative bronchospasm refractory to simple measures and is of particular concern.

Poor weight gain suggests other causes for wheezing, such as gastroesophageal reflux disease, cystic fibrosis, or immunodeficiency.

The child with chronic pulmonary disease, such as bronchopulmonary dysplasia, needs to be assessed with regard to optimization. Parental assessment of the child's current status and a history of recent respiratory infection or productive cough are important. The requirement for home oxygen therapy in the past or currently should be noted as an indicator of significant disease. An objective measure, such as pulse oximetry breathing air, is useful and may be compared with previous readings. The question that must be asked is, "Is this child in the best possible condition?" If so, it is appropriate to proceed with caution.

On physical examination, the anesthesiologist should decide if the child looks unwell. The temperature should be checked and the work of breathing should be assessed. Transient wheezers generally do not have significant respiratory distress and hypoxia. Tachypnea and the use of intercostal and supraclavicular muscles are indicative of more severe asthma. Unilateral wheezing suggests aspiration of a foreign body or bronchomalacia. Wheezing together with crackles suggests an interstitial lung disease such as infection, bronchopulmonary dysplasia, or pulmonary edema (e.g., in a child with congenital heart disease). Wheezing together with stridor and noises transmitted from upper airway narrowing would suggest an upper and lower airway process such as croup, tracheomalacia, or bronchomalacia.

4. How is intraoperative wheezing managed?

A rapid diagnosis of the cause of intraoperative wheezing must be made. Wheezing usually occurs under light anesthesia as a result of bronchial or carinal stimulation. It may also result from bronchospasm subsequent to aspiration or **anaphylaxis** or might be drug-related via a variety of other mechanisms. The clinical context will help ascertain the cause. Mechanical causes of **airway obstruction** (e.g., kinking or mucous plugging of the ETT) need to be recognized by inspecting the circuit and inserting a suction catheter to the tip of the ETT. Other mechanical causes are rare but may include incidental inhaled foreign body (this may not have been witnessed or suspected), obstructive mass, vascular ring, and vocal cord dysfunction.

Anaphylaxis is likely when all of the following three criteria are met:

- Sudden onset and rapid progression of symptoms
- Life-threatening airway and/or circulation problems
- Skin and/or mucosal changes (flushing, urticaria, angioedema)

In the child in this scenario, a mechanical cause was excluded and anaphylaxis was thought to be unlikely. The child had *persistent wheezing*. This is best managed by deepening the anesthesia with a bolus of propofol (1–2 mg/kg) or by increasing the inspired sevoflurane concentration. **Desflurane** causes a marked increase in airway resistance, particularly in children with airway irritability, and should have been avoided (Von Ungern-Sternberg et al., 2008). In this scenario, a beta-2 agonist was also given to treat acute bronchospasm via the inhalational route. Short-acting agents such as **albuterol** (salbutamol) may be given through the breathing circuit. One puff is equivalent to 100 mcg. Alternatively, a 0.5% solution (5 mg/mL) may be nebulized, either diluted (0.5 mL in 4 mL) or undiluted. Other beta-2 agonists include terbutaline and metoproterenol. In life-threatening bronchospasm, a bolus of epinephrine (adrenaline) 1 to 2 mcg/kg intravenously (one-tenth the resuscitation dose) or an IV infusion of a beta-2 agonist is indicated.

Systemic corticosteroids are used in more severe attacks than seen in this scenario. They are slower in onset than the beta-2 agonists. Methylprednisolone 0.5 to 1 mg/kg or hydrocortisone 2 to 4 mg/kg may be given intravenously. Corticosteroids enhance and prolong the response to beta-adrenergic agents within 1 hour, while 4 to 6 hours are required for the anti-inflammatory effects. Lidocaine (lignocaine; 1.5 mg/kg IV) may reduce the airway response to instrumentation and drug-induced bronchospasm. However, paradoxically, lidocaine can itself also cause a significant increase in airway tone and narrowing when given by inhalation or intravenously (Chang et al., 2007). Magnesium may also be used in severe asthma attacks (Cheuk et al., 2005). Aminophylline is not recommended as a therapy under anesthesia because it may cause cardiac dysrhythmias (Streetman et al., 2002).

The wheezing child should be observed closely in the PACU for increasing work of breathing, respiratory distress, and changing oxygen requirement. Children with a past history of reactive airways disease may develop wheezing as they emerge from anesthesia. Volatile agents are good bronchodilators; an effect that wanes on emergence. The possibility of nonsteroidal anti-inflammatory drugs triggering asthma should be remembered, although this phenomenon is more common in adults.

Persistent oxygen dependence may indicate a need for arterial blood gas measurement. A chest radiograph may be normal in reactive airways disease; however, typical findings include peribronchial thickening, subsegmental atelectasis, and hyperinflation. Unusual causes of wheeze such as congenital lung malformations or vascular malformations may be detected. A pulmonologist (respiratory pediatrician) may be consulted if symptoms do not resolve.

5. How can intraoperative wheezing be avoided?

Elective surgery should be postponed in children at high risk (i.e., those with concurrent respiratory infection or poorly controlled asthma and those with preoperative wheezing). A careful anesthetic plan is required for the child considered to be at risk if surgery is to proceed. All asthma medications should be continued until surgery. *Premedication with a beta-2 agonist* (e.g., albuterol) decreases the incidence of perioperative bronchospasm and should be considered in high-risk children. A course of preoperative *corticosteroids* might also be considered in high-risk children.

Inhalational induction with sevoflurane may be preferred, as volatile agents generally are bronchodilators and the mask is often familiar and well tolerated. IV induction may be safely performed, bearing in mind the effects of the different agents on bronchomotor tone. Propofol causes significant upper airway relaxation, while ketamine has weak sympathomimetic actions and causes bronchodilation; however, the disadvantage is that it increases secretions.

For maintenance of anesthesia, desflurane should be avoided, and sevoflurane may be superior to isoflurane (Rooke et al., 1997). Adequate depth of anesthesia is critical before airway instrumentation is attempted. Endotracheal intubation is associated with a lower incidence of respiratory events but is more likely to provoke bronchospasm than placement of a laryngeal mask airway (Kim & Bishop, 1999; Mamie et al., 2004). Extubation of the trachea under deep anesthesia is often recommended. Emergence in patients with irritable airways is associated with laryngospasm and bronchospasm.

A number of drugs routinely used in anesthesia can induce bronchospasm through histamine release or muscarinic activity or by provoking allergic reactions. Atracurium has histamine-releasing effects, while cisatracurium does not. Rocuronium may be used for rapid sequence intubation, although succinylcholine is not contraindicated in those at risk of bronchospasm. As for all cases, care must be taken that nondepolarizing neuromuscular block is fully reversed. The use of morphine in asthmatics has been controversial, although there is little objective evidence to validate these concerns (Eschenbacher et al., 1984).

SUMMARY

1. Wheezing is common and has many potential causes.
2. Risk factors for developing intraoperative wheezing include intercurrent respiratory infection and poorly controlled asthma. In these cases, consider postponing surgery.
3. A careful anesthetic plan will decrease the risk of intraoperative wheezing. Premedication with albuterol, avoidance of desflurane, and maintenance of a deep plane of anesthesia minimize the likelihood of wheezing.
4. In cases of intraoperative wheezing due to bronchospasm, cease triggering agents, deepen anesthesia, and administer inhaled beta-2 agonists. Exclude anaphylaxis, aspiration, and mechanical obstruction of the ETT.

ACKNOWLEDGMENT

The author wishes to acknowledge the first edition author, Dr. Lindy Cass.

ANNOTATED REFERENCES

Von Ungern-Sternberg BS, Boda K, Chambers NA, Rebmann C, Johnson C, Sly PD, Habre W. Risk assessment for respiratory complications in paediatric anaesthesia: a prospective cohort study. *Lancet* 2010;376:773–783.

This paper outlines the risk factors for perioperative respiratory complications in children, including asthma.

Von Ungern-Sternberg BS, Saudan S, Petak F, Hantos Z, Habre W. Desflurane but not sevoflurane impairs respiratory tissue mechanics in children with susceptible airways. *Anesthesiology.* 2008;108:216–224.

This excellent article demonstrates the adverse effect that desflurane has on the respiratory mechanics of children with recent respiratory infection or asthma.

Woods BD, Sladen RN. Perioperative considerations for the patient with asthma and bronchospasm. *Br J Anaesth.* 2009;103(Suppl 1) i57–i65.

This comprehensive review of asthma and anesthesia is essential reading.

BIBLIOGRAPHY

Chang HY, Togias A, Brown RH. The effects of systemic lidocaine on airway tone and pulmonary function in asthmatic subjects. *Anesth Analg.* 2007;104:1109–1115.

Cheuk DKL, Chau TCH, Lee SL. A meta-analysis on intravenous magnesium sulphate for treating acute asthma. *Arch Dis Child.* 2005;90:74–77.

Eschenbacher WL, Bethel RA, Boushey HA, Sheppard D. Morphine sulfate inhibits bronchoconstriction in subjects with mild asthma whose responses are inhibited by atropine. *Am Rev Respir Dis.* 1984;130(3):363–367.

Henry R. Wheezing disorders other than asthma. In: Roberton DM, South M, eds. *Practical Paediatrics.* 6th ed. Edinburgh, UK: Churchill Livingstone; 2007:459–463.

Kilbaugh TJ, Zwass M, Ross P. Pediatric and neonatal intensive care. In: Miller RD, ed. *Miller's Anesthesia.* 8th ed. Philadelphia: Elsevier; 2015:2854–2922.

Kim ES, Bishop MJ. Endotracheal intubation, but not laryngeal mask airway insertion, produces reversible bronchoconstriction. *Anesthesiology.* 1999;90:391–394.

Mamie C, Habre W, Delhumeau C, Argiroffo CB, Morabia A. Incidence and risk factors of perioperative respiratory adverse events in children undergoing elective surgery. *Paediatr Anaesth.* 2004;14:218–224.

Rooke GA, Choi JH, Bishop MJ. The effect of isoflurane, halothane, sevoflurane, and thiopental/nitrous oxide on respiratory system resistance after tracheal intubation. *Anesthesiology.* 1997;86:1294–1299.

Streetman DD, Bhatt-Mehta V, Johnson CE. Management of acute, severe asthma in children. *Ann Pharmacother.* 2002;36:1249–1260.

Von Ungern-Sternberg BS, Saudan S, Petak F, Hantos Z, Habre W. Desflurane but not sevoflurane impairs respiratory tissue mechanics in children with susceptible airways. *Anesthesiology.* 2008;108:216–224.

18

Cystic Fibrosis

BRIAN TINCH, DAVID MARTIN, AND JUNZHENG WU

INTRODUCTION

Cystic fibrosis (CF) is autosomal recessive disorder with numerous mutations in the cystic fibrosis transmembrane conductance regulator (CFTR). This inherited disease has an incidence of 1 in 2,000 births in Caucasians and 1 in 17,000 in African Americans. It is the most common fatal inherited disorder affecting Caucasians. Penetrance can vary in severity; the most common clinical manifestations involve progressive lung damage and chronic digestive problems due to exocrine gland dysfunction and the production of thick viscous mucus caused by defect of CFTR. Careful perioperative management is important to avoid respiratory complications.

LEARNING OBJECTIVES

1. Understand the pathophysiology of CF and its clinical implications.
2. Know how to evaluate and optimize the patient with CF preoperatively.
3. Explain the key principles of intraoperative management.
4. Develop a plan to avoid postoperative respiratory complications.

CASE PRESENTATION

A 14-year-old girl with CF is scheduled for endoscopic sinus surgery with polypectomy and elective flexible bronchoscopy with alveolar lavage due to a worsening ***productive cough****. Her history is significant for* ***meconium ileus*** *requiring bowel resection in infancy. Her chest x-ray shows* ***hyperinflation*** *and diffuse interstitial disease with* ***bronchiectasis*** *and nodular densities of mucoid impaction. She is on oral supplementation of pancreatic enzymes and fat-soluble vitamins. She is in the less than 10th percentile for weight and height. She has an extensive pulmonary clearance routine and numerous medications:*

Pulmonary clearance/medications

Percussion vest therapy 4 times a day
Mucomyst nebulizer with albuterol twice a day
Hypertonic saline with albuterol twice a day
Inhaled gentamicin once a day every other month
Albuterol inhaled as needed
Fluticasone inhaled twice a day
Ipratropium inhaled 4 times a day
Pancreatic enzymes before meals and snacks
Fat-soluble (A, D, E, K) vitamins
Prednisone burst currently
Regular insulin
Insulin glargine
Note: The patient's compliance to pulmonary clearance routine has been less since becoming a teenager.

Labs

FEV_1- Decline 60% -40% over last 12 months
Creatinine 1.1
Glucose 202
Coagulation within normal limits
Liver Function Tests (LFTs) within normal limits

In the operating room (OR), propofol, fentanyl, and rocuronium are used to induce anesthesia after thorough preoxygenation. Upon intubation, the peripheral capillary oxygen saturation (SpO_2) quickly drops from 97% to 65% and ***bilateral wheezing and rhonchi*** *are heard on auscultation. She is given multiple puffs of an albuterol using an aerosolizing chamber inserted into the anesthesia circuit and deepening of anesthetic with some improvement in wheezing but rhonchi are worse. A 14 French soft catheter is utilized to suction the endotracheal* *tube (ETT) with removal of a large volume of viscous secretions. She is given positive-pressure ventilation with a FiO_2 of 1.0. The SpO_2 returns slowly to 96% over a several minutes and the wheezing is minimal and rhonchi are absent. The patient was maintained on propofol and remifentanil invenous anesthetic secondary to her poor pulmonary status and to guarantee an adequate plane of anesthesia during the bronchoscopy. The pulmonologist proceeds first with flexible bronchoscopy. A thick, yellow layer of mucus is seen throughout the bronchial tree. After lavage and* ***extensive*** *suction of visible* ***secretions,*** *the procedure is completed. After completion of bronchoscopy, a heat and moisture exchanger is placed to optimize humidification and avoid drying out secretions. The otolaryngologist begins the endoscopic sinus surgery with removal of multiple polyps and clearing of viscous secretions from sinuses. Hemostasis is achieved and procedure is completed. The patient required frequent suctioning during the procedure. The patient's plane of anesthesia is lightened and she is given full reversal after confirming train of four is 3/4. The patient is given prophylactic albuterol prior to extubation.*

In the postanesthesia care unit (PACU), the first set of vital signs are within the normal limits, but over the next 30 minutes the patient develops an increased frequency of a productive cough. The PACU nurse initiates manual ***chest physiotherapy*** *with postural drainage and albuterol with hypertonic saline. The patient expectorates copious thick mucus from the respiratory tract and maintains SpO_2 at 96% on room air. She is encouraged to sit up in the PACU as soon as possible. The patient is sent to the floor for overnight observation.*

DISCUSSION

1. What are the genetic and molecular abnormalities in CF?

CF is an autosomal recessive disorder caused by a genetic mutation on chromosome 7 that alters the function of CFTR. The CFTR is a protein that controls the flux of ions across the cell membrane in particular chloride among others. The CFTR, which is widely localized on the surface of the epithelium lining the respiratory tract, pancreas, intestine, sweat and salivary glands, and reproductive tract, is responsible for the pathophysiologic process of this disease. Up to 1,200 mutations on a gene that directs the synthesis of CFTR have been identified on the long arm of chromosome 7 in CF patients (Boucher et al., 2010; Davis, 2006). CFTR loses its chloride-regulating mechanism, resulting in the impermeability of epithelial cells to chloride ions. Diagnostic tests for CF include DNA sequencing to identify mutations and sweat testing, which demonstrates an excessive amount of sodium and chloride in the sweat.

2. What are the pathophysiologic features and the clinical manifestations of CF in the respiratory and gastrointestinal (GI) system?

Respiratory system: Pulmonary involvement accounts for more than 90% of the morbidity and mortality in CF patients. In the normal airway epithelium, chloride ions are actively transported into the airway lumen with sodium and water to hydrate the airway secretions. In CF, the abnormal CFTR protein causes an inability to actively secrete Cl^- ions. As a result, sodium and water are attracted into the epithelial cells from the airway lumen, leading to the thick, viscous airway secretions that are the hallmark of the disease. This thick mucus leads to airway inflammation and mucociliary dysfunction. The resulting inability to clear secretions causes mucus plugging and increased bacterial colonization. The upper airway involvement includes an increased volume of thick mucus, hyperactive mucus-secreting glands, edema and hypertrophy of the mucous membranes, chronic nasal congestion, sinusitis, and nasal polyps. CF patients have frequent anesthetics secondary to chronic sinusitis. The involvement of the lower respiratory tract in CF usually dominates the clinical picture. Small airway obstruction by thick secretions causes progressive **bronchiectasis** and **hyperinflation** of the lungs due to air trapping, **atelectasis**, and frequent pulmonary infection with a wide variety of pathogens (most commonly *Staphylococcus aureus* and *Pseudomonas aeruginosa*). Wheezing is the result of airway hyperreactivity, especially accompanying pulmonary infection. Over time, pulmonary function deteriorates as measured by decreases in forced expiratory volume in the first second (FEV_1) and exercise tolerance, which are inversely proportional to mortality. Hypoxia and respiratory failure result from acute exacerbation, pulmonary infections, or progressive loss of lung function due to chronic lung disease. With advanced disease, hypoxemia leads to pulmonary hypertension, cor pulmonale, and right ventricular failure. Pneumothorax and hemoptysis may occur in advanced stages (Boucher et al., 2010; Davis, 2006).

GI system: GI complications of CF have several implications for the anesthesiologist. **Meconium ileus** in neonates results in intestinal obstruction in 15% to 20%; the babies can present to the OR with volvulus, and/or peritonitis from perforation. Infants who do not pass their first meconium within 48 hours of birth have concern for bowel obstruction. Pancreatic duct blocked by thick exocrine secretions results in two major consequences: first the enzymes are prevented from reaching the intestine, leading to malabsorption of protein, fat, and the fat-soluble vitamins A, D, E, and K. Vitamin K deficiency is closely associated with coagulopathy and bone disease, frequently seen in CF patients. Delayed puberty and vitamin D and calcium deficiencies also contribute to osteoporosis. Second, duct plugging causes progressive pancreatic fibrosis (Farrell et al., 2008). This eventually leads to pancreatic endocrine dysfunction and insulin-dependent diabetes in about 8% of patients after age of 10. Biliary cirrhosis, portal hypertension, and cholelithiasis can develop in the late stages of this disease (Firth et al., 2013).

3. How should one assess and optimize the patient for elective surgery?

CF is a lifelong chronic and progressive disease. CF patients coming to the OR may therefore have different issues depending on when and why they present. Preanesthetic assessment of the CF patient should account for the dynamics of the disease and focus on the most commonly affected organs and systems. CF patients have frequent pulmonary function test to compare to baseline. Pulmonary function test, exercise tolerance, peak flow meter, mucus production, history of patient compliance to pulmonary regimen, recent sputum cultures, and oxygen saturation (Firth et al., 2013) are often considered. About 40% of patients are responsive to bronchodilators, but in some "paradoxical responders," the FEV_1 may in fact deteriorate. The most likely explanation is that albuterol reduces smooth airway tone; CF patients who have damaged, bronchiectatic airways require this tone to prevent airway collapse (Firth et al., 2013). One should inquire about recent fever and pulmonary infection. Pulmonary function tests and chest x-rays should be reviewed. An electrocardiogram and echocardiogram should be obtained when cor pulmonale, pulmonary hypertension, or other cardiac abnormalities are suspected. Arterial blood gas analysis should be considered to analyze the baseline of partial pressure of oxygen and partial pressure of carbon dioxide prior to any major and prolonged surgery. Clinical measures that can be taken (in consultation with the a pulmonologist) to optimize the patient for surgery include (a) *a full course of antibiotics* for ongoing active pulmonary infection prior to elective surgery; (b) *oral and inhaled corticosteroids* to treat coexistent allergic pulmonary aspergillosis and reactive airway disease; (c) *daily bronchodilators* and/or steroid for active wheezing if a good response to the drug is observed; (d) *intensive pulmonary therapy* including incentive spirometry, daily regimens of postural drainage, and manual and mechanical chest physiotherapy (percussion, clapping, and vibration) to facilitate bronchial airway drainage; and (e) *aerosol therapy* with inhaled mucolytic agents (N-acetylcysteine), hypertonic saline, or inhaled DNAase. *Mucolytic agents* decrease sputum viscosity and improve mucus clearance; inhaled tobramycin has the benefit of reaching distal sites of lung infection in high concentrations. Inhalation of hypertonic saline (7% NaCl) accelerates mucus clearance and improves lung function and is now part of the routine management of CF patients. A strict compliance to a pulmonary regimen is also vital. It should be continued throughout the perioperative period (Della Rocca, 2002; Elkins et al., 2006). When possible, surgery should be scheduled later in the day to allow enough time for ambulation and chest physiotherapy in the morning to facilitate expectoration of secretions retained overnight.

Review of the GI system should focus on nutritional status and gastroesophageal acid reflux disease (GERD), which can be seen in nearly 50% of pediatric patients. Insulin-dependent diabetes and coagulopathy should be suspected and evaluated with preoperative testing if indicated. Clinical optimization of the CF patient includes acid suppression to control GERD, blood sugar management regimens if indicated (see Chapter 46), preoperative administration of oral or intramuscular vitamin K to reduce the risk of coagulopathy, nutritional therapy such as pancreatic enzymes, and vitamin replacement to increase immune function (Randell & Boucher, 2006).

Numerous metabolic disturbances are seen in patients with CF, including *decreased plasma albumin levels* (which may affect drug binding and wound healing), *intravascular volume depletion* (due to chronic diarrhea, poor oral intake, and diuretic therapy), and *electrolyte imbalances*, which may be caused by excessive chloride and sodium loss from sweat (Huffmyer et al., 2009).

Patients with CF are often malnourished from malabsorption secondary to the loss of the exocrine function of the pancreas. The patient's weight percentile and trend are important indicators of overall health.

4. What are key points of intraoperative management?

The anesthetic plan for the CF patient depends upon the nature of the operation and the condition of the patient. If the surgery is elective and patient is not at baseline, consider postponing surgery until he or she is optimized. The goal is to provide minimal long-term ventilatory depression and to enhance clearance of secretions.

Premedication: Daily medications, particularly bronchodilators, corticosteroids, and cardiotonic drugs, should be continued into the perioperative period. Preoperative oral benzodiazepines have been used successfully to treat the anxiety that may be seen in children with chronic diseases such as CF. Prophylactic treatment with bronchodilators should be considered before induction if reactive airways and bronchospasm are significant components of the disease. Anticholinergics offer little advantage, and their use should be avoided in CF patients. The use of H_2 receptor antagonists and antacid premedication is recommended in patients with poorly controlled GERD. Provided that coagulation is normal, regional anesthesia can be considered when appropriate as a method of reducing the systemic side effects of anesthetic drugs, especially opioids (Huffmyer et al., 2009).

Induction/intubation: If general anesthesia is selected, preoxygenation to maximize hemoglobin saturation before induction is especially important. CF patients with moderate to severe lung disease may have an altered hypoxic respiratory drive, so close attention should be paid to the adequacy of respiration during preoxygenation. Inhalation induction may be used in young CF patients; however, use caution with inhalational induction if patient is having a CF exacerbation or decline in pulmonary function. Pronounced ventilation/perfusion mismatch and large functional residual capacity and small tidal volumes may significantly prolong inhalation induction (Karlet, 2000). Intravenous induction may be the best option for patients not at baseline or severe pulmonary disease. In patients with poorly controlled GERD, rapid sequence induction and intubation should be considered to reduce the risk of aspiration. Propofol is favored for intravenous induction due to its bronchodilating effect and minimal airway irritation. Ketamine, despite its bronchodilating properties, is less desirable as it tends to increase bronchial secretions and may promote laryngospasm. Intubation should be performed at a deep plane of anesthesia to avoid coughing, breath holding, and bronchospasm. Cuffed ETTs offer the advantage over uncuffed tubes for permitting higher ventilation pressure, if required. Humidification of inspired gases is important to reduce desiccation and inspissation of already thick secretions. One should be prepared to suction thick secretions from the ETT, which can become plugged or narrowed by mucus. Intravenous fentanyl and the application of lidocaine spray to the upper airway may smooth the intubation process. Nasal polyps causing nasal obstruction may complicate mask ventilation and present a relative contraindication to nasotracheal intubation. Muscle relaxation is preferred in CF patients with severe respiratory involvement; note that concurrent use of aminoglycoside antibiotics (gentamicin) may prolong the duration of action of a nondepolarizing muscle relaxant. Short-acting muscle relaxants are preferred so that recovery of strength is not delayed postoperatively. Stress-dose steroids and parenteral vitamin K can be administered if indicated (Fitzgerald & Ryan, 2011).

Maintenance of general anesthesia: Inhalation agents, particularly sevoflurane, are advantageous in producing bronchodilation with minimal airway irritation. Most anesthesiologists will avoid desflurane in CF patients secondary to the increased risk of airway reactivity. Isoflurane is typically avoided due to the high solubility hence increased time to achieve a MAC and risk of prolonged emergence. **Even though some anesthesiologists have safely used nitrous oxide, it should be used cautiously because of the potential risk of sudden rupture of emphysematous bullae, resulting in pneumothorax.** If patient's FEV_1 is less than 40% or the patient is having an acute exacerbation, a total intravenous technique may be beneficial for maintenance and emergence. A total intravenous anesthetic will not rely on minute ventilation, airway resistance, and so on for elimination. To reduce the risk of pneumothorax, adequate ventilation should be achieved with minimal peak ventilatory pressures. Adequate intravenous hydration and humidified and warmed inspired gases are important in preventing intraoperative inspissation of secretions. Frequent suctioning through the ETT or by bronchoscopy reduces the risk of mucous plugging and helps to maintain adequate oxygenation and ventilation. Although the laryngeal mask airway

(LMA) is an option for short cases, disadvantages include the inability to suction, obstruction of the LMA by thick secretions, and the risk of laryngospasm and aspiration. Attention to maintaining euthermia is important since CF patients have less subcutaneous fat and tend to develop hypothermia during and after surgery (Fitzgerald & Ryan, 2011). Blood sugar should be monitored in patients with diabetes. Lastly, due to sweat chloride losses, patients can dehydrate easily. Careful attention must be paid to the patient's volume status, starting preoperatively. Patient's pulmonary secretions are vicious and difficult to clear at baseline and considerably worsen with exposure to dry gases during anesthesia. It is important to deliver humidified gases to the patients to optimize pulmonary clearance intra- and postoperatively (Hedley & Allt-Graham, 1994; Shelly et al., 1988).

Extubation: Avoidance of prolonged intubation and mechanical ventilation reduces the risk of postoperative pulmonary infection. The ETT should be thoroughly suctioned and lung recruitment maneuvers should be performed prior to extubation. Complete reversal of neuromuscular blockade should be confirmed, and the patient should be extubated fully awake, meeting standard extubation criteria.

5. What postanesthetic interventions facilitate patient recovery?

Postanesthetic care must be directed toward continued *aggressive respiratory therapy, oxygen supplementation,* and *clearance of respiratory secretions.* Good pain management is important in reducing the effect of splinting on pulmonary function and sputum clearance. Patient-controlled analgesia may be particularly useful to allow patients to time administration of analgesia along with their need to cough. Either opioid- or regional anesthesia-based techniques can be used. Care must be used when considering nonsteroidal anti-inflammatory drugs in patients with a history of hemoptysis. Opioids must be administered very carefully and titrated to effect to minimize respiratory depression. The effect of opiates on bowel motility should also be monitored. **Chest physiotherapy** should be included in the perioperative care of the CF patient. Treatment with bronchodilators and prolonged oxygen supplementation are expected in the recovery room for many postoperative CF patients (Liou et al., 2010). Patients should be restarted on their maintenance pulmonary regimen as soon as possible. Admission to the hospital for overnight observation or even an intensive care unit stay may be required, depending on baseline pulmonary status and perioperative changes.

SUMMARY

1. CF manifests from birth with a number of medical problems that require surgery or complicate anesthesia. Optimal preoperative preparation of the patient is important and differs at varying stages of the disease.
2. Be aware of CF patient's baseline and most recent PFTs; assess a detailed history of compliance, exercise tolerance, and sputum production.
3. Adequate depth of anesthesia for intubation is important to reduce coughing, bronchospasm, and desaturation. Volatile agents promote bronchodilation and frequent suctioning is helpful in removing copious thick secretions.
4. CF patients with severely diminished function or during exacerbation may be more easily maintained with total intravenous anesthesia versus a volatile agent.
5. Postoperative care emphasizes chest physiotherapy and pain control to optimize pulmonary function.

BIBLIOGRAPHY

Baum VC, O'Flaherty JE. Cystic fibrosis. In: *Anesthesia for Genetic, Metabolic, and Dysmorphic Syndromes of Childhood.* 2nd ed. Philadelphia: Lippincott Williams and Wilkins; 2007:94–96.

Boucher R, Knowles M, Yankaskas J. Cystic fibrosis. In: Mason R, Broaddus VC, Martin T, King T, Schraufnagel D, Murray J, Nadel J, eds. *Murray and Nadel's Textbook of Respiratory Medicine.* 5th ed. Philadelphia: Saunders; 2010.

Cowl CT, Prakash UB, Kruger BR. The role of anticholinergics in bronchoscopy: a randomized clinical trial. *Chest.* 2000;118:188–192.

Davis PB. Cystic fibrosis since 1938. *Am J Respir Crit Care Med.* 2006;173:475–482.

Della Rocca G. Anaesthesia in patients with cystic fibrosis. *Curr Opin Anaesthesiol.* 2002;15:95–101.

Elkins MR, Robinson M, Rose BR, et al. A controlled trial of long-term inhaled hypertonic saline in patients with cystic fibrosis. *N Engl J Med.* 2006;354:229–240.

Farrell PM, Rosenstein BJ, White TB, et al. Guidelines for diagnosis of cystic fibrosis in newborns through older adults: Cystic Fibrosis Foundation consensus report. *J Pediatr*. 2008;153(2):S4–S14.

Firth P, Kinane, T Bernard. Essentials of pulmonology. In: Coté C, Lerman J, Anderson BJ, eds. *Coté and Lerman's A Practice of Anesthesia for Infants and Children*. Philadelphia: Saunders; 2013:233–235.

Fitzgerald M, Ryan D. Cystic fibrosis and anaesthesia. Continuing Education in Anaesthesia. *Crit Care Pain*. 2011;11(6):204–209.

Hedley RM, Allt-Graham J. Heat and moisture exchangers and breathing filters. *Br J Anaesth*. 1994;73:227–236.

Huffmyer JL, Littlewood KE, Nemergut EC. Perioperative management of the adult with cystic fibrosis. *Anesth Analg*. 2009;109(6):1949–1961.

Karlet M. An update on cystic fibrosis and implications for anesthesia. *AANA J*. 2000;68:141–146.

Liou T, Elkin E, Pasta D, et al. Year-to-year changes in lung function in individuals with cystic fibrosis. *J Cystic Fibrosis*. 2010;9(4):250–256.

Randell SH, Boucher RC. Effective mucus clearance is essential for respiratory health. *Am J Respir Cell Mol Biol*. 2006;35:20–28.

Sanchez I, Holbrow J, Chernick V. Acute bronchodilator response to a combination of beta-adrenergic and anticholinergic agents in patients with cystic fibrosis. *J Pediatr*. 1992;120:486–488.

Shelly MP, Lloyd GM, Park GR: A review of the mechanisms and methods of humidification of inspired gases. *Intensive Care Med*. 1988;14:1–9.

19

Anesthetic Implications for Surgical Correction of Pectus Excavatum

CHRIS D. GLOVER AND WALLIS T. MUHLY

INTRODUCTION

Pectus excavatum is the most common congenital chest wall deformity in children and it is characterized by a posterior depression of the sternum (Fig. 19.1). This deformity is usually well tolerated in younger children but with increasing skeletal rigidity and aerobic activity, older children with this deformity can experience dyspnea, decreased exercise tolerance, and shortness of breath reflecting a restrictive pulmonary insufficiency. Cardiac manifestations can include mitral valve prolapse and cardiac compression. In addition to physical limitations, patients can also experience depression and/or anxiety secondary to body image concerns.

Surgical repair has been correlated with enhanced quality of life and improvement in body image with recent studies indicating improved pulmonary function and cardiac output as well as decreased strain on both the left and right ventricles. Early surgical approaches to this deformity involved an open surgical repair with rib cartilage resection and sternal osteotomy which was refined and popularized by Ravitch. The Ravitch procedure was the primary surgical approach for 40 years until Nuss and colleagues introduced a minimally invasive approach that did not involve rib resection. The minimally invasive repair of pectus excavatum (MIRPE) or Nuss procedure involves placing a convex bar through small lateral chest wall incisions aided by thoracoscopy under the sternum in order to produce anterior displacement of the chest wall without rib cartilage resection (Nuss et al., 2008). MIRPE has become the most common procedure used to correct pectus excavatum.

Complications from MIRPE can occur in anywhere from 7% to 25% of patients and can occur for as long as the bar is in place. Pain control remains a major issue in the perioperative period as patients may require weeks to months of oral opioids before becoming pain-free after surgical correction. After a period of 2 to 4 years, the bar or bars are usually removed.

LEARNING OBJECTIVES

- Understand the preoperative issues that need to be addressed prior to undergoing pectus repair.
- Develop a comprehensive understanding of the potential intraoperative complications that can occur with MIRPE.
- Discuss available options for pain control and formulate a strategy of multimodal analgesia for managing patients undergoing MIRPE.

CASE PRESENTATION

A 15-year-old male with severe pectus excavatum deformity, reactive airway disease, and anxiety presents for repair via the Nuss procedure. While he has always had the defect, it was only over the last 2 years that the patient began to develop cardiorespiratory symptoms. The patient reports shortness of breath during physical exertion, and he is having trouble participating in athletic activities. His history is otherwise significant for intermittent albuterol use. He has a computed tomography (CT) scan, which shows a Haller index of 4.3.

After oral versed administration in the perioperative area, the patient has a 20G intravenous line placed. In the operating room, standard American Society of Anesthesiologists monitors are applied and general anesthesia is induced with

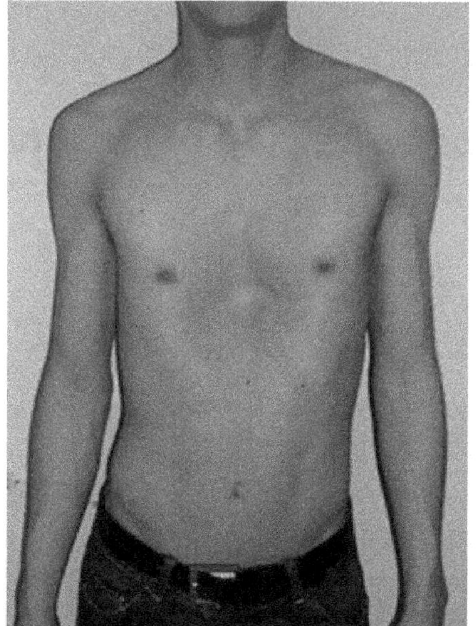
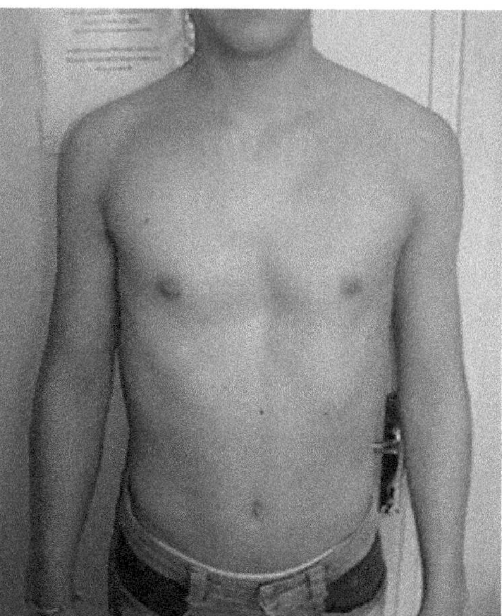

FIGURE 19.1: Pectus excavatum before and after surgical correction.

propofol, fentanyl, and vecuronium. After securing the airway with an endotracheal tube, the surgeon positions the patient in the left lateral decubitus position for placement of a thoracic epidural. The epidural is placed in the T6-T7 interspace, and position is confirmed following epidural injection of contrast with fluoroscopic visualization. The patient is returned to the supine position with arms extended to allow for lateral access to the thorax. The surgeon proceeds to make lateral chest wall incisions and a convex stainless steel bar is passed under the sternum using thoracoscopic visualization. The bar is then flipped and secured with stabilizers to anchor the bar to the chest wall. Prior to surgical closure, the surgeon requests application of continuous positive pressure up to 30 mmHg to decompress the air in the chest cavity and to minimize the presence of a residual pneumothorax. The patient is then extubated and transported to recovery where he complains of significant pressure in his chest. The pain service is paged to the bedside for implementation of a perioperative pain strategy.

DISCUSSION

1. What are the indications for surgical correction of pectus excavatum? Is there an optimal time for repair?

Surgical repair is indicated when patients present with severe pectus excavatum and associated physical impairment. Severe pectus is generally defined as a Haller index greater than 3.1. Physical impairment is primarily related to pulmonary limitations with patients often reporting dyspnea on exertion or reduced aerobic capacity. Cardiac compression, mitral valve prolapse, and conduction abnormalities can also be indications for surgical intervention. MIRPE may be technically easier and associated with less pain if performed prior to puberty as the chest wall is more malleable. However, pulmonary symptoms often do not present until after skeletal maturity, so patients often seek care later in adolescence.

2. How do you calculate a Haller index? Is the index in this patient severe?

The Haller index is calculated by dividing the transverse dimension of the chest by the anterior-posterior distance between the sternum and the vertebral body. In Figure 19.2, the Haller index is calculated by dividing 268.8 mm by 62.1 mm, which equals 4.33. As noted previously, a Haller index greater than 3.1 is considered severe with surgical correction indicated in the presence of associated physical symptoms. For reference, a normal Haller index is approximately 2.5.

3. What preoperative concerns do you have for this patient?

Preoperative evaluation should focus on an assessment of the patient's cardiopulmonary function.

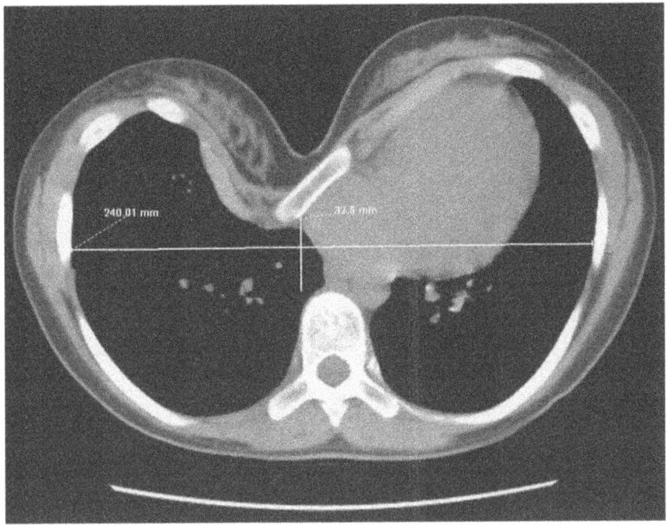

FIGURE 19.2: Example CT scan for patient with pectus excavatum.

Preoperative history should focus on presenting symptoms such as dyspnea on exertion, decreased exercise tolerance, and palpitations as well as identifying any other comorbidities. There is an association with pectus excavatum and some connective tissue disorders including Marfan's syndrome and Ehlers-Danlos syndrome. If a connective disease is suspected or present in the patient, further cardiac evaluation may be indicated. However, it should be noted that most patients with pectus excavatum deformity are relatively healthy.

Preoperative testing should include CT to enable calculation of the patient's Haller index and assessment of chest wall asymmetry and cardiac compression. Depending on the severity of the deformity and the presence of associated medical problems, preoperative evaluation with an electrocardiogram, echocardiogram, and pulmonary function testing may be indicated.

While preoperative lab testing is not indicated in otherwise healthy patients, obtaining a type and screen may be worthwhile as there is a potential for catastrophic blood loss in the event of cardiac perforation with bar placement. Additionally, there have been reports of metal allergy (nickel or chromium) complicating recovery following MIRPE with stainless steel bar placement. Thus some surgeons proceed with metal allergy testing prior to surgery. If patients test positive, a titanium bar may be indicated.

Postoperative pain can be significant following MIRPE. Thus pain control methods should be discussed at length during the preoperative period in an effort to better communicate the perioperative expectation and inform the patient and the family about the pain management plans for the recovery period. In institutions with an acute pain service, this patient population may benefit from a pain service consult to aid in the assessment and management postoperative pain.

4. What complications may occur with MIRPE?

While MIRPE is a minimally invasive approach, it can be associated with serious complications. First, careful attention must be paid to patient positioning. Patients are positioned in the supine position with the arms abducted to 90 degrees. This potentially places the patient at risk for developing brachial plexus injury. Brachial plexus pressure can be relieved with padding under the elbow and hand to reduce shoulder tension (Fig. 19.3).

The procedure can result in pneumothorax via insufflation of the thoracic cavity and injury to the heart or other mediastinal structures as the pectus bar traverses across the thorax. The introduction of thoracoscopic guidance has improved the technique as it allows for careful evaluation of the retrosternal space prior to passage of the bar. However, cases of cardiac injury and death from massive hemorrhage, while rare, have been reported. Thus extreme vigilance on the part of the anesthesiology team is required. An arterial line is generally not indicated but

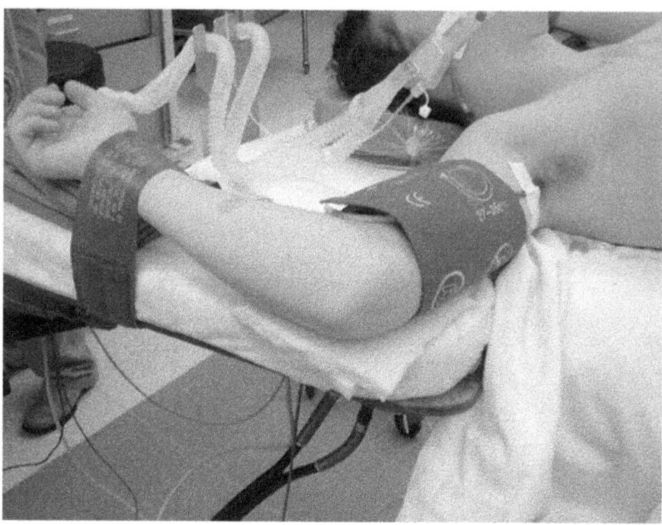

FIGURE 19.3: Arm positioning for minimally invasive repair of pectus excavatum.

adequate intravenous access is, in the event that resuscitation is required. Other complications include bar dislodgement or rotation, skin infection or reaction to the bar, and arrhythmias.

While pneumothorax following thoracoscopy is common, most centers now try to mitigate this via a small tube in the thorax as positive pressure and positive end-expiratory pressure is applied though ventilation. The majority of pneumothoraces in the perioperative period resolve spontaneously. Most surgeons will obtain a chest x-ray during the recovery period to ensure that any pneumothorax is resolved prior to discharge.

Finally, smooth emergence from anesthesia is important to ensure that the patient does not cough on the endotracheal tube, which can lead to worsening of pneumothorax or even bar displacement. Careful consideration should be given to proceeding with a deep extubation or use of adjuvants like dexmedetomidine or propofol, which facilitate smooth emergence from anesthesia.

5. What options are available for pain control in this patient?

Despite being minimally invasive, MIRPE is associated with considerable postoperative pain, which can last for weeks after surgery. The mechanism of the pain response is complex and involves inflammatory pain from the costal incisions as well as neuropathic pain from the stretching of intercostal nerves during correction. In addition, the acute change in the architecture of the thoracic cavity likely results in muscle stretch and postoperative spasmodic pain. As a result, strategies for managing pain are quite variable, and a consensus on the optimal strategy for pain control remains elusive. Thoracic epidurals, intravenous opioids via patient-controlled analgesia, and regional blockade such as paravertebral and intercostal catheters have all been used with success by case report. It is, however, becoming increasingly clear that a comprehensive multimodal treatment strategy is needed for this surgical population (Table 19.1).

Incorporation of regional anesthesia via epidural placement or through the use of paravertebral or intercostal catheters should be offered for every patient undergoing MIRPE. Epidural analgesia has proven to be effective for thoracic procedures. Local anesthetics combined with opioids block spinal nociceptive pathways with epidural administration, providing pain relief while reducing the dose-related adverse effects of both classes of drugs. This offering is not without its detractors as a recent analysis reported two instances of lower extremity paralysis following epidural placement. Some institutions have transitioned from offering epidurals to placement of paravertebral catheters given their equal efficacy when compared to epidurals.

Intravenous patient-controlled analgesia can be used to supplement the regional anesthesia modalities discussed or be used as the primary adjunct for pain control following MIRPE. A basal

TABLE 19.1. POSTOPERATIVE ANALGESIA PROTOCOL FOR PECTUS EXCAVATUM REPAIR

Education

Pain is significant despite "minimally invasive" approach.

The chest will feel tight and breathing will feel different from preoperatively. Patients need to know this is normal.

Transition from epidural to oral regimen may be challenging.

Epidural/PCA

Epidural:

- T5–T6 entry
- Optimal mixture of local anesthetic and opioid is unclear; consider a hydrophilic opioid as multiple dermatomes are involved

PCA:

- Consider basal infusion.
- Opioid choice as per local preference

Intravenous Regimen

Methocarbamol scheduled, for continuous relief of spasmodic pain

Ketorolac scheduled, for general musculoskeletal pain

Diazepam: for acute muscle spasm

Oral Regimen

Start prior to discontinuing the epidural to smooth the transition:

- Ibuprofen
- Methocarbamol scheduled
- Diazepam as needed for muscle spasm
- Oxycodone: scheduled long-acting form with immediate release as needed for breakthrough pain

Duration of Treatment

Epidural/PCA regimen:

- Run until POD 3 for single bar
- Run until POD 3–4 for double bar
- Older patients may need longer

PO regimen:

- Up to 2–4 weeks
- Older patients may need longer

Note: PCA = patient-controlled analgesia; POD = postoperative day; PO = oral.

infusion is warranted with weaning performed as oral intake improves. This modality is not without its own set of issues centered on opioid-related adverse drug events.

Adjuncts such as benzodiazepines, nonsteroidal anti-inflammatory drugs, and GABA analogues all play a role in improving pain control post-MIRPE. Benzodiazepines are commonly used for a wide range of conditions and are known to have sedative, hypnotic, anticonvulsant, muscle relaxant, and amnesic properties, making them useful in treating anxiety and muscle spasm. Clinical research supports a correlation between psychological factors like anxiety and pain. In this context, anxiolytic drugs may have a beneficial role by giving the patient a reduced sensation of pain in the postoperative period. Adjuncts for muscle spasms such as diazepam should be scheduled as needed.

The anti-inflammatory agents via their inhibition of cyclooxygenase 1 and 2 decrease the formation of prostaglandin precursors, which play a role in the inflammatory cascade. Agents such as ketorolac should be scheduled, but optimal timing is not known. Some centers use this agent in a limited fashion in conjunction with the transition to oral medications while others use this through recovery. The benefits of using these agents should be weighed against their potential for causing gastric ulceration.

Gabapentin is thought to mitigate propagation of neuropathic pain through action on voltage-dependent calcium channels in the dorsal horn, limiting calcium influx during nociception. Gabapentin should be discussed as an adjunct given the potential for long-term pain issues following MIRPE.

The transition to oral medications for discharge usually occurs within the first 5 days. This has been noted to be particularly stressful and difficult time for patients. Oral medications such as oxycodone or hydrocodone combined with ibuprofen should facilitate pain control following discharge. Medications for breakthrough, such as morphine or hydromorphone, should readily be available and accessible for families during this time. Oftentimes patients also need to continue their antispasmodics through recovery, and this should be included for every patient. Following the previously outlined process should allow for a smoother recovery for patients undergoing MIRPE.

In conclusion, while the procedure to correct pectus deformity is now largely minimally invasive, anesthesiologists must be cognizant of the inherent risks associated with this technique. Outside of the intraoperative concerns discussed, postoperative pain and developing a strategy that is multimodal in nature ensures the best pathway for patients undergoing MIRPE.

SUMMARY

- While the Nuss procedure is considered minimally invasive, pain can be severe.
- Cardiac and respiratory dysfunction has been associated with severe pectus excavatum as evidenced by cardiac magnetic resonance imaging and pulmonary function testing.
- Postoperative pain management for pectus repair remains challenging, and multimodal analgesia should be incorporated for all patients undergoing repair.

ANNOTATED REFERENCES

Nuss D, Kelly R, Croitoru D, Katz M. A 10-year review of a minimally invasive technique for the correction of pectus excavatum. *J Pediatr Surg.* 1998;33(4):545–552.

This landmark article assessed the results of a minimally invasive repair for pectus over a 10-year period, which ushered the transition from the open Ravitch procedure to the Nuss procedure.

Stroud AM, Tulanont DD, Coates TE, Goodney PP, Croitoru DP. Epidural analgesia versus intravenous patient-controlled analgesia following minimally invasive pectus excavatum repair: a systematic review and meta-analysis. *J Pediatr Surg.* 2014;49(5):798–806.

This meta-analysis searched for randomized controlled trials comparing epidurals to patient-controlled analgesia for postoperative pain management following Nuss bar placement from 1946 to 2012. Six total studies met inclusion criteria, and they noted pain scores were lower with an epidural in the time periods immediately following surgery and through time points of 12, 24, and 48 hours. No differences were noted in secondary outcomes between the two methods of pain control.

FURTHER READING

Butkovic D, S, Matolic M, Kralik M, Toljan S, Radesic L. Postoperative analgesia with intravenous fentanyl PCA vs epidural block after thoracoscopic pectus excavatum repair in children. *Br J Anaesth.* 2007;98(5):677–681.

Densmore JC, Peterson DB, Stahovic LL, Czamecki ML, Hainsworth KR, Davies HW, et al. Initial surgical and pain management outcomes after Nuss procedure. *J Pediatr Surg.* 2010;45(9):1767–1771.

Kelly RE Jr, Lawson ML, Paidas CN, Hruban RH. Pectus excavatum in a 112-year autopsy series: anatomic findings and the effect on survival. *J Pediatr Surg.* 2005;40(8):1275–1278.

Kelly RE Jr, Shamberger RC, Mellins RB, Mitchell KK, Lawson ML, Oldham K, et al. Prospective multicenter study of surgical correction of pectus excavatum: design, perioperative complications, pain, and baseline pulmonary function facilitated by Internet-based data collection. *J Am Coll Surg.* 2007;205(2):205–216.

Kelly RE, Goretsky MJ, Obermeyer R, et al. Twenty-one years of experience with minimally invasive repair of pectus excavatum by the Nuss procedure in 1215 patients. *Annals Surg.* 2010;252(6):1072–1081.

Krasopoulos G, Dusmet M, Ladas G, Goldstraw P. Nuss procedure improves the quality of life in young male adults with pectus excavatum deformity. *Eur J Cardiothorac Surg.* 2006;29(1):1–5.

Malek MH, Berger DE, Housh TJ, Marelich WD, Coburn JW, Beck TW, et al. Cardiovascular function following surgical repair of pectus excavatum: a metaanalysis. *Chest.* 2006;130(2):506–516.

Nuss D, Kelly RE Jr. Minimally invasive surgical correction of chest wall deformities in children (Nuss procedure). *Adv Pediatr*. 2008;55:395–410.

Nuss D, Kelly RE Jr. Indications and technique of Nuss procedure for pectus excavatum. *Thorac Surg Clin*. 2010;20(4):583–597.

Ravitch MM. The operative treatment of pectus excavatum. *J Pediatr*. 1956;48(4):465–472.

St. Peter SD, Weesner KA, Weissend EE, et al. Epidural vs patient-controlled analgesia for postoperative pain after pectus excavatum repair: a prospective, randomized trial. *J Pediatr Surg*. 2012;47(1):148–153.

Weber T, Mätzl J, Rokitansky A, et al. Superior postoperative pain relief with thoracic epidural analgesia versus intravenous patient-controlled analgesia after minimally invasive pectus excavatum repair. *J Thorac Cardiovasc Surg*. 2007;134(4):865–870.

PART 5

Challenges in Blood and Fluid Management

20

Massive Transfusion in a Child

RACHEL CHAPMAN AND STEFANO SABATO

INTRODUCTION

The traditional early management of hemorrhagic shock is currently being challenged, and many centers around the world have already changed their practice. Damage-control resuscitation, in conjunction with damage-control surgery, has been shown to improve major morbidity and mortality outcomes in adults. In children there is little direct evidence for these new approaches, but supporting evidence is accumulating. This chapter introduces these concepts while also reinforcing the core principles of managing acute hemorrhage in the trauma setting.

LEARNING OBJECTIVES

1. Appreciate the principles of preparation for and early assessment and management of a major pediatric trauma involving major hemorrhage.
2. Understand the concepts of damage-control resuscitation and damage-control surgery.
3. Know how to avoid the complications of a massive transfusion.
4. Understand the basics of acute trauma coagulopathy.

CASE PRESENTATION

*The **trauma team** arrives to the emergency bay to receive a 4-year-old who has been in a motor vehicle accident. The paramedics have failed to obtain intravenous (IV) access. The initial assessment reveals hypovolemic shock due to intra-abdominal hemorrhage. An 18-gauge IV cannula is sited in the right antecubital fossa, blood is sent to the laboratory and for point of care testing with thromboelastography (TEG). An O-negative packed red blood cell (PRBC) transfusion commences, and tranexemic acid (TXA) is loaded at 15 mg/kg over 10 minutes, with a subsequent ongoing infusion of 2 mg/kg/hr. The hospital's **massive transfusion protocol** (MTP) is activated, and a focused secondary survey and trauma series of radiographs are performed. The abdomen continues to become more distended, the patient remains hypotensive, and transfusion continues with a unit of thawed fresh frozen plasma (FFP). Fibrinogen deficiency is demonstrated on the TEG and 5ml/kg cryoprecipitate is administered. The hemodynamic aim is for a palpable pulse, improved conscious state, and **systolic blood pressure within the lower limit of the normal range**. The decision is made to take the child to the operating room (OR) without further investigation and transfusion of a unit of platelets commences en route (Table 20.1).*

In preparation, the OR has been warmed to 24°C, a rapid infuser has been primed, and the cell salvage machine is available. Blood products have been placed in the OR refrigerator as per the MTP. An arterial line is inserted, but it is difficult to obtain further large-bore venous access. After induction with manual in-line stabilization of the cervical spine, the surgeon performs a cutdown to gain large-bore venous access in the left antecubital fossa.

*While preparing for surgery, ventilation becomes more difficult due to increasing abdominal distention. The surgeon incises the abdomen and blood immediately pours from the wound. Worsening hypotension ensues. The child is transfused with sequential units of PRBCs/salvaged blood, FFP, and platelets. The surgeon identifies a laceration in the inferior vena cava and clamps the vessel to control the hemorrhage. Further exploration reveals a lacerated liver and perforated transverse colon. The surgeon then places **packs** in the abdominal cavity to allow the patient to be stabilized.*

TABLE 20.1. PATIENT'S APPEARANCE IN THE EMERGENCY DEPARTMENT

Primary and Secondary Survey
Patent airway and spontaneous respiration
Heart rate 190
Blood pressure 50/-
Child's Glasgow Coma Scale score 10
Distended abdomen
Evidence of abrasion to right upper quadrant
No external bleeding
No apparent head injury
No other obvious evidence of trauma

The initial coagulation tests taken earlier demonstrate that the patient was ***coagulopathic upon arrival*** *to the hospital. Approximately 2 blood volumes have been transfused prior to clamping, and further transfusion continues to be is now guided by laboratory assessment and* ***TEG****; 0.5 mL/kg calcium gluconate is given to* ***correct hypocalcemia,*** *and a further 5 mL/kg cryoprecipitate is transfused to treat* ***hypofibrinogenemia****. To avoid* ***hypothermia*** *and* ***acidosis,*** *the patient is actively warmed, and sodium bicarbonate is slowly titrated to achieve a pH of >7.2. Ongoing microvascular bleeding is observed despite normalization of temperature and the TEG; therefore, 100 IU/kg of activated* ***recombinant factor VIIa*** *(rFVIIa) is administered. The surgery is completed with a defunctioning colostomy, placing packs around the lacerated liver and in the abdominal cavity, and forming a temporary laparostomy.*

DISCUSSION

1. What are the key aspects of the assessment and management of a major pediatric trauma where major hemorrhage is suspected or possible?

Advance notice prior to a major trauma patient arriving in the hospital is crucial. This allows mobilization of the trauma team and time to ensure that the appropriate locations, such as the computed tomography (CT) scanner and an OR, are vacant. The **trauma team** consists of the emergency physician, general/trauma surgeon, anesthesiologist, intensivist, nursing staff, radiographers, and support staff. It is important that the role of the team leader and each individual is clearly defined. The anesthesiologist warms the OR, calculates the estimated body weight and blood volume of the patient, and prepares the correct drugs, rapid infusion device, and cell saver. Continued communication with the paramedics also facilitates preparation.

Most trauma patients will not require a massive transfusion, and existing advanced trauma life support guidelines of crystalloid transfusion followed by PRBCs will suffice. However, in major trauma, if death from hemorrhage does occur, it is usually within 6 hours of the injury. Therefore it is important to identify which patients are likely to require massive transfusion early and in these cases facilitate the delivery of blood products. A narrow pulse pressure may be the most sensitive sign of hypovolaemia in children, and up to 40% blood volume may be lost before hypotension ensues. Unlike the adult population, there is currently no commonly utilized scoring system in pediatrics to trigger activation of a MTP protocol, with most institutions relying on either estimation of total blood loss, transfusion requirements, or evidence of severe biochemical derangement. Coagulopathy on arrival (international normalized ratio [INR] >1.5) is associated with an increased risk of mortality in children independent of their injury severity (Patregnani et al., 2012).

Institution of a **MTP** in pediatric trauma has been shown to reduce time to transfusion, although clear evidence of a reduction in morbidity and mortality is currently lacking (Blain & Paterson, 2016). A MTP allows the treating team to focus on the patient's physiology instead of ordering blood products based on laboratory values that may no longer be relevant by the time the result is available (Dressler et al., 2010). The MTP streamlines communication with the blood bank, expedites the delivery of blood products, and engages the support of a hematologist. Inadequate communication between treating physicians and the blood bank is a consistent cause of transfusion-related adverse outcomes (Stainsby et al., 2008).

In this case, the initial assessment revealed hemodynamic instability from intra-abdominal bleeding. Therefore, supradiaphragmatic IV access was obtained. The decision on whether to CT scan the child will depend on the stability of the patient and the location of the scanner. If the CT is within the emergency room, then the scan may be performed efficiently while resuscitation continues. In this scenario the child went straight to the OR due to ongoing instability. The focused abdominal ultrasound scan is limited in children: intra-abdominal free fluid does not mandate laparotomy, nor does the absence of free fluid rule out significant intra-abdominal bleeding. As a rule, the decision to operate is based on hemodynamics rather than imaging.

2. What are the components of damage-control resuscitation?

Damage-control resuscitation includes rapid control of surgical bleeding, avoidance of the complications of massive transfusion (hemodulition, acidosis, hypothermia, and hypocalcemia), and hemostatic resuscitation (Spinella & Holcomb, 2009). Hemostatic resuscitation is aggressive *volume resuscitation with a physiological balance of PRBC, FFP, platelets, coagulation factors, and antifibrinolytics,* and is associated with a 2.5-fold increase in 30-day survival (Stephens et al., 2016). The aim is to deliver "reconstituted whole blood" in a simple manner that is easy in a crisis. Utilization of a fixed ratio of blood products is the standard approach of most MTPs. More recently, several European trauma centers have introduced goal directed therapy algorithms based on vesicoelastic testing (VET) results such as TEG/rotational thromboelastometry (ROTEM; Schochl et al., 2016); however, this approach depends on the availability and training in the use of VET, which may not be possible or practical. A ratio of PRBC:FFP:platelets of 1:1:1 has been mathematically modeled to have a hematocrit of 29%, coagulation factor activity of 65%, and platelet count of 90,000 μl (Armand & Hess, 2003). This combination avoids exacerbating coagulopathy with excessive crystalloid and PRBC transfusions and helps address consumptive coagulopathy.

Subsequent transfusion should be guided by the hematocrit, coagulation profile, platelet count, **VET if available,** and the clinical scenario. Laboratory-based coagulation assessment with prothrombin and activated partial thromboplastin may take up to 40 minutes to provide a result and thus is not always helpful in guiding transfusion practice in the actively bleeding patient. The limited evidence concerning the use of VET in adult massive transfusion is encouraging (primarily in liver, cardiac, and trauma surgery) and supports its use to reduce transfusion requirements and overall mortality compared to conventional testing (Stephens et al., 2016; Wikkelsø et al., 2016). Within 5 minutes, VET provides rapid assessment of coagulation, fibrinolysis, and platelet function at the patient's current temperature. In addition to providing "real-time" assessment of hemostasis, VET can also predict potentially large blood loss (Hsu et al., 2016).

Timely deactivation of the MTP is important to limit resource wastage and overtransfusion (Hsu et al., 2016). After hemostasis is achieved, the aim is to minimize total transfusion volume and number of donor exposures. Data from the United Kingdom has shown that children have higher rates of adverse outcomes from transfusion than adults, and infants have almost triple the adult rate (Stainsby et al., 2008). Complications relate to both the volume administered and the number of units to which the child is exposed. Evidence for the theoretical benefits of "young" versus "old" blood in massive transfusion is conflicting and further research is required; however, transfusing the most recently donated products seems prudent (Pham & Shaz, 2013).

It is important to avoid the "lethal triad" of **hypothermia, acidosis**, and **coagulopathy**. This triad results in further bleeding and hence transfusion, which in turn worsens the hypothermia, acidosis, and coagulopathy, resulting in a "vicious cycle" that may eventually lead to death from hyperkalemia- and hypocalcaemia-induced cardiac arrhythmia. Acidosis prolongs clotting time by impairing enzyme activity and depleting fibrinogen levels and platelet counts (Fries & Martini, 2010). It is more important to fix the cause of the acidosis (i.e., hypoperfusion) rather than treating the acidosis itself (Ganter & Pittet, 2010), but if acidosis becomes severe (<7.2), consider administering bicarbonate or tromethamine (Rossaint et al., 2010). Hypothermia affects coagulation protease function below 33°C and worsens coagulopathy, especially in acidosis (Ganter & Pittet, 2010). Hypothermia below 34°C is associated with increased mortality in trauma patients (Fries & Martini, 2010).

Some authors also include permissive hypotension as part of damage control; however, this has been demonstrated to improve morbidity and mortality outcomes only in penetrating torso trauma in adults. Some guidelines recommend moderate hypotension in adult trauma in the absence of central nervous system injury. Given the lack of evidence in children, and as children are able to maintain normotension with moderate hypovolemia, normotension should be the goal of resuscitation (Blain & Paterson, 2016).

3. What does a 1:1:1 transfusion ratio mean in pediatrics?

Evidence for the optimal ratio of PRBC:platelets:FFP in adult trauma and nontrauma resuscitation supports a "high" ratio of 1:1:1. The PROPPR trial, comparing PRBC:platelets:FFP 1:1:1 to 2:1:1, demonstrated more hemostasis and decreased death due to exsanguination in the first 24 hours in the 1:1:1 group, with no increased incidence of transfusion related complications (i.e., less blood products used overall with an initial aggressive resuscitation approach). However, there was no significant difference between mortality at 24 hours and 30 days (Holcombe et al., 2015). At present there is no evidence that a 1:1:1 ratio reduces morbidity and mortality in the pediatric population. Practical difficulties in rapidly obtaining FFP likely also contribute to individual pediatric MTPs variably recommending ratios of 1:1:1 or 2:1:1 for PRBC:platelets:FFP (Blain & Paterson, 2016; Duchesne et al., 2008; Holcomb et al., 2008; Rossaint et al., 2010).

When considering the use of "reconstituted whole blood" transfusion in children, it is important to be aware that the literature describes a ratio of 1 adult unit of PRBCs to 1 adult unit of FFP to 1 buffy coat-derived single-random-donor platelet unit. In the setting of massive transfusion, it is easier to keep track of what should be given if the team thinks in terms of the number of units transfused rather than volume or mL/kg., as the mass of blood product in each unit should be relatively consistent. Doctors should be aware of the different units of bloods products available. Some centers offer both adult and neonatal sized units of PRBCs and FFP, and some blood banks pool platelets into a single bag of 5 units (~300 mL) from 3 or 4 donors to reduce the total donor exposure to the recipient. Also, platelets may be collected from the buffy coat of spun donated whole blood or obtained by apheresis. One unit of apheresis-derived platelets (~180 mL) is equivalent to a pooled bag of buffy coat-derived platelets.

Plasma, traditionally administered as (unmatched) universal group AB FFP initially in massive transfusion, may also be administered from readily available thawed plasma (derived from FFP), which has a further 5 days shelf life (but less factor V and factor VIII). Lyophilized plasma, available in Germany and currently undergoing clinical trials elsewhere, is a promising future alternative, with a shelf life at room temperature of 15 months and lower risk of transfusion-related acute lung injury (TRALI) than FFP (Hsu et al, 2016).

4. What are the adjuncts to reconstituted whole blood?

CRASH-2 (CRASH-2 Trial Collaborators, 2010), a large multicenter prospective randomized controlled trial, demonstrated a small improvement in the rate of survival with the use of **tranexamic acid** (TXA) in adult trauma with significant hemorrhage. The improved survival was seen without an increase in thrombotic complications. In pediatric trauma, most protocols recommend a TXA load be administered within 3 hours of injury, and ideally within the first hour, and an infusion continued for 8 hours postinjury or until bleeding ceases (Blain & Paterson, 2016). Importantly, a profibrinolytic state may exist even with a normal TEG, so TXA should be given on a clinical basis (Schochl et al, 2016). In the case presentation, TXA was commenced as part of damage-control resuscitation, as soon as IV access was obtained.

During resuscitation, **fibrinogen** levels may fall as a result of dilution, hypothermia, and acidosis (Fries & Martini, 2010). It is increasingly recognized that fibrinogen deficiency in hemorrhage occurs early in particular patient groups, including pediatric trauma and burns. Neonates are also particularly susceptible to relative fibrinogen deficiency due to hematological immaturity. Fibrin is crucial in the formation of a stable blood clot; early administration of fibrinogen may even partially compensate for inadequate platelet numbers or function (Schochl et al., 2016). Plasma transfusion alone is inadequate for replacement of fibrinogen deficiency. Published guidelines recommend cryoprecipitate if bleeding occurs with TEG signs of functional fibrinogen deficit or a plasma fibrinogen level of less than 1.5 to 2 g/L (Rossaint et al., 2010). Fibrinogen concentrate, a lyophilized powder for reconstitution, presents a promising alternative to cryoprecipitate, although at present it is only Food and Drug Administration approved for congenital fibrinogen deficiency. Fibrinogen concentrate contains 0.9 to 1.6 3g fibrinogen per ampoule, with 1 gram of administered fibrinogen increasing plasma fibrinogen by around 2.5 g/L. It is important to note that in states of hyperfibrinolysis or disseminated intravascular coagulation (DIC), an antifibrinolytic such as TXA must be coadministered for fibrinogen replacement to be effective (Blain & Paterson, 2016). In the case presentation, the child received cryoprecipitate early in resuscitation as guided by the TEG.

Prothrombin complex concentrate (PCC) contains vitamin K dependent coagulation factors, does not require cross-matching, and has been used in the reversal of congenital or acquired vitamin K coagulation factor deficiency. Although there is a lack of evidence in the use of PCC for traumatic hemorrhage in children, it may be an alternative to FFP where volume overload is an issue. PCC is contraindicated in DIC and hyperfibrinolysis due to increased risk of thromboembolism, so it is therefore not routinely included as part of MTPs (Blain & Paterson, 2016, Hsu et al 2016).

Massive transfusion can lead to **hypocalcaemia** because blood products are preserved with a citrate-containing solution that chelates calcium. FFP and platelets have the highest citrate concentrations. As the liver rapidly metabolizes citrate, citrate-induced hypocalcemia is generally transient, but it can affect hemostasis during resuscitation. Current recommendations are to maintain an ionized calcium level of above 0.9 mmol/L (Rossaint et al., 2010).

Most guidelines suggest consideration of **recombinant activated factor VII** (rFVIIa) in blunt abdominal trauma in adults, with evidence supporting improved coagulopathy and decreased transfusion requirements but no improved mortality (Blain & Paterson, 2016). To be effective, rFVIIa requires adequate platelets and fibrinogen, normothermia, and a normal pH. In trauma, there are reduced levels of *anti*-coagulant factors along with increased *pro*-coagulant factors, and thus there may be a risk of thrombosis with rFVIIa. rFVIIa has a short half-life, with an average of 2.7 hours for adults and 1.3 hours for children. The clearance is faster for pediatric patients (67 mL/kg/hr) compared to adults (33 mL/kg/hr). Varying doses have been described in children, but it seems that 80 to 100 IU/kg is sufficient as an initial dose, with a second dose 1 hour later. TEG may guide therapy administration as rFVIIa normalizes the in vitro prothrombin time (PT) and INR.

Acute traumatic coagulopathy

The child in the case presentation was already **coagulopathic on arrival** prior to the administration of any IV fluid. 30% of major trauma patients are coagulopathic upon arrival to the emergency department prior to any aggressive IV crystalloid or colloid resuscitation or the onset of any hypothermia and acidosis. Trauma-induced coagulopathy may be described as a combination of acute trauma coagulopathy (ATC) in addition to dilutional coagulopathy, hypothermia, and acidosis (Davenport & Brohi, 2016). ATC is a state of endothelial dysfunction, systemic anticoagulation, hyperfibrinolysis, and impaired platelet function. With shock, there is increased plasma-soluble thrombomodulin expressed by the endothelium. Thrombomodulin binds with thrombin, resulting in less available thrombin to cleave fibrinogen into fibrin. Also, the thrombin–thrombomodulin complex activates protein C, which in turn irreversibly inactivates factors Va and VIIIa and deactivates plasminogen activator inhibitor (PAI-1). Inhibition of these coagulation factors further impairs the ability to cleave fibrinogen to fibrin, and deactivation of PAI-1 promotes fibrinolysis (Ganter & Pittet, 2010). This phenomenon may be a protective mechanism to prevent thrombosis in isolated tissues with hypoperfusion, but it is counterproductive in the bleeding patient. Raised tissue plasminogen activator levels from injured vessel walls and reduced thrombin activatable fibrinolysis inhibitor also contribute to fibrinolysis (Ganter & Pittet, 2010). Lastly, tissue injury also activates the complement cascade, which in turn affects coagulation.

The possible presence of ATC is one reason why coagulation factors, particularly fibrinogen, and an antifibrinolytic such as TXA, should be given early, and the possibility of developing ATC highlights the importance of correcting tissue hypoperfusion as early as possible. Research is currently addressing the potential benefits of prehospital transfusion of plasma and PRBC in limiting the development of ATC in adults (Stephens et al., 2016).

5. What are the elements of damage-control surgery?

Communication between the surgeon and the anesthesiologist is important in any emergency operation. The case presentation illustrates how good teamwork improves patient outcome. The surgeon assisted in obtaining large-bore IV access prior to incising the abdomen and releasing the tamponade. Damage-control surgery is an abbreviated resuscitative laparotomy for control of bleeding, restitution of blood flow where necessary, and control of contamination (Rossaint et al., 2010). Once the inferior vena cava was clamped, controlling the hemorrhage, **packing the abdomen** allowed the anesthesiologist to stabilize the patient. The packs will remain in situ for 24 to 48 hours, allowing normalization of the coagulation profile, intravascular volume, and electrolytes in the intensive care unit. Then the patient will have definitive surgical repair of the viscera, if necessary, and closure of the abdomen.

SUMMARY

1. Establishing appropriate trauma procedures and protocols such as MTPs streamlines the institution's management of trauma patients and can improve patient outcomes.
2. In cases of trauma with major hemorrhage, blood products should be given early in a high ratio of FFP:platelets:PRBC.
3. Massive transfusion may cause coagulopathy, hypothermia, and acidosis. These can result in further bleeding and should be treated aggressively. Hyperkalemia and hypocalcaemia should also be treated early.
4. Coagulopathy may develop early after trauma. Along with FFP and platelets, TXA, fibrinogen, and rFVIIa should be considered as ways to reverse coagulopathy.

ANNOTATED REFERENCES

Holcomb JB, Wade CE, Michalek JE, et al. Increased plasma and platelet to red blood cell ratios improves outcome in 466 massively transfused civilian trauma patients. *Ann Surg.* 2008;248:447–458.

The best evidence in a civilian population for a 1:1:1 ratio of blood products.

Riskin DJ, Tsai TC, Riskin L, et al. Massive transfusion protocols: the role of aggressive resuscitation versus product ratio in mortality reduction. *J Am Coll Surg* 2009;209:198–205.

An excellent illustration of the beneficial impact of an MTP.

Spinella PC, Holcomb JB. Resuscitation and transfusion principles for traumatic hemorrhagic shock. *Blood Rev.* 2009;23:231–240.

An excellent recent summary of both acute coagulopathy of trauma shock (ACoTS) and damage-control resuscitation.

BIBLIOGRAPHY

Armand R, Hess JR. Treating coagulopathy in trauma patients. *Transfus Med Rev.* 2003;17:223–231.

Barcelona SL, Thompson AA, Cote CJ. Intraoperative pediatric blood transfusion therapy: a review of common issues. Part II: transfusion therapy, special consideration, and reduction of allogenic blood transfusions. *Pediatr Anesth.* 2005;15:814–830.

Blain S, Paterson N. Paediatric massive transfusion. *BJA Educ.* 2016;16(8):269–275.

CRASH-2 Trial Collaborators. Effects of tranexamic acid on death, vascular occlusive events, and blood transfusion in trauma patients with significant hemorrhage (CRASH-2): a randomised, placebo-controlled trial. *Lancet.* 2010;376:23–32.

Davenport RA, Brohi K. Causes of trauma induced coagulopathy. *Curr Opin Anesthesiol.* 2016;29:212–219.

Dressler AM, Finck CM, Carroll CL, Bonanni CC, Spinella PC. Use of a massive transfusion protocol with hemostatic resuscitation for severe intraoperative bleeding in a child. *J Pediatr Surg.* 2010;45:1530–1533.

Duchesne JC, Hunt JP, Wahl G, et al. Review of current blood transfusion strategies in a mature level 1 trauma center: were we wrong for the last 60 years? *J Trauma.* 2008;65:272–276.

Fries D, Martini WZ. Role of fibrinogen in trauma-induced coagulopathy. *Br J Anaesth.* 2010;105:116–121.

Ganter MT, Pittet J-F. New insights into acute coagulopathy in trauma patients. *Best Pract Res Clin Anaesthesiol.* 2010;24:15–25.

Holcomb JB, Tilley BC, Baraniuk S, et al. Transfusion of plasma, platelets and red blood cells in a 1:1:1 vs a 1:1:2 ratio and mortality in patients with severe trauma: the PROPPR randomized clinical trial. *JAMA.* 2015;313(5):471–482.

Hsu YM, Haas T, Cushing MM. Massive transfusion protocols: current best practice. *Int J Clin Transfus Med.* 2016;4:15–27.

Hunt H, Stanworth S, Curry N, et al. Thromboelastography (TEG) and rotational thromboelastometry (ROTEM) for trauma induced coagulopathy in adult trauma patients with bleeding. *Cochrane Database Syst Rev.* 2015;2:CD010438.

Patregnani JT, Borgman MA, Maegele M, Wade CE, Blackbourne LH, Spinella PC. Coagulopathy and shock on admission is associated with mortality for children with traumatic injuries at combat support hospitals. *Pediatr Crit Care Med.* 2012;13(3):273–277.

Pham HP, Shaz BH. Update on massive transfusion. *Br J Anaesth.* 2013;111(Suppl 1):i71–i82.

Rossaint R, Bouillon B, Cerny V. Management of bleeding following major trauma: an updated European guideline. *Crit Care.* 2010;14:R52.

Schochol H, Maegele M, Voelckel W. Fixed ratio vs goal directed therapy in trauma. *Curr Opin Anesthesiol.* 2016;29(2):234–244.

Stainsby D, Jones H, Wells AW, Gibson B, Cohen H, SHOT Steering Group. Adverse outcome of blood transfusion in children: analysis of UK reports to the serious hazards of transfusion scheme 1996–2005. *Br J Haematol.* 2008;141:73–79.

Stephens, CT, Gumbert S, Holcomb JB. Trauma associated bleeding: management of massive transfusion. *Curr Opin Anesthesiol.* 2016;29:250–255.

Wikkelsø A, Wetterslev J, Møller AM, Afshari A. Thromboelastography (TEG) or thromboelastometry (ROTEM) to monitor haemostatic treatment versus usual care in adults or children with bleeding. *Cochrane Database Syst Rev.* 2016;8:CD007871.

21

Management of Acutely Burned Children

ROBERT MCDOUGALL

INTRODUCTION

The resuscitation of the child with burns poses a number of challenges to the anesthesiologist. It is vital that there is a systematic approach to managing the airway, breathing, and circulation. This requires an understanding of the pathophysiology of burn injury. Particular attention must be paid to the timing and technique of securing the airway. Appropriate vascular access and pain management are also of high priority in the burned child.

> LEARNING OBJECTIVES
>
> 1. Understand the approach to resuscitation of the child with acute burn injuries.
> 2. Review the key issues in developing a plan to secure the airway.
> 3. Describe effective pain management in the setting of an acute burn.

CASE PRESENTATION

A 3-year-old, 15-kg boy is brought to the emergency department with face, neck, and trunk burns sustained when he pulled a pot of boiling soup from the stove. The incident occurred 2 hours ago. First aid, in the form of cold running water, was administered to the burn immediately after injury. The ambulance service has placed ***an intraosseous line*** *and has administered 300 mL 0.9% saline and morphine 1.5 mg. He appears to be in severe distress and has obvious facial burns and swelling.*

Oxygen is administered via a non-rebreathing mask and his airway is assessed. There is no evidence of stridor and his cry sounds normal. His ***lips and anterior tongue*** *are* ***swollen****. On auscultation, his chest is clear. His* ***respiratory rate is 40****, peripheral capillary oxygen saturation (SpO_2) 100%,* ***heart rate 190/minute****. It is impossible to get a blood pressure reading but he has strong peripheral pulses.* ***Capillary refill time*** *is 2 seconds. An intravenous cannula is placed in the saphenous vein at the ankle and an additional dose of 0.75 mg morphine is administered while preparations are made for intubation. Five minutes later he is still distressed and another dose of morphine 0.75 mg is repeated. His mother is now present and she confirms the history of the injury and states that he is otherwise healthy. The heart rate has now settled to 130/minute and respiratory rate to 25/minute.*

A ***secondary survey*** *confirms that he has no other injuries. It is estimated that the size of the burn is 20% to 25% of* ***body surface area (BSA)****. The burn on the right upper arm appears to be circumferential. A radial pulse is still present. A urinary catheter is inserted and the patient is taken to the operating room for elective intubation, as his facial swelling has continued to worsen, and for escharotomy of his right arm.*

There is some debate between the senior anesthesiologist and the trainee as to the type of induction, particularly the merits of inhalational versus intravenous techniques. Anesthesia is induced with sevoflurane and oxygen and the trachea is intubated with a size 4.0 ***cuffed endotracheal tube*** *(ETT). At laryngoscopy, the tongue is swollen but the larynx appears normal. The cuff is gently inflated to a pressure of 20 cmH_2O. Ketamine 30 mg is administered and the burn surgeon performs an escharotomy to the right upper arm. The burns are dressed and the patient is transferred to the intensive care unit.*

DISCUSSION

1. How should the young child with burns be assessed?

The general approach for the burned child, as for any injured child, should be assessment and management of airway, breathing, and circulation (ABC). Intubation may be necessary due to respiratory distress or, more commonly, may be instituted early, in the absence of current symptoms of distress, when facial burns or airway swelling is evident and it is suspected that intubation may become urgent at a later stage. This is because as increased swelling of the face and airway occur, it becomes increasingly difficult to secure the airway due to distorted anatomy. Flame burns may involve a significant intraoral and laryngeal burn leading directly to increasing swelling and obstruction. In patients with scalds, it is rare for the larynx and pharynx to be swollen directly from the burn, or for the laryngeal anatomy to become significantly distorted. However, scalds may still result in significant **facial, lip, and tongue swelling**, making intubation and airway management difficult.

This child had significant **facial burns,** and in the hours following the burn it would be expected that the **face, lips, and tongue** would **swell**; possibly leading to upper airway obstruction. Early intubation was indicated in this patient primarily because of this risk. Eventual intubation of the airway may also have become necessary due to decreased pulmonary function secondary to burn-induced systemic inflammatory response resulting in pulmonary edema and pulmonary hypertension. Lastly, in this child intubation would likely be needed for anesthesia for the escharotomy, and securing the airway early on would allow for liberal use of opioid analgesia without fear of respiratory depression.

Assessment of the circulation is challenging in the distressed child. **Heart rate** and **respiratory rate** will be elevated due to pain and anxiety, as well as due to any hypovolemia. There is a wide range of normal blood pressure for a 3-year-old child. **Capillary refill time** is highly variable between patients and therefore on its own is an *unreliable sign* to diagnose hypovolemia. Also, *it is unusual for a burn patient to be profoundly hypovolemic secondary to dehydration in the first 2 hours after a burn. Significant hypovolemia immediately postinjury is more likely due to another injury.* In this child the presence of strong peripheral pulses indicates that circulatory compromise was not severe at this stage.

It is important that other injuries are identified during the assessment. Burns often occur in the setting of other injuries. A careful **secondary survey**, looking at each organ system, should be undertaken once ABCs have been stabilized. The severity of the burn based on surface area affected can be assessed at this point. Accurate assessment of burn size is important as it is the main determinant in the calculation of resuscitation fluids. Overestimation of burn size may lead to over-resuscitation and secondary complications due to "fluid creep" (Rogers et al., 2010).

2. What is the correct approach to securing the airway in a burn patient?

A patient who has suffered burns with associated facial, neck, and airway injury should be treated similar to the patient with a potentially difficult airway. If airway obstruction is impending, then preparations for intubation should be expedited. In this case, both intravenous and inhalational induction may be considered. An intravenous induction may be quicker and less distressing for the child but may lead to apnea and hypoventilation. Hypoxia may be accentuated in this situation, if bag and mask ventilation is not possible. If bag and mask ventilation can be employed, slow intravenous supplemental sedatives may be administered in addition to inhaled induction of anesthesia. Succinylcholine (suxamethonium) may be administered as part of a rapid sequence induction within 48 hours of a burn injury. After this time, proliferation of extrajunctional nicotinic-acetylcholine receptors can lead to significant hyperkalemia when succinylcholine is administered. In the clinical case described, an inhalational induction was chosen because it allowed greater control over a potentially difficult airway. Awake, fiberoptic bronchoscopy is often used to secure the airway in adults with burns; however, this technique is of limited use in the pediatric patient.

Burn injuries trigger inflammatory responses which may result in poor lung compliance. The use of an uncuffed ETT may lead to increasing air leak, which may make ventilation difficult; while it is possible to change ETTs, increasing facial edema will make this difficult. A **cuffed ETT** typically avoids these problems and was therefore the first option in this case described.

Securing an ETT in a patient with facial burns is challenging. Conventional adhesive tapes do not stick and may cause further damage to burned tissue. Tracheostomy tapes may be useful but can put pressure on the facial area. A novel way of securing a tube is the use of orthodontic brackets, which are bonded to the maxillary incisors (Sakata et al., 2009). The oral ETT can then be secured to the brackets with wire. This avoids the use of tapes and allows oral and facial hygiene to be maintained.

3. What are the options for intravenous access in the child with burns?

Intravenous access in the child with burns may present a challenge to the anesthesiologist; particularly if there have been numerous previous unsuccessful attempts. If possible, intravenous lines should not be placed through burned tissue. An intravenous cannula placed in the burned area may increase the risk of infection and may be difficult to secure. The dorsum of the hand, cubital fossae, and the long saphenous veins at the medial ankle are the most reliable sites. In this case, an **intraosseous needle** was placed. This is an excellent emergency option if peripheral veins cannot be accessed. The usual site is at the anteromedial aspect of the proximal tibia, taking care to avoid the growth plate. Resuscitation fluids and drugs can be administered safely and rapidly through the intraosseous needle. Complications such as osteomyelitis are rare, but compartment syndrome can occur if the needle becomes displaced. It can be difficult to secure intraosseous needles, so after initial resuscitation, peripheral access should be attempted again. Central venous access may be attempted after attempts at peripheral access have failed or other indications for central access exist (e.g., inotropic support).

4. How should resuscitation fluids be managed in the child with burns?

As part of the ABC approach, most children with burns of more than 10% **BSA** require intravenous fluid resuscitation. In estimating the amount of fluid required, the size of the burn is more important than the depth. The size of the burn should be estimated using a burn estimation tool (e.g., Lund and Browder chart, Wallace's rule of nines). Fluid loss from burns is predominantly from the extracellular compartment; therefore, an isotonic fluid (such as Ringer's lactate) should be utilized for resuscitation. The *Parkland formula* is a useful guide to calculating total fluid resuscitation for the first 24 hours: 4 × % burn area × weight (kg). Fifty percent of this amount should be given in the first 8 hours (after burn injury) and the remainder over the next 16 hours. This formula is a guide only and may lead to over-resuscitation in smaller burns. This calculation *does not include maintenance requirements*. In this patient, part of the calculated resuscitation volume was administered as a fluid bolus of 20 mL/kg by the ambulance service, presumably because there was clinical evidence of hypovolemia (**tachycardia**, **tachypnea**, **prolonged capillary refill**).

Most burn patients retain gut activity, and oral intake should be encouraged. Urine output should be closely monitored, aiming for an hourly output of more than 0.75 mL/kg/hr. In large burns, blood electrolytes should be checked regularly (every 6 to 12 hours) as Na^+ and K^+ abnormalities are not uncommon.

5. What are the options for analgesia in the acutely burned patient?

Pain from thermal injury is particularly severe. Strong pain relief should be administered as soon as the primary survey has been completed. In this case morphine was administered and titrated to effect. The correct total dose is the dose that leads to adequate pain relief. Other opioids (e.g., fentanyl) may be used with equal effect. This child is likely to need a continuous opioid infusion for some days. *Multimodal analgesia* is also useful during the acute phase of pain management, and agents such as ketamine, tramadol, acetaminophen (paracetamol), dexmedetomidine infusions, and nonsteroidal anti-inflammatory drugs may be used as adjuncts to opioids.

This patient required escharotomy for a circumferential burn to his arm. Traditional teaching has been that escharotomy requires minimal analgesia or anesthesia because most of the burns causing limb constriction are considered full thickness and therefore have little sensation. In practice, most scald burns have a significant component of partial-thickness burn, and escharotomy will be a painful procedure as sensory nerves in the burned area will be intact. Escharotomy for children is generally performed under general anesthesia. In this case ketamine was used as it provides anesthesia as well as postprocedure analgesia.

Over the medium term of care, multimodal analgesia will help minimize some of the side effects of opioid administration, such as the development of opioid tolerance. Aggressive pain control in the pediatric burn patient is mandatory as improved pain control in this patient population may reduce the risk for future psychiatric problems and chronic pain.

SUMMARY

1. In resuscitating the acutely burned child, assessment of airway, breathing, and circulation are priorities. A careful secondary survey should be performed to exclude other injuries and assess the size of the burn. Fluid management depends on the size of the burn and the time of injury.
2. The airway should be secured early if there is a risk of airway obstruction. Inhalational or intravenous induction techniques may be appropriate. Securing the ETT can be challenging.
3. Burn pain is severe and requires strong analgesics. Multimodal analgesia may reduce the side effects from opioids.

ANNOTATED REFERENCES

Fuzaylov G, Fidkowski CW. Anesthetic considerations for major burn injury in pediatric patients. *Pediatr Anesth.* 2009;19(3):202–211.

This paper gives a good summary of the pathophysiology of thermal injury and outlines the major complications that must be managed by the anesthesiologist.

Jeschke MJ, Herndon DN. Burns in children: standard and new treatments. *Lancet.* 2014;383:1168–1178.

This summary of current surgical management of children with burns is useful for understanding the overall management of these children.

Rogers AD, Karpelowsky J, Millar AJW, Argent A, Rode H. Fluid creep in major pediatric burns. *Eur J Pediatr Surg.* 2010;20:133–138.

This case highlights the problems with over-resuscitation with fluids in paediatric burns.

Sakata S, Hallett B, Brandon MS, McBride CA. Easy come, easy go: a simple and effective orthodontic enamel anchor for endotracheal tube stabilization in a child with extensive facial burns. *Burns.* 2009;35:983–986.

This gives instructions on securing an ETT with an orthodontic bracket.

FURTHER READING

Light TD, Latenser BA, Heinle JA, et al. Demographics of pediatric burns in Vellore, India. *J Burn Care Res.* 2009;30(1):50–54.

Pardesi O, Gennadiy R. Pain management in pediatric burn patients: review of literature and future directions. *J Burn Care Res.* 2017;38(6):335–347.

Quinlan KP, O'Connor A, Robinson M, Gottlieb LJ. Protecting children from fires and burns. *Pediatr Ann.* 2010;39(11):709–713.

22

Liver Transplant

CARLOS J. CAMPOS AND RAHUL BAIJAL

INTRODUCTION

There are many challenges in anesthetizing a child with pediatric end-stage liver disease (ESLD). The treatment of choice for ESLD is orthotopic liver transplant. Adequate preparation and an exquisite understanding of the patient's pathophysiology are critical to anticipating all the potential complications for each stage of the transplant. Even with all this preparation, being flexible with the anesthetic plan is imperative, in order to deliver the child in hepatic failure to hepatic physiology normalcy.

LEARNING OBJECTIVES

1. Direct the preoperative assessment of the pediatric patient for liver transplantation.
2. Define the stages of liver transplantation.
3. Discuss the anesthetic management issues associated with each of the stages.
4. Describe the surgical options for anastomosing the new liver and the impact on anesthetic management.
5. Understand the etiology and management of the liver reperfusion syndrome.

CASE PRESENTATION

A 1-year-old, 8-kg male presents for orthotopic liver transplantation. Past medical and surgical history is significant for biliary atresia treated with a hepatoportoenterostomy (Kasai procedure) at 2 months of age when he presented with acute onset abdominal pain with lethargy, nausea, and vomiting. He recovered well from the procedure but over the past months developed chronic portal hypertension and worsening liver failure with a decline in renal function as well.

During this hospitalization, physical examination reveals an awake and alert, anxious child in the semi-recumbent position with a moderate protuberant abdomen. Oxygen saturation on room air is 93%. He has no known drug allergies and his current medications include furosemide, pantoprazole, spironolactone, and ursodiol. Total parenteral nutrition and intralipids are infusing via a right subclavian porta Cath. His Pediatric End-stage Liver Disease (PELD) score is 25.

DISCUSSION

1. What is biliary atresia? Are there associated congenital anomalies?

Biliary atresia is an inflammatory sclerosing cholangiopathy with an incidence between 1 in 8,000 to 1 in 18,000 live births. Biliary atresia is the most common cause of neonatal cholestasis and is the most frequent indication for pediatric transplantation. Biliary atresia progresses over time. At the onset, the child is often of normal weight. However, the infant soon develops clinical signs and laboratory abnormalities over the ensuing weeks. Pale stools, dark urine, and icterus are apparent by the age of 4 to 6 weeks.

In addition to the clinical findings, the patient will have abnormal laboratory values including moderate conjugated hyperbilirubinemia, elevated gamma-glutamyl transferase, and mildly to moderate elevated serum transaminases. Associated congenital anomalies include polysplenia, situs inversus, absent vena cava, malrotation, and cardiac anomalies.

Without surgical intervention, biliary cirrhosis, portal hypertension and ESLD will occur in 50% of patients by 2 years of age.

2. What is a Kasai procedure? What are the implications of the previous Kasai procedure in this patient?

The Kasai procedure (hepatic portoenterostomy), named after Dr. Kasai who first developed the technique in 1959, consists of the excision of all extrahepatic fibrous biliary remnants at the point where the portal vein enters the hepatic parenchyma. The fibrous surface is then anastomosed to a Roux-en-Y loop of proximal jejunum. The timing of the procedure is linked to success. Between 65% and 80% of neonates will have flow of bile when operated on at less than 60 days of life. Even though results decrease with increasing age, most centers will recommend any type of hepatoportoenterostomy regardless of the time of diagnosis of the biliary atresia.

The Kasai procedure remains an important bridge until transplant. A previous Kasai procedure, however, may make dissection of the native liver difficult secondary to scarring and adhesions.

3. What is the PELD score?

The PELD was developed to establish a scoring system to allow for appropriate allocation of donor grafts. It is an objective tool used to prioritize children aged 12 years and younger awaiting liver transplantation. Higher PELD scores are associated with increased pre-liver transplant mortality. However, high PELD scores are not associated with worsening outcome post-liver transplant. This helps substantiate the current adopted "sickest child first" allocation policy.

The PELD includes albumin (g/dl), bilirubin (mg/dl), international normalized ratio (INR), presence of growth failure, and age at placement on transplant list.

4. Why did this patient develop portal hypertension?

Most children with biliary atresia will ultimately go on to develop cirrhosis and portal hypertension secondary to an increased resistance to portal flow and an increased portal venous inflow. There is also an apparent deficiency of nitric oxide contributing to portal vein venoconstriction. Portal hypertension is defined as portal venous pressures above 10 to 20 mmHg. While portal hypertension may be silent, its manifestations are not. Bleeding from esophageal varices is the most common presentation. Collateral vessels form prominently in areas in which absorptive epithelium joins stratified epithelium, especially in the esophagus or anorectal region. While increased pressure gradient leads to the formation of the varices, it is the increased flow that leads to variceal expansion and eventual rupture.

As portal pressure increases, collateral vessels form. These collaterals should compensate for increased resistance within the liver and decrease portal pressure. However, the increased portal pressure is maintained by an increased splanchnic blood inflow secondary to vasodilation. This splanchnic vasodilatation is the beginning of the hyperdynamic state that aggravates many of the complications of cirrhosis. Vasodilator mediators are most likely the cause of this high outflow state.

5. Is the infant at risk for hepatorenal syndrome?

While there are multiple causes of renal failure in the setting of advanced liver disease such as volume depletion, shock, exposure to nephrotoxic drugs, or intrinsic renal disease, acute renal failure typically occurs in the absence of these factors. The common pathway for hepatorenal syndrome is the splanchnic arterial vasodilation which triggers compensatory vasoconstriction and activation of the antinatriuretic system in the kidneys. Renal perfusion cannot be maintained because of extreme arterial underfilling causing maximal activation of vasoconstrictor systems.

There are no specific clinical findings in hepatorenal syndrome. Acute renal failure present in a cirrhotic patient needs to be worked up fully. However, renal failure in hepatorenal syndrome is often associated with severe oliguria (<500 ml/24h), intense urinary sodium retention (urine Na <10mEq/L), and spontaneous dilutional hyponatremia (serum Na <130 mEq/L). Creatinine levels depend on which of the two types of hepatorenal syndrome is present. Type 1 happens rapidly with doubling of the creatinine within 2 weeks. Practically all patients die within 8 to 10 weeks after onset of this renal failure. Type 2 has a more insidious course and is more benign. Patients' median survival time is approximately 6 months. The patient presented in our case falls into this type.

6. Why is his oxygen saturation on room air 93%?

The renal system is not the only organ affected by portal hypertension. The pulmonary system may be affected as well. Both portopulmonary hypertension and hepatopulmonary syndrome are caused by portal hypertension. In portopulmonary hypertension, high cardiac output and hyperdynamic circulation causes an increase in shear stress on the pulmonary circulation. The pulmonary vascular bed responds by increasing pulmonary resistance eventually leading to pulmonary vascular remodeling and smooth muscle proliferation. In portopulmonary syndrome, the same factors that produce splanchnic vasodilatation cause pulmonary vasculature dilatation. This ultimately leads to perfusion/ventilation mismatch and eventually hypoxemia.

7. What additional preoperative work-up, if any, would you order prior to the procedure?

Preoperative labs include:

Hemoglobin: 9.7, hematocrit: 29.8, platelets: 80K, PT: 19.6, INR: 1.9,
Na: 131, K: 3.1, CI: 105, HCO3: 27, BUN: 30, Cr: 0.9, glucose 71, Ca: 8.1, Mg: 1.9, albumin: 3.2, total bilirubin: 3.9

Additional preoperative work-up may include liver transaminases, chest x-ray to evaluate appropriate placement of port-a-cath and echocardiogram. Eighty-five percent of patients with ESLD present with a significant degree of diastolic or lusotropic dysfunction.

The evaluation and possible findings in the pediatric liver patient with liver failure includes the following:

1. Neurological = hepatic encephalopathy; cerebral edema and increased intracranial pressure (ICP)
2. Cardiovascular= hyperdynamic circulation; congestive heart failure
3. Pulmonary = restrictive lung function due to ascites; multiple causes of hypoxemia
4. Gastrointestinal = portal hypertension; delayed gastric emptying; malnutrition
5. Renal = acute and chronic renal failure
6. Hematologic = coagulopathy, disseminated intravascular coagulation, anemia, thrombocytopenia
7. Immunologic = decreased gamma globulins
8. Electrolytes = hyponatremia, hypo/hyperglycemia
9. Prior surgical procedures
10. Other associated pathologies

8. Would you give premedication to this patient?

Separation anxiety may be managed with intravenous short-acting benzodiazepines like midazolam 0.1 mg/kg. This patient age and weight may not make him a good candidate for an early extubation postoperatively, but some centers are also utilizing centrally acting alpha 2-adrenoceptor agonists like dexmedetomidine which have sedative and anesthetic properties possible by activating G-proteins in the brainstem, which results in the inhibition of norepinephrine release.

9. How would you induce anesthesia?

A rapid sequence induction with cricoid pressure should be strongly considered due to the patient's ascitic abdomen. Propofol can be administered in low doses to preserve systemic arterial pressure, and succinylcholine or rocuronium are commonly used to facilitate intubation; the utilization of short-acting highly potent opioids such as fentanyl are also desired. The physiologic principle should be to maintain adequate organ perfusion during this stage in the procedure.

10. What kinds of monitoring will you place? Is his port-a-cath adequate for the procedure?

One to two large-bore peripheral intravenous vein catheters should be inserted in the upper extremities (as the inferior vena cava [IVC] may be cross-clamped). Even though the port-a-cath could be accessed preoperatively and used for anesthesia induction, its uses for the procedure are inadequate for aggressive volume resuscitation and a supradiaphragmatic central line should be inserted to guide fluid management and may also be used to administer vasoactive medications. An upper extremity arterial line is placed, as the aorta may also be cross-clamped occasionally. An infusion of dextrose or continuation of total parenteral nutrition should be considered to maintain normoglycemia secondary to impaired gluconeogenesis and glycogenolysis.

11. How would you maintain anesthesia?

Maintenance of anesthesia can be accomplished in a variety of ways; no technique has been shown to be the best. More important is the need to provide hemodynamic stability, along with fluid resuscitation, temperature homeostasis, and correction of metabolic and coagulation abnormalities.

12. What is the initial phase of liver transplantation, and what are your anesthetic concerns?

There are three separate stages during liver transplantation. Anesthetic concerns vary with the stage of the procedure.

The pre anhepatic stage (the "dissection") is characterized by the potential for large volume blood loss due to coagulopathy and a difficult dissection, especially in those patients who have undergone a Kasai procedure or previous liver transplantation.

Maintenance of hemodynamic stability by adequate fluid and blood product administration and correction of coagulation and metabolic abnormalities is essential. Glucose homeostasis and temperature control is also of importance. Manipulation of the liver may obstruct major vessels and produce hypotension by decreasing venous return.

The anhepatic stage begins with clamping of the IVC and portal vein, decreasing venous return. Most pediatric patients tolerate this well because of adequate collateral blood flow that has developed secondary to the portal hypertension. After the IVC has been cross-clamped, the preload is significantly decreased and is now dependent on superior vena cava flow rates. Careful fluid resuscitation to a central venous pressure (CVP) of 5 to 10 cm H2O before the IVC is cross-clamped, together with the use of vasoactive drugs, will help prevent significant hypotension.

12. The surgeon encounters a difficult dissection while removing the old liver. There is noticeable oozing, and the removal lasts 3 hours. The hepatic artery is ligated and the surgeon clamps the IVC and portal vein. What are your anesthetic concerns?

Coagulopathy is common in liver disease, and the difficult dissection was not unexpected in this patient. Fresh frozen plasma (FFP) is most commonly utilized to correct coagulopathies. FFP is administered at our institution only if clinically necessary and not based on a laboratory value.

Metabolic abnormalities may occur following cross-clamping. Ionized calcium may decrease because the liver does not metabolize the citrate; metabolic acidosis may worsen because the liver does not metabolize lactate to bicarbonate. Monitoring and correction of the pH, electrolytes, calcium, and glucose is therefore required. Hyperventilation with adequate volume resuscitation will improve the metabolic acidosis and hyperkalemia. Volume resuscitation should be guided by the CVP, arterial pressure waveform, and urine output. This may be challenging in patients who have pre-existing renal impairment, portopulmonary hypertension, intracardiac shunts, or high ICP.

13. An hour later the surgeon states that he will reperfuse the new liver within 5 minutes. What preparations should you make prior to reperfusion?

Reperfusion completes the anhepatic stage. This stage starts with release of the suprahepatic clamp followed by removal of the portal vein and infrahepatic clamps. Inadequate fluid resuscitation, insufficient flushing of the cold preservative solution, and release of vasoactive substances into the central circulation may cause hemodynamic instability during this phase due to elevated pulmonary vascular resistance, decreased cardiac output, and decreased systemic vascular resistance.

Hyperkalemia, hypocalcemia, and acidosis may develop necessitating sodium bicarbonate and calcium chloride or gluconate. The cold solution may directly decrease cardiac output, necessitating warm infusion solution in the surgical field.

In anticipation of the electrolyte changes that may occur following reperfusion, sodium bicarbonate is given to normalize serum pH. Calcium should be maintained around 1.1 to 1.2 mmol/l to mitigate the adverse effects of hyperkalemia and to maintain optimal cardiac output. Incremental doses of 10 to 20 mg/kg of calcium chloride or 30 to 60 mg/kg calcium gluconate may be required.

Body temperature should be increased to 36.5° to 37°C if possible. Vigorous flushing of the liver with colloid solution followed by retrograde flushing with the recipient's blood prior to reperfusion reduces the potassium concentration and acid content of the effluent. In addition, the fraction of inspired oxygen (FiO2) should be increased to 1.0 and volatile agents should be discontinued or decreased 3 to 5 minutes prior to reperfusion. Epinephrine and atropine should be available to treat bradycardia.

The circulatory changes associated with reperfusion usually subside within 10 minutes, provided that appropriate therapeutic measures are implemented. Blood must be ready for immediate transfusion in the event of hemorrhage following removal of vascular clamps.

14. The vascular clamps are removed. Within 1 minute a prolonged QT interval, peaked T wages, and slowing of the heart rate are noted on the electrocardiogram (EKG), along with a decrease in blood pressure. What is the differential diagnosis, and how will you manage these changes?

The EKG changes are provoked by the rapid intravenous infusion of effluent from the transplanted liver. It has a low pH and temperature and is high in potassium. In addition, infusion of air and/or microthrombi into the heart may precipitate acute pulmonary hypertension.

The acute treatment of hyperkalemia post-liver transplant reperfusion syndrome includes epinephrine 10 mcg/kg to support the right ventricle, calcium chloride 10 mg/kg or calcium gluconate 30 to 50 mg/kg to stabilize the cardiac membrane, and regular insulin 0.1 to 0.2 units/kg to drive the potassium intracellularly followed by 1 cc/kg of dextrose 50% to avoid hypoglycemia. In addition, sodium bicarbonate 1 to 2 mEq/kg or based on acid-base arterial blood gas and hyperventilation with 100% oxygen (1.0 FiO2) is used to treat the acidosis. If the serum K+ concentration remains greater than 5 mmol/1 despite an alkaline pH, furosemide 0.5 to 1.0 mg/kg should be administered although its efficacy may be reduced if the vena cava is cross-clamped.

15. What is the final phase of liver transplantation, and what are your anesthetic concerns?

Intraoperative labs are now:
Hemoglobin: 9.2, hematocrit: 27.8, platelets: 85K, PT: 20.4, INR: 2.2, PTT: 39.5

The postanhepatic stage or neohepatic is characterized by completion of the hepatic artery anastomosis and creation of the biliary drainage system. There may be additional blood loss with split-liver grafts, but it is not known until reperfusion how much bleeding there will be from the raw edge of the liver graft. It is important during this stage to avoid congestion of the new graft with too aggressive fluid resuscitation and to maintain a hematocrit below 30% to minimize blood viscosity and decrease the risk of hepatic artery thrombosis. Patients may be started on heparin (5–10 units/kg/hr) or dopamine (3–5 mcg/kg/min) infusion to maintain hepatic artery patency as hepatic artery thrombosis (HAT) is the most common reason for graft failure. HAT is directly related to the size of the vessel and thus is most likely in the smallest pediatric recipients. HAT is a serious postoperative complication that can result in bacteremia, biliary stricture, and hepatic necrosis with resultant loss of the graft. The incidence has been found to be as high as 25% with children younger than 3 years at greater risk. Transplant recipients with HAT have a 50% survival rate (and most undergo retransplant) compared to the 80% survival rate of those without HAT.

Surgical factors that may play a role include technique of anastomosis, vessel size less than 3 mm, use of grafts, and donor anatomy. Medical factors include use of procoagulants and hyperviscosity from packed red blood cells. Early suspicion and evaluation with duplex sonography, magnetic resonance angiography, or contrast angiography, and immediate exploration and successful thrombectomy may salvage the graft. Bile leaks resulting from bile duct ischemia secondary to early HAT requires retransplantation.

16. Would you extubate this patient in the operating room?

Patients less than 10 kg are commonly ventilated 12 to 24 hours or more following the surgery. Those less than 5 kg may require longer ventilation due to compromised respiratory mechanics and, in many cases, greater restriction of lung expansion because of a proportionally larger liver graft. Pleural or epicardial effusions and splenomegaly can reduce lung volume in children with liver failure. Intrapulmonary right-to-left shunting through abnormally dilated pulmonary arterioles and impaired hypoxic pulmonary vasoconstriction may cause severe hypoxemia. A decrease in pulmonary diffusing capacity has also been described, further contributing to hypoxemia. When large amounts of blood products have been transfused, there is the possibility of transfusion related-acute lung injury. Large fluids shifts will occur in the transplanted patient because of hypoalbuminemia and aggressive fluid resuscitation, making pulmonary edema a postoperative risk. In addition, the decreased hepatic clearance of opioids and the increased free fraction of benzodiazepines will result in significant postoperative sedation.

17. What are other forms of orthotopic liver transplant in pediatric patients?

Surgical innovations based on standard techniques for partial hepatectomy has led to the use of reduced-sized liver grafts, cadaveric split liver transplantation, and live donor liver transplantation. Recipients of lobar or segmental grafts are at an increased risk of bleeding from the transected surface of the liver. Left or right lobe liver transplantation preserves the vena cava of the living donor so the donor hepatic vein is anastomosed directly to the recipient vena cava or hepatic vein.

A lower rate of arterial thrombosis has been achieved by using microvascular techniques to perform an end-to-end arterial anastomosis. A portion of saphenous vein may be harvested from the donor to provide extension of the hepatic artery. The biliary anastomosis depends on the underlying diagnosis and the relative sizes of the recipient and donor liver. A Roux-en-Y anastomosis is obviously necessary in patients with biliary atresia because there is no native biliary tree. In addition, the donor duct will be implanted into a Roux-en-Y limb in babies receiving segmental grafts and in older children with an abnormal native biliary system (primary sclerosing cholangitis).

SUMMARY

1. A full understanding of a patient's current illness (portal hypertension and liver failure) and risk factors for coagulopathy and bleeding will help determine the intraoperative management of a pediatric liver transplant.
2. Reperfusion syndrome and electrolyte abnormalities (hyperkalemia, hypocalcemia, and hypomagnesemia) can contribute to procedure instability.
3. Minimize the risk of thrombotic events, specifically hepatic artery thrombosis, due to increased blood viscosity.
4. Avoid aggressive fluid resuscitation and volume overload that may lead to graft congestion and bleeding from surgical anastomosis as well as biventricular dysfunction and pulmonary edema. Keep the CVP 5 to 10.

ANNOTATED REFERENCES

Massicote L, Lenis S. Effect of low central venous pressure and phlebotomy on blood products transfusion requirements during liver transplantation. *Liver Transplant.* 2005;12:117–123.

Reduced transfusion of red blood cells and coagulation factors occurred when the CVP was kept below the controls levels. It demonstrated a viable alternative to decrease blood loss during liver transplantation.

Ozier Y, Le Cam B. Intraoperative blood loss in pediatric liver transplantation: analysis of preoperative risk factors. *Anesth Analg.* 1995;81:1142–1147.

This analysis of 14 preoperative risk factors studied in 95 patients undergoing orthotopic liver transplant demonstrated that reduced-sized liver graft and increased portal pressure were found to be significant risk factors for blood loss.

FURTHER READING

Barshes NR, Lee TC, Balkrishnan R, Karpen SJ, Carter BA, Goss JA. Orthotopic liver transplantation for biliary atresia: the US experience. Liver *Transplant.* 2005;11:1193–1200.

Bezerra JA. Potential etiologies of biliary atresia. *Pediatr Transplant.* 2005;9:646–651.

Davenport M. Biliary atresia. *Semin Pediatr Surg.* 2005;14:42–48.

Gerstle JT, Superina R. Liver transplantation: surgical considerations. In Bissonnette B, Dalens B, eds. *Pediatric Anesthesia: Principles and Practice.* New York: McGraw-Hill; 2002:1299–1308.

Hammer GB, Krane EJ. Anesthesia for liver transplantation in children. *Pediatr Anesth.* 2001;11:318.

Kim TW, Harbott M. The use of caudal morphine for pediatric liver transplantation. *Anesth Analg.* 2004;99:373–374.

Neidecker J, Lehot J. Organ transplantation: anesthesia considerations and postoperative management. In Bissonnette B, Dalens B, eds. *Pediatric Anesthesia: Principles and Practice.* New York: McGraw-Hill; 2002:1326–1329.

Rand EB, Olthoff K. Overview of pediatric liver transplantation. *Gastroenterol Clin North Am.* 2003;32:913–929.

Schumann R. Intraoperative resource utilization in anesthesia for liver transplantation in the United States: a survey. *Anesth Analg.* 2003;97:21–28.

Yudkowitz FS, Chietero M. Anesthetic issues in pediatric liver transplantation. *Pediatr Transplant.* 2005;9:666–672.

23

Craniosynostosis Repair

HELENA KARLBERG

INTRODUCTION

Craniosynostosis is a condition where one or more of the fibrous sutures in an infant skull fuse prematurely. This may lead to restricted skull and brain growth, elevated intracranial pressure, and visual complications. Many children with craniosynostosis undergo corrective cranioplasty in infancy, an age when the skull is relatively large in proportion to the rest of the body. Depending on the operation, blood loss is usually substantial, sometimes exceeding the child's estimated blood volume. Managing this blood loss is challenging and requires careful planning for fluid and blood product administration. Children with syndromic craniosynostosis should also be evaluated for associated critical issues, such as airway obstruction, difficult intubation, and obstructive and/or central apnea.

LEARNING OBJECTIVES

1. Analyze the threshold for initiating blood transfusion.
2. Develop a strategy to minimize blood loss and the need for red blood cell transfusion.
3. Describe the risks of massive blood transfusion that are particularly relevant in an infant.
4. Explain the risks and necessary precautions associated with the prone position.
5. Review the information from the arterial line tracing that suggests hypovolemia.
6. Understand, recognize, and treat venous air embolism (VAE).

CASE PRESENTATION

An otherwise healthy, 7-month-old boy with sagittal synostosis presents for cranial vault reconstruction. He weighs 7.1 kg. His preoperative hemoglobin (Hb) is 10 g/dL, equivalent to a hematocrit (Hct) of 30%. His estimated blood volume is approximately 70 mL/kg, or 500 mL. Anesthesia is induced, the endotracheal tube is secured, and 2 large-bore peripheral intravenous lines are inserted. Monitoring includes: a radial arterial line, a femoral central venous catheter, a urinary catheter, and a rectal temperature probe. The child is carefully placed in the prone position, pressure areas are padded, the endotracheal tube position is reconfirmed, and the child is kept warm.

His allowable blood loss to reach a Hb of 8 g/dL (Hct 24%) is 2/10 × 500 mL, or 100 mL. The fluid management plan includes an initial bolus of 20 mL/kg of crystalloid solution and thereafter utilizing a mixture of a colloid solutions, 20 mL/kg and red blood cells.

Bleeding is minimal at first but increases with the craniotomy. Once 200 mL crystalloid has been given, the Hb is 8 g/dL (Hct 24%) and a transfusion with packed cells and albumin 5% in a 1:1 ratio is started. Bleeding increases further while the bone flaps are removed. Arterial blood gases, including Hb, Hct, electrolytes, ionized Ca, and lactate levels are followed every 30 minutes during periods of intraoperative blood loss. Once blood loss reaches 500 mL, Hb, platelets, and clotting parameters are checked and packed red blood cells and fresh frozen plasma are administered in a 1:1 ratio.

Suddenly, the end-tidal carbon dioxide (ETCO$_2$) falls from 37 to 15 mmHg and the mean blood pressure falls from 45 to 30 mmHg. VAE is suspected. The sevoflurane is immediately discontinued, and the inspired oxygen fraction (FiO$_2$) is increased to 1.0. A fluid bolus is administered, the table is tilted so the patient is head-down, and the surgeon floods the operative field with saline, while using bone wax for bone hemostasis.

After the patient's condition stabilizes, the surgeon removes the last bone flap and controls the bleeding. The operation proceeds uneventfully thereafter, with the patient in a slight Trendelenburg position.

DISCUSSION

1. What is the lowest acceptable Hb/Hct in an otherwise healthy infant undergoing cranioplasty?

There is little clinical evidence to guide transfusion triggers which are directly relevant to healthy infants and neonates undergoing acute, massive blood loss. Most guidelines are based on basic physiology and clinical studies of adults as well as critically ill patients. The crucial issue with brisk ongoing blood loss is maintaining adequate oxygenation to vital organs. Oxygen delivery is determined by the product of Hb concentration, cardiac output, and the arterial oxygen saturation. As the Hb falls, oxygen delivery to the tissues is maintained by increasing cardiac output. When cardiac output reaches a maximum, any further fall in Hb will result in insufficient oxygen delivery to meet tissue demand, and tissue hypoxia occurs. Accepting a lower than normal Hb should be considered only if the patient's cardiac output and oxygen saturation are satisfactory.

Under conditions of isovolemic hemodilution, healthy resting adults can tolerate a Hb of 5 g/dL without evidence of inadequate oxygen delivery; however, myocardial oxygen supply at these levels is borderline and may become inadequate if the subject's activity level or heart rate increases (Weiskopf et al., 1998). In a study of healthy children undergoing repair of idiopathic scoliosis, patients were hemodiluted to Hb of 7 g/dL before the start of surgery. The volume state was closely monitored with arterial and pulmonary arterial catheters, and the FiO_2 remained 1.0 throughout anesthesia. Blood was not retransfused until the end of surgery unless the intraoperative mixed venous oxygenation fell below 60%. This occurred in only 1 patient, who developed transient ST-segment depression at a Hb of 2.2 g/dL (Fontana et al., 1995). This small study suggests that if circulatory volume and oxygenation are closely monitored, otherwise healthy children may be able to tolerate low levels of Hb without apparent harm.

During critical illness, many of the compensatory mechanisms for anemia are impaired. Despite this, data in both adult and pediatric critical care have not shown that a liberal transfusion strategy (target Hb 10–12 g/dL) is associated with a better outcome than a restrictive strategy (target Hb 7–9 g/dL). However, transfusion strategies in the intensive care patient population cannot be extrapolated to a hemodynamically unstable scenario, such as an acute massive intraoperative blood loss in infants. A Cochrane review of transfusion thresholds concluded, "for most patients, blood transfusion is probably not essential until Hb levels drop below 7.0 g/dl" (Hill et al., 2000). This threshold has been applied in the craniofacial surgical context, albeit without much evidence-based data. More recent institutional pediatric blood use and transfusion guidelines, however, recommend red cell blood transfusion in infants with acute blood loss of >10% to 15% of their blood volume in certain instances: when signs of hypovolemia are not responding to fluid administration and when Hb is < 8.0 g/dl (Hct 24%) (Nguyen et al., 2015). In order to not "get behind" at stages of the operation where sudden bleeding is anticipated or most likely, a higher threshold is justified. When there is blood left over from a partially infused unit at the end of surgery, it is common practice to transfuse additional blood to reach a targeted Hb of 10 to 12 in the postoperative care unit and a Hb of >8.0 at discharge. This practice significantly reduces the need for additional postoperative transfusions to correct postoperative anemia caused by continued postoperative bleeding.

2. What are the techniques to minimize intraoperative blood loss and the need for red blood cell transfusion?

Significant intraoperative bleeding, with dilution coagulopathy and continued postoperative bleeding, is expected in patients undergoing craniosynostosis repair. Measures implemented to reduce the need for transfusion of blood products and to reduce the blood loss include intraoperative antifibrinolytic therapy and acceptance of lower transfusion targets. Early consideration to transfuse products, such as fresh frozen plasma, platelets, and fibrinogen, will reduce blood loss from coagulation abnormalities.

3. Which risks of blood transfusion are particularly relevant to an otherwise healthy infant undergoing cranioplasty?

Clerical error leading to the transfusion of the wrong blood is the most common cause of adverse events related to transfusion. This risk may be higher amid the anxiety and haste created by uncontrolled hemorrhage. Where possible, check blood products before major bleeding starts. Potassium levels in stored blood increase in proportion to the duration of storage, and, in old blood, they may be greater than 18 mEq/L. One unit of old stored blood is unlikely to cause hyperkalemia when transfused to an adult, but in an infant, one unit may represent half the circulating blood volume, and if transfused rapidly may precipitate arrhythmias. If fresh blood is unavailable, older blood can be washed in a cell saver to reduce the potassium concentration.

4. What risks and necessary precautions should be addressed to prevent complications associated with the prone position?

Airway management, physiological changes, position-related complications, and equipment-related issues are of concern in patients in the prone position. Ensuring the optimal position of the endotracheal tube (ETT) requires auscultation of breath sounds in neck flexion and extension. Additionally, securing the ETT with submandibular sutures placed by the surgeon further helps to secure the ETT in place. Intraoperative ETT dislodgement, migration, disconnection, kinking, or obstruction can have serious consequences, since resuscitation and airway rescue is often delayed and less effective in the prone position.

Changing from supine to prone position is associated with a temporary absence of vital signs monitoring; risk of desaturation from a temporary interruption of mechanical ventilation; and risk of dislodgement of the ETT, intravenous lines, arterial lines, and urinary catheter. Discontinuation of inhalation agents during repositioning may require intravenous anesthesia supplementation in order to avoid untimely emergence of the patient from anesthesia. Pressure-related injury to skin, soft tissue, and peripheral nerves may occur, in spite of optimal positioning and padding. An example of surgical positioning considerations is included here (Figure 23.1). Prophylaxis against corneal abrasions includes eye lubrication, corneal protectors, or eyelids sutured closed by the surgeon. The effects of the prone position on the cardiovascular and respiratory system are minimal in young and otherwise healthy patients compared to adult patients who may have pre-existing cardiovascular and respiratory comorbidities. Postoperative visual loss does not seem to be a major risk in infants undergoing craniofacial procedures in the prone position.

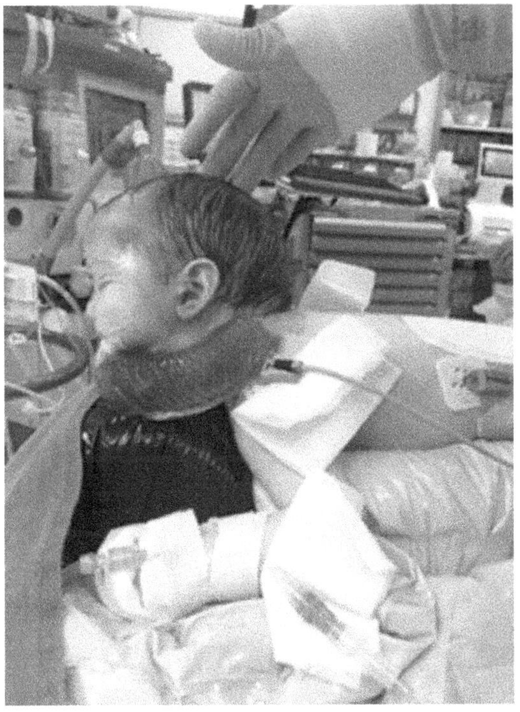

FIGURE 23.1: Surgical positioning.

5. What information from the arterial line trace is suggestive of hypovolemia in the infant?

The mean arterial pressure (MAP) is considered the driving pressure for the perfusion of most vital organs. When MAP falls below the lower limit of autoregulation (LLA), regional blood flow becomes linearly dependent on MAP. The cerebral LLA in adults is generally considered to be a MAP of 60 mmHg. Although there are no conclusive data regarding the lowest MAP that patients can tolerate without neurologic sequelae, a sustained intraoperative MAP below 60 mmHg is generally considered undesirable. In children, the cerebral LLA is not clearly known. Baseline MAP is lower in children than in adults, and it is often assumed that the LLA is also lower in children, but there are limited data to support this assumption.

MAP will fall when a child is significantly hypovolemic, but it is preferable to detect hypovolemia before a fall in MAP. The arterial pressure tracing is suggestive of hypovolemia when the tracing varies with the respiratory cycle. During the inspiratory phase of positive-pressure ventilation, ventricular preload decreases and stroke volume falls, causing a decrease in both pulse pressure and systolic pressure. A large change in pulse pressure indicates that the cardiac output is likely to increase in response to fluid. A variation of more than 10 mmHg in the peak systolic pressure during the respiratory cycle of a patient on positive-pressure ventilation is indicative of at least a 10% reduction in circulating volume.

Although the appearance of the waveform may differ between patients, due to damping, trends in the same patient may be useful. The slope of the systolic upstroke gives some indication of the contractile state of the myocardium. The diastolic downstroke is a combination of forward pressure from the heart and reflected pressure from the circulation. The slope of the diastolic decay indicates resistance to outflow; a slow fall is seen in vasoconstriction. A flat or low dicrotic notch is seen in hypovolemia. The general pattern is shown in Figure 23.2.

6. What is the pathophysiology, diagnosis, and initial management of VAE?

VAE occurs when air at a pressure higher than venous pressure comes into contact with the venous circulation. During cranioplasty, air may enter the circulation either through an open dural venous sinus or through exposed cancellous bone. An air embolus can be potentially fatal, both from mechanical obstruction of the right ventricular outflow tract and pulmonary arterial tree and from platelet aggregation, inflammation, and pulmonary edema. As the obstruction to the right heart progresses, left ventricular filling decreases and cardiovascular collapse may ensue. Air may also pass through intracardiac shunts and occlude systemic arteries, leading to focal ischemia.

In an anesthetized patient, physical signs of VAE include *raised central venous pressure, tachycardia, hypotension,* and *signs of ventilation–perfusion mismatch*; resulting in a *fall in both* $ETCO_2$ and *arterial oxygen saturation.* Pulmonary artery pressure may be elevated or decreased, depending on the site of obstruction. Bronchoconstriction may cause airway pressures to rise. The mill-wheel murmur, a loud, continuous slapping noise heard best at the left sternal border, is probably attributable to the right ventricle beating against subpulmonic air and is specific to a VAE. These signs may be difficult to differentiate from low right ventricular output due to sudden, major blood loss, especially if central venous pressure is not being monitored. In pediatric cranioplasty, both VAE and massive hemorrhage may occur, especially when cranial bone flaps are raised. They may also occur simultaneously.

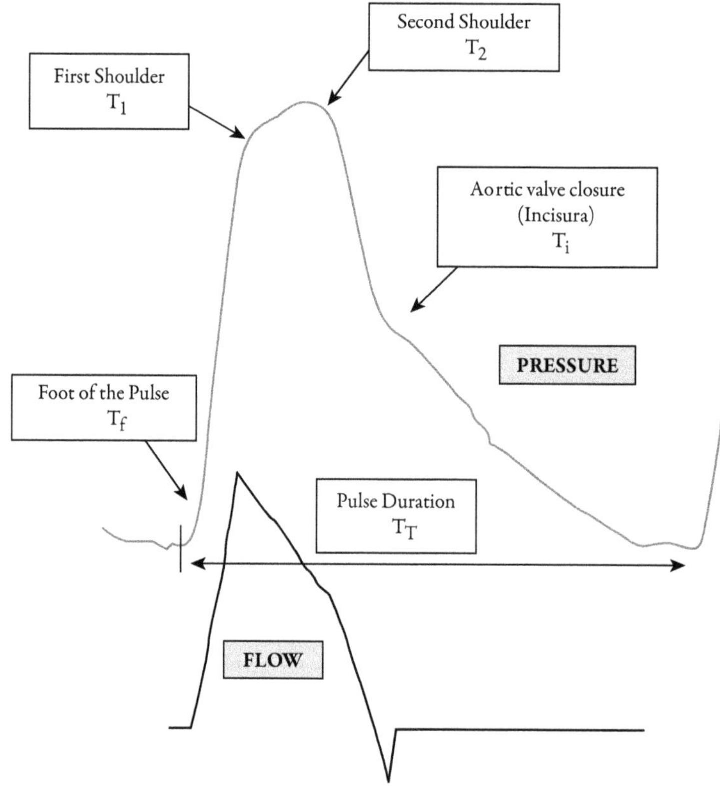

FIGURE 23.2: Arterial waveform.

If VAE is suspected, the first priority is to prevent further air entry by repositioning the patient and flooding the surgical field. Both the Trendelenburg position and placing the patient in the left lateral position have been shown to divert air from the right ventricular outflow tract. The patient should be ventilated with 100% O_2 and the circulation supported with fluid and vasopressors, as appropriate. Administering 100% O_2 helps to reabsorb nitrogen from smaller bubbles. Aspirating air from a central venous line has been more successful in animal studies than in humans and is probably best considered a last resort. A fluid bolus should always be considered in the management algorithm of VAE, because VAE is not only often associated with major blood loss but may be difficult to differentiate from major blood loss.

SUMMARY

1. A transfusion threshold of Hb 8g/dL is justifiable in a hemodynamically stable, well-oxygenated infant.
2. Blood units for surgery should be verified by 2 individuals prior to the beginning of surgery. If fresh blood is unavailable, consider washing red cells before transfusion to decrease hyperkalemia.
3. Major bleeding may occur suddenly and may be difficult to distinguish from VAE. The initial management of both conditions is similar, and resuscitation efforts are challenging in a prone position.
4. Prone positioning requires special attention to the airway, securing intravascular lines, and avoidance of pressure points. It is associated with an increased risk of disruption of ventilation due to dislodgement, disconnection, migration, and kinking of the ETT and therefore requires continual intraoperative vigilance.
5. Signs of VAE are: a sudden drop in $ETCO_2$, oxygen saturation, and/or blood pressure; and possibly elevated central venous pressure and airway pressures.
6. Emergency management of VAE is as follows: Informing the surgeon, flooding of the operative field by surgeons, placing the patient head-down. Call for help. Administer 100% O2, intravenous fluid, vasopressors. Consider left lateral position.

ACKNOWLEDGMENT

The author wishes to acknowledge the first edition author, Peter Howe.

ANNOTATED REFERENCES

Barcelona SL, Thompson AA, Cote CJ. Intraoperative pediatric blood transfusion therapy: a review of common issues. Part I: hematologic and physiologic differences from adults. *Pediatr Anesth.* 2005;15(9):716–726.

Barcelona SL, Thompson AA, Cote CJ. Intraoperative pediatric blood transfusion therapy: a review of common issues. Part II: transfusion therapy, special considerations, and reduction of allogenic blood transfusions. *Pediatr Anesth.* 2005;15(10):814–830.

A succinct but thorough guide to understanding the complications of blood transfusion (Part I) and the management of massive transfusion in the operating room (Part II).

Morris LM. Nonsyndromic craniosynostosis and deformational head shape disorders. *Facial Plast Surg Clin North Am.* 2016;24:517–530.

A thorough description of the classification of craniosynostosis and its management.

Nguyen TT, Lam HV, Phillips M, Edwards C, Austin TM. Intraoperative optimization to decrease postoperative PRBC transfusion in children undergoing craniofacial reconstruction. *Pediatr Anesth.* 2015;25:294–300.

A retrospective analysis of patients who underwent craniosynostosis repair and thorough discussion of factors that can decrease the need for postoperative transfusion.

Reiles E, Van der Linden P. Transfusion trigger in critically ill patients: has the puzzle been completed? *Crit Care.* 2007;11:142.

A helpful summary of studies that have compared restrictive and liberal transfusion strategies in critically ill adults and children.

Weiskopf RB, Viele MK, Feiner J, et al. Human cardiovascular and metabolic response to acute, severe isovolemic anemia. *JAMA.* 1998;279(3):217–221.

A remarkable paper that explores the effects of acute hemodilution on conscious healthy adults at rest.

BIBLIOGRAPHY

Fontana JL, Welborn L, Mongan PD, Sturm P, Martin G, Bünger R. Oxygen consumption and cardiovascular function in children during profound intraoperative normovolemic hemodilution. *Anesth Analg.* 1995;80(2):219–225.

Hill SR, Carless PA, Henry DA, Carson JL, Hebert PC, McClelland DB, and Henderson KM. Transfusion thresholds and other strategies for guiding allogeneic red blood cell transfusion. *Cochrane Database Syst Rev* 2000;1:CD002042. doi:10.1002/14651858

Orebaugh SL. Venous air embolism: clinical and experimental considerations. *Crit Care Med.* 1992;20(8):1169–1177.

van Woerkens, ECSM, Trouwborst A, van Lanschot JJB. Profound hemodilution: what is the critical level of hemodilution at which oxygen delivery-dependent oxygen consumption starts in an anesthetized human? *Anesth Analg.* 1992;75:818–821.

Vavilala MS, Lee LA, Lam AM. The lower limit of cerebral autoregulation in children during sevoflurane anesthesia. *J Neurosurg Anesth.* 2003;15(4):307–312.

24

Kidney Transplantation

TITILOPEMI A. O. AINA AND MIGUEL PRADA

INTRODUCTION

Kidney transplantation is the treatment of choice for patients with end-stage renal disease (ESRD). The other therapeutic options for ESRD are hemodialysis (HD) and peritoneal dialysis (PD), with HD being more common (United States Renal Data System, 2016). There are two main types of kidney transplants: living donor or deceased donor. Kidneys are the most frequently transplanted organs. In 2014, over 17,000 renal transplants were performed; a distant second place was the approximately 7,000 liver transplants performed (UNOS Transplant Trends, 2014). The success rate of a renal transplant is improved with adequate management of perioperative fluid balance, electrolyte anomalies, anemia, blood pressure, and comorbidities. Also critical is the appropriate utilization of immunosuppressive agents, and close communication is required between the pediatric nephrologist, transplant surgeon, and anesthesiologist.

LEARNING OBJECTIVES

1. Describe the key steps in the preoperative assessment.
2. Explain the features of intraoperative anesthetic management.
3. Review the risk factors for reintubation.
4. Identify the optimal plan for postoperative pain management.

CASE PRESENTATION

A 4-year-old girl with anuric ESRD is scheduled for an intra-abdominal ***deceased-donor kidney transplantation****. Her medical history is significant for congenital nephrotic syndrome status post bilateral nephrectomies. She is currently maintained on PD but had previously been on HD. The rest of her medical history is significant for hypothyroidism, anemia, hypotension, epilepsy, and gastroesophageal reflux disease. Her medications include lansoprazole, levetiracetam, levothyroxine, midodrine, oral vitamin D, calcium, and intermittent erythropoietin. She is listed as allergic to ibuprofen. On examination, she is a thin child with a post-dialysis weight of 14.5 kg, heart rate 135 bpm, blood pressure 110/70, peripheral capillary oxygen saturation (SpO_2) 100%. Cardiorespiratory and airway examinations are otherwise normal, and she is afebrile. Blood tests show hemoglobin (Hb) 10.6 g/dL (white cell count and platelets are normal), Na^+ 143 mM/L, K^+ 3.1 mM/L, Ca^{2+} 9.2 mg/dL, PO_4^{2-} 7.6 mg/dL, Mg^{2+} 2.5 mg/dL, blood urea nitrogen (BUN) 56 mg/dL, creatinine 8.0 mg/dL, and albumin 3.3 g/dL.* ***Echocardiography*** *shows* ***mild left ventricular hypertrophy*** *with* ***good biventricular systolic function*** *and no evidence of a* ***pericardial effusion****. She is cross-matched for blood. A central venous line is in situ and is used for overnight hydration and infusion of anti-thymocyte globulin (rabbit).*

Anesthesia is induced with propofol, and rocuronium and maintained with sevoflurane in an O_2/air mixture. The ***central venous pressure (CVP)*** *transducer is connected and reads 4 mmHg. A urethral catheter is inserted. Fentanyl 5 mcg/kg and antibiotics are given before skin incision. Intravenous hydration (30 mL/kg saline 0.9% and 15 mL/kg albumin 5%) is given prior to donor graft revascularization. This increases the CVP to 15 mmHg. A venous blood gas shows the Hb has fallen to 7 g/dL. Warmed, irradiated packed red cells (20 mL/kg) are transfused; this increases the CVP to 18 mmHg. The Hb increases to 12 g/dL* *and the K^+ is 5.2 mmol/L. The electrocardiogram (ECG) shows no changes suggestive of hyperkalemia throughout surgery. Methylprednisolone 10 mg/kg is administered on release of the venous anastomosis. Following reperfusion, urine production is confirmed by inspection of the ureter from the donor kidney (before its connection to the bladder). At this stage, the blood pressure target is in the "low normal" adult pressure range. The CVP target is 10 to 15 mmHg. The estimated blood loss is 300 mL and urine output is 160 mL. Anastomoses are made on to the aorta and vena cava. By the conclusion of the case, the patient has received fentanyl 13mcg/kg, rocuronium 2mg/kg, and albumin 15mL/kg, packed red blood cells 20mL/kg, and crystalloid 90mL/kg. At the conclusion of the surgery, she was extubated awake to continuous positive airway pressure. On arrival to the recovery room, the patient becomes increasingly somnolent with decreased respiratory effort. She is reintubated and transferred to the intensive care unit.*

DISCUSSION

1. What are the key comorbidities to consider in the preoperative assessment?

Common comorbidities in pediatric patients with ESRD include, but are not limited to, hypertension, dyslipidemia, acidosis, renal osteodystrophy, vasculopathy, and anemia. Cardiovascular disease is a leading cause of mortality. It accounts for 57% of deaths for pediatric patients on HD, 43% for those on PD, and 30% for those who have received a transplant. Some of the exact causes of mortality are cardiac arrest, myocardial ischemia, stroke, and pulmonary edema (McDonald et al., 2004).

A preoperative **echocardiogram** is helpful to evaluate for **ventricular hypertrophy** and dilatation and systolic and **diastolic ventricular dysfunction** and to **exclude a uremic pericardial effusion.** Continuation of antihypertensive medications before surgery is recommended; although this could lead to intraoperative hypotension, it may prevent rebound hypertension.

The current volume status is best assessed by reference to the child's weight. Patients may be hypovolemic following dialysis. Also, mild anemia is often present but is well tolerated, and per the Kidney Disease Improving Global Outcomes clinical practice guidelines, the target Hb in pediatric ESRD patients should be 10 to 12 g/dL. Severe azotemia with a BUN greater than 80 mg/dL may be associated with pericardial and pleural effusions. Platelet dysfunction may also occur and may influence the decision to place an epidural catheter. Common electrolyte anomalies include hypernatremia, hyperkalemia, hypocalcemia, acidosis, and hypermagnesemia. Severe hyperkalemia should be treated by dialysis before surgery, when possible, in patients who are chronically on HD or PD.

However, not every transplant patient is on dialysis. Some patients undergo a pre-emptive kidney transplant instead of dialysis. In these patients, severe symptomatic hyperkalemia should be treated medically, and, if not corrected, the case should be postponed.

Furthermore, the underlying cause of **renal failure** could influence the assessment and perioperative management. For example, Takayasu's arteritis may affect the coronary circulation, and systemic lupus erythematosus results in immune complex deposition and cellular proliferation in the glomeruli. Finally, high-dose, chronic steroid therapy given to patients with diverse types of glomerulonephritis and patients with nephrotic syndrome may require perioperative stress-dose steroids.

2. What level of intraoperative monitoring is appropriate?

Routine intraoperative monitors would include five-lead ECG, SpO_2 (pulse oximetry), noninvasive blood pressure, end-tidal carbon dioxide, and core temperature. Placing the blood pressure cuff on the upper limb is preferable in the event that the great vessels need to be clamped during the procedure. Additionally, if an arteriovenous (AV) fistula is present, the blood cuff should be placed on the opposite arm. However, regarding AV fistulas, these are generally not surgically constructed until after the patient is about 12 years of age. Intra-arterial blood pressure should be reserved for small children undergoing an anastomosis of the allograft directly to the great vessels (aorta and inferior vena cava), or when cardiac dysfunction is present (e.g., severe hypertensive cardiomyopathy). Avoidance of the brachial vessels is prudent as damage to these may preclude the future construction of AV fistulas. Also, an indwelling Foley catheter is helpful for monitoring urine output.

The CVP may be monitored by using an existing central venous dialysis catheter or a newly inserted central venous line in the internal jugular or subclavian veins. A multilumen catheter is helpful, especially with likely difficulty with peripheral intravenous access. Careful asepsis is required during line insertion and access due to the immunosuppressed state of the child.

Intraoperative transthoracic (TTE) or transesophageal echocardiography (TEE) may be indicated if severe coexisting heart disease is present.

3. What are the intraoperative stages of a renal transplant?

See Table 24.1. The technical aspects of surgery depend on a number of factors. For example, the size of recipient and donor kidney as well as the size of recipient blood vessels will determine the position of graft implantation. The incision is usually in the right lower quadrant; however, in smaller children a large live donor kidney may be too big to insert extraperitoneally. In this case, a midline incision may be performed and the kidney inserted into the right paravertebral gutter. Depending on the cause of **renal failure**, the diseased kidney may also need to be removed (e.g., nephrotic syndrome, severe hypertension, or polycystic kidneys).

4. What is the management of intraoperative hypotension?

The first intervention is volume resuscitation, guided by the CVP. Isotonic fluid without added potassium (e.g., 0.9% saline) is ideal for resuscitation. The aim is to have the patient "well filled" before unclamping the renal vein and artery. However, large amounts of isotonic fluids may lead to a dilutional anemia. This may in turn lead to a lower blood pressure for a given cardiac output secondary to the reduction in blood viscosity. If the hemoglobin is less than 7g/dL, blood transfusion is recommended. In order to reduce the chance of developing hyperkalemia, packed red blood cells should be washed or less than 7 days old.

In cases of intractable hypotension, intraoperative TEE or TTE could provide a rapid, noninvasive assessment of cardiac filling and function. Always consider other causes of hypotension, including cardiac tamponade (from a pericardial effusion) and anaphylaxis. In this context, the latter is most likely to occur with neuromuscular blockers, antibiotics, or immunosuppressive drugs like basiliximab (monoclonal anti-IL-2Rα receptor antibody) or rabbit anti-thymocyte globulin. Inotropic support of the circulation is sometimes required to maintain the systemic blood pressure in the target range after anastomosis of the graft vessels.

5. What is the management of intraoperative hypertension?

The patient's baseline blood pressure should be determined and hypertension noted only if significantly elevated from baseline. A higher blood pressure relative to an age-matched population without renal failure may be present at baseline. The therapeutic choices for hypertension are to ensure adequate depth of anesthesia and analgesia, nicardipine, and beta-blockers, among others. The ideal pharmacologic agent will be easily titratable and short-acting in order to avoid intractable hypotension following

TABLE 24.1. INTRAOPERATIVE STAGES, TIME COURSE, AND METHOD OF OPTIMIZING THE PHYSIOLOGY DURING PEDIATRIC RENAL TRANSPLANTATION

Event	Duration	Comments
Induction	40 minutes	Avoid long-acting neuromuscular blockers (e.g., pancuronium)
Incision/dissection vessels	2 hours	Perioperative antibiotics and immunosuppressive medications
Cross-clamp vessels	NA	Heparin (as per surgical request)
Vascular anastomosis	30 minutes	IV fluids to raise CVP to 12–15 mmHg
Unclamping vein and artery	NA	Maintain intravascular volume. Mannitol/furosemide as per local protocol.
Ureter anastomosis to bladder	30 minutes	Initial urine output from the graft can be observed in the surgical field.
Closing	30 minutes	Maintain intravascular volume. Monitor urine output. Replace urine output (ml for ml) with a balanced salt solution (e.g., 0.9% saline).
Extubation	15 minutes	Ensure adequate (low normal adult) perfusion pressure and neuromuscular blockade reversal. Ensure patient is warm.

Note: IV = intravenous; CVP = central venous pressure.

reperfusion of the donor kidney. The target blood pressure following transplant of an adult-sized donor kidney will be higher than the child's usual blood pressure.

6. How should one manage intraoperative hyperkalemia?

Symptomatic hyperkalemia should be considered if the typical ECG changes of peaked T waves, widening of the QRS complex, and bradycardia occur. The therapeutic options are listed in Table 24.2. Symptomatic hyperkalemia can occur intraoperatively in association with a blood transfusion. Initial management would depend on the severity of clinical features and the degree of suspicion. For example, if there is cardiovascular compromise with suspicion of hyperkalemia, resuscitation needs should be assessed and managed as per the pediatric advanced life support guidelines, in addition to targeted hyperkalemia therapy.

7. Which patients should remain intubated at the end of the procedure?

The majority of patients are extubated following renal transplantation. However, a subgroup may require postoperative ventilation. Patients who may benefit from postoperative ventilation are those patients who weigh less than 12 kg (due to patient size to kidney size discordance). Also, patients with severe coexisting heart disease may benefit from a period of postoperative ventilation because the efforts to maintain the perfusion pressure in the setting of limited cardiac reserve may result in significant pulmonary edema.

TABLE 24.2. THERAPEUTIC OPTIONS FOR INTRAOPERATIVE TREATMENT OF HYPERKALEMIA

- Increase minute ventilation to decrease $PaCO_2$ (and induce a respiratory alkalosis), which will promote intracellular uptake of K^+.
- Ca^{++} (0.1 mM/kg IV) to protect the myocardium from the arrhythmogenic effects of hyperkalemia. Preferably given into a central vein.
- Sodium bicarbonate IV: Dose (mEq/L) = Base excess (mEq/L) × Weight (kg)/6
- IV insulin (0.1 unit/kg IV) with 2 mL/kg dextrose 50% to increase the intracellular uptake of K^+
- Low-dose epinephrine (adrenaline) infusion (0.02 mcg/kg/min) to stimulate β_2-receptor–mediated cellular uptake of K^+
- Nasogastric calcium polystyrene sulfonate: Dose = 0.6 g/kg to absorb K^+.
- Intraoperative hemofiltration or dialysis. This will take time to implement and extra help will be required.
- ECMO if severe cardiovascular instability is present and the hyperkalemia is refractory to treatment.

Note: IV = intravenous; ECMO = extracorporeal membrane oxygenation.

8. What are the risk factors for reintubation?

The following are **case-specific risk factors**: volume overload, size discrepancy of transplanted kidney (resulting in increased intra-abdominal pressure, decreased pulmonary compliance), and sensitivity to opioids.

In general, **patient-related factors** for reintubation in all-comers include age < 1 year, chronic pulmonary disease, preoperative hypoalbuminemia, and renal insufficiency. **Procedure-related factors** include emergency case, type of surgery (e.g., head and neck, cardiothoracic, airway), and operative time >3 hours. **Anesthesia-related factors** include American Society of Anesthesiologists PS III classification, use of neuromuscular blocking agents, and presence of residual neuromuscular blockade.

9. What are the options for postoperative analgesia?

The therapeutic options include systemic analgesics (intravenous or oral), wound infiltration with local anesthesia, and epidural analgesia/anesthesia. Systemic care also could be opioid or non-opioid. Fentanyl is usually the preferred analgesic because there are no active metabolites that may accumulate in the context of renal failure. However, for morphine, the metabolites of morphine-6-glucuronide and morphine-3-glucuronide accumulate. Increased levels of morphine-6-glucuronide may cause increased sedation and respiratory depression, and morphine-3-glucuronide can cause neuroexcitation. With hydromorphone, the metabolite hydromorphone-3-glucuronide can also accumulate in renal failure and cause neuroexcitation. Meperidine is also avoided because the metabolite normeperidine can decrease the seizure threshold.

Non-opioids, such as acetaminophen and tramadol, are useful coanalgesics. However, it is advisable to wait for satisfactory renal function in the graft kidney before starting tramadol. When oral intake is established, an opioid analgesic such as oxycodone is appropriate. Hydrocodone, which is metabolized into hydromorphone, should be used with caution due to the potential for accumulation of hydromorphone-3-glucuronide.

In theory, an epidural block can provide good analgesia for kidney transplantation. However, it is not commonly used, and this may be attributable to concern for mild coagulation disturbance in ESRD and the potential for hypotension leading to decreased graft perfusion.

SUMMARY

1. The preoperative assessment should focus on cardiorespiratory comorbidity, fluid status, and electrolyte balance
2. Carefully consider the method and type of invasive and noninvasive monitoring needed.
3. Optimize perfusion of the donor organ through volume resuscitation guided by CVP. Remember the likely causes of hemodynamic instability.
4. In general, reintubation rates are low following kidney transplant.
5. The optimal postoperative analgesic plan should be multimodal.

ACKNOWLEDGMENT

The authors would like to thank Ian Smith for his contributions to the first edition.

ANNOTATED REFERENCES

Chavers B, Najarian JS, Humar A. Kidney transplantation in infants and small children. *Pediatr Transplant.* 2007;11:702–708.

This article reviews the factors that support a successful outcome for pediatric kidney transplantation.

Lemmens HJM. Kidney transplantation: recent developments and recommendations for anesthetic management. *Anesthsiol Clin North Am.* 2004;22:651–662.

A review article on perioperative anesthetic considerations for patients presenting for kidney transplantation.

Taylor K, Kim WT, Maharramova M, et al. Intraoperative management and early postoperative outcomes of pediatric renal transplants. *Pediatr Anesth.* 2016;26:987–991.

Retrospective study examining the intraoperative anesthetic and surgical factors, as well as postoperative management, that impact early graft function.

BIBLIOGRAPHY

Coupe N, O'Brien M, Gibson P, de Lima J. Anesthesia for pediatric renal transplantation with and without epidural analgesia—a review of 7 years experience. *Pediatr Anesth.* 2005;15(3):220–228.

Davis ID, Bunchman TE, Grimm PC, et al. Pediatric renal transplantation: Indications and special considerations. *Pediatr Transplant.* 1998;2:117–124.

Della Rocca G, Costa MG, et al. Pediatric renal transplantation: anesthesia and perioperative complications. *Pediatr Surg Int.* 2001;17(2–3):175–179.

Goodman WG, Goldin J, Kuizon BD, et al. Coronary-artery calcification in young adults with end-stage renal disease who are undergoing dialysis. *N Engl J Med.* 2000;342:1478–1483.

Kim MS, Jabs K, Harmon WE. Long-term patient survival in a pediatric renal transplantation program. *Transplantation.* 1991;51(2): 413–416.

McDonald SP, Craig JC. Long-term survival of children with end-stage renal disease. *N Engl J Med.* 2004;350:2654–2662.

Othman MM, Ismael AZ, Hammouda GE. The impact of timing of maximal crystalloid hydration on early graft function during kidney transplantation. *Anesth Analg.* 2010;110:1440–1446.

Rujirojindakul P, Geater AF, McNeil EB, et al. Risk factors for reintubation in the post-anaesthetic care unit: a case-control study. *Br J Anaesth.* 2012;109(4):636–642.

United States Renal Data System. 2016 USRDS annual data report: Epidemiology of kidney disease in the United States. National Institutes of Health. National Institute of Diabetes and Digestive and Kidney Disease, Bethesda, MD; 2016. https://www.usrds.org/adr.aspx

UNOS Transplant Trends. 2014. https://www.unos.org/data/transplant-trends

PART 6

Challenges in Congenital Heart Disease

25

Management of Children with Congenital Heart Disease for Noncardiac Surgery

DEAN B. ANDROPOULOS

INTRODUCTION

Congenital heart disease (CHD) affects approximately 8 neonates per 1,000 live births and is the most common birth defect requiring surgery in the first year of life. Survival for congenital heart surgery has increased dramatically in recent decades, and current surgical mortality as reported in the Society for Thoracic Surgeons' Congenital Heart Surgery Database is now at 3%; neonatal surgical mortality is 8.8%. Over 1 million children in the United States have CHD, and these patients frequently require anesthetics for a variety of noncardiac procedures and present with a broad range of cardiac pathophysiology. This ranges from a completely normal, two-ventricle, fully repaired state to poorly compensated, palliated single-ventricle patients. These patients also often have other comorbidities, including genetic and dysmorphic syndromes, that present extracardiac challenges as well. The pediatric anesthesiologist needs to understand the pathophysiology of the major cardiac lesions, perform a focused preanesthetic evaluation, and devise an appropriate anesthetic plan that includes recovery from the procedure.

LEARNING OBJECTIVES

1. Describe major categories of CHD and understand the unrepaired, palliated, or repaired status in each.
2. Identify the 4 highest risk categories of CHD for noncardiac anesthetics.
3. Know the major considerations for a thorough preoperative evaluation for noncardiac procedures in patients with CHD.
4. Describe approach to the anesthetic plan, including postoperative intensive care unit (ICU) admissions.

CASE PRESENTATION

A 3-day-old, 3.2-kg full-term male presents for right thoracotomy for repair of esophageal atresia (EA) and tracheoesophageal fistula (TEF). He also has Trisomy 21 and a balanced complete atrioventricular canal. He does not have respiratory distress; chest radiograph reveals normal cardiac silhouette and normal lung fields. Room air peripheral capillary oxygen saturation (SpO_2) is 85%, and echocardiogram reveals normal-sized right and left ventricles with good systolic function, a common atrioventricular valve with mild left-sided regurgitation, a large inlet ventricular septal defect (VSD), primum atrial septal defect (ASD), and a small patent ductus arteriosus (PDA). Color Doppler indicates bidirectional shunting at the PDA, ASD, and VSD levels. Umbilical artery and vein catheters are in place and in good position.

Induction of anesthesia is accomplished with FiO_2 1.0 and sevoflurane inhalation, increasing inspired concentration to 5%; gentle manual assisted ventilation is well tolerated without gastric distension. Tracheal intubation is accomplished with direct laryngoscopy and a 3.5 mm ID uncuffed endotracheal tube, which is passed intentionally into the right mainstem bronchus and withdrawn slowly until the carina is identified by auscultation of bilateral breath sounds and secured 0.5 cm above the carina. Manual ventilation is accomplished with peak pressures of about 25 cm H_2O, and there is no gastric distension. After intubation the SpO_2 progressively decreases to 60% to 70%, and arterial blood gas reveals PaO_2 of

35 mmHg and PaCO2 of 55 mmHg. Inhaled nitric oxide (iNO) is started at 20 ppm, as well as low-dose epinephrine at 0.03 mcg/kg/min. SpO_2 gradually increases to 90% to 95% and PaO_2 to 55 mmHg; $PaCO_2$ decreases to 35 mmHg. The thoracotomy and repair of EA and TEF are performed without major ventilation issues; the TEF is about 1.5 cm above the carina and 2 mm in diameter. SpO_2 varies from 85% to 95%; mean arterial pressure is in the 40 to 50 range, and heart rate is 130 to 150. The patient remains intubated and is transferred to the neonatal ICU on epinephrine and iNO.

DISCUSSION

1. What are the major categories of CHD, and what are the considerations for unrepaired, palliated, and repaired CHD?

A functional classification of CHD is presented in Table 25.1. Two-ventricle CHD without obstruction to either outflow tract is common, with VSD, ASD, PDA with left-to-right shunting, and normal oxygen saturations the largest group. Depending on the size of the defect and the relative pressures/resistances of left and right heart, usually these patients will develop heart failure symptoms over time as pulmonary vascular resistance (PVR) decreases in the first months of life. Two-ventricle CHD with outflow tract obstruction is categorized as right-sided, as in pulmonary stenosis or tetralogy of Fallot, or left-sided, as in aortic stenosis. Right-sided obstruction can lead to right-to-left shunting and cyanosis. Left-sided obstruction, if severe, may result in left ventricular hypertrophy and coronary ischemia. Single-ventricle lesions without obstruction, such as tricuspid atresia, are by definition "mixing lesions" where blood return from the systemic and pulmonary circulations mixes in the single systemic ventricle, causing cyanosis. Unrestricted pulmonary blood flow, over time, will result first in congestive heart failure symptoms and then in fixed pulmonary hypertension and increasing cyanosis. Single-ventricle lesions with outflow tract obstruction often depend on a PDA for adequate pulmonary blood flow for right-sided obstruction or systemic blood flow for left-sided obstruction such as in hypoplastic left heart syndrome (HLHS).

TABLE 25.1. MAJOR CATEGORIES OF CHD

Category of CHD	Example
Two-ventricle, no outflow tract obstruction	ASD, VSD, PDA
Two-ventricle with outflow tract obstruction	Pulmonary: tetralogy of Fallot, Aortic: aortic stenosis
Single ventricle, no outflow tract obstruction	Tricuspid atresia without pulmonic stenosis
Single ventricle with outflow tract obstruction	Hypoplastic left heart syndrome

Note: CHD = congenital heart disease; ASD = atrial septal defect; VSD = ventricular septal defect; PDA = patent ductus arteriosus.

The major surgical classifications are unrepaired, palliated, and repaired. Examples of surgical stages in CHD correction are included in Table 25.2.

Unrepaired patients with CHD can range from asymptomatic with small VSD, ASD, or PDA, to severely affected physiology such as in unrepaired truncus arteriosus with truncal valve regurgitation, very low diastolic pressure, and coronary ischemia. Unrepaired patients generally are at highest risk for anesthetic complications. Palliation refers to cardiac surgery that does not correct the anatomy of the heart to a normal, two-ventricle circulation without residual shunting or mixing lesions. All single-ventricle patients by definition can only undergo palliation; they will never have a two-ventricle circulation. Prominent examples are superior cavopulmonary connection and Fontan completion for nearly all patients with a single functional right or left ventricle. Other common examples are pulmonary artery banding to restrict pulmonary blood flow or systemic to pulmonary artery shunts to provide pulmonary blood flow. The term "repaired" refers to anatomic correction to a two-ventricle state with no residual shunting defects and normal blood flow patterns. However, many patients, although undergoing corrective surgery, have residual defects that must be identified and understood. Examples are residual left-sided atrioventricular valve regurgitation, or residual aortic regurgitation, after repair of these valves.

2. What are the 4 highest risk categories of CHD for noncardiac anesthetics?

In large retrospective multicenter registry studies, 4 lesions stand out as highest risk: the shunt-dependent single-ventricle patient, severe left ventricular outflow tract obstruction, pulmonary hypertension at the systemic or suprasystemic level, and cardiomyopathy with severely depressed systemic ventricular function. The shunt-dependent single-ventricle

TABLE 25.2. EXAMPLES OF SURGICAL STAGES IN CHD CORRECTION

Unrepaired	Palliated	Repaired
Unoperated truncus arteriosus	Pulmonary artery banding in single ventricle anatomy	Complete repair of tetralogy of Fallot
Complete atrioventricular canal	Norwood stage I palliation for HLHS	Ross-Konno operation
HLHS	Bidirectional cavopulmonary anastomosis	TAPVR repair
TAPVR	Fontan completion (total cavopulmonary anastomosis)	Complete AV canal repair
Aortic stenosis	Systemic to pulmonary artery shunt for pulmonary atresia	Coarctation of aorta

Note: CHD = congenital heart disease; HLHS = hypoplastic left heart syndrome; TAPVR = total anomalous pulmonary venous return; AV = atrioventricular.

patient, such as after HLHS stage I palliation with a systemic to pulmonary artery shunt, has a delicate balance between the systemic and pulmonary circulations, which are arranged in series. Lowering PVR excessively, as with high FiO_2 and hyperventilation, shunts blood flow away from the systemic circulation and causes hypotension and coronary ischemia. Raising PVR acutely, such as with inadequate ventilation with hypoxemia and hypercarbia, increases right-to-left shunt and leads to progressive cyanosis. Left ventricular outflow tract obstruction, such as in sub-, valvar-, or supravalvar aortic stenosis, is exacerbated by systemic hypotension, as with high doses of volatile anesthetics, or hypovolemia. This can lead to coronary ischemia, which can be especially severe in Williams syndrome, which is an elastin gene defect that also involves coronary artery ostia. Pulmonary hypertension has a number of causes but is often seen in unrepaired cardiac lesions such as complete atrioventricular canal; the large increase in flow and pressure causes muscularization of the pulmonary arterioles, resulting eventually in right-to-left shunting. These patients often have very reactive pulmonary vascular beds that constrict severely to stimuli such as hypoxia, hypercarbia, acidosis, and catecholamine surge from inadequate anesthetic depth. Neonatal PVR is high in the first days of life; the stimuli noted here can lead to a reversion to transitional or fetal circulation; in the case of a complete atrioventricular canal, this can result in profound cyanosis. Suprasytemic pulmonary hypertension is considered the highest risk condition for anesthetic complications and is diagnosed by echocardiography (tricuspid regurgitation jet velocity, depressed right ventricular function, right ventricular dilation, right-to-left shift of the intraventricular septum) or cardiac catheterization. iNO has become the mainstay of treatment of an intraoperative pulmonary hypertensive crisis. Finally, dilated cardiomyopathy can be the result of CHD, viral myocarditis, chemotherapy, or familial cardiomyopathy. These patients also often have atrial and ventricular arrhythmias. Ejection fraction in the 10% to 20% range is often observed; left ventricular end-diastolic volume is huge, and stroke volume can be relatively maintained. However, any decrease in preload or sudden vasodilation is poorly tolerated.

3. What are the major considerations for a thorough preoperative evaluation for noncardiac procedures in patients with CHD?

A paradigm named "The Ten Fingers of CHD Diagnosis" can be very useful in systematically evaluating any patient with CHD for noncardiac surgery (Fig. 25.1). The first 5 are the classical elements used for many decades: History, Physical Exam, Chest Radiograph, Electrocardiogram (ECG), and Hemoglobin. The history reveals signs and symptoms of CHD, as well as surgical history and complications. Physical exam reveals cyanosis, murmurs, congestive heart failure, and sternotomy and thoracotomy scars and assess pulses and peripheral circulation. Chest radiograph assesses heart size and configuration and the state of the pulmonary vasculature: normal, oligemic as in decreased pulmonary blood flow, or hyperemic as in congestive heart failure. An ECG will diagnose arrhythmias, pacemaker function, chamber

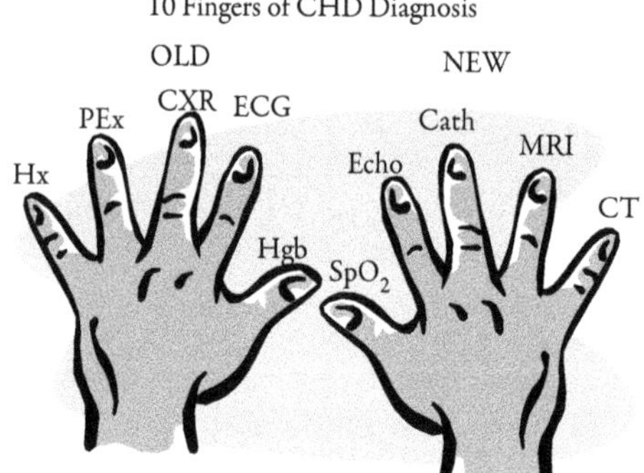

FIGURE 25.1: Hx, history; PEx, physical examination; CXR, chest radiograph; ECG, electrocardiogram; hgb, hemoglobin; SpO_2, peripheral oxygen saturation; echo, echocardiography; cath, cardiac catheterization; MRI, cardiac magnetic resonance imaging; CT, cardiac computed tomography. See text for explanation.

enlargement, and myocardial ischemia. Hemoglobin is elevated in cyanosis and the degree of elevation correlates with significant, chronic hypoxemia. The newer 5 elements are SpO_2, echocardiography, cardiac catheterization, and cardiac magnetic resonance imaging (MRI) and computed tomography (CT) scanning. Resting oxygen saturation accurately measures the degree of cyanosis—right-to-left shunting, or mixing. Echocardiography is the noninvasive mainstay of CHD diagnosis: anatomy and function, with newer high-resolution techniques including 3-dimensional echo greatly enhancing diagnostic tools and supplanting cardiac catheterization for pure anatomic diagnosis. Cardiac catheterization has been performed for over 60 years; in modern practice most catheterizations are for interventional procedures, but the anatomic information gained is invaluable. Pulmonary hypertension studies in the catheterization laboratory are instrumental to understand baseline state, response to therapy, and anesthetic risk. Cardiac MRI has evolved into a high-resolution diagnostic modality for anatomy but also function and can assess the myocardium, ejection fraction, shunt fraction, and regurgitant fraction. Modern multislice CT scanning can make accurate anatomic diagnoses of even tiny structures, and radiation exposure has been dramatically reduced with new technology and scanning sequences. The modern electronic medical record is invaluable to quickly access the data for the 10 Fingers of CHD approach and help practitioners rapidly understand the most important features when planning the anesthetic approach.

4. What is the best approach to the anesthetic plan, including postoperative ICU admissions?

Each patient's unique needs should be accounted for when planning, including the anatomy, pathophysiology, and effect of the surgical procedure. Thoroughly understanding the hemodynamic effects of anesthetic drugs and ventilatory maneuvers is a crucial component of the anesthetic plan. A useful approach is to construct a set of hemodynamic consequences resulting from the patient's pathophysiology and then a set of hemodynamic and ventilatory goals. An example for left ventricular outflow tract obstruction is presented in Table 25.3.

The need for invasive monitoring of arterial and central venous pressure, and secure access for inotropic infusions, varies significantly with the underlying anatomy and pathophysiology, invasive nature of the surgery and anticipated blood loss,

TABLE 25.3. HEMODYNAMIC CONSEQUENCES AND GOALS FOR LEFT-SIDED OBSTRUCTIVE LESIONS: AORTIC STENOSIS

Hemodynamic Consequences:
- Decreased blood pressure/systemic perfusion
- Decreased cardiac output
- Decreased coronary perfusion
- Left ventricular failure

Hemodynamic/Ventilatory Goals:

Parameter	**HR**	**Contractility**[a]	Preload[b]	SVR	PVR	FiO_2	$PaCO_2$
Goal	↓	↓	↑↑	↑↑	NC	NC	NC

Note: HR = heart rate; SVR = systemic vascular resistance; PVR = pulmonary vascular resistance; NC = no change.

[a]Do not decrease if depressed at baseline. [b]Do not increase with depressed baseline contractility with high preload.

and anticipated hemodynamic instability and need for inotropic support. Generally, the threshold for invasive monitoring is lower than for patients without CHD and should be considered when significant instability and intravascular volume shifts are anticipated. Blood transfusion goals also may be very different, especially in cyanotic CHD, where elevated hemoglobin is needed to increase oxygen-carrying capacity. Transfusion triggers are often considerably higher (i.e., at no lower than 30%–35% in patients whose baseline hematocrit is >40%). ICU admission should be discussed and planned preoperatively; it should not be decided upon mid-procedure. Patients with significant physiological derangements undergoing invasive surgery should be considered for ICU monitoring, even if extubated at the end of the case. Caregivers in the ICU need to be familiar with the pathophysiology of CHD, and a thorough handoff report must be given by the anesthesiologist and intraoperative team to the ICU team.

Infective endocarditis prophylaxis (IEP) is indicated only if the patient has a cardiac condition that warrants IEP and is undergoing a surgical procedure that warrants IEP. Major categories of cardiac indications for IEP are prosthetic cardiac valve, previous IE, CHD: cyanotic unrepaired, completely repaired with patch or prosthetic material for 6 months after procedure, repaired CHD with residual defects, and heart transplant with valvulopathy. Surgical procedures where IEP is indicated are dental procedures, procedures where respiratory or gastrointestinal mucosal barriers are disrupted, (i.e. tonsillectomy), and procedures on infected skin or musculoskeletal tissue. IEP is not recommended for simple bronchoscopy, laryngoscopy, gastrointestinal tract endoscopy, or cystoscopy.

Pacemakers and defibrillators are increasingly implanted in patients with CHD, and indications for their implantation must be understood, as well as the patient's underlying cardiac rhythm and functioning of the device. Whenever possible, evaluation and advice from an expert (i.e., cardiologist or pacemaker manufacturer's representative) should be sought before anesthesia. Electrocautery often interferes with pacemaker functioning, and the mode of the device may need to be converted to asynchronous pacing only for the operating room period. Defibrillators also may be activated unintentionally, and this function often needs to be turned off for the operating room period.

SUMMARY

1. CHD patients are increasingly presenting for noncardiac surgery, and the anesthesiologist must possess an understanding of the major classes of CHD and their pathophysiology, as well as surgical approaches for correction or palliation.
2. A thorough preoperative evaluation and anesthetic plan, including invasive monitoring, inotropic support, blood transfusion, endocarditis prophylaxis, pacemaker/defibrillator functioning, and ICU admission, must be developed, and include a multidisciplinary team. Each patient has a unique pathophysiology and a systematic approach to understanding hemodynamic consequences, and developing hemodynamic goals for the anesthetic will improve the potential to minimize anesthetic complications and ensure the best possible outcomes.

BIBLIOGRAPHY

American Society of Anesthesiologists. Practice advisory for the perioperative management of patients with cardiac implantable electronic devices: pacemakers and implantable cardioverter-defibrillators: an updated report by the American Society of Anesthesiologists Task Force on Perioperative Management of Patients with Cardiac Implantable Electronic Devices. *Anesthesiology*. 2011;114:247–261.

Andropoulos DB, Gottlieb EA. Congenital heart disease. In: Fleisher LA, ed. *Anesthesia and Uncommon Diseases*. 6th ed. Philadelphia: Elsevier; 2012:75–136.

Gottlieb EA, Andropoulos DB. Anesthesia for the patient with congenital heart disease presenting for noncardiac surgery. *Curr Opin Anaesthesiol*. 2013;26:318–326.

Gottlieb EA, Stayer SA. Anesthesia for non-cardiac surgery and magnetic resonance imaging. In: Andropoulos DB, Stayer SA, Mossad EB, Miller-Hance WH, eds. *Anesthesia for Congenital Heart Disease*. 3rd ed. Oxford: Wiley; 2015:705–719.

Ramamoorthy C, Haberkern CM, Bhananker SM, et al. Anesthesia-related cardiac arrest in children with heart disease: data from the Pediatric Perioperative Cardiac Arrest (POCA) registry. *Anesth Analg*. 2010;110:1376–1382.

Society of Thoracic Surgeons Congenital Heart Surgery Database. 2017. http://www.sts.org/national-database/database-managers/congenital-heart-surgery-databas

Wilson W, Taubert KA, Gewitz M, et al. Prevention of infective endocarditis: guidelines from the American

Heart Association: a guideline from the American Heart Association Rheumatic Fever, Endocarditis, and Kawasaki Disease Committee, Council on Cardiovascular Disease in the Young, and the Council on Clinical Cardiology, Council on Cardiovascular Surgery and Anesthesia, and the Quality of Care and Outcomes Research Interdisciplinary Working Group. *Circulation*. 2007;116:1736–1754.

26

Single-Ventricle Physiology

ERIN A. GOTTLIEB AND DAVID F. VENER

INTRODUCTION

Single-ventricle palliation is now a common pathway for a wide variety of congenital heart defects, including hypoplastic left heart syndrome (HLHS), double inlet left ventricle, double outlet right ventricle, tricuspid atresia, unbalanced forms of atrioventricular canal defects, and others. The surgical palliation of these defects takes place over a series of operations that typically occur in 2 to 3 stages over a 4- to 5-year period, depending upon the defect and the patient's physiologic status.

Pediatric anesthesiologists may be asked to care for these children at any stage of single-ventricle palliation for various elective noncardiac procedures including gastrostomy tube placement, Ladd's procedure, and radiologic imaging, as well as other common pediatric surgeries, both elective and emergent (e.g., appendectomy). Failure to appreciate this physiology and the impact of anesthesia may lead to cardiovascular collapse and patient injury or death. Multiple studies have shown that children with underlying congenital heart defects, particularly single-ventricle defects, have among the highest incidence of cardiac arrest and death during the perianesthetic period (Ramamoorthy et al., 2010).

Depending upon the staging, pulmonary blood flow will be supplied by a shunt from a systemic artery, a conduit from the systemic ventricle, the systemic ventricle into the native pulmonary artery with a band restricting pulmonary arterial flow, or passive flow from the systemic venous system. Appropriate management of the patient requires a clear understanding of the source of pulmonary blood flow and the functional status of the single ventricle, as well as the common problems associated with single-ventricle physiology. There are terms related to congenital heart disease that all practicing pediatric anesthesiologists should be familiar with in order to understand the current functional anatomy of their patients. At a minimum, these include modified Blalock-Taussig shunt (MBTS), right ventricle to pulmonary artery conduit (RV-PA conduit, Sano shunt), bidirectional Glenn (BDG), and Fontan circulation.

LEARNING OBJECTIVES

1. Understand the anatomy and physiology of each stage of single-ventricle palliation.
2. Become familiar with the ventilation and oxygenation strategy for each stage of single-ventricle palliation.
3. Recognize the risks associated with anesthetizing the single-ventricle patient with a modified Blalock-Taussig shunt.
4. Discuss the rationale for performing elective noncardiac surgery during the Glenn stage of the single-ventricle pathway.
5. Describe the effects of positive-pressure ventilation on the patient with Fontan physiology.
6. Formulate a perioperative plan for caring for single-ventricle patients undergoing noncardiac procedures.

CASE PRESENTATION

A 7-week-old, 4.0 kg male infant with HLHS who has undergone a Norwood operation with placement of a right MBTS presents for placement of a gastrostomy tube due to poor weight gain. The infant is an inpatient. He takes enalapril and aspirin, and his vital signs are as follows:

Heart rate: 138

Noninvasive blood pressure: 73/28

Temperature: 37.1°C

SpO_2: 89% on room air

Physical exam is remarkable for a continuous murmur in the right upper sternal border. He has a single lumen peripherally inserted central catheter in the right lower extremity and a 24-gauge peripheral intravenous (IV) line in his left hand. Transthoracic echo shows features of HLHS with a mildly dilated right ventricle with mild depression in systolic function, minimal atrioventricular valve (AVV) regurgitation, and a patent right MBTS. He has a preoperative hematocrit of 32%. The patient has been nil per os (NPO) for breast milk for 4 hours and is receiving maintenance IV fluids.

DISCUSSION

1. What is HLHS, and what does stage I palliation/the Norwood operation involve?

Patients with HLHS present either prenatally or in the immediate newborn period. These patients have a single right ventricle and a hypoplastic left ventricle. The different variations of left ventricular hypoplasia are aortic valve atresia (no prograde flow across the aortic valve), severe aortic stenosis, mitral atresia or severe mitral stenosis, or a combination of these defects along with a diminutive ascending aorta. The right ventricle supports both pulmonary blood flow through the pulmonary outflow tract and systemic blood flow through the patent ductus arteriosus (PDA) (Fig. 26.1), potentially including retrograde flow into the coronary arteries. Normal physiologic closure of the PDA in the hours after birth results in rapid hemodynamic collapse and death due to loss of systemic and coronary perfusion; for this reason, a prostaglandin E_1 infusion is immediately started after delivery or postnatal diagnosis to prevent or reverse duct closure. The neonate then undergoes stage I palliation, most commonly the Norwood operation or one of its variants, or the hybrid procedure for HLHS. This operation is generally performed by day of life 5. The "Hybrid" is a newer technique which

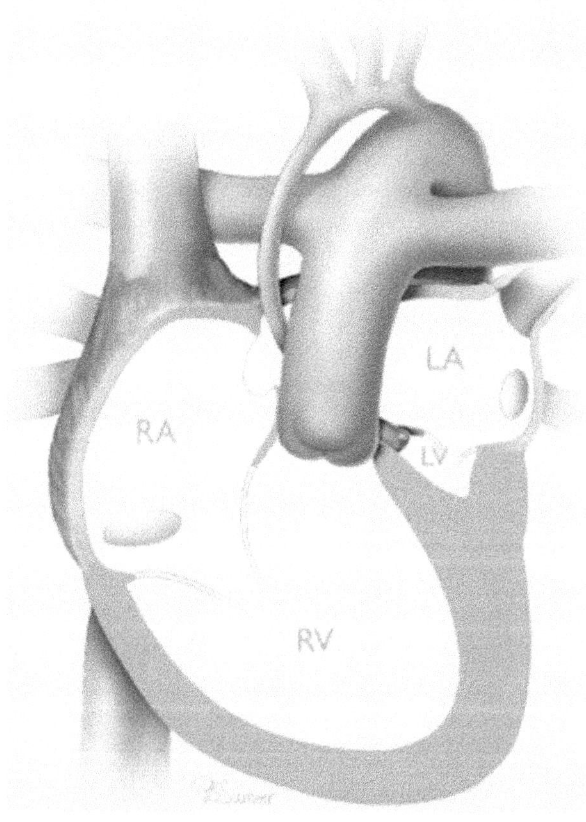

FIGURE 26.1: HLHS (CHS 111409).

combines placement of a stent into the ductus arteriosus to prevent closure combined with bilateral pulmonary artery banding to prevent excess pulmonary blood flow and augment systemic blood flow through the stented ductus arteriosus. Its use is variable depending upon center preference and patient anatomy.

Norwood stage I palliation consists of the creation of a neoaorta using the native pulmonary outflow tract, an atrial septectomy to create an unobstructed route for pulmonary venous flow from the left atrium to the right atrium and right ventricle, ligation and division of the PDA, and the creation of a stable source of pulmonary blood flow. Pulmonary blood flow can either be supplied via a MBTS (Fig. 26.2) from the right innominate or subclavian artery to the right pulmonary artery or a RV-PA conduit (Fig. 26.3). The choice of the source of pulmonary blood flow, shunt versus RV-PA conduit, is surgeon and institution specific as there does not appear to be any mortality benefit long term for one source versus the other.

2. What is the physiology of a shunted single ventricle? What are the risks associated with anesthetizing this type of patient for a noncardiac procedure?

A patient with a MBTS has a 3.5 or 4 mm GORE-TEX® tube graft from the right subclavian or innominate artery to the pulmonary artery. This shunt provides systemic arterial blood into the pulmonary circuit throughout the cardiac cycle. The continuous flow through the shunt can lead to coronary hypoperfusion and ischemia due to preferential diastolic runoff through the shunt into the low-resistance pulmonary circuit away from the systemic circulation. Evidence of this phenomenon includes low diastolic blood pressure and electrocardiographic evidence of ischemia (ST segment changes). In addition to the potential for coronary ischemia, the right ventricle is significantly volume loaded, supporting both systemic and pulmonary blood flow.

The balance between systemic and pulmonary blood flow is influenced by the systemic vascular resistance (SVR), the pulmonary vascular resistance (PVR), the hematocrit, and the size and location

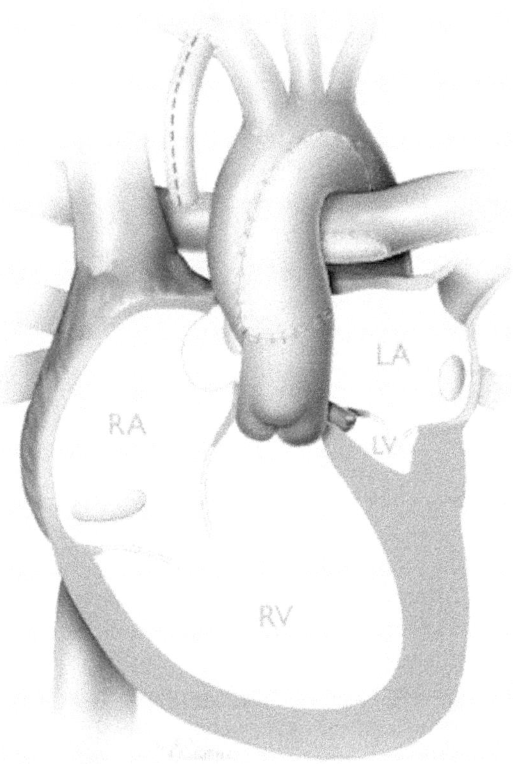

FIGURE 26.2: MBTS (CHS 111405).

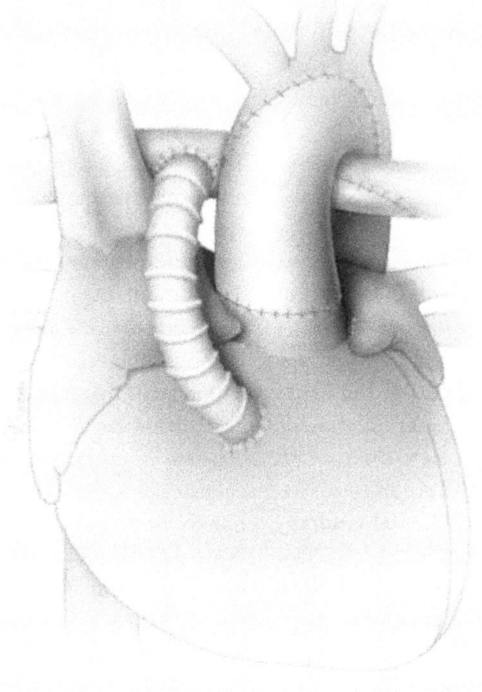

FIGURE 26.3: RV to PA conduit (CHS 111405, 111406).

of the MBTS. The size and location of the shunt are fixed. Larger and shorter shunts will have more flow through them, as do more proximal shunts. Hematocrit has an effect on blood viscosity. A lower hematocrit is associated with lower viscosity of blood and more flow through the shunt. Manipulation of the PVR is the main strategy for increasing or decreasing pulmonary blood flow. Increasing PVR decreases relative flow through the shunt into the pulmonary vascular bed, and decreasing PVR increases flow through the shunt. Strategies for increasing and decreasing PVR can be found in Table 26.1.

Shunted single-ventricle patients have delicate physiologies, placing them at increased risk of morbidity and mortality when undergoing anesthesia for cardiac and noncardiac surgery. The combination of an anesthetic-related decrease in SVR, hypovolemia, and diastolic runoff from a relatively large MBTS can quickly result in coronary ischemia, decreased cardiac output, and cardiac arrest. In addition, the MBTS can also become acutely occluded, leading to hypoxemia, decreased cardiac output, and cardiac arrest. Constant vigilance and early recognition of these conditions is critical to avoiding morbidity and mortality in this patient population (Holtby, 2014).

TABLE 26.1. MECHANISMS FOR PVR MANIPULATION

Actions to Decrease PVR	Actions to Increase PVR
Increase FiO_2	Decrease FiO_2
Decrease $PaCO_2$	Increase $PaCO_2$
Optimize ventilation (decrease atelectasis, lower airway pressures)	Mechanical (pulmonary artery banding)
Medications (nitric oxide, PGE-5 inhibitors)	

Note: PVR = pulmonary vascular resistance.

3. How can one evaluate a shunted single ventricle such as this one for this type of case?

Shunted single-ventricle patients are closely followed by their cardiologists, and a review of their most recent visit at a minimum is important to understand the patient's current status. Unless the procedure is an emergency, a perioperative consultation with the cardiology team is generally prudent.

It is crucial to get an idea of the amount of flow through the shunt preoperatively. Higher baseline oxygen saturations (i.e., greater than 88%) may suggest this. In addition, knowledge of the size of the shunt and its relative position can give more information. Lower than age-appropriate diastolic blood pressures may indicate higher flow through the shunt. In patients with a large amount of flow through the shunt, intraoperative instability can be predicted, and preparations, including the intraoperative availability of vasoactive medications such as epinephrine and vasopressin, should be made.

It is important to appreciate how the systemic ventricle is handling the volume and pressure loads preoperatively. If the ventricle is dilated and function is depressed, inotropic support with either epinephrine or dopamine should be immediately available. Some practitioners advocate the administration of a low-dose prophylactic epinephrine infusion (0.01–0.02 mcg/kg/min) prior to induction to maintain optimal hemodynamics during this dangerous period. Additionally, arrhythmias are very poorly tolerated in this population, as the loss of atrial "kick" may significantly worsen cardiac output and elevate atrial pressures. Appropriately sized equipment for defibrillation should be readily available.

The optimal hematocrit for a shunted single ventricle maximizes oxygen-carrying capacity while not overly increasing blood viscosity. This balance is typically thought to be in the 40% to 45% range. Relative anemia decreases oxygen-carrying capacity and increases shunt flow through a decrease in viscosity. Too high of hematocrit, however, can increase viscosity to the point of being thrombogenic. Most shunt-dependent patients are on some form of anticoagulant such as aspirin to minimize the risk of shunt thrombosis. Patients may be transfused preoperatively, and blood should be available in the operating room if the hematocrit needs to be further optimized.

Prolonged fasting without IV fluids should also be avoided in these patients. Many shunted patients undergoing noncardiac surgery are admitted preoperatively for IV hydration while NPO. If the patient is not admitted for preoperative hydration, clear fluids should be encouraged until 2 hours prior to the procedure. Hypovolemia is poorly tolerated in these patients, and cardiac arrest can occur solely due to poor oral intake (Brown et al., 2007; Stockton et al., 2012).

Invasive monitoring of arterial blood pressure should be strongly considered depending upon patient status, the projected length of surgery, the possibility of blood loss, and whether the surgical procedure might impact cardiac and pulmonary hemodynamics such as laparoscopy with CO_2 insufflation.

4. What is the preoperative status of this single-ventricle patient with a shunt? What preoperative preparations should be considered, and what is the best approach to induction, ventilation, and oxygenation?

This patient with HLHS who has undergone a Norwood operation with MBTS placement is scheduled for a gastrostomy tube placement. On transthoracic echocardiography, his cardiac function is reasonable; his systemic right ventricle is mildly depressed and mildly dilated with minimal AVV regurgitation. It is not uncommon for a single right ventricle that is handling both the pulmonary and systemic blood flow to have some mild ventricular dysfunction. He has adequate flow through the MBTS; in fact, one would infer that his pulmonary blood flow might be somewhat generous, as his room air oxygen saturation is in the high 80s and his diastolic blood pressure is relatively low.

To avoid hypovolemia, this patient has a peripheral IV and is receiving maintenance fluids while NPO. His preoperative hematocrit is 32%, however, which is low for a cyanotic single ventricle. The anemia could be a result of a combination of physiologic nadir, insufficient iron intake, and the effect of multiple blood samples. Ideally, this patient should be transfused preoperatively to a hematocrit of 40% to 45% over the course of 1 to 2 days to avoid acute volume overload. Alternatively, he could be transfused in the operating room after induction, depending on the comfort of the anesthesiologist, with careful monitoring of his relative volume status. Many of these patients are on chronic diuretic therapy, and preoperative electrolyte evaluation is an additional important consideration.

Preoperatively, vasoactive medications (e.g., epinephrine and vasopressin infusions) should be prepared, and blood products should be in the room. An intensive care unit bed should be strongly considered for postoperative recovery. A defibrillator and appropriately sized pads should also be available. It is also reasonable to let the surgeons and operating room staff know that the patient is at particularly high risk for anesthesia-related morbidity and mortality; the team should be focused, and distractions should be kept to a minimum.

The goal of induction should be to anesthetize the patient without a large drop in SVR or myocardial function. This can be accomplished in a number of ways and with different pharmacologic agents, including narcotics, ketamine, and judicious use of volatile agents. Induction with a bolus of propofol or a high concentration of sevoflurane is best avoided. The effects of hyperventilation and high FiO_2 should be considered throughout this period. Mask ventilation with a high FiO_2 and high minute ventilation can quickly lead to a decrease in PVR and increased shunt flow, leading to diastolic runoff and coronary ischemia. This spiral of events can quickly lead to cardiac arrest. The oxygen saturation should be a rough guide to shunt flow, and PVR may be manipulated by adjustments in FiO_2 and minute ventilation (Table 26.1). After induction and intubation, the FiO_2 should be decreased to room air as tolerated, to avoid a dangerous drop in PVR. The goal oxygen saturation should be approximately 85%, which would indicate an appropriate balance between SVR and PVR. Near-infrared spectroscopy monitoring through induction in this case is strongly suggested, as it typically has a much faster response time to critical changes than relying solely on pulse oximetry, which may lag by as much as 45 seconds or more, is less accurate at lower saturations, and relies on adequate pulse perfusion. Loss of pulse oximetry where previously present should immediately be a cause for concern and addressed; changing out probes and locations and "blaming" the equipment can lose valuable seconds.

5. What is the anatomy and physiology of the Glenn circulation? What is the rationale for performing elective noncardiac surgery at this stage of single-ventricle palliation?

The bidirectional cavopulmonary anastomosis or Glenn operation is the second stage of single-ventricle palliation and is generally performed after approximately 3 months of age. The MBTS or RV-PA conduit is taken down, and the superior vena cava is anastomosed to the pulmonary artery (Fig. 26.4). Blood from the inferior vena cava still returns to the right atrium where it mixes with pulmonary venous blood. Oxygenation relies on passive pulmonary blood flow from the superior vena cava. In centers performing the hybrid procedure, this second stage is also the period where the neoaorta is constructed out of the pulmonary artery, the comprehensive stage II procedure for HLHS, sometimes referred to as the "Glenn-Wood."

A successful Glenn circulation is always preferable to the shunted circulation and relies on low to normal PVR. The takedown of the shunt removes the threat of diastolic runoff and resulting coronary ischemia. It also relieves the volume burden from the systemic ventricle. The patient still remains cyanotic with a predicted oxygen saturation of around 85%. It also has the advantage of preserving cardiac output in the event of an increase in PVR, unlike the Fontan circulation (see later discussion), due to the venous return to the heart via the inferior vena cava. It is because of the relative stability of this stage that elective procedures are frequently postponed until after the Glenn. This patient, however, is in the catch-22 of needing sufficient caloric intake to grow to an appropriate age and weight to undergo the bidirectional Glenn procedure.

6. Describe the anatomy and physiology of the Fontan circulation, the complications associated with Fontan physiology, and the effects of positive pressure on the patient with a Fontan circulation

The third stage of single-ventricle palliation is the Fontan procedure where the inferior vena cava is connected to the pulmonary artery with either an "extra-cardiac" GORE-TEX® conduit (Fig. 26.5) or an intracardiac baffle separating systemic venous blood from the arterial circulation and routing up to the pulmonary artery (a "lateral tunnel"). In this circulation, all systemic venous blood passively enters the pulmonary arteries where it is oxygenated and returns to the heart via the pulmonary veins. This circulation relies on adequate preload, normal or low PVR, and low atrial pressure to facilitate blood flow across the pulmonary bed. The oxygen saturation of a patient with a completed Fontan is expected to be close to 100%. Occasionally, a fenestration between the venous return and the atrium is made so that in the event of high PVR, systemic venous blood can return to the heart and augment cardiac output. Fenestrations are generally placed in situations where the patient has relatively high baseline PVR or atrial pressure, though some institutions will utilize a fenestrated Fontan as a matter of routine. Patients with a fenestrated Fontan will have an oxygen saturation close to 100% when there is no blood moving across the fenestration but a lower oxygen saturation when blood is moving across the fenestration and bypassing the pulmonary bed. A fenestration can help to maintain cardiac output in the event of unfavorable physiology at the expense of oxygen saturation. However, the fenestration may also serve

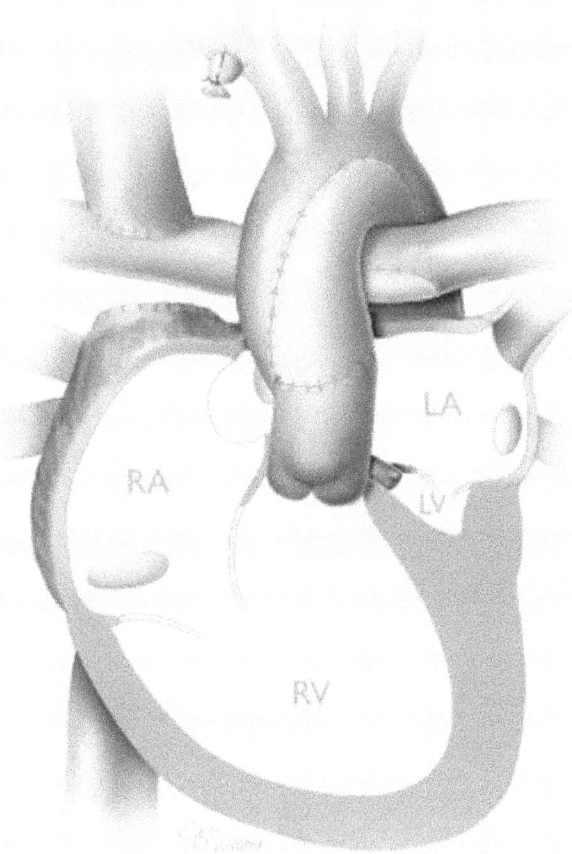

FIGURE 26.4: Glenn (CHS 111407).

as a site for right-to-left shunting. Air and thrombi may potentially cross the fenestration, entering into the systemic arterial circulation.

Complications arising in patients with a Fontan circulation include protein-losing enteropathy, hepatic congestion and dysfunction, pleural effusions, and plastic bronchitis. Presence of these complications may alter anesthetic management and should be considered when formulating an anesthetic plan (Christensen et al., 2012).

The switch from spontaneous ventilation to positive-pressure ventilation in the patient with a Fontan may be poorly tolerated, and a potential decrease in cardiac output should be anticipated. Volume administration and low-dose vasoconstrictor or inotrope administration can be helpful in maintaining central venous pressure and cardiac output. Some advocate maintenance of spontaneous ventilation to avoid the negative effect of positive-pressure ventilation on PVR and the beneficial effects on venous return of negative intrathoracic pressure "drawing in" venous blood. However, care should be taken to avoid hypoventilation, hypercarbia, and a resultant increase in PVR.

7. What are the steps for formulating a perioperative plan for single-ventricle patients undergoing noncardiac procedures?

Preparation for anesthesia for a single-ventricle patient begins preoperatively. First, a multidisciplinary discussion should take place regarding the risks and benefits of the timing of the noncardiac procedure. For example, completely elective procedures should generally not be done on the shunted patient. These procedures should wait for the relatively more stable patient with a Glenn circulation.

Plans for preoperative fasting and hydration should also be considered. Patients for whom hypovolemia may not be tolerated (e.g., shunted single ventricle) should always be scheduled early in the day to minimize NPO time, and clear fluids should

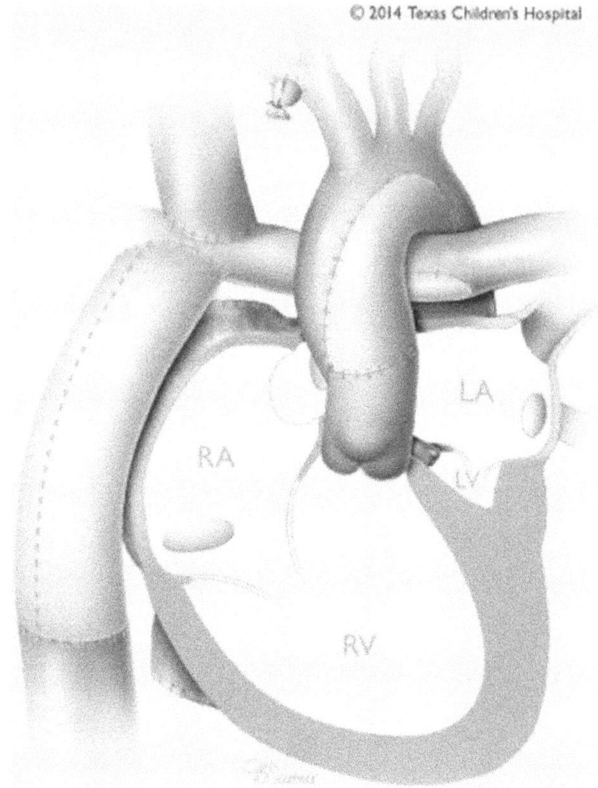

FIGURE 26.5: Fontan (CHS 111408).

be encouraged until 2 hours prior to the procedure. In addition, preoperative admission and IV hydration is encouraged to avoid hypovolemia, especially in shunted single-ventricle patients and regardless of the procedure being performed. For cardiac magnetic resonance imaging, for example, it is routine at some centers to admit the patient the night before the procedure for IV fluids and possible heparin infusion to avoid instability due to hypovolemia and shunt thrombosis (Brown et al., 2007; Stockton et al., 2012).

Preoperative preparation should also include the plan for postoperative recovery. These complex patients with fragile physiology are rarely suitable for same-day discharge. Overnight observation may be more appropriate. When single-ventricle patients undergo noncardiac procedures, observation in the intensive care unit is often warranted, and an intensive care unit bed should be reserved prior to anesthetic care.

Intraoperative instability should be anticipated when caring for these patients. Inotropic and vasopressor support should be readily available in the operating room and appropriate emergency medications and doses reviewed and available. Blood products should be in the operating room, and a defibrillator and appropriately sized pads should be present. Invasive monitors may be indicated if the patient is at high risk for instability and to guide vasoactive administration.

SUMMARY

1. Pediatric anesthesiologists should have a basic knowledge of anatomy and physiology of the 3 stages of single ventricle palliation.
2. Preoperative assessment should include the stage of palliation, the functional condition of the single ventricle, the preoperative volume status of the patient, and laboratory values including hematocrit.
3. Hemodynamic instability should be anticipated in shunted single-ventricle patients, and preparations should be made to manage it in advance.
4. Care must be taken to avoid decreases in PVR in shunted patients as a decrease in PVR can lead to diastolic runoff, coronary ischemia, and cardiac arrest.

5. Shunted single-ventricle patients are at high risk for anesthetic morbidity and mortality. Purely elective procedures should be postponed until after the Glenn operation.
6. The 3 stages of single ventricle palliation are quite different physiologically, and the pediatric anesthesiologist should understand the basic approach to anesthesia for each stage.

ACKNOWLEDGMENT

The authors wish to acknowledge the first edition author, Dr. Ian McKenzie.

ANNOTATED REFERENCES

Christensen RE, Gholami AS, Reynold PI, Malviya S. Anaesthetic management and outcomes after noncardiac surgery in patients with hypoplastic left heart syndrome: a retrospective review. *Eur J Anaesthesiol.* 2012;29:425–430.

An extensive review of the physiology of all stages of single-ventricle palliation undergoing noncardiac surgery.

Holtby HM. Anesthetic considerations for neonates undergoing modified Blalock-Taussig shunt and variations. *Pediatr Anesth.* 2014;24:114–119.

A complete review of shunt physiology focusing on the perioperative management of patients for shunt placement and the fragile physiology of the patient with a shunt.

Ohye RG, Sleeper LA, Mahony L, et al. Comparison of shunt types in the Norwood procedure for single-ventricle lesions. *N Engl J Med.* 2010;362:1980–1992.

An excellent description of stage I palliation and the 2 options for sources of pulmonary blood flow.

BIBLIOGRAPHY

Brown DW, Gauvreau K, Powell AJ, et al. Cardiac magnetic resonance versus routine cardiac catheterization before bidirectional Glenn anastomosis in infants with functional single ventricle. *Circulation.* 2007;116:2718–2725.

Ramamoorthy C, Haberkern CM, Bhananker SM, et al. Anesthesia-related cardiac arrest in children with heart disease: data from the Pediatric Perioperative Cardiac Arrest (POCA) Registry. *Anesth Analg.* 2010;110:1376–1382.

Stockton E, Hughes M, Broadhead M, et al. A prospective audit of safety issues associated with general anesthesia for pediatric cardiac magnetic resonance imaging. *Pediatr Anesth.* 2012;22:1087–1093.

27

Tetralogy of Fallot

PREMAL M. TRIVEDI AND PABLO MOTTA

INTRODUCTION

Tetralogy of Fallot (TOF) is the most common cause of the cyanotic congenital heart disease, affecting 3 to 6 infants per 10,000 live births. Due to its frequent association with syndromes and other anomalies, surgical intervention and anesthesia may be needed prior to a complete repair. Anesthetic management in such situations is predicated on knowledge of the basic anatomy and pathophysiology of this lesion and what factors can exacerbate or improve the patient's hemodynamics. This chapter reviews these concerns as well as provides additional detail regarding unique anatomic variants of tetralogy, the management of a "TET spell," and considerations in the individual presenting following palliation as well as complete repair.

LEARNING OBJECTIVES

1. Identify the anatomic features of TOF and its variants.
2. Discuss the different and evolving clinical presentations that can be encountered depending on the patient's anatomy.
3. Recognize the risk factors for the development of a TET spell, and cite the steps in its management.
4. Apply knowledge of the anatomy, pathophysiology, and associated syndromes of TOF to develop a perioperative plan for noncardiac surgery.

CASE PRESENTATION

A-4-day-old term neonate presents with imperforate anus, malrotation of the intestine, and duodenal atresia necessitating urgent surgical repair. Prenatally, the patient was also diagnosed with TOF, confirmed postnatally by transthoracic echocardiography demonstrating an overriding aorta, ventricular septal defect, and pulmonary stenosis (V Max 2.49 m/sec, peak gradient 24.9 mmHg) (Figs. 27.1, 27.2, and 27.3). *On physical exam, the patient is cyanotic with saturations in the 80s on room air and has a distended abdomen despite having a nasogastric tube in place. The patient has been nil per os (NPO) since birth and has one 24-g peripheral intravenous line as well as a neonatal peripherally inserted central catheter with total parenteral nutrition (TPN) and lipids infusing. The labs are within normal limits with the exception of relative anemia (H/H of 14.9 g/dl and 41.9%, respectively). Blood has been made available for surgery.*

Following communication with cardiology, surgery, and neonatology, the patient is brought to the operating room. Standard monitors are applied and a modified rapid sequence induction is performed with midazolam, fentanyl, and rocuronium. Induction and intubation are well-tolerated. An arterial line is placed subsequently and an additional peripheral IV is added. TPN is continued to maintain normoglycemia, and a manifold is added as an entry point for vasoactive infusions.

As surgery begins, the patient becomes progressively tachycardic, hypotensive, and desaturates to the lower 70s despite unchanged lung compliance. Temporizing measures include increasing ***FiO_2 to 1.0****, deepening the anesthetic using additional doses of* ***fentanyl****, giving* ***volume*** *(10 cc/kg of crystalloid), and increasing the systemic vascular resistance (SVR) with* ***phenylephrine****. While the hemodynamics and saturations improve with these interventions, the response is only temporary. A* ***vasopressin*** *infusion is started to maintain SVR and an arterial blood gas is checked to assess the hemoglobin level. The H/H results are 12 g/dl and 35%. Transfusion is thus initiated to improve oxygen-carrying capacity as well as to increase preload to the right ventricle. The remainder of the procedure proceeds uneventfully, and the patient is taken to the neonatal intensive care unit intubated and on a low-dose vasopressin infusion for postoperative care.*

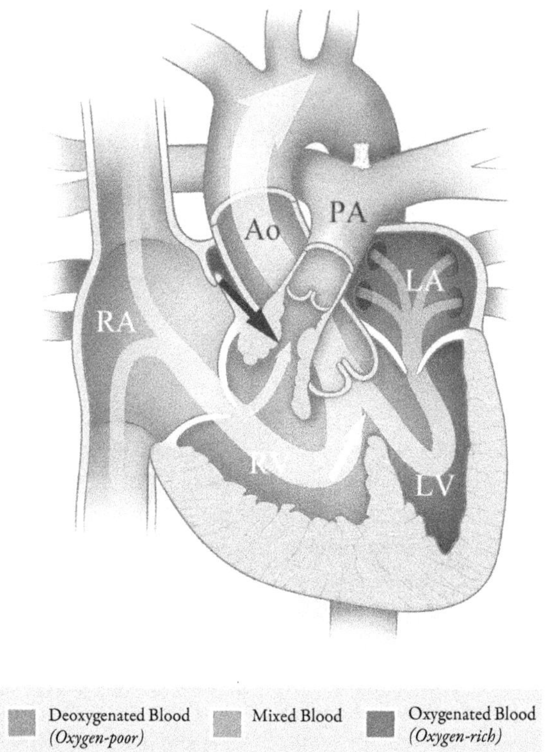

FIGURE 27.1: Color illustration of tetralogy of Fallot showing the right ventricular hypertrophy, ventricular septal defect (white arrow), overriding aorta, and right ventricular outflow stenosis (black arrow). RA, right atrium; RV, right ventricle; LA, left atrium; LV, left ventricle; Ao, aorta; PA, pulmonary artery.

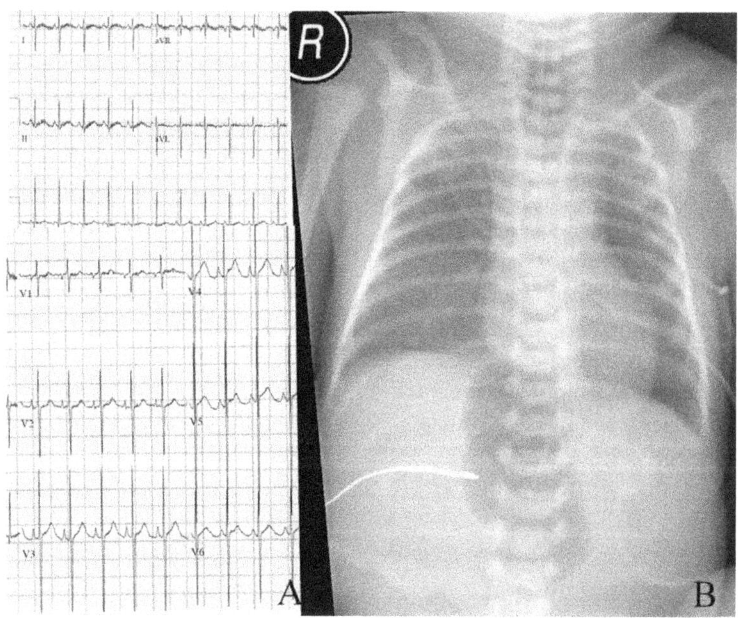

FIGURE 27.2: A. **EKG** shows a normal sinus rhythm with right axis deviation and right ventricular hyperthrophy. B. **Antero-posterior chest X-ray** shows a "boot shape" cardiac silhouette with pulmonary oligemia. The abdomen shows gaseous distention of the stomach abnormally positioned in the midline of the upper abdomen. The distal tip of an enteric tube is visualized in the stomach.

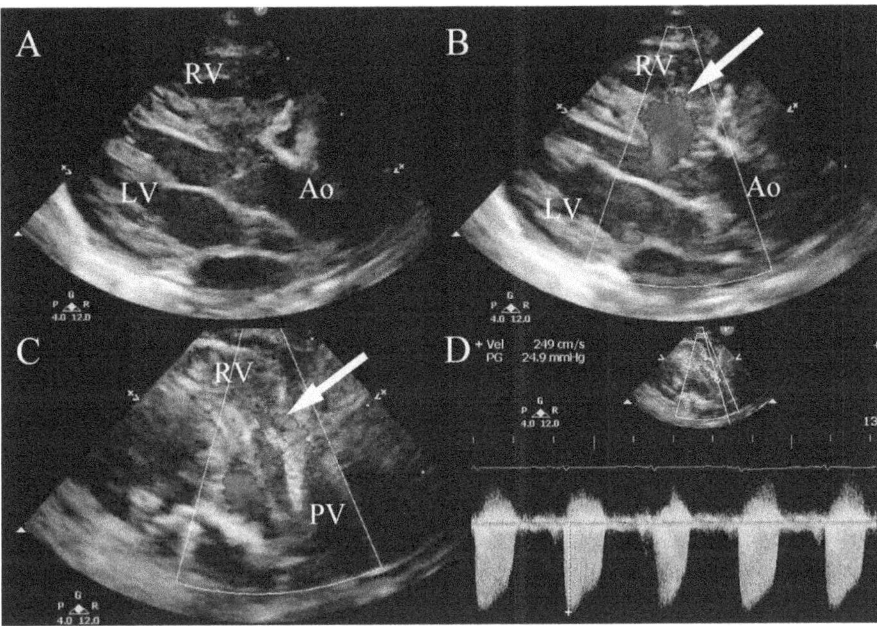

FIGURE 27.3: Preoperative transthoracic echocardiography images. A. Parasternal long axis view showing the right ventricular hypertrophy ventricular septal defect and overriding aorta. B. Color flow Doppler of the parasternal long axis illustrating the ventricular septal defect (white arrow) and the right-to-left shunt (dark gray flow). C. Parasternal long axis view sweep to show the pulmonary outflow tract (white arrow) showing flow acceleration through the right ventricular outflow tract and pulmonary valve (light gray turbulent flow). D. In the same window continuous wave Doppler shows the acceleration at the right ventricular outflow tract with a peak velocity of 2.49 m/sec and a peak gradient of 24.9 mmHg at rest.

DISCUSSION

1. What are the anatomic features of TOF?

The hallmarks of Fallot's tetralogy include (i) a large, unrestrictive ventricular septal defect (VSD); (ii) narrowing or atresia of the pulmonary outflow; (iii) aortic override of the VSD and right ventricle; and (iv) right ventricular hypertrophy that develops in response to the outflow tract obstruction (Fig. 27.1).

2. Where in the right ventricular outflow tract can obstruction occur?

While some amount of obstruction is almost always present at the subvalvar level, both the valvar and supravalvar levels of the right ventricular outflow tract can also contribute to the stenosis observed in tetralogy. At the subvalvar level, narrowing is due to both to an anterior deviation of the infundibular septum and prominent muscle bands that hypertrophy secondary to an increased afterload. Abnormalities of the pulmonary valve or hypoplasia of the pulmonary annulus account for obstruction at the valvar level. Above the valve, stenosis or diffuse hypoplasia can occur at the main pulmonary trunk and/or the branch pulmonary arteries.

3. Can obstruction worsen over time?

Yes. This **dynamic** component of obstruction is attributed to the progressive hypertrophy of muscular bands within the right ventricle. Exposure to the **fixed obstruction** at the valvar and supravalvar levels provides the stimulus for hypertrophy, and so a patient who may not have been symptomatic early in life may become symptomatic only months later.

4. How does this anatomy lead to the observed pathophysiology?

The combination of multilevel obstruction to pulmonary blood flow and a large ventricular septal defect can result in **right-to-left shunting** with subsequent **cyanosis**. The extent of cyanosis is dictated by the severity of obstruction present and whether or not the child continues to have a patent ductus arteriosus (PDA). An infant with severe stenosis and a closed ductus would have limited pulmonary blood flow and would thus be markedly cyanotic. On the other hand, a patient with only minimal pulmonary stenosis could behave as a child with pulmonary overcirculation due to predominantly left-to-right shunting across the VSD. Such a patient would be normally saturated and could also be in heart failure due to excessive pulmonary blood flow. Between these two extremes are those patients who are acyanotic or only mildly cyanotic initially but who develop progressive desaturation due to worsening subvalvar obstruction. Colloquially, those who are acyanotic are referred to as "pink TETs," indicating minimal obstruction, whereas those with more significant obstruction and cyanosis are termed "blue TETs."

5. What is the pathophysiology of a TET spell, or hypercyanotic episode?

An acute and severe increase in right-to-left shunting across the VSD can produce a **TET spell.** Such spells are manifest by a profound decrease in saturation (**hypercyanosis**), which, if unchecked, can lead to a sequence of myocardial ischemia, bradycardia, and hypotension that would further reduce pulmonary blood flow and ultimately result in cardiac arrest.

The mechanism underlying these spells is either an acute increase in the resistance to pulmonary blood flow or an acute decrease in SVR. The former is thought to be manifest by catecholamine-induced muscle spasm of the right ventricular infundibulum. Muscle contraction of an already narrowed outflow tract further limits pulmonary blood flow and promotes right-to-left shunting. Pain, anxiety, or agitation may stimulate such a crisis. Decreases in SVR can be observed in the setting of an anesthetic in which both arterial vasodilation and venous pooling can occur. In this scenario, even in the absence of a change in resistance to pulmonary outflow, the decrease in SVR would promote right-to-left shunting by allowing blood to follow the path of least resistance.

Factors that may play a role in exacerbating spells include tachycardia and hypovolemia. The tachycardia that can initially accompany a catecholamine surge decreases ventricular-filling in diastole, making right ventricular outflow tract obstruction more likely. The same process occurs in the hypovolemic patient, whose right ventricle is subsequently underfilled.

6. What associated anomalies are relevant to the anesthesiologist?

Genetic syndromes or associations with **major extracardiac malformations** are present in at least 20% of patients with TOF. The most common is DiGeorge syndrome, which is the result of a chromosome 22q11 deletion. Other clinical names for this entity are velocardiofacial syndrome and conotruncal anomaly face syndrome. Alagille syndrome, trisomy 21, VACTERL, and CHARGE are also observed with tetralogy.

Vessel abnormalities of note that can influence line placement include the potential for an aberrant origin of the subclavian artery or a persistent left superior vena cava (LSVC). The origin of the subclavian is considered aberrant if it arises from the side opposite its final position (i.e., a left subclavian artery arising from the rightward aspect of the aorta or vice versa). Most often it courses posterior to the esophagus to reach its appropriate location. As such, a temperature probe or suction catheter placed deep in the esophagus or into the stomach may compress the artery and affect blood pressure measurement on that side. If a left subclavian central line is attempted in a patient with a LSVC, it should be noted that the line will end not at the junction of the superior vena cava and the right atrium but at the coronary sinus.

7. What are the anatomic variants of TOF?

Common variants include (i) TOF with an atrioventricular septal defect, (ii) TOF with double outlet right ventricle, (iii) TOF absent pulmonary valve, and (iv) TOF with pulmonary atresia (also known as pulmonary atresia with a VSD). The latter two diagnoses merit additional discussion.

Those with **TOF absent pulmonary valve** have near absence of the pulmonary valve leaflets as well as annular hypoplasia, producing a combined stenotic and regurgitant pulmonary outflow. The severe pulmonary regurgitation that occurs *in utero* can result in **aneurysmal dilation of the main and branch pulmonary arteries**, which can be so large as to compress the tracheobronchial tree. This can manifest as severe respiratory distress at birth requiring intubation. In such cases, prone positioning is often needed to alleviate the compression. Even following repair, in which the size of the pulmonary arteries is reduced surgically, tracheo- and bronchomalacia often persist.

TOF pulmonary atresia is an entity in which the pulmonary valve fails to develop. In its place, a plate of tissue forms which completely separates the right ventricle from the pulmonary vasculature. Pulmonary blood flow is thus dependent on a PDA and/or the presence of **major aortopulmonary collateral arteries (MAPCAs)**. Importantly, those with PDAs tend to have branch pulmonary arteries which arborize to perfuse most segments of the lung. In contrast, patients whose pulmonary blood flow is provided mainly by MAPCAs may not have a well-developed pulmonary arterial system. Indeed, the native pulmonary arteries may be completely absent. This distinction is relevant because MAPCAs do not possess the same growth potential as the true pulmonary arteries and also develop stenoses which lead to complete occlusion over time. Because of these significant variations in pulmonary arterial anatomy and sources of pulmonary blood flow, TOF pulmonary atresia has a different presentation, natural history, and management compared to classical TOF.

8. What should the preoperative evaluation of a patient with *unrepaired* tetralogy entail?

Key elements to identify include the child's baseline saturations, history of "spells," and echocardiography results. Knowledge of the child's saturation trend and history of hypercyanotic episodes can relay the severity of the pulmonary outflow tract obstruction and propensity to "spell" intraoperatively. Echo can serve to confirm such suspicions, indicate the presence or absence of a PDA, and identify other associated cardiac anomalies.

The child's **volume status** preoperatively is also significant as dehydration predisposes toward increased obstruction and right-to-left shunting. Ideally, the NPO time should be minimized and consideration should be given to preoperative admission for intravenous hydration the evening prior to surgery.

Labs to be reviewed independent of the reason for surgery include hemoglobin and parameters of coagulation including platelet count, prothrombin time, partial thromboplastin time, international normalized ratio, and fibrinogen. **Secondary erythrocytosis** develops in response to long-standing cyanosis resulting in an elevated hematocrit. Patients who are cyanotic yet anemic preoperatively may need a blood transfusion to increase their oxygen-carrying capacity and optimize oxygen delivery to end organs. In older children or adults with uncorrected cyanotic congenital heart disease, a **hyperviscosity syndrome** can be observed in which oxygen delivery is actually impaired by the markedly elevated hematocrit. Coagulation is often abnormal in patients with persistent cyanosis. Thrombocytopenia may be present, fibrinogen activity may be impaired, and factor levels may be abnormal. These effects are compounded in the neonate or infant with an immature coagulation system.

Additional data to consider include medications and the airway exam. Infants who have had episodes of hypercyanosis may be placed on a **beta-blocker** by their cardiologist to minimize obstruction. Such therapy should be continued perioperatively. In the neonatal period, the patient with severe obstruction and cyanosis may be on an infusion of **prostaglandin E1** to maintain ductal patency to provide a stable source of pulmonary blood flow. This should also be continued intraoperatively; an extra syringe should be readily available in the event the infusing prostaglandin empties. Given the high incidence of associated syndromes that can influence airway anatomy and thus intraoperative management, particular attention should be given to the airway exam preoperatively.

9. What are the intraoperative goals in managing such a patient?

Central to intraoperative management is avoiding increases in right-to-left shunting that could precipitate a hypercyanotic episode. Factors that would increase this risk include (i) increased resistance to pulmonary blood flow as may occur with infundibular spasm due to anxiety preoperatively or with pain during surgery, (ii) decreased SVR or hypotension, (iii) tachycardia, and (iv) decreased preload to the right heart.

While having intravenous access prior to induction is preferred, an inhalational induction can be performed safely assuming high doses are not used and intravenous access is obtained quickly. Alternatively, an intramuscular induction can be performed using ketamine and rocuronium. For the older infant, oral premedication may be helpful in allowing access to be obtained without causing significant agitation.

When access is present, one may consider induction with ketamine, fentanyl, and/or midazolam in junction with a low-dose inhalational agent. While ketamine may theoretically increase the risk of infundibular muscle spasm, the effects on increasing SVR appear to predominate clinically.

Goal-inspired oxygen concentration varies depending on the patient's physiology and the patient's response to surgery and anesthesia. In patients with severe obstruction and an absent ductus, there is little risk of pulmonary overcirculation, and so using a higher FiO_2 may be reasonable to guard against the risk of a spell. For those patients with only minimal stenosis, however, using a lower FiO_2 may be appropriate. Regardless, if conditions change such that the patient begins to desaturate, the FiO_2 should be increased.

Adequate analgesia and hydration are critical, as noted. If volume is needed and the patient's hematocrit is less than 40, consideration should be given to transfusing blood to optimize oxygen delivery. Surgical bleeding or insensible losses should be treated promptly to maintain intravascular volume.

As such infants would qualify as having cyanotic and unrepaired congenital heart disease, **infectious endocarditis antibiotic prophylaxis** should also be administered if indicated by the procedure.

10. What monitors should be placed?

Monitor choice is informed by the patient's physiology and the procedure to be performed. At a minimum, American Society of Anesthesiologists standard monitors in addition to a 5-lead electrocardiogram should be used. Additional monitors to consider would include an arterial line, a central venous line if vasoactive infusions are anticipated, and cerebral near-infrared spectroscopy as a trend of cardiac output.

11. How would you treat a TET spell?

Several steps can be taken, often concurrently, to reverse the right-to-left shunt of a TET spell. Goals of management and specific actions are as follows (see also Table 27.1):

- Reduce hypoxic pulmonary vasoconstriction
  - o Increase FiO_2
- Increase SVR
  - o Administer phenylephrine 5 to 10 mcg/kg
  - o Bring the knees to the chest or manually compress the abdomen
- Increase preload to the right ventricle
  - o Administer volume, 10 to 20 mL/kg
  - o Bring the knees to the chest or manually compress the abdomen
- Decrease myocardial contractility and heart rate
  - o Increase the concentration of sevoflurane administered
    - Be aware that high doses of sevoflurane will also decrease SVR
    - Isoflurane is more likely to cause vasodilation with rebound tachycardia and hypercontractility and so should be avoided
  - o Administer esmolol 50 to 200 mcg/kg
  - o Administer fentanyl, assuming that the etiology was inadequate analgesia
    - Morphine is not preferred under anesthesia due its propensity to decrease SVR
- If these measures fail, call for extracorporeal membrane oxygenation

12. What should one assess in patients presenting for noncardiac surgery *status post-repair?*

Patients with TOF may undergo either a **single-stage or two-stage repair**. Depending on the center, single-stage repairs may be performed in the neonatal period or later in infancy if the patient is acyanotic and without spells. A two-stage repair is often reserved for those patients who are highly cyanotic or who have spells early in life. This involves first the placement of a palliative shunt, the **modified Blalock-Taussig shunt (mBTS)**, to provide a secure source of pulmonary blood flow followed by a complete repair later in infancy. In either scenario, a complete repair includes (i) closure of the VSD, (ii) resection of hypertrophied right ventricular muscle bundles, and (iii) relief of the valvar and/or supravalvar pulmonary stenosis. The latter can be accomplished by a pulmonary valvotomy or the placement of a small patch across the pulmonary annulus to increase the cross-sectional area.

TABLE 27.1. STEP-WISE APPROACH FOR THE TREATMENT OF A "TET SPELL"

Pathophysiology	Treatment Regimen
Increased PVR	100% FiO_2
Decreased SVR	Phenylephrine
	Vasopressin
	Manual compression of the abdomen/aorta
Increased Infundibular Spasm	Increase the depth of anesthesia
	Beta-blockers
Decreased RV preload	Volume
	Manual compression of the abdomen/aorta

Note: PVR = pulmonary vascular resistance; SVR = systemic vascular resistance; RV = right ventricle.
If these measures fail, consider extracorporeal membrane oxygenation.

In patients who present following placement of a mBTS, the physiology is essentially that of a ductal-dependent child. Perioperative concerns would focus on maintaining the patency of the shunt and avoiding extended increases in FiO_2 that would serve to increase pulmonary blood flow at the expense of systemic and coronary perfusion.

Following complete repair, almost all patients develop some element of **pulmonary insufficiency** and/or stenosis. While both are generally well-tolerated, severe insufficiency over time can cause right ventricular enlargement, depressed function, and atrial or ventricular arrhythmias. Routine surveillance allows patients at risk to be identified and put forward for pulmonary valve replacement before irreversible changes occur. For the anesthesiologist caring for the patient post-complete repair, an assessment of the patient's functional status and the results of echocardiography, cardiac magnetic resonance imaging, and the Holter monitor can give the necessary information to risk-stratify the individual and plan an appropriate anesthetic.

SUMMARY

1. TOF is the most common cause of the cyanotic congenital heart defects and accounts for nearly 10% of all congenital cardiac disease.
2. Presentation can range from those with severe cyanosis early in life to those with symptoms consistent with pulmonary overcirculation. Most often, patients are acyanotic and develop cyanosis over time as the right ventricular progressively hypertrophies.
3. Determinants of presentation are the degree of pulmonary obstruction present and whether or not there is a PDA. Patients with moderate to severe obstruction are more likely to "spell," but even those with minimal obstruction can "spell" should SVR decrease or the resistance to pulmonary blood flow increase acutely.
4. Management of a "spell" focuses on efforts to reverse right-to-left shunting across the VSD. This entails increasing FiO_2 and SVR, giving volume, and decreasing myocardial contractility and heart rate.
5. Preoperative evaluation should include an assessment of baseline saturations, history of "spells," echocardiography findings, hydration status, use of beta-blockade, and the presence of associated syndromes/associations with attention to their influence on the airway.

ANNOTATED REFERENCES

Schmitz ML, Ullah S, Dasgupta R, Thompson LL. Anesthesia for right-sided obstructive lesions. In: Andropoulos DB, Stayer S, Mossad EB, Miller-Hance WC, eds. *Anesthesia for Congenital Heart Disease*. 3rd ed. Hoboken, NJ: Wiley-Blackwell; 2015:524–531.

An excellent and concise overview on the anesthetic management of patients with TOF.

Stewart RD, Mavroudis C, Backer CL. Tetralogy of Fallot. In: Mavroudis C, Backer CL, eds. *Pediatric Cardiac Surgery*. 4th ed. Chichester, UK: Wiley-Blackwell; 2013:410–427.

Provides further insight into the anatomy, clinical presentation, and surgical management and outcomes in TOF.

Twite MD, Ing RJ. Tetralogy of Fallot: perioperative anesthetic management of children and adults. *Semin Cardiothorac Vasc Anesth*. 2012;16(2):97–105.

An excellent review of the anatomy, physiology, and anesthetic considerations in infants, children, and adults with tetralogy.

Sharkey AM, Sharma A. Tetralogy of Fallot: anatomic variants and their impact on surgical management. *Semin Cardiothorac Vasc Anesth*. 2012;16(2):88–96.

Focuses on the anatomic, and thus clinical variability, seen in TOF and how this can influence anesthetic management.

FURTHER READING

Motta P, Miller-Hance WC. Transesophageal echocardiography in tetralogy of Fallot. *Semin Cardiothorac Vasc Anesth*. 2012;16;70–87.

Prevention of infective endocarditis: Guidelines from the American Heart Association: A Guideline from the American Heart Association Rheumatic Fever, Endocarditis, and Kawasaki Disease Committee, Council on Cardiovascular Disease in the Young, and the Council on Clinical Cardiology, Council on Cardiovascular Surgery and Anesthesia, and the Quality of Care and Outcomes Research Interdisciplinary Working Group. *Circulation*. 2007;116:1736–1754.

Zabala LM, Guzzetta NA. Cyanotic congenital heart disease (CCHD): focus on hypoxemia, secondary erythrocytosis, and coagulation alterations. *Pediatr Anesth*. 2015;25:981–989.

28

Cardiac Catheterization

ERICA P. LIN, ANDREAS W. LOEPKE, AND EMAD B. MOSSAD

INTRODUCTION

With continued technological advancements in the management of congenital heart disease, the scope of procedures performed in the cardiac catheterization laboratory has evolved from historically being primarily diagnostic to now including several therapeutic interventions. Importantly, these complex, nonsurgical, catheter-based procedures can entail substantially increased risks of adverse events, especially in younger and/or sicker patients. Hence, it is crucial for anesthesia providers in the cardiac catheterization laboratory to have a good understanding of each patient's underlying cardiac physiology, the implications of the anesthetic technique on this physiology, as well as the inherent risks and potential complications of the procedure to be performed in a satellite location that poses its own challenges.

LEARNING OBJECTIVES

1. Be familiar with the limitations of the cardiac catheterization lab and the risk of radiation exposure.
2. Understand the general goals for cardiac catheterization and the implications of the anesthetic technique.
3. Appreciate the commonly encountered complications in this setting.

CASE PRESENTATION

A 14-month-old, 8.5-kg girl with ***hypoplastic left heart syndrome (HLHS)*** *presents for cardiac catheterization to evaluate her frequent cyanotic spells and poor growth. The patient was born at 35 weeks' gestation with an antenatal diagnosis of HLHS. As a neonate, she underwent a* ***hybrid procedure*** *in the catheterization laboratory with stenting of the ductus arteriosus and pulmonary artery banding. At 5 months of age, she underwent a comprehensive stage II procedure that included aortic arch reconstruction, removal of a pulmonary artery band, and creation of a bidirectional superior cavopulmonary anastomosis (bidirectional Glenn shunt). Her medications include aspirin, furosemide, and enalapril. Her most recent echocardiogram showed no neo-aortic stenosis or insufficiency, a patent bidirectional Glenn shunt, questionable narrowing of distal branch pulmonary arteries (right > left), and low-normal right ventricular function. Baseline hemoglobin is 16.8 g/dL. During an attempt to examine her preoperatively, she becomes agitated and notably cyanotic. Oxygen saturation at this time drops from a baseline in the mid-70s to the 50s, and supplemental oxygen via nasal cannula is provided.* ***Oral midazolam*** *is administered prior to beginning the procedure.*

In the catheterization laboratory, noninvasive monitors are placed and the patient tolerates an inhalational induction with sevoflurane in oxygen. A peripheral 22-g cannula is inserted with some difficulty due to multiple previous attempts. A ***laryngeal mask airway*** *size 1½ is placed, and the patient is allowed to breathe spontaneously to facilitate negative intrathoracic pressure and improve venous return. Anesthesia is maintained with sevoflurane and intermittent boluses of fentanyl. Body temperature is maintained with a forced-air warmer. The cardiologist obtains procedural access to the pulmonary arteries through the right internal jugular vein, to the systemic ventricle via the femoral vein, and to the femoral artery for blood pressure monitoring. The first arterial blood gas reflects* ***hypercarbia*** *($PaCO_2$ 76 mmHg) consistent with* ***hypoventilation.*** *The decision is made to convert to mechanical ventilation, so a nondepolarizing muscle relaxant is given to facilitate* ***endotracheal intubation.***

Hemodynamic data, obtained while the patient is normoventilated on room air, demonstrates moderate ***pulmonary hypertension****. Pulmonary angiography reveals several stenotic areas in the peripheral pulmonary arteries. Heparin is administered and the interventional cardiologist dilates the stenotic lesions with repeated balloon angioplasties. During the intervention, the patient experiences sudden worsening of* ***hypoxemia*** *(SpO_2 decreases from 78% to 45%) with* ***hypotension*** *(systolic blood pressure decreasing from 75 mmHg to 30 mmHg). However, vital signs improve with removal of the catheter from the pulmonary artery. After hemostasis is obtained at the catheter sites, the patient is extubated awake and is transported to the postanesthesia care unit, where she recovers uneventfully.*

DISCUSSION

1. What are some of the challenges for the anesthesiologist working in the cardiac catheterization laboratory environment?

Catheterization laboratories are often located in remote areas of the hospital, away from the main operating room suite. Furthermore, appropriate recovery facilities may be some distance away, as catheterization laboratories have historically not been designed with anesthesiologists' input. It is imperative that monitoring, oxygen supply, resuscitation equipment, and drugs, as well as sufficient personnel, be available both during the procedure and also for transport to the recovery area.

Regardless of the physical dimensions of the room, functional space is often limited, with bulky fluoroscopy equipment hindering access to the patient and the airway. During continuous fluoroscopy, higher doses of ionizing radiation in close proximity to the patient discourage immediate access to the patient to check positioning or to administer medications. Subdued lighting, while necessary for the cardiologist, further impairs the anesthesiologist's ability to visually monitor the patient. Intravenous lines, monitor cables, and breathing circuits often require additional length to reach the patient and must be secured in an organized fashion to not be snared by the frequent movement of the procedure table and fluoroscopy arms, especially during rotational angiography.

Effective communication among all team members is of the utmost importance to ensure situational awareness of both the progression of the procedure and the hemodynamic state of the patient. Especially for high-risk procedures, a prebriefing conversation before the procedure begins can focus the entire team on the details of each patient, the procedure and need for special equipment and/or implantable devices, specific risks and any mitigating strategies, and disposition plan. Cardiologists and anesthesiologists must function as partners in decision-making and work effectively not only with each other but also with the cardiac catheterization team and the operating and surgical team in hybrid scenarios. Optimal care relies on close collaboration and coordination among all present and the promotion of a teamwork culture.

When an anesthesiologist is working as the sole anesthesia provider in these remote locations, the value of skilled personnel to provide support (assistance with venous access, airway management, and equipment) cannot be overstated, especially in crisis situations. Furthermore, the practitioner must be aware of other available personnel resources that can be mobilized during an emergency, such as cardiac intensivists, surgeons, and the extracorporeal membrane oxygenation team. Despite the most detailed planning, serious complications can occur suddenly and unexpectedly during the procedure, which may necessitate the rapid preparation and administration of potent medications, such as bronchodilators, antiarrhythmic drugs, vasopressors, and inotropes.

2. What is the radiation exposure risk for patients and personnel associated with the catheterization laboratory?

Fluoroscopy use in congenital cardiac catheterization can result in significant radiation exposure to the patient. Doses vary by age and procedure type. Overall, radiation dose from diagnostic exams increases with advancing age and body mass, and interventional procedures incur greater exposures than diagnostic studies. By some estimates, interventional therapies, especially pulmonary angioplasty procedures, are associated with some of the greatest radiation exposures observed across all age groups (Verghese et al., 2012). However, reduced body size, smaller cardiovascular structures, and complicated anatomic variations may necessitate lengthier procedures and can result in a higher average radiation dose in newborns compared with older patients (Rassow et al., 2000). Furthermore, children with congenital heart disease are at unique risk of considerable cumulative lifetime exposure because they are frequently subject to repeated catheterization procedures both for diagnostic surveillance and interventional therapies. Given their improved life expectancy with advanced therapies, they may be more likely to develop subsequent sequelae from ionizing radiation exposure, including dermatologic effects, carcinogenic effects, and heritable changes in reproductive cells.

Personnel working in the catheterization laboratory are also inevitably subject to higher levels of radiation exposure compared with other medical specialties (Venneri et al., 2009). Dosimeters should be worn to track cumulative radiation exposure, and since there is no "safe dose" of radiation, every effort should be made to minimize occupational exposure. The goal of the ALARA principle (as low as reasonably achievable), as advocated by the Centers for Disease Control and Prevention, is to provide the maximal diagnostic and/or therapeutic benefit while using the lowest possible radiation dose during diagnostic procedures involving ionizing radiation (Justino, 2006). To minimize exposure, anesthesiologists should strictly adhere to *three radiation safety principles:* (i) *maximize the distance* from the radiation source, as radiation dose varies with the inverse square of that distance (i.e., doubling the distance results in a 4-fold dose reduction); (ii) *minimize exposure time*; and (iii) always use *proper shielding* (e.g., lead aprons, thyroid collars, acrylic shields, and protective eyeglasses).

3. Should every child undergoing a pediatric cardiac catheterization receive a general anesthetic?

Since pediatric cardiac catheterizations can be complicated, lengthy, and require relative patient immobility, most children, especially younger ones, do require sedation or anesthesia. An expert consensus statement on anesthesia and sedation practices in the pediatric and congenital cardiac catheterization laboratory, jointly presented by the Society for Cardiovascular Angiography and Intervention, the Society for Pediatric Anesthesia, and the Congenital Cardiac Anesthesia Society, widely acknowledges that there is no singular anesthetic technique that is universally applicable to all patients (Odegard et al., 2016). Instead, the recommendations focus more on aspects of patient management and monitoring that are important irrespective of whether no or light sedation versus full general anesthesia are used.

Regardless of which modality is utilized, there should be a dedicated practitioner, not involved in the cardiac catheterization procedure itself, managing the patient's sedation or anesthesia. A recent multicenter survey demonstrated anesthesiology participation in the majority (>80%) of cases in most institutions (Vincent et al., 2016). The skill set required includes the ability to manage the continuum from sedation to general anesthesia; to understand the cardiac pathophysiology; to securely manage the airway; and to prevent, rapidly recognize, and treat complications related to both the procedure and the anesthesia/sedation. Pediatric cardiac anesthesiologists are specifically trained in this unique skill set. When it is not feasible for a pediatric cardiac anesthesiologist to staff every congenital cardiac catheterization procedure, it is paramount that the expertise of the care providers be matched to the level of risk posed by each individual patient and the procedure he or she is to undergo (Odegard et al., 2016).

4. How does one match the anesthetic technique and the procedural goals?

The ultimate goal of a safe cardiac catheterization procedure is to acquire accurate hemodynamic information and to facilitate therapeutic interventions while maintaining hemodynamic stability and patient comfort. For diagnostic studies, measurements are usually taken with the patient breathing 21% oxygen, while the pH and partial pressure of carbon dioxide are maintained at preoperative levels. Unfortunately, there is no single technique that guarantees this goal, and the choice of anesthetic agent or airway management may considerably affect these variables. For instance, while **spontaneous breathing** may promote venous return, it increases the risk for hypoventilation, hypercarbia, and airway obstruction. The resulting respiratory acidosis can increase pulmonary vascular resistance, altering shunt physiology and hemodynamic measurements. On the other hand, **tracheal intubation** and positive-pressure ventilation, while providing a secure airway, may decrease venous return, cardiac output, and hemodynamic stability. This is particularly noticeable in patients with right heart failure, hypovolemia, or Fontan physiology.

Each patient with congenital heart disease has a unique physiologic state. A thorough preoperative assessment should review diagnosis and current symptoms and take previous interventions/repairs/

palliations into consideration to determine the safest anesthetic technique for each particular patient. Anxious patients may benefit from **preoperative sedation.** The choice of sedative and anesthetic medications will depend on the patient's hemodynamic status and cardiac reserve. For anesthetic maintenance, inhalational and intravenous agents are commonly combined to minimize their respective adverse effects.

5. What vascular access points do interventional cardiologists commonly use, and what are the concomitant risks?

The necessary vascular access for congenital cardiac catheterization is generally obtained percutaneously. However, surgical cutdown may sometimes be necessary, for example, in extremely small infants to access the carotid artery or internal jugular vein or to access the axillary artery (Radtke, 2005). The most frequent vessels used for percutaneous access are the femoral arteries and veins, with the right side accessed more often than the left. The internal jugular vein is also a favored site for myocardial biopsies and in patients with interrupted inferior vena cava or in those with Glenn or Fontan physiology. Additionally, newborns within the first few days of life may still have patency of the umbilical vessels, which can be accessed for procedures. The carotid artery is the preferred nonfemoral arterial access in children, while the radial artery is favored in adults (Vincent et al., 2016). The axillary and brachial arteries are additional alternative sites. Transhepatic venous access is often considered when other, traditional sites have been occluded or thrombosed from prior interventions or need to be preserved for future surgeries, like Glenn or Fontan operations. This route, however, can carry higher risks of bleeding that can manifest as hemothorax or hemoperitoneum; thus there must be a high index of suspicion during postprocedural care. While rare, retroperitoneal bleeding can also occur following very proximal cannulation of the femoral vessels. Alternative routes of vascular access may be deliberately chosen to avoid acute angles and tortuous courses and to accommodate larger sheaths, based on the intervention performed.

Loss of pulsation, in spite of prophylactic heparin administration, is the most common access-related complication of cardiac catheterization, with mostly younger and smaller patients accounting for this morbidity. Risk factors include the use of large catheters, the need to perform an intervention through arterial access, repeat catheterizations, and multiple attempts to establish access. Anticoagulation and thrombolytic therapies can be employed to restore patency. Another vascular complication is external bleeding, which can be quickly recognized and treated with manual compression. Pressure should be held just enough to prevent bleeding without completely occluding the vessel; this can be judged by perfusion and color of the leg. Retroperitoneal bleeding and hemoperitoneum are more challenging to diagnose but should be considered when patients who had femoral or transhepatic access are unstable postprocedure or who have symptoms of pallor, malaise, abdominal discomfort, tachycardia, and/or diminished blood pressure. Hemothorax can similarly complicate internal jugular and carotid access and may require chest tube placement.

6. What are some of the potential complications of cardiac catheterization?

Other than vascular access complications, adverse events occur more commonly during pediatric cardiac catheterization than during pediatric anesthesia in general (Bennett et al., 2005), and the overall incidence distributes rather evenly between diagnostic and interventional procedures at 10% and 11.1%, respectively (Vincent et al., 2016). Life-threatening events are rare, occurring in 1% to 2% of cases (Lin et al., 2014; Vincent et al., 2016), and are lower in centers with higher case volumes (Jayaram et al., 2017). Catheterization related mortality rates remain low at <1%. Predictors for major adverse events include age <1 year, hemodynamic instability, and high-risk procedures including ventricular septal defect device closure, interventions for intact atrial septum or restricted atrial septal flow in children requiring mixing of the circulation, mitral valve balloon valvuloplasty, aortic balloon valvuloplasty, and pulmonary vascular dilations (Lin et al., 2014; Odegard et al., 2014). Severe **pulmonary hypertension**, not infrequently encountered in the cardiac catheterization laboratory, dramatically increases the risk of morbidity and mortality (Carmosino et al., 2007).

Arrhythmias and vascular damage are the two most common complications encountered. Dysrhythmias are usually transient; the vast majority result from mechanical stimulation by intracardiac wires and catheters and respond to cessation of manipulation and correction of any contributing metabolic or electrolyte abnormalities. Nevertheless, pacing capabilities and equipment for defibrillation must be immediately available for treatment of more persistent, potentially fatal dysrhythmias. Indeed, in a study reviewing cardiac arrests in congenital heart catheterizations, arrhythmias preceded cardiac arrest in 54% of cases (Odegard et al., 2014).

The insertion of intraluminal catheters or wires may cause obstruction of blood vessels, distortion of cardiac chambers, or create incompetence of cardiac valves, potentially reducing pulmonary or systemic blood flow and/or cardiac output and resulting in **hypotension, oxygen desaturation**, or both. These issues are more prominent in younger patients with significant comorbidities, as exemplified by the case scenario. Other catheter-related complications include vascular damage and bleeding at the access sites, vascular thrombosis, air embolus, catheter fragment embolus, bleeding, pericardial effusion, cardiac tamponade, and perforation or rupture of vessels of the heart. Cross-matched blood products should therefore be immediately available during all complex interventions.

Sedation-, anesthesia-, and airway-related adverse events are also rare. **Hypotension** on initiation/induction of anesthesia is the most common complication and is usually managed with volume infusion and/or low-dose vasoactive infusions that can be weaned and discontinued following normalization of vital signs toward the completion of the procedure. Airway obstruction, hypoxia, respiratory acidosis, and unplanned extubation, when not recognized promptly, can progress to a major event requiring cardiopulmonary resuscitation. Furthermore, patients converted from spontaneous respiration to intubation with mechanical ventilation have a higher rate of serious adverse events (Lin et al., 2015). Infants undergoing high-risk procedures and patients requiring inotropic support are more apt to require conversion to general anesthesia and intubation (Lin et al., 2015).

7. What are some of the emerging applications involving the catheterization laboratory?

The number of interventional catheterizations continues to escalate, with increasing heterogeneity in procedure type and patient complexity (Table 28.1). There exists a particular growth in the number of palliative procedures performed, both in neonates and in adult patients with congenital heart disease (Arnold & Shah, 2015). In neonates, both traditional endovascular approaches and **hybrid procedures** that combine open surgical and interventional catheterization techniques are being increasingly utilized. Through direct cardiac access facilitated by surgical colleagues, stenting of the ductus arteriosus or right ventricular outflow tract have become valid cardiopulmonary bypass-sparing alternatives in select patients. For older patients with congenital right heart lesions, percutaneous

TABLE 28.1. PROCEDURES CONDUCTED IN THE CARDIAC CATHETERIZATION LABORATORY

Procedure	Purpose and Comment
Endocardial biopsy	Surveillance, assessment for rejection after cardiac transplant
Diagnosis of myocarditis and cardiomyopathy	
Valvotomy	Balloon dilation of stenotic aortic, pulmonary, mitral, or bioprosthetic valves
Angioplasty	Treatment of stenosis in native blood vessels (aorta, pulmonary artery) and surgical conduits
Endovascular stents	Applied to pulmonary artery stenosis, systemic venous stenosis, aortic coarctation
Closure of shunts	Patent ductus arteriosus, aortopulmonary collaterals, coronary artery fistulas, arteriovenous malformations: helical wire coils
	Atrial septal defect, ventricular septal defect: umbrella device comprising two discs
Electrophysiology study and ablation	Delineate mechanism of arrhythmia and destroy abnormal pathways and automatic foci, most commonly with radiofrequency energy and cryotherapy
Implantation of pacemakers and defibrillators	Placement of transvenous leads with tunneling to a subcutaneous pocket

valve replacement has been a revolutionary development that potentially precludes the need for repetitive surgeries for valve replacement. The Melody® Transcatheter Pulmonary Valve (Medtronic, Inc., Minneapolis, MN) is designed for use in patients with a surgically implanted right ventricular-to-pulmonary artery conduit with at least moderate regurgitation or stenosis. Patients must be of adequate size, such that their venous anatomy can accommodate the large 22 French delivery system. Follow-up in the US Investigational Device Exemption trial has shown good outcomes up to 7 years, with rare valve failure (Cheatham et al., 2015). Furthermore, the practice of conduit pre-stenting has reduced the incidence of stenosis secondary to stent fracture (Cheatham et al., 2015). Expanding on the concept of a hybrid approach, cardiothoracic surgeons have recently reported on the surgical implantation of a modified Melody valve at a compressed diameter in aortic, mitral, pulmonary, and tricuspid positions in neonates and young children, with the intent for subsequent catheter-based expansion after somatic growth to provide durable valve function and delay the need for reoperation (Emani et al., 2016).

Angiography remains a mainstay of cardiac catheterization laboratory, guiding interventions. The use of rotational angiography with the capacity for 3-dimensional angiographic reconstruction addresses the limitations of traditional biplane angiography by providing additional anatomic information, specifically for complex vascular structures including the pulmonary vascular tree, the coronary arteries, and surgically placed shunts with a single image acquisition. It also provides the ability to visualize the anatomy from multiple vantage points, including those not possible with fixed-plane angiography (Aldoss et al., 2016). Collectively, this allows subsequent fixed-plane angiography for interventions to be performed in optimal projections.

SUMMARY

1. Preparation, clear communication, and situational awareness in the remote environment of the cardiac catheterization lab are essential.
2. Minimize radiation exposure for both the patient and the providers.
3. The anesthesia providers must be familiar with the specific patient's cardiac pathophysiology and prepared to recognize and immediately treat serious complications related to cardiac catheterization, including arrhythmias, hypotension, hypoxia, and bleeding.
4. Complex therapeutic cardiac catheterization procedures increasingly replace open surgical procedures in higher risk patients, ranging from the younger and smaller neonates/infants to adults with congenital heart disease. This will even further increase the already significantly elevated patient acuity in the cardiac catheterization laboratory.

ANNOTATED REFERENCES

Arnold P, Shah A. 2015. Anesthesia for the cardiac catheterization laboratory. In: Andropoulos DB, Stayer S, Mossad EB, Miller-Hance WC, eds. *Anesthesia for Congenital Heart Disease.* 3rd ed. Hoboken, NJ: Wiley-Blackwell; 2015:677–704.

A thorough overview of anesthetic considerations in the cardiac catheterization laboratory. Sections are organized based on type of procedure: diagnostic catheterization, interventional cardiology, electrophysiology procedures.

Odegard KC, Vincent R, Baijal RG, et al. SCAI/CCAS/SPA expert consensus statement for anesthesia and sedation practice: recommendations for patients undergoing diagnostic and therapeutic procedures in the pediatric and congenital cardiac catheterization laboratory. *Anesth Analg.* 2016;123:1201–1209.

This consensus statement makes recommendations for the optimal management of patients requiring sedation and anesthesia in the congenital catheterization laboratory.

Justino H. The ALARA concept in pediatric cardiac catheterization: techniques and tactics for managing radiation dose. *Pediatr Radiol.* 2006;36:146–153.

This article provides a list of strategies to improve radiation safety in the pediatric cardiac catheterization lab.

Radtke WAK. Vascular access and the management of its complications. *Pediatr Cardiol.* 2005;26:140–146.

This article summarizes the various vascular access sites, strategies for vessel protection and restoration, and management of complications.

BIBLIOGRAPHY

Aldoss O, Fonseca BM, Truong UT, et al. Diagnostic utility of three-dimensional rotational angiography in congenital cardiac catheterization. *Pediatr Cardiol.* 2016;37:1211–1221.

Bennett D, Marcus R, Stokes M. Incidents and complications during pediatric cardiac catheterization. *Pediatr Anesth.* 2005;15:1083–1088.

Carmosino MJ, Friesen RH, Doran A, et al. Perioperative complications in children with pulmonary hypertension undergoing noncardiac surgery or cardiac catheterization. *Anesth Analg.* 2007;104:521–527.

Cheatham JP, Hellenbrand WE, Zahn EM, et al. Clinical and hemodynamic outcomes up to 7 years after the transcatheter pulmonary valve replacement in the US Melody Valve Investigational Device Exemption trial. *Circulation.* 2015;131:1960–1970.

Emani SM, Piekarski BL, Zurakowski D, et al. Concept of an expandable cardiac valve for surgical implantation in infants and children. *J Thorac Cardiovasc Surg.* 2016;152:1514–1523.

Jayaram N, Spertus JA, O'Byrne ML, et al. Relationship between hospital procedure volume and complications following congenital cardiac catheterization: a report from the Improving Pediatric and Adult Congenital Treatment (IMPACT) Registry. *Am Heart J.* 2017;183:118–128.

Lin CH, Hegde S, Marshall AC, et al. Incidence and management of life-threatening adverse events during cardiac catheterization for congenital heart disease. *Pediatr Cardiol.* 2014;35:140–148.

Lin CH, Desai S, Nicolas R, et al. Sedation and anesthesia in pediatric and congenital cardiac catheterization: a prospective multicenter experience. *Pediatr Cardiol.* 2015;36:1363–1375.

Odegard KC, Bergersen L, Thiagarajan R, et al. The frequency of cardiac arrest in patients with congenital heart disease undergoing cardiac catheterization. *Anesth Analg.* 2014;118:175–182.

Rassow J, Schmaltz AA, Hentrich F, et al. Effective doses to patients from paediatric cardiac catheterization. *Br J Radiol.* 2000;73:172–183.

Venneri L, Rossi F, Botto N, et al. Cancer risk from professional exposure in staff working in cardiac catheterization laboratory: insights from the National Research Council's Biological Effects of Ionizing Radiation VII Report. *Am Heart J.* 2009;157:118–124.

Verghese GR, McElhinney DB, Strauss KJ, et al. Characterization of radiation exposure and effect of a radiation monitoring policy in a large volume pediatric cardiac catheterization lab. *Cathet Cardiovasc Intervent.* 2012;79:294–301.

Vincent RN, Moore J, Beekman RH, et al. Procedural characteristics and adverse events in diagnostic and interventional catheterisations in paediatric and adult CHD: initial report from the IMPACT Registry. *Cardiol Young.* 2016;26:70–78.

29

Pulmonary Hypertension

ERIN S. WILLIAMS

INTRODUCTION

Pediatric pulmonary arterial hypertension (PAH) is characterized by a pathologically elevated pulmonary artery pressure in children. The etiology of PAH is multifactorial, and while its prognosis is closely related to the reversibility of the underlying disease process, much progress has recently been made in its diagnosis and treatment, significantly decreasing the associated morbidity and mortality.

LEARNING OBJECTIVES

1. Identify etiologies of PAH in young children.
2. Recognize risk factors for exacerbation of PAH.
3. Identify and describe the management of a pulmonary hypertensive crisis.
4. Identify the best setting for postanesthesia care in the patient with PAH.

CASE PRESENTATION

A 16-year-old girl with past medical history significant for autism, cystic fibrosis, and secondary pulmonary hypertension presents with her parents to the preoperative assessment clinic in preparation for dental restorations. She is sitting calmly watching a movie on her mother's phone and appears to be in no distress. Her mother tells you that she takes all of her pulmonary medications and her dose of sildenafil has been decreased. She also mentions that the patient had a procedure 6 months ago and during the surgery the doctors measured the pressures in her heart. She saw her cardiologist later the same week. The mother states that she thinks everything is okay but she is most concerned about her daughter's cavities since she appears to be uncomfortable. She also wants to know if her daughter will be able to go home after the dental procedure.

DISCUSSION

1. What is PAH?

PAH is defined as mean pulmonary artery pressures greater than or equal to 25 mmHg (Pilkington et al., 2015). This measurement is obtained at rest during a right heart catheterization. The overall pathophysiology of PAH involves the pulmonary blood vessels constricting, leading to increased pressure. This increased tone of the pulmonary vasculature can be idiopathic or secondary to another disease state.

2. How is pediatric PAH diagnosed?

As in adults, pediatric PAH is defined as a mean pulmonary artery pressure of (i) higher than 25 mmHg at rest with normal pulmonary capillary wedge pressure or (ii) higher than 30 mmHg during exercise (Carmosino et al., 2007).

Clinically, PAH has to be considered in children with a history of respiratory complications or cardiac abnormalities when hypoxemia is refractory to oxygen therapy or alveolar recruitment strategies (Roberts et al., 1997) or when the neonatal preductal to postductal oxygen gradient exceeds 20 mmHg (Walsh-Sukys et al., 2000). The suspected diagnosis can be confirmed by echocardiography when tricuspid regurgitation is present or by direct measurement of pulmonary artery pressures during cardiac catheterization.

3. Overall, how is pulmonary hypertension classified?

Causes of PAH in children are shown in Table 29.1. In 1998 the decision was made to assign a consistent classification of PAH. This was the Evian classification. Then, in 2003, the Third World Symposium of Pulmonary Arterial Hypertension (in Venice)

TABLE 29.1. UPDATED CLASSIFICATION OF PULMONARY HYPERTENSION*

1. Pulmonary arterial hypertension
    1.1 Idiopathic PAH
    1.2 Heritable PAH
        1.2.1 BMPR2
        1.2.2 ALK-1, ENG, **SMAD9, CAV1, KCNK3**
        1.2.3 Unknown
    1.3 Drug and toxin induced
    1.4 Associated with:
        1.4.1 Connective tissue disease
        1.4.2 HIV infection
        1.4.3 Portal hypertension
        1.4.4 Congenital heart diseases
        1.4.5 Schistosomiasis

1′ Pulmonary veno-occlusive disease and/or pulmonary capillary hemangiomatosis

1″. Persistent pulmonary hypertension of the newborn (PPHN)

2. Pulmonary hypertension due to left heart disease
    2.1 Left ventricular systolic dysfunction
    2.2 Left ventricular diastolic dysfunction
    2.3 Valvular disease
    2.4 Congenital/acquired left heart inflow/outflow tract obstruction and congenital cardiomyopathies
3. Pulmonary hypertension due to lung diseases and/or hypoxia
    3.1 Chronic obstructive pulmonary disease
    3.2 Interstitial lung disease
    3.3 Other pulmonary diseases with mixed restrictive and obstructive pattern
    3.4 Sleep-disordered breathing
    3.5 Alveolar hypoventilation disorders
    3.6 Chronic exposure to high altitude
    3.7 Developmental lung diseases
4. Chronic thromboembolic pulmonary hypertension (CTEPH)
5. Pulmonary hypertension with unclear multifactorial mechanisms
    5.1 Hematologic disorders: **chronic hemolytic anemia**, myeloproliferative disorders, splenectomy
    5.2 Systemic disorders: sarcoidosis, pulmonary histiocytosis, lymphangioleiomyomatosis
    5.3 Metabolic disorders: glycogen storage disease, Gaucher disease, thyroid disorders
    5.4 Others: tumoral obstruction, fibrosing mediastinitis, chronic renal failure, **segmental PH**

BMPR = bone morphogenic protein receptor type II; CAV1 = caveolin-1; ENG = endoglin; HIV = human immunodeficiency virus; PAH = pulmonary arterial hypertension.

*Updated classification from the 5th WSPH, Nice, 2013.

Reprinted from Simonneau G, Gatzoulis MA, Adatia I, et al. Updated clinical classification of pulmonary hypertension. *J Am Coll Cardiol.* 2013;62(25):D34–D41. With permission from Elsevier.

reclassified pulmonary hypertension. Most recently, at the Fifth World Symposium (in Nice, France), modifications and updates were made to the current classification system. The overall changes include moving persistent pulmonary hypertension of the newborn to its own category as well as adding more information regarding pediatric pulmonary hypertension. In general, this new classification places pulmonary hypertension into 5 main categories (Table 29.1).

PAH can be further categorized by its responsiveness to a drug or oxygen challenge (reactive) or lack of response (fixed), which has significant implications for patient outcome (Sarkar et al., 2005).

4. What are the etiologies leading to persistent pulmonary hypertension of the newborn (PPHN)?

PAH is physiologic during fetal life, but pressures decrease to normal adult levels soon after birth. Generally, 3 types of developmental defects can lead to PPHN that are not associated with congenital cardiac anomalies (Walsh-Sukys et al., 2000).

- *Underdevelopment* of pulmonary parenchymal tissue, leading to hypoplastic pulmonary vasculature, such as in: congenital diaphragmatic hernia, oligohydramnios with obstructive uropathy, cystic malformations of the lungs, or intrauterine growth restriction
- Peripartum *maladaptation* with constricted pulmonary vasculature due to adverse pulmonary conditions such as infections (especially group B streptococcus), meconium aspiration, or sepsis with respiratory distress syndrome
- Genetic predisposition leading to maldevelopment of pulmonary parenchyma

5. What is the significance of increased pulmonary artery pressures, and what factors may precipitate a crisis?

Pulmonary hypertension is an independent predictor of morbidity in both children and adults with congenital heart disease undergoing noncardiac surgery. Moreover, the incidence of pulmonary hypertensive crisis (PHC) and cardiac arrest is significantly increased in children with PAH undergoing noncardiac surgery or cardiac catheterization; and it may occur suddenly without overt warning signs (Carmosino et al., 2007; Morray et al., 2000).

Physiological derangements such as hypoxemia, hypercarbia, acidosis, or increased sympathetic tone can lead to a sudden, dramatic increase in pulmonary vascular resistance (PVR). This increase in PVR will lead to a rise in right ventricular pressure, right-to-left intracardiac shunt, and a decrease in myocardial oxygen delivery, which will further diminish cardiac output and worsen hypoxemia and hypercarbia and increase PVR, ultimately leading to cardiac arrest (Fig. 29.1).

6. What are the preferred anesthetic agents for patients with PAH?

Adverse events have not been found to be significantly associated with any particular type of anesthetic, procedure, or method of airway management (Carmosino et al., 2007). The overriding goal in the design of an anesthetic for patients with elevated pulmonary artery pressure is the avoidance of sudden increases in pulmonary artery pressures due to sympathetic stimulation. Anxiolytics help to decrease sympathetic tone, thus avoiding elevated oxygen consumption and arrhythmias. However, combinations of benzodiazepines and narcotics can cause hypotension, producing a reactive increase in sympathetic tone that is counterproductive.

Similarly, inhaled anesthetics can cause a dose-dependent reduction of systemic vascular resistance (SVR) and cardiac contractility, which may lead to an increase in sympathetic tone. However, both isoflurane and sevoflurane have been shown to promote pulmonary vasodilation, whereas nitrous oxide

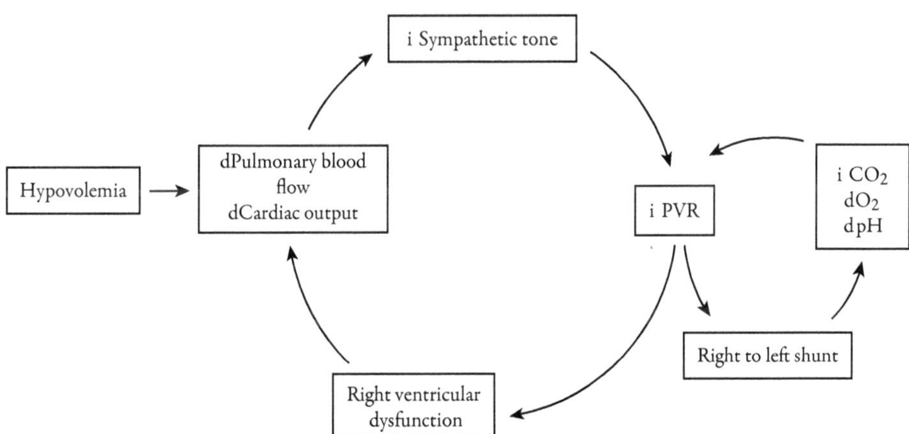

FIGURE 29.1: Cycle of events in pulmonary hypertensive episode.

has very little effect on pulmonary hemodynamics in children with PAH.

Opioids are favored in PAH because of their minimal pulmonary and systemic hemodynamic effects and the advantageous blunting of increases in PVR due to noxious stimulation. Propofol has also been used successfully in children with PAH; however, it should be administered with caution as boluses may cause precipitous reduction in cardiac output and SVR. Etomidate provides hemodynamic stability during induction of anesthesia. It also has demonstrated a relaxant effect on pulmonary arteries in normoxic rats (Rich et al., 1994). However, opioids should still be used as adjuncts to etomidate in order to blunt spikes in sympathetic tone, such as during endotracheal intubation. Conversely, ketamine has not been commonly used in pediatric PAH because of concerns about its ability to increase sympathetic tone and PVR (Hickey et al., 1985; Morray et al., 1984). This effect is less problematic when patients are mechanically ventilated and hypoxia and hypercarbia are avoided (Hickey et al., 1985).

7. What are the strategies to treat a PHC?

Avoidance: Avoid factors that may precipitate an increase in PVR, such as hypoxemia, hypercarbia, acidosis, systemic hypotension, and increased sympathetic tone.

Treatment: Prompt diagnosis and treatment of PHC are paramount for successful resuscitation. First in line are the administration of 100% oxygen, treatment of hypercarbia by hyperventilation, and alkalization of blood by administering sodium bicarbonate. Chest compressions and epinephrine may be required if there are signs of significantly diminished cardiac output or cardiac arrest. Muscle relaxants may help in controlling ventilation. Remove any noxious stimulus and consider giving narcotics. Support cardiac output by augmenting preload with fluids and inotropic drugs, such as dobutamine or milrinone, which may also reduce PVR, or dopamine, which will maintain SVR and therefore help to optimize coronary perfusion. Start pulmonary vasodilators.

8. What is the role of pulmonary vasodilators in the treatment of PHC?

Inhaled nitric oxide (iNO): iNO is a selective pulmonary vasodilator that activates guanylate cyclase in pulmonary vascular smooth muscle cells and decreases intracellular calcium (Roberts et al., 1997). Its rapid onset and pulmonary selectivity make it the first-line pulmonary vasodilator therapy during a PHC in children and adults. iNO has also been demonstrated to be safe in the treatment of PPHN. iNO is inactivated by rapidly binding to hemoglobin, thereby avoiding any systemic effects.

Phosphodiesterase-5 inhibitors: Inhibitors of phosphodiesterase-5, including dipyridamole, zaprinast, pentoxifylline, and sildenafil, lead to vascular smooth muscle relaxation and pulmonary artery vasodilation. Dipyridamole has significant systemic vasodilatory effects and should be used with caution in patients with limited cardiac reserve. Sildenafil has been shown to lead to marked reductions in PVR in neonates and adults and can be used to ameliorate rebound PAH after cessation of iNO. However, it may precipitate severe hypotension when coadministered with iNO. Sildenafil is available in intravenous, oral, and inhaled forms.

Endothelin inhibitors: The smooth muscle mediator endothelin-1 has been implicated in the etiology of PAH because of its potent vasoconstrictive effects. Bosentan is an antagonist at the dual receptors endothelin A and endothelin B. It is available in oral form with a half-life of 5 hours. Its use in children with PAH has been shown to decrease pulmonary artery pressure (mPAP) and PVR and to increase cardiac output.

Calcium channel blockers: Calcium channel blockers have been used in the treatment of PAH due to their pulmonary vasodilatory effects, as well as their ability to reverse smooth muscle cell hypertrophy occurring in PAH. Challenges with this class of drugs are their negative inotropic effects, which are least with nifedipine.

Prostacyclins: Patients with PAH have a reduced capacity for producing vasodilatory prostacyclins in pulmonary arteries. Epoprostenol, the most commonly used prostacyclin analog, leads to improved exercise capacity, hemodynamics, and survival in patients with severe pulmonary hypertension who suffer from symptoms during less-than-ordinary life tasks or at rest (New York Heart Association class III and IV; Badesch et al., 2007). It is used as a continuous infusion due to its extremely short half-life (2–5 minutes) or via a nebulizer into the breathing circuit of ventilated patients.

9. Where is the most ideal postanesthesia setting for the patient with PAH?

In order to determine the most ideal place for the patient after surgery, the anesthesiologist must first be aware of the severity of the patient's PAH along

TABLE 29.2. DELINEATION OF PULMONARY HYPERTENSION SEVERITY

Classification	Description
Subsystemic	<70%
Systemic	70%–100%
Suprasystemic	>100%

with other comorbidities. Typically, the severity of illness along with the type and length of procedure will help predict the potential for complications. Typically, the ratio of mean mPAP to mean systemic blood pressure (mSAP) or [mPAP/mSAP] written in percentages will help identify severity of this dynamic disease process (Chau et al., 2016). The classification of PAH severity is included in Table 29.2.

Other anesthetic factors risk that can increase risks include emergency surgery, age <1 year, large intraoperative opioid doses, oxygenation, and ventilation issues during the case. Thus the ideal location for the patient after anesthesia again lies in a multiplicity of factors ranging from the preoperative comorbidities, severity of pulmonary hypertension, as well as intraoperative happenings. The overall goal is to prevent complications such as PHC. This can only be done with a well-formulated plan based on multidisciplinary team discussion among anesthesiologist, surgeon, pulmonologist, and cardiologist. Additionally, expertise in the care of such patients is imperative. However, ensuring the availability of a pediatric intensive care unit bed is prudent. It is always better to be conservative and not deescalate care too hastily since complications have occurred many hours after procedures.

SUMMARY

1. Risk factors for PAH are hypoxemia, hypercarbia, acidosis, and increases in sympathetic tone.
2. Developmental abnormalities that lead to persistent fetal circulation include underdevelopment of the pulmonary system (e.g., congenital heart disease, polyhydramnios), genetic predisposition leading to abnormally thickened pulmonary arterioles, and events such as aspiration of meconium or premature closure of a patent ductus arteriosus.
3. Signs of PAH include tachypnea, tachycardia, cyanosis, arrhythmias, and cardiac arrest.
4. For management of PAH, focus on avoiding or treating hypoxemia, counteracting hypercarbia and acidemia, preventing dehydration/hypovolemia, treating dysrhythmias, and maintaining cardiac output. Avoid increases in sympathetic tone by aggressively treating agitation, noxious stimuli, and pain. Use iNO for direct vasodilation of the pulmonary vasculature, then transition to oral sildenafil.
5. The ideal location for the patient after anesthesia depends on a multiplicity of factors ranging from the preoperative comorbidities, severity of pulmonary hypertension, as well as intraoperative happenings.

ACKNOWLEDGMENTS

The author wishes to acknowledge the first edition authors, George Istaphanous and Andreas Loepke.

ANNOTATED REFERENCES

Carmosino MJ, Friesen RH, Doran A, Ivy DD. Perioperative complications in children with pulmonary hypertension undergoing noncardiac surgery or cardiac catheterization. *Anesth Analg.* 2007;104(3):521–527.

A review of medical records of children with PAH who underwent anesthesia or sedation for noncardiac procedures and cardiac catheterizations. Significant predictor of major complications (cardiac arrest and/or PHC) was baseline suprasystemic PAH but not age, etiology of PAH, or anesthetic type.

Roberts JD, Fineman JR, Morin FC, et al. Inhaled nitric oxide and persistent pulmonary hypertension of the newborn. The Inhaled Nitric Oxide Study Group. *N Engl J Med.* 1997;336(9):605–610.

A prospective, randomized, multicenter study of infants with severe hypoxemia and persistent PAH. iNO improved systemic oxygenation and decreased the need for extracorporeal membrane oxygenation when compared to nitrogen without causing systemic hypotension or methemoglobinemia.

BIBLIOGRAPHY

Adams JM, Stark AR. Persistent pulmonary hypertension of the newborn. In: Garcia-Prats JA, ed. *UpToDate.* Waltham, MA: UpToDate; 2011.

Badesch DB, Abman SH, Simonneau G, Rubin LJ, McLaughlin VV. Medical therapy for pulmonary arterial hypertension: updated ACCP evidence-based clinical practice guidelines. *Chest.* 2007;131:1917–1928.

Chau DF, Gangadharan M, Hartke LP, Twite MD. The Post-Anesthetic Care of Pediatric Patients with Pulmonary Hypertension. *Semin Cardiothorac Vasc Anesth.* 2016;20(1):63–73.

Hickey PR, Hansen DD, Cramolini GM, Vincent RN, Lang P. Pulmonary and systemic hemodynamic responses to ketamine in infants with normal and elevated pulmonary vascular resistance. *Anesthesiology.* 1985;62(3):287–293.

Morray JP, Geiduschek JM, Ramamoorthy C, et al. Anesthesia-related cardiac arrest in children: initial findings of the Pediatric Perioperative Cardiac Arrest (POCA) Registry. *Anesthesiology.* 2000;93(1):6–14.

Morray JP, Lynn AM, Stamm SJ, Herndon PS, Kawabori I, Stevenson JG. Hemodynamic effects of ketamine in children with congenital heart disease. *Anesth Analg.* 1984;63(10):895–899.

Pilkington SA, Taboada D, Martinez G. Pulmonary hypertension and its management in patients undergoing non-cardiac surgery. *Anaesthesia.* 2015;70(1):56–70.

Rich GF, Roos CM, Anderson SM, Daugherty MO, Uncles DR. Direct effects of intravenous anesthetics on pulmonary vascular resistance in the isolated rat lung. *Anesth Analg.* 1994;78(5):961–966.

Sarkar M, Laussen PC, Zurakowski D, Shukla A, Kussman B, Odegard KC. Hemodynamic responses to etomidate on induction of anesthesia in pediatric patients. *Anesth Analg.* 2005;101(3):645–650.

Simonneau G, Galiè N, Rubin LJ, et al. Clinical classification of pulmonary hypertension. *J Am Coll Cardiol.* 2004;43(12 Suppl S):5S–12S.

Simonneau G, Gatzoulis MA, Adatia I, et al. Updated clinical classification of pulmonary hypertension. *J Am Coll Cardiol.* 2013;62(25):D34–D41.

Walsh-Sukys MC, Tyson JE, Wright LL, et al. Persistent pulmonary hypertension of the newborn in the era before nitric oxide. *Pediatrics.* 2000;105:14–20.

PART 7

Challenges in Ophthalmology

30

Open Globe Repair

MICHAEL LIN AND ERIN S. WILLIAMS

INTRODUCTION

Ocular trauma in childhood is common and may cause transient or permanent visual impairment. Approximately 840,000 eye injuries occur in children annually in the United States. Open globe injuries, compared to closed globe injuries, generally lead to more complications and a worse visual outcome. The anesthetic management of children with penetrating eye injuries presents several unique challenges, including potential associated injuries that may take precedence over the treatment of the eye injury, the prevention of aspiration of gastric contents, the regulation of intraocular pressure (IOP), the prevention of the oculocardiac reflex (OCR), and the preservation of vision in the affected eye. An understanding of the mechanisms and management of these potential problems can favorably influence anesthetic and surgical outcomes.

LEARNING OBJECTIVES

1. Review the definition, assessment, and potential complications of open globe injury.
2. Explain the anesthetic management of patients with open globe injury and full stomach.
3. Discuss contributing factors and management of the OCR.
4. Analyze the determinants of IOP and anesthetic effects on IOP.
5. Outline anesthetic goals to help reduce any further injury or complications.

CASE PRESENTATION

A previously healthy 4-year-old girl presents to the emergency department after slipping and falling in the bath tub. Unfortunately during the fall, her right eye hit the end of the faucet. She weighs 14 kg and has no other injuries. She ate dinner 2 hours ago and currently does not have intravenous (IV) access.

DISCUSSION

1. What is an open globe injury?

An open globe injury is a full-thickness injury of the cornea and/or sclera that is caused by rupture or laceration of the globe of the eye. Globe rupture is typically caused by blunt eye force leading to a tear near the equator of the globe and behind the insertion of the rectus muscle. Globe laceration is caused by penetrating injury and may have an associated exit wound or intraocular foreign body. Open globe injuries can further be categorized by the extent of the injury: Zone 1 occurs in the cornea and limbus, Zone 2 extends from limbus to anterior 5 mm of sclera, and Zone 3 extends posteriorly to Zone 2. An open globe injury may present with decreased visual acuity, visible laceration, decreased volume of the eye, defect of the iris, or an afferent pupillary defect. Evaluation of the injury may include a computed tomography scan and any other evaluation necessary to assess for any accompanying trauma that may have occurred in addition to the globe injury. If an open globe injury is suspected, actions and medications that may increase IOP should be avoided to prevent further injury and extrusion of vitreous fluid.

2. What are the determinants of IOP?

Normal IOP is 16 ± 5 mmHg in the upright position and increases by 2 to 4 mmHg when supine. IOP maintains the shape and optical properties of the eye. It is determined by the balance between production

TABLE 30.1. EFFECT OF CARDIAC AND PULMONARY VARIABLES ON IOP

Variable	Effect on IOP
Central venous pressure	
Increase	↑↑↑
Decrease	↓↓↓
Arterial blood pressure	
Increase	↑
Decrease	↓
PaO_2	
Increase	0
Decrease	↑
$PaCO_2$	
Increase (hypoventilation)	↑↑
Decrease (hyperventilation)	↓↓

↓ = decrease (mild, moderate, marked); ↑ = increase (mild, moderate, marked); 0 = no effect.

Reprinted with permission from Butterworth JF. Mackey DC, Wasnick JD. Anesthesia for ophthalmic surgery. In: Butterworth JF. Mackey DC, Wasnick JD, eds. *Morgan & Mikhail's Clinical Anesthesiology*. 5th ed., p. 760: Table 36-1. Copyright The McGraw-Hill Companies, 2013.

and drainage of aqueous humor, change in choroidal blood volume, vitreous volume, and extraocular muscle tone. Temporary variations in pressure are usually well tolerated in normal eyes. However, when the globe is ruptured, IOP is lowered and may be as low as ambient pressure. Any factor that normally increases IOP will cause drainage or extrusion of vitreous fluid through the wound resulting in decreased intraocular volume. This is a serious complication that can permanently impair vision.

Several cardiac and pulmonary variables affect IOP (Table 30.1). Increase in central venous or systolic blood pressure, hypoxia, hypercarbia, and increased tension within the extraocular muscles all raise IOP. The opposite physiological parameters lower it (Seidel & Dorman, 2006). Hypoxemia and hypercapnia may increase IOP through choroidal arteriole vasodilatation; sustained hypertension raises IOP by increasing choroidal blood volume. The most significant impact on IOP is *changes in central venous pressure*. Actions that cause congestion in the venous system impede outflow of aqueous humor and increase the volume of choroidal blood. *Coughing, straining, bucking on the endotracheal tube, vomiting, excessive cricoid pressure, and the Valsalva maneuver can all elicit a dramatic elevation in IOP, as high as 30 to 40 mmHg.*

3. What anesthetic effects increase the risk of vitreous herniation?

Any of the factors above that increase IOP can result in vitreous herniation. Additionally, external pressure on the eye from a tightly fitted mask, improper positioning, coughing, straining, bucking, vomiting, or retrobulbar hemorrhage may result in extravasation of intraocular contents. Other factors include extraocular muscle spasm induced by depolarizing muscle relaxants, surgical stimulation during light anesthesia, or poorly applied cricoid pressure. Choroidal congestion from hypoxia, hypercapnia, osmotic diuretics, laryngoscopy, intubation, or increases in blood pressure also play a role.

Most anesthetic agents either lower or have no effect on IOP (Table 30.2). This occurs either directly, by alteration in aqueous humor flow or extra- and intraocular muscle tone, or indirectly, by altering cardiovascular parameters. All IV induction agents (except ketamine) and inhalational agents reduce IOP by direct effects. Sedative agents such as benzodiazepines and opioids also lower IOP. Lidocaine 2 mg/kg blunts IOP response to laryngoscopy and intubation by attenuating airway response and the cough reflex (Yukioka et al., 1985).

Succinylcholine (suxamethonium) is the muscle relaxant of choice in patients with a full stomach.

TABLE 30.2. EFFECT OF ANESTHETICS ON IOP

Drug	Effect on IOP
Inhaled Anesthetics	
Volatile agents	↓↓
Nitrous oxide	↓
Intravenous Anesthetics	
Barbiturates	↓↓
Benzodiazepines	↓↓
Ketamine	?
Opioids	↓
Propofol	↓↓
Muscle Relaxants	
Succinylcholine	↑↑
Nondepolarizers	0/↓

↓ = decrease (mild, moderate); ↑ = increase (mild, moderate); 0/↓ = no change or mild decrease;? = conflicting reports

Reprinted with permission from Butterworth, et al. Anesthesia for ophthalmic surgery. In: Morgan GE, Mikhail MS, Murray MJ, eds. *Clinical Anesthesiology*, 5th ed., pp. 760: Table 36-3. Copyright The McGraw-Hill Companies, 2013.

However, its effect on IOP produces the possibility of ocular content extrusion. Succinylcholine raises IOP by 6 to 8 mmHg by increasing extraocular muscle tension and by contracting orbital smooth muscle, which reduces outflow of aqueous humor. The alteration in IOP begins at 1 minute, peaks at 2 to 4 minutes, and lasts up to 6 minutes. Although two large reviews have shown the safety of succinylcholine with no reports of vitreous herniation (Donlon, 1986; Libonati et al., 1985), the use of succinylcholine in patients with open globe injuries remains widely debated. The decision on whether to use succinylcholine in open globe surgeries should be based on the potential for a difficult airway and the viability of the eye. In the setting of an easy airway, regardless of the patient's aspiration risk and regardless of the viability of the eye, succinylcholine can be avoided and replaced with the currently available short- or intermediate-acting nondepolarizing muscle relaxants. Ideal intubation conditions can be achieved rapidly with large-dose rocuronium (1–1.2 mg/kg, 60 seconds), vecuronium (0.25 mg/kg, 60 to 90 seconds), or cisatracurium (0.25 mg/kg, 60 to 90 seconds; Doenicke et al., 1998). *If the airway is difficult and the eye is viable,* succinylcholine may be favored because the nondepolarizing agents may have a prolonged effect that may result in increases in IOP from mask application, hypercarbia, and a longer time with an unprotected airway. *If the risk of aspiration is considered high,* succinylcholine may be used. It is better to avoid aspiration by using succinylcholine than to have aspiration occur and have subsequent increases in IOP from hypoxia and hypercarbia.

Studies that examined techniques to prevent the increase in IOP due to succinylcholine have shown that a greater increase in IOP occurs from the stimulation of laryngoscopy and endotracheal intubation (Zimmerman et al., 1996). If succinylcholine will be administered, it is imperative to *blunt the IOP response to laryngoscopy and endotracheal intubation* by ensuring adequate depth of anesthesia with appropriate induction agents, which will also suppress laryngeal airway reflexes, such as opioids or lidocaine.

The use of dexmedetomidine, an α2-agonist, may be helpful not only as a premedication for anxiolysis but also in decreasing IOP throughout the perioperative course. However, the anesthesia provider should be extra vigilant when administering dexmedetomidine as bradycardia may occur when it is rapidly administered. Hypertension may also occur with dexmedetomidine administration especially at higher doses.

4. What are the triggers for the OCR, and how is it managed?

The trigemino-vagal OCR is characterized by bradycardia and cardiac dysrhythmias, including ectopy, junctional rhythm, atrioventricular block, ventricular fibrillation, and cardiac arrest. The reflex is induced by mechanical stimulation, such as traction on the extraocular muscles (especially medial rectus), pressure on the eye or on the empty orbit, and intraorbital injections or hematomas. OCR is thus frequently encountered during ocular procedures and can be evoked in all age groups. Contributing factors include a light plane of general anesthesia, hypoxia, hypercarbia, and increased vagal tone.

The OCR consists of an initial parasympathetic phase, followed by a sympathetic phase. Anticholinergic medication may be helpful in preventing this reflex, but the need for routine prophylaxis is controversial. The hemodynamic response to OCR is of fast onset and short duration. The reflex typically fatigues itself with repeated stimulation. In severe cases of OCR requiring pharmacological intervention, IV atropine or glycopyrrolate immediately prior to surgery is more effective than intramuscular premedication. Also, a retrobulbar block is unreliable in preventing OCR and may actually precipitate OCR, cause cardiac arrest, or cause retrobulbar hemorrhage.

Management of OCR includes the following:

- Immediate notification of the surgeon and temporary cessation of surgical stimulation or traction until heart rate increases
- Confirmation of adequate ventilation, oxygenation, and depth of anesthesia
- Administration of IV atropine if conduction disturbance persists
- In recalcitrant episodes, infiltration of the rectus muscles with local anesthetic

5. How should one manage patients with an open globe injury and a full stomach?

Initial management of an open globe injury prior to surgery should be to limit the risk of further injury by minimizing any increase in IOP that may lead to a secondary injury from vitreous herniation.

Measurements of IOP and pupillary dilation should not be performed. Pain medications should be administered as needed along with antiemetics. The patient should be positioned upright to lower the IOP as well. Patients who have a full stomach at the time of surgery will also need precautions to minimize the risk of aspiration during anesthesia induction. Prophylaxis with an H_2 receptor antagonist, proton pump inhibitor, or nonparticulate antacid should be considered. An IV should be placed prior to induction of anesthesia. IV placement can be facilitated with oral midazolam and application of topical anesthetic to the area where the IV will be placed. Once an IV is secured, dexmedetomidine may be administered in addition to midazolam in order to facilitate separation from the parents and aid in a smooth anesthesia induction.

General anesthesia is the preferred method for the pediatric patient undergoing an ocular procedure. Gentle placement of the face mask during the preoxygenation period will avoid pressure on the eye. If the patient has a full stomach and an easy airway, rapid sequence induction can be accomplished without succinylcholine using a large dose of nondepolarizing agent after induction with propofol and properly applied cricoid pressure. Succinylcholine with its shorter duration of action may be the safer choice if there is doubt about the ability to ventilate and/or intubate the patient, even if the eye is viable. In fasted patients, the use of nondepolarizing muscle relaxants is recommended. For either situation, prior administration of IV opioids and/or lidocaine (2 mg/kg) is recommended to attenuate the hypertensive response to laryngoscopy and intubation.

Intraoperative administration of antiemetic medications, such as dexamethasone, prior to the start of surgery and ondansetron at the completion of the operation will minimize the risk of postoperative nausea and vomiting. Decompression of the stomach may decrease the incidence of postoperative emesis, although it does not guarantee an empty stomach. Intravenous lidocaine (1.5 mg/kg) may be administered 1 to 2 minutes prior to extubation to reduce coughing during emergence. Multimodal analgesia with opioids, nonsteroidal anti-inflammatory drugs, and acetaminophen will help with a smooth emergence and minimize straining in the recovery room. Extubation should be delayed until the child is awake and has intact airway reflexes. Additional dexmedetomidine (0.3–0.5 μg/kg IV) may also be administered to facilitate emergence and the postanesthesia care.

SUMMARY

1. Overall anesthetic goals are to avoid increasing IOP and to prevent aspiration.
2. Premedicate judiciously; minimize coughing, crying, and vomiting preoperatively.
3. Succinylcholine has been used safely in patients with a full stomach and open globe injury, but high-dose nondepolarizing muscle relaxants offer an attractive alternative. Consider succinylcholine when the risk of aspiration is high, the eye is not salvageable, or a difficult intubation is anticipated.
4. Administer drugs to minimize postoperative nausea and vomiting, and extubate awake.
5. Successful treatment of an open globe injury involves an anesthetic that minimizes vitreous herniation and assists in swift treatment to minimize the risk of infection (endophthalmitis.)
6. Perioperative management of pain, anxiety, and nausea can minimize the risk of vitreous herniation.
7. Treatment of other life-threatening injuries take precedence over surgery for an open globe injury; however, urgent treatment should be undertaken as soon as possible.
8. Full-stomach precautions should be taken if the patient has a full stomach, and rapid sequence induction is strongly recommended.

ACKNOWLEDGMENTS

The authors wish to acknowledge the first edition authors, J. Fay Jou and Judith O. Margolis.

ANNOTATED REFERENCES

Butterworth JF. Mackey DC, Wasnick JD. Anesthesia for ophthalmic surgery. In Butterworth JF. Mackey DC, Wasnick JD, eds. *Morgan & Mikhail's Clinical Anesthesiology*. 5th ed. New York: Lange McGraw-Hill; 2013:826–836.

A solid discussion of basic principles and anesthesia considerations involved in the management of a patient presenting for ophthalmic surgery.

Kudlak TT. Open-eye injury. In: Yao FF, Malhotra V, Fontes ML, eds. *Yao & Artusio's Anesthesiology: Problem-Oriented Patient Management.* 6th ed. Philadelphia: Lippincott Williams & Wilkins; 2008:1007–1024.

A case-based, problem-oriented overview of the topic with comprehensive practical explanations and references.

Seidel J, Dorman T. Anesthetic management of preschool children with penetrating eye injuries: postal survey of pediatric anesthetists and a review of the available evidence. *Pediatr Anesth.* 2006;16:769–779.

This paper discusses the practice of anesthetists in Great Britain and Ireland based on a survey pertaining to the care of the child with an open globe injury and full stomach. The paper also discusses the evidence regarding management of the patient with a penetrating eye injury.

Yukioka H, Yoshimoto N, Nishimura K, Fujimori M. Intravenous lidocaine as a suppressant of coughing during tracheal intubation. *Anesth Analg.* 1985;64:1189–1192.

Coughing was suppressed completely when 2 mg/kg of lidocaine IV was administered between 1 and 5 minutes before intubation compared with partial cough suppression with 1- and 1.5-mg/kg doses.

BIBLIOGRAPHY

Allen SL, Duncan E. Open globe injury. In: Atlee J, ed. *Complications in Anesthesia.* 2nd ed. Philadelphia: Saunders; 2007:745–746.

Chidiac EJ. Succinylcholine and the open globe: questions unanswered. *Anesthesiology.* 2004;100:1035–1036.

Doenicke AW, Czeslick E, Moss J, Hoernecke R. Onset time, endotracheal intubating conditions, and plasma histamine after cisatracurium and vecuronium administration. *Anesth Analg.* 1998;87:434–438.

Donlon JV Jr. Succinylcholine and open eye injury II [letter]. *Anesthesiology.* 1986;64:525–526.

Hahnenkamp K, Honemann CW, Fischer LG, Durieux ME, Muehlendyck H, Braun U. Effect of different anaesthetic regimes on the oculocardiac reflex during paediatric strabismus surgery. *Pediatr Anesth.* 2000;10:601–608.

Libonati MM, Leahy JJ, Ellison N. The use of succinylcholine in open eye surgery. *Anesthesiology.* 1985;62:637–640.

Zimmerman AA, Funk KJ, Tidwell JL. Propofol and alfentanil prevent the increase in intraocular pressure caused by succinylcholine and endotracheal intubation during a rapid sequence induction of anesthesia. *Anesth Analg.* 1996;83:814–817.

PART 8

Challenges in Neurosurgical Conditions and Neuromonitoring

31

Prone Positioning for Posterior Fossa Tumor Resection

MATTHIAS W. KÖNIG, MOHAMED A. MAHMOUD, JOHN J. MCAULIFFE III, AND MATTHEW D. JAMES

INTRODUCTION

Brain tumors are the second most common malignancy in children. About one-third occur in toddlers under the age of 3, and about two-thirds are located in the posterior fossa. Resection of posterior fossa tumors is often a lengthy procedure that is commonly performed in the prone position. The prone position is associated with physiological changes and predisposes the patient to certain types of injuries.

LEARNING OBJECTIVES

1. Appreciate the logistic challenges of turning a small patient into the prone position.
2. Be aware of potential complications unique to prone positioning.
3. List strategies to avoid position-related injuries.
4. Consider cardiopulmonary resuscitation (CPR) in the prone position.

CASE PRESENTATION

A 3-year-old girl is scheduled for elective resection of a posterior fossa medulloblastoma. She initially presented with nausea, vomiting, lethargy, and problems keeping her balance. Her weight is 14.2 kg, vital signs are within normal range, and preoperative blood counts, electrolytes, and coagulation studies are unremarkable. Anesthesia is induced through an existing intravenous line, the airway is secured with a cuffed 4.5 endotracheal tube (ETT), and a second intravenous line and a radial artery catheter are placed. The procedure proceeds uneventfully and after ***almost 5 hours*** *the patient is turned supine. At this time,* ***marked swelling is noted in the face,*** *both eyes are swollen shut; the* ***tongue appears swollen*** *and protrudes from the mouth.*

DISCUSSION

1. What are common logistic issues of positioning the pediatric patient prone?

The list of potential "mishaps" during the turning maneuver is long, but the anesthesia provider should vigilantly watch for the following issues.

Airway: The ETT needs to be securely taped to prevent dislodgement. Due to the patient's oral secretions in the prone position, the tape securing the ETT may get moist and gradually loosen. For this reason, some practitioners use skin adhesives (e.g., tincture of benzoin, Mastisol® liquid adhesive) to increase adherence of the tape to the skin, apply clear tape or Tegaderm® on the cheeks on top of the primary ETT tape, and/or administer anticholinergics to minimize salivation. Access to the airway will be limited once the patient is positioned prone, and a dislodged or kinked ETT will be more difficult to reposition. Some practitioners advocate armored/spiral ETTs to reduce the risk of kinking; others intubate nasally. Whatever technique is used, bilateral breath sounds, adequate ventilation, and proper positioning and taping of the ETT must be confirmed after turning into prone position and before surgery commences. During skin preparation for surgery, ensure the prep fluid does not drip down over the tape securing the ETT, as alcoholic prep can dissolve tape adhesive. The laryngeal mask airway is probably the best immediate rescue option if the ETT is accidentally pulled out in the prone position and thus should be immediately available.

Prolonged "blackout" period: It is tempting to simplify the turning maneuver by temporarily disconnecting monitors and intravenous and arterial lines to avoid having to disentangle them later. However, this frequently leads to periods of prolonged monitoring "blackout" where the patient's vital signs are not properly monitored. When positioning, it is critical for the anesthesia provider to avoid being distracted by other tasks that delay adequate monitoring, ventilation, and provision of anesthesia. Some would argue to keep at least the pulse oximetry probe attached while turning, since it will provide basic information on oxygenation and perfusion. End-tidal carbon dioxide monitoring should be restored with ventilation once the patient is prone. The configuration of the trace should be examined for evidence of airway obstruction or bronchospasm that may have been precipitated by the movement of the child.

Positioning and padding: Numerous devices, tables, and frames are utilized to position the patient prone position. However, some common precautions apply to all of them:

- Bony prominences should be padded to limit and diffuse pressure.
- There should be no direct pressure on genitals and breasts.
- The chest and pelvis are typically supported by foam/gel rolls or pillows to allow the abdomen to "hang" free in order to minimize venous congestion and maximize diaphragmatic excursion. Ensure chest rolls do not extend down to the groin and place pressure on femoral vessels.
- There should be padding under the knees and support under the ankles/feet such that the toes are elevated off of the bed.
- Direct pressure to eyes and nose is avoided by using suitably cut-out foam pillows, using commercially available pillows/headrests, or securing the head in a holder with pins.
- The neck should stay close to the neutral position. Acute flexion of the head or neck should be done carefully to avoid impeding drainage of the neck veins and to avoid strain on the neck ligaments and cervical nerve roots.
- Consider a Tegaderm® over the eyes instead of tape as the prep solution can enter the eye around or through saturated tape.
- Arms can be positioned neutrally alongside the body or be abducted less than 90 degrees to avoid traction on the brachial plexus.
- Before the patient is covered with surgical drapes, make sure that no monitoring or fluid lines are under the patient's extremities or torso, where they may cause pressure points. Likewise, the ETT, ETT pilot balloon, anesthesia breathing circuit, and oro/nasogastric tube should not put any pressure on the face.
- Verify proper function of all intravenous and arterial lines and monitoring equipment before the patient is draped. Be sure there is easy access to injection sites and access ports to be able to draw blood samples without competing with the surgeon for space.
- Address the risk for venous stasis and deep vein thrombosis. Consider elevation of the limbs, elastic wrappings, or compression devices.
- Patient position changes should be done slowly so that physiologic effects may be noticed and then the anesthetic adjusted.

Temperature: During line placement, the child is frequently left uncovered, and a significant drop in body temperature may occur. To avoid/minimize hypothermia, the patient's body should be covered as much as is practical during this phase; forced-air warming blankets should be used, and the ambient temperature of the operating room should be raised. For small patients, radiant heat loss is the predominant type of heat loss. Raising the operating room temperature well ahead of surgical start time is important in order to warm the walls and major objects in the room to reduce the heat gradient, which would enhance such losses.

2. What are the effects of the prone position on major organ systems?

The pathophysiological consequences of prone positioning are well researched in adults, but data in small children are not available. However, several points can probably be extrapolated from adult studies (Table 31.1). Prone positioning may accentuate the physiologic challenges of intracranial surgery. A posterior fossa tumor may cause obstruction to the free flow of cerebrospinal fluid. A proper understanding of the pressure-volume curve and

TABLE 31.1. PATHOPHYSIOLOGICAL EFFECTS OF THE PRONE POSITION

Cardiovascular	Respiratory	Central Nervous
Venous return ↓	Functional residual capacity ↑; ⇔	Jugular venous flow↑; ⇔
Stroke volume ↓	Total lung capacity↑; ⇔	Jugular venous resistance ↓ ⇔
Cardiac output ↓ ⇔	V/Q mismatch ↓	Intracranial pressure ↑; (if head lower than heart)
Heart rate ↑		
Systemic vascular resistance ↑		
Systolic blood pressure ↑ ⇔		
Mean arterial pressure ↑ ⇔		

This table was published in Rozet I, Vavilala MS. Risks and benefits of patient positioning during neurosurgical care. *Anesthesiol Clin.* 2007;25:631–653. Copyright Elsevier, 2007.

careful intracranial pressure control are essential in managing these cases.

3. What are typical position-related injuries during and after prolonged prone positioning for surgery?

Although severe long-term morbidity is fortunately rare as a consequence of prolonged prone positioning, the anesthesia provider must be aware of several uncommon but potentially disastrous complications. It is good practice to explain these potential risks when obtaining consent for anesthesia. Preoperative warning usually helps simplify postoperative discussions.

Pressure sores/abrasions: These are usually found overlying bony prominences and are rarely a significant clinical problem. Careful padding can help avoid most of these.

Facial/intraoral swelling: After prolonged face-down position, some degree of facial swelling is common. Seeing their child with the eyes swollen shut after surgery may be distressing to parents, but usually reassurance is all that will be required in cases of facial swelling. Several cases have been reported where significant ***tongue swelling*** led to *partial or complete airway obstruction* after extubation. In cases of significant tongue swelling, it may be prudent to delay extubation until the swelling subsides. If proceeding with extubation then a nasal airway may be useful at this time.

Neurologic injury: Peripheral nerve injury, most commonly due to *overstretching of the brachial plexus,* has been described after prone surgeries. Abduction of the arms more than 90 degrees should be avoided, as well as using overly thick padding under the arms in small children, which may stretch the plexus by forcing an abducted arm backwards/posteriorly. Rare cases of vascular *injury to the cervical spinal cord* have been reported, and avoidance of excessive neck flexion and hypotension has been recommended to maintain adequate cord perfusion.

Postoperative visual loss: This is probably the most feared complication by surgeons and anesthesiologists in this setting. Although mostly reported in posterior spine surgery, it has also been reported in a child undergoing sagittal synostosis repair in the prone position (Lee et al., 2005). The exact pathophysiology is still somewhat elusive, but intraoperative *hypotension, anemia, prone position,* and *duration of procedure (>6 hr)* are the most consistently identified risk factors. Direct pressure on the eye is responsible for only a minority of cases. The most common (~90%) ophthalmologic diagnoses are *anterior and posterior optic nerve ischemia*. Much less common is retinal artery/vein occlusion (the only diagnosis that is related to pressure on the eye) and cortical blindness.

Preventive strategies include

- Hemodynamic stability
- Adequate hemoglobin/hematocrit
- Avoiding excessive crystalloid infusion to minimize risk of edema
- Meticulous positioning of the head and frequent checks to make sure nothing presses on the eyes

4. Can one perform CPR in the prone position?

Conventionally, CPR is performed in the supine position in all age groups. However, successful CPR in the prone position, including cardiac compressions, has been described in a number of cases, both in operating rooms and intensive care units (e.g. Tobias et al., 1994). There are several considerations when conducting CPR of the prone patient:

Speed: Resuscitation relies on rapid initiation of CPR. Taking the time to pack and cover a wound and flip the patient supine may cause deleterious delays in starting chest compressions. In some cases, the anesthesiologist placed his or her clenched fist under the sternum of the patient while the surgeon gave cardiac compressions. CPR can therefore be started while a stretcher is brought into the operating room so that the patient can be turned supine for ongoing resuscitation.

Protecting intravenous access and invasive monitoring: Turning a patient supine under emergency conditions to perform CPR poses the substantial risk of losing intravenous access and the arterial line when they are needed most.

Contamination of surgical field: Depending on the nature of the surgery, turning the patient supine may risk infection and/or trauma to exposed tissue.

SUMMARY

1. Turning an anesthetized child prone requires the undivided attention of the anesthesia provider to protect the airway and intravenous and arterial access.
2. Reestablishing ventilation and complete monitoring—if it has been disconnected before turning—should have highest priority.
3. Closely attend to padding and positioning; frequently recheck the face and eyes.
4. Avoid hypotension and anemia.
5. Not all facial swelling after long prone surgeries is benign, and airway compromise may occur in cases of tongue swelling.
6. CPR is possible in the prone position and may be safer than hastily turning the patient.

ACKNOWLEDGMENT

This chapter was updated and edited by Matthew D. James, MD.

ANNOTATED REFERENCES

American Society of Anesthesiologists Task Force on Perioperative Blindness: practice advisory for perioperative visual loss associated with spine surgery. *Anesthesiology*. 2012;116:274–285.

Summary of the current knowledge and expert/evidence-based recommendations on prevention and treatment of perioperative visual loss. Initially published in 2006 and then revised in 2012 but with no significant changes.

Edgcombe H, Carter K, Yarrow S. Anaesthesia in the prone position. *Br J Anaesth*. 2008;100:165–185.

Excellent and comprehensive review of physiological effects of the prone position and potential complications.

Tobias JD. Anesthesia for spinal surgery in children. In: Gregory G, Andropoulos D, eds. *Pediatric Anesthesia*. 5th ed, pp. 654–677. Chichester, UK: Wiley; 2012.

Textbook chapter about spinal surgery that covers relevant topics of prone positioning and CPR and eye injuries.

Tobias JD, Mencio GA, Atwood R, Gurwitz GS. Intraoperative cardiopulmonary resuscitation in the prone position. *J Pediatr Surg*. 1994;29:1537–1538.

Case report of successful CPR in a 12-year-old in the prone position after cardiac arrest during posterior spine surgery.

BIBLIOGRAPHY

Lee J, Crawford MW, Drake J, Buncic JR, Forrest C. Anterior ischemic optic neuropathy complicating cranial vault reconstruction for sagittal synostosis in a child. *J Craniofac Surg*. 2005;16(4):559–562.

Martínez-Lage JF, Almagro MJ, Izura V, Serrano C, Ruiz-Espejo AM, Sánchez-Del-Rincón I. Cervical spinal cord infarction after posterior fossa surgery: a case-based update. *Child's Nerv Syst*. 2009;25:1541–1546.

Sinha A, Agarwal A, Gaur A, Pandey CK. Oropharyngeal swelling and macroglossia after cervical spine surgery in the prone position. *J Neurosurg Anesth*. 2001;13:237–239.

32

Anesthetic Considerations for Scoliosis Repair

KIM-PHUONG NGUYEN AND CHRIS D. GLOVER

INTRODUCTION

Scoliosis is a multidimensional deformity caused by a lateral and rotational deformity of the thoracolumbar spine that has an incidence of 1% to 2%. Scoliosis can be categorized as idiopathic, congenital, or neuromuscular. Despite extensive research, the cause and pathogenesis remain unknown, although leading hypotheses center on a multifactorial origin (Owen, 1999; Sloan et al., 2002). Adolescent idiopathic scoliosis is the most common variant seen with an incidence of 1% to 3% in children aged 10 to 16 years. Many of these patients can be managed with conservative therapy via bracing; however, surgical intervention is usually warranted for those with significant curvature. Surgical correction involves wide exposure of the spine for placement of stabilizing rods along a pedicle screw framework. These procedures can result in significant complications from excessive blood loss and neurologic impairments, requiring vigilance to acid-base status, hemodynamic fluctuations, coagulation, temperature maintenance, and neurologic monitoring from anesthesiologists.

Anesthetic concerns for this procedure include maintaining the integrity of perfusion to the spinal cord, positioning concerns, optimal technique for neuromonitoring, and pain control in the perioperative period.

LEARNING OBJECTIVES

- Define scoliosis and list indications for scoliosis repair with a background in relevant anatomical concerns.
- Describe the types of intraoperative neurophysiologic monitoring (IONM) commonly used in scoliosis repair.
- Summarize how varying anesthetic techniques affect evoked potentials in those undergoing scoliosis repair.
- Review the risk factors associated with potential complications for scoliosis repair.

CASE PRESENTATION

A 14-year-old girl with adolescent idiopathic scoliosis presents for posterior spinal instrumentation and fusion from T4-L4 with autologous bone graft.

Her past medical history is significant for obesity, back pain, and dyspnea on exertion. She weighs 85 kg and is 155 cm tall. Laboratory tests are within normal limits. Her preoperative hemoglobin (Hgb) is 13.2 g/dl. Her chest x-ray (Figure 32.1) revealed a Cobb angle >40 degrees.

Two intravenous (IV) lines are started after an uneventful inhalational induction. An endotracheal tube, orogastric tube, and bite block are placed following intubating doses of propofol and opioids. An arterial line is also placed for intraoperative assessment of blood pressure and facilitation of lab draws. The inhalation agents are then discontinued and the patient is started on an infusion of propofol and sufentanil as part of a total IV anesthetic plan. Tranexamic acid is the institution-specific antifibrinolytic which is bolused at the start of the case and infused throughout. After assessing a baseline set of evoked potentials, the patient is turned in the prone position for the procedure. With adequate exposure, pedicle screws are placed and the first bar is attached along the spine. Estimated blood loss is now 3 L, which has been replaced with 4 units of packed red blood cells, 1 L of albumin, and 2,500 ml of crystalloid fluids. Her Hgb is now at 9.8 g/dl and the mean arterial pressures have been trending

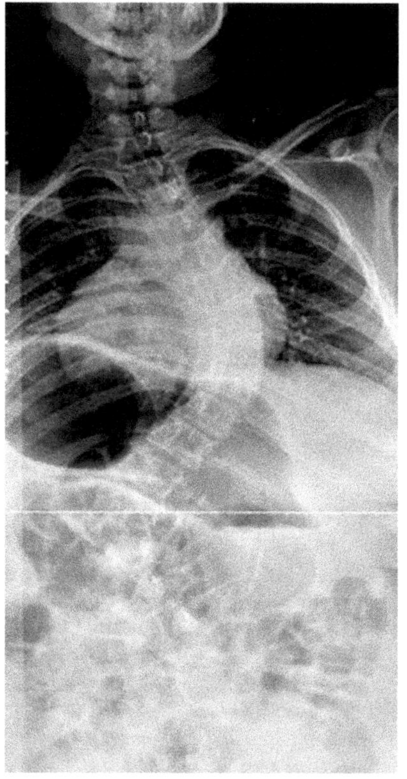

FIGURE 32.1: Chest x-ray exhibiting severe scoliosis.

in the 50s. With the placement of the second bar, the neurophysiologist reports a decrease in his signals on testing of the transcranial motor evoked potentials. The patient is placed on 100% oxygen and the mean arterial pressure is raised using a combination of vasopressors and fluids. The second bar is removed by the surgeon and the neurophysiologist now reports complete loss of signals. The surgeon requests a wakeup test be performed. All anesthetic agents are discontinued and the patient emerges from anesthesia briefly moving all extremities. The operative team consults together and decides to proceed with placing the second rod with elevated mean pressures. Total intravenous anesthesia (TIVA) is reinstituted and the subsequent attempt at rod placement goes well with no discernible changes in evoked potentials. After completion of the case, the patient is extubated and taken to recovery. A patient-controlled analgesia device is set up for managing postoperative pain. When you stop by to reevaluate the patient in recovery, she reports some discomfort with facial swelling and pain associated along her thorax. Physical exam reveals a grade 1 pressure ulcer, which slowly resolves over the course of her hospitalization.

DISCUSSION

1. Define scoliosis and delineate the different types of scoliosis encountered in anesthetic practice. What are the presenting findings associated with this disease? What are indications for repair?

Scoliosis is an anatomic defect of the thoracolumbar spine caused by lateral and rotational deformation of the spine with rib cage abnormalities. Scoliosis can be categorized as idiopathic, congenital, or neuromuscular. Idiopathic is the most common variant seen and occurs more frequently in females. Congenital scoliosis is a defect noted at birth that occurs from vertebral or costal maldevelopment thought to occur in 1 out of every 1,000 live births (Ravish et al., 2012). The etiology extrapolated from mice research points to maternal toxin exposure as likely. The rate of progression is quite rapid in the first 5 years of life and again during puberty, which coincide with stages of rapid spine growth. Neuromuscular scoliosis is commonly associated with the patient conditions listed in Table 32.1.

Left uncorrected, scoliosis can result in back pain, dyspnea on exertion, and restrictive lung disease. Progression from these symptoms can lead to the development of pulmonary hypertension, respiratory failure, and right heart failure.

TABLE 32.1. CLASSIFICATION OF SCOLIOSIS

Idiopathic	Congenital	Neuromuscular
Infantile (0–3 yrs)	Bony deformity	Cerebral palsy
Juvenile (4–10 yrs)	Neural tube defects	Poliomyelitis
Adolescent idiopathic (>10 yrs)		Muscular dystrophy
		Spinal muscular atrophy
		Neurofibramotosis

As symptom severity is associated with disease progression, repair is usually undertaken when the Cobb angle is greater than 50 degrees in those considered skeletally mature and >40 degrees in those with skeletal immaturity.

2. What is a Cobb angle and what is its utility?

The Cobb angle is a way of quantifying the degree of scoliosis in a patient. It is measured by the intersection of perpendicular lines extending from lines along the vertebral body at the superior and inferior margins of the spine deformity (Fig. 32.2). While any lateral curvature >10 degrees is considered abnormal, repair is usually undertaken once this angle becomes greater than 40 degrees. Severe scoliosis is usually defined as a Cobb angle greater than 50 degrees.

3. How is blood supplied to the spinal cord? What are the different types of IONM available for use in scoliosis repair, and how do they correlate with the blood supply for the spinal cord?

The spinal cord blood supply is derived from paired posterior spinal arteries supplying the posterior third of the spinal cord with a single anterior spinal artery supplying the anterior two-thirds of the spinal cord.

Segmental medullary and radicular arteries arising from the aorta facilitate perfusion for the anterior portion of the lower thoracic and lumbar spinal. Of significance is the artery of Adamkiewicz, which is instrumental for perfusion of the lower spinal cord. This relationship puts the thoracolumbar area at increased risk with manipulation associated with scoliosis repair. Cord blood flow follows the same principles with regards to autoregulation as cerebral blood flow.

Amplitude and latency are the measures used for all evoked potential monitoring. Somatosensory-evoked potential (SSEP) monitoring became widely adopted in the 1980s and allows for monitoring of the dorsal column-medial lemniscus pathway, which mediates proprioception, vibration, and tactile discrimination. This correlates with the paired posterior spinal arteries. Pain and temperature are not mediated by this assessment as they are mediated through the spinothalamic tract. SSEP monitoring stimulates the extremities at fixed intervals, which leads to a signal being recorded via scalp electrodes.

Changes are considered significant if the amplitude is decreased by more than 50% and/or the latency is increased by 10%. In addition, testing at the level of the brachial plexus can give insight into potential brachial plexus injury from positioning issues.

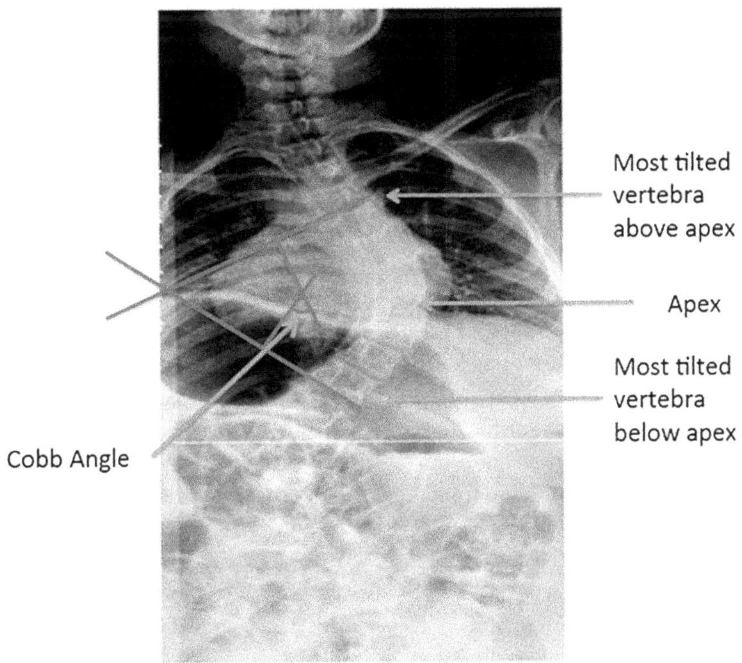

FIGURE 32.2: Cobb angle.

TABLE 32.2. ELECTROMYOGRAPHY AND DERMATOMAL LEVEL ASSESSED

Nerve root	Muscles Monitored
C8-T1	Adductor pollicis
T2-T6	Intercostals
T6-T12	Rectus abdominus
L3-L4	Vastus lateralis
L4-L5	Anterior tibialis
S1-S2	Gastrocnemius

TABLE 32.3. ANESTHETIC AGENTS ON EVOKED POTENTIALS

Modality	Significant Finding
SSEP	Amplitude—decrease >50%
	Latency—increase >10%
TcMEP	Amplitude—decrease >75%80%
EMG	Sustained neurotonic discharges

Note. SSEP = somatosensory-evoked potential; TcMEP = transcranial motor evoked potentials; EMG = electromyography.

However, SSEPs do not have the sensitivity to identify individual nerve root injury.

Motor-evoked potentials (MEPs) can be recorded at multiple levels and are more commonly recorded as compound muscle action potentials via surface electrodes or via subdermal needles placed in peripheral muscles. Monitoring primarily occurs in adductor pollicus, adductor hallucis, and the tibialis anterior. The control is the upper extremity with a comparison to the lower extremity to assess amplitudes between the two. Amplitude decreases of 75% are considered significant. Monitoring of transcranial motor evoked potentials (TcMEPs) are advantageous for a couple of reasons. TcMEPs are exquisitely sensitive to spinal cord impairment, with TcMEPs detecting spinal cord impairment an average of 5 minutes before SSEPs in a study by Schwartz et al. (2007). TcMEPs are also quite sensitive to blood pressure changes given the anterior blood supply described earlier. There are limitations with this monitoring modality given the patient movement associated with testing.

Free running electromyography (EMG) tracks spontaneous electrical discharges from muscles in effort to assess potential nerve injury. These spontaneous sustained discharges usually result when nerves are irritated. Recordings occur via placement of electrodes in specific muscles associated with nerve roots (see Table 32.2). Nerve root injuries are quite common in spine surgery, accounting for 65% of all new neurologic deficits. SSEPs do not have the specificity or sensitivity to identify individual nerve root injury as they assess multiple nerve roots simultaneously. A normal EMG has low-amplitude, high-frequency activity. EMG can be classified as free running or triggered EMG. EMG is relatively resistant to anesthetics' effects, and as such there are relatively few limitations to maintain adequate monitoring conditions outside of limiting or avoiding altogether the use of muscle relaxants.

4. How do the anesthetics commonly used affect evoked potentials?

Most anesthetics through their lipid solubility decrease amplitude and increase latency (see Table 32.3). The commonly used volatile anesthetics all produce a dose-dependent decrease in amplitude and increase in latency for SSEPs. The volatile anesthetics can be used for cortical SSEP monitoring in concentrations less than 0.5 MAC, but concentrations as low as 0.2 MAC have been noted to abolish TcMEPS. Nitrous oxide causes profound reduction in amplitude with increased latency in all neurophysiologic monitoring as well.

IV opioids produce limited depression of evoked potentials. Ketamine differs from other agents in that it increases amplitudes. Etomidate can be used as a constant infusion to enhance SSEP cortical recordings, but lack of analgesia, potential for enhanced seizure activity, and potential for adrenal suppression are factors to consider with its use.

Benzodiazepines can be used in IONM as they minimally affect evoked potentials.

Propofol produces amplitude depression with large doses. Given its rapid metabolism, the depression noted is transient. In fact, this rapid metabolism makes propofol a superb agent as part of a TIVA regimen for those undergoing scoliosis repair. Table 32.3 covers what is considered a significant change with the types of IONM used in practice. A summary of anesthetic agents and their effects on evoked potentials is listed in Table 32.4.

5. What is a wake-up test?

The wake-up test is credited to Stagnara and Vazuelle (1973) and remains the gold standard for assessing spinal cord integrity. Assessing function via the movement with emergence allows for an evaluation of global motor function. A major limitation of this form of testing is that it can localize injury along the motor

TABLE 32.4. EVOKED POTENTIAL SIGNIFICANT FINDINGS

Anesthetic Agents	Amplitude	Latency
Volatile agents		
• Isoflurane		
• Desflurane		
• Sevoflurane	↓	↑
Barbiturates	↓	↑
Nitrous oxide	↓	↔
Midazolam	↓	↔
Propofol	↔	↔
Dexmedetomidine	↔	↔
Opioids	↔	↔
Etomidate	↑	↔
Ketamine	↑	↔

pathway only for a single point in time. Accidental extubation, intraoperative recall, and increased surgical time are all possible risks during a wake-up test.

6. What strategies are available to decrease potential blood loss in scoliosis repair?

There are various strategies that can be implemented to reduce intraoperative blood loss. Holistically, things like positioning, controlled hypotension, and normothermia are ways to mitigate blood loss. Blood conservation strategies via preoperative autologous donation, use of intraoperative cell salvage, and the hemodilution are other methods to decrease blood loss. Antifibrinolytics have been shown to decrease blood loss for these cases and should be part of the anesthetic regimen.

7. What are your anesthetic goals during surgery? What specific concerns do you have with a patient in the prone position?

Anesthetic goals should encompass the following:

- Neuroprotection via an anesthetic strategy that allows for uninterrupted IONM. Although <0.5 MAC inhaled agents have been used successfully at many institutions, a comparison of the energy required to elicit MEPs in those receiving desflurane versus TIVA revealed the need for higher voltage and more frequent pulses to elicit comparable MEP amplitudes. Consequently, TIVA techniques with propofol as a central component have been advocated to optimize neuromonitoring during spine surgery. This usually entails a TIVA strategy of propofol and an institutional choice of opioid.
- Blood conservation as described.
  - o Proper positioning has been noted to decrease total blood loss via decreases in intra-abdominal pressure.
  - o Avoidance of hypothermia. Temperatures <35°C should be avoided given their association with coagulopathy and increased blood loss.
  - o Use of antifibrinolytics given findings of decreased blood loss and need for transfusion.
- Maintenance of volume status
- Moderate induced hypotension (reduction of systolic blood pressure 20 mmHg from baseline or lowering mean arterial pressure to 65 mmHg in the normotensive adolescent patient) has been shown to decrease blood loss and reduce transfusion requirements.

Concerns during and following scoliosis repair include bleeding, pain control, and catastrophic complications such as postoperative visual loss and paraplegia. Dental guards and soft bite blocks are necessary as evoked potentials can result in significant muscle contractions, which may cause dental and tongue injury.

Induced hypotension is not without risk and has been reported to increase the risk of *neurologic deficits such as vision loss and spinal cord ischemia*. Visual loss following nonocular surgery is an infrequent but disastrous complication with an estimated incidence ranging from 0.001% to 0.2%. The three recognized causes of postoperative visual loss are ischemic optic neuropathy, central retinal artery or vein occlusion, and cerebral ischemia. Intraoperative risk factors that may precipitate development of postoperative vision loss include anemia and hypotension during spine surgery.

Neurologic injuries following spine fusion occur at an incidence between 1% to 2% when procedures involve anterior and posterior repair. A review by the Scoliosis Research Society found that patients with kyphoscoliosis, severe scoliosis, and congenital scoliosis were at increased risk of developing postoperative neurologic injury (Burton et al., 2016). Methods to mitigate this complication would center on discussions with surgeons on the need for controlled hypotension in high-risk patients, maintaining volume status, and being vigilant with monitoring blood loss during surgery. Of those patients who developed neurologic deficits, approximately 60% fully recovered from their injury, while the remainder had partial or no improvement.

8. Describe a treatment algorithm to treat a loss in evoked potentials

An algorithm should be readily available and staff should be trained on their responsibilities in a situation where evoked potentials are lost. Immediate steps should be undertaken to elicit the etiology of the signal loss. From an anesthesiologist perspective, the immediate aims center on improving perfusion to the spinal cord. This includes administering 100% oxygen and raising the mean arterial pressure to >90 mmHg. This can be accomplished by reducing anesthetic agent exposure, expanding the intravascular volume, and/or using a vasoactive agent. Oxygen-carrying capacity can be increased by raising the hematocrit and physiologic factors such as temperature. Acid base status should be assessed and optimized as well. Recent rod or pedicle screws should be removed by the surgeon, and any action that may have precipitated loss of evoked potentials should be reversed. The neurophysiology technician should ensure that machine error is not contributing to this scenario. The use of steroids remains controversial, but some centers do include this agent as part of a spinal cord injury protocol.

The recommended protocol is methylprednisolone 30 mg/kg IV as a loading dose, followed by an infusion of methylprednisolone at 5.4 mg/kg/hour for the next 23 hours. If improvement in potentials is not seen with attempts to correct hemodynamics and perfusion, an **intraoperative wake-up** test should be performed. Imaging via computed tomography scan may further elucidate etiology from a surgical standpoint.

9. What options for postoperative pain control are available for patients undergoing scoliosis repair?

Consensus is currently lacking with regards to optimal postoperative pain management. All strategies are multimodal in nature. Options are primarily opioid based but vary on route of administration. Methods described in the literature include patient-controlled analgesia, intrathecal opioid administration, and placement of epidural catheters under direct vision. Patient-controlled analgesia seems to be the most commonly used method. Most centers allow for a continuous rate over the first postoperative day (POD) with transition to oral medications occurring over POD 2 to 5. Intrathecal administration of morphine has been reported to result in decreased blood loss and pain relief over the course of 14 hours. Single and double epidural catheters with infusions have also been used. Comparisons between the methods are limited but trend toward lower pain scores in those receiving medications in the neuraxial space. Adjuncts include the use of benzodiazepines to combat muscle spasms and anxiety in the postoperative period. Ketorolac has shown benefit in the immediate period, but its use should be discussed with surgical colleagues due to perioperative concerns of bleeding and development of pseudoarthrosis.

SUMMARY

1. SSEPs are more sensitive to inhalation agents with decreases in amplitude and increases in latency compared to IV agents such as propofol, ketamine, dexmedetomidine, and opioids.
2. Ketamine and etomidate may be used to try to augment SSEPs.
3. MEPs are the modality of choice for monitoring motor tract function, are easily abolished by inhalational agents, and negate the use of full neuromuscular blockade.
4. Patients with immature neural pathways or pre-existing neuromuscular disease may have abnormal baseline SSEP recordings.
5. Maintenance of adequate physiological parameters for normal neuronal functioning is critical to IONM during scoliosis repair.

ACKNOWLEDGMENTS

The authors wish to acknowledge the first edition authors, Mohamed A. Mahmoud, Matthew W. Konig, and John J. McAuliffe.

ANNOTATED REFERENCES

Merton PA, Morton HB. Stimulation of the cerebral cortex in the intact human subject. *Nature.* 1980;285(5762):227.

1980 article demonstrating that single-pulse voltage applied transcranially could result in contralateral motor activity, marking the first time the integrity of the corticospinal tract could be assessed.

Soundararajan N, Cunliffe M. Anaesthesia for spinal surgery in children. *Br J Anaesth*. 2007;99:86–94.

This review article provides a comprehensive discussion of the anesthetic issues in children undergoing spine surgery. It also goes into a very good discussion on issues associated with prone positioning.

Schwartz DM, Auerbach JD, Dormans JP, et al. Neurophysiological detection of impending spinal cord injury during scoliosis surgery. *J Bone Joint Surg Am*. 2007;89(11):2440–2449.

Report that details the sensitivity of TcMEPs to spinal cord impairment with TcMEPs detecting spinal cord impairment an average of 5 minutes before SSEPs.

Sethna NF, Zurakowski D, Brustowicz RM, Bacsik J, Sullivan LJ, Shapiro F. Tranexamic acid reduces intraoperative blood loss in pediatric patients undergoing scoliosis surgery. *Anesthesiology*. 2005;102(4):727–732.

The study concludes that intraoperative administration of tranexamic acid significantly reduces blood loss during spinal surgery in children with scoliosis.

Vauzelle C, Stagnara P, Jouvinroux P. Functional monitoring of spinal cord activity during spinal surgery. *Clin Orthop Relat Res*. 1973;93:173–178.

Article with significance describing the wake-up test to assess functional integrity of the spinal cord.

BIBLIOGRAPHY

Altaf F, Gibson A, Dannawi Z, Noordeen H. Adolescent idiopathic scoliosis. *BMJ*. 2013;30(346).

Burton DC, Carlson BB, Place HM, et al. Results of the Scoliosis Research Society Morbidity and Mortality Database 2009–2012: A Report from the Morbidity and Mortality Committee. *Spine Deform*. 2016;4(5):338–343.

Giampietro PF, Blank RD, Raggio CL, et al. Congenital and idiopathic scoliosis: clinical and genetic aspects. *Clin Med Res*. 2003;1(2):125–136.

Hamilton DK, Smith JS, Sansur CA, et al. Rates of new neurological deficit associated with spine surgery based on 108,419 procedures: a report of the scoliosis research society morbidity and mortality committee. *Spine*.2011;36(15):1218–1228.

Machida M. Cause of idiopathic scoliosis. *Spine*. 1999;24(24):2576–2583.

McNicol ED, Tzortzopoulou A, Schumann R, Carr DB, Kalra A. Antifibrinolytic agents for reducing blood loss in scoliosis surgery in children. *Cochrane Database Syst Rev*. 2016 Sep 19;9.

Owen JH. The application of intraoperative monitoring during surgery for spinal deformity. *Spine*. 1999;24(24):2649–2662.

Patil CG, Lad EM, Lad SP, Ho C, Boakye M. Visual loss after spine surgery: a population-based study. *Spine*. 2008 Jun 1;33(13):1491–1496.

Ravish M, et al. Pain management in patients with adolescent idiopathic scoliosis undergoing posterior spinal fusion: combined intrathecal morphine and continuous epidural versus PCA. *J Pediatr Orthop*. 2012 Dec;32(8):799–804.

Sloan TB, Heyer EJ. Anesthesia for intraoperative neurophysiologic monitoring of the spinal cord. *J Clin Neurophysiol*. 2002;19(5):430–443.

Vauzelle C, Stagnara P, Jouvinroux P. Functional monitoring of spinal cord activity during spinal surgery. *Clin Orthop Relat Res*. 1973;93:173–178.

Yamada K, Yamamoto H, Nakagawa Y, Tezuka A, Tamura T, Kawata S. Etiology of idiopathic scoliosis. *Clin Orthop Relat Res*. 1984;184:50–57.

PART 9

Challenges in Patients with Hematologic and Oncologic Disorders

33

Sickle Cell Disease

ANN NG AND ERIN S. WILLIAMS

INTRODUCTION

Sickle cell anemia (sickle cell disease [SCD]) is a common hemoglobinopathy with predominance in populations of African descent; approximately 0.2% of African Americans have sickle cell anemia, while 8% to 10% have sickle cell trait. This chapter provides an overview of the etiology, pathophysiology, and treatment of sickle cell anemia and the perioperative management of affected patients.

LEARNING OBJECTIVES

1. Review the etiology and pathophysiology of SCD.
2. Understand the specifics of the preoperative evaluation of a sickle cell patient and indications for preoperative blood transfusion.
3. Explain the intraoperative management of patients with SCD.
4. Understand the issues in postoperative management.
5. Consider alternatives, such as ketamine, for managing painful vaso-occlusive crises.

CASE PRESENTATION

A 4-year-old boy with sickle cell anemia presents to the hospital for inguinal hernia repair. He has not had any recent infections or issues with pain. He has never had a true pain crisis or acute chest syndrome. His mother states that he has done well with his diagnosis and has been transfused only one time in the last year.

His last hemoglobin was 10 from 1 month ago. You ask about his nil per os status and find out that he last ate 8 hours ago and drank clears 2 hours earlier. You discuss your anesthetic plan which includes general anesthesia and a caudal block. To ensure that the patient remains adequately calm, you introduce the child life therapist to the patient and family. Once the consent is obtained, you proceed to the operating room (OR) with the child.

You enter the OR, which has been warmed to 80ºF, and perform a smooth inhaled induction after application of monitors. Once the peripheral venous catheter and the laryngeal mask airway have been placed, the patient is turned to the left lateral decubitus position for the caudal block.

The block is performed successfully, and the patient is returned to the supine position. You allow the patient to breathe spontaneously and give additional parenteral opioids as needed prior to incision. The case proceeds uneventfully, and you notice an increase in the end-tidal carbon dioxide (ETCO$_2$) increased from 40 to 55mmHg. You adjust the ventilator accordingly and utilize the pressure support setting. The ETCO$_2$ subsequently decreases to 42 mmHg. The surgery is completed successfully and the patient emerges from anesthesia without complication.

DISCUSSION

1. What is SCD or anemia, and what are the preoperative concerns for a patient with SCD?

SCD is an autosomal recessive disease whereby the normal hemoglobin A is replaced by hemoglobin S. The normal hemoglobin molecule is a tetramer consisting of four subunits—two alpha and two beta. Hemoglobin S consists of two normal alpha subunits and two abnormal beta subunits; where valine substitutes for glutamic acid at the sixth position on the beta chain. Sickling occurs due to hemoglobin polymer formation when the arterial oxygen content drops below 20 mmHg in heterozygotes and below 40 mmHg in homozygous patients. Polymerized hemoglobin increases blood viscosity and obstructs microcirculation. This further increases hypoxia and sickling, and a vicious cycle results in tissue infarction, release of inflammatory mediators, and pain. ***Acidosis, cold, dehydration, trauma, infection, fever, and stress all predispose to sickling.*** Protective factors may include the presence of fetal hemoglobin (hemoglobin F—two alpha and two gamma subunits), which has higher affinity for oxygen. Hemoglobin F is the main hemoglobin present at birth, but its levels decrease significantly after 6 months of age. Around this time the symptoms of sickle cell anemia become apparent. Disease severity can range from mild, with sickle cell *trait* (40% hemoglobin S), to severe (and potentially fatal) sickle cell *anemia* (70%–98% hemoglobin S).

Diagnosis is made by hemoglobin electrophoresis. Table 33.1 presents an overview of the clinical issues seen in SCD.

Clinically, sickle cell anemia presents as chronic hemolysis with acute exacerbations (crises). Acute exacerbations themselves can manifest as painful (vaso-occlusive) crises (e.g., abdominal pain mimicking surgical condition or musculoskeletal pain), infarctive crisis, sequestration crisis (with blood pooling in the spleen or liver), and aplastic crisis with complete bone marrow suppression. **Acute chest syndrome** is a medical emergency (mortality up to 10%), the cause of which is not fully understood.

TABLE 33.1. OVERVIEW OF CLINICAL ISSUES IN SICKLE CELL DISEASE

Causes of Sickling
Hypoxemia
Hypotension
Hypovolemia
Hyperviscosity
Vasoconstriction
Acidosis
Fever
Increases in 2,3-diphosphoglyceride
Shivering or increased metabolic rate
Clinical Syndromes of Sickle Cell Disease
Chronic pain
Painful or vaso-occlusive crises
Aplastic
Sequestration
Hemolysis (chronic or acute)
Acute chest syndrome
Systemic Effects of Sickle Cell Anemia
Constitutional: Delayed growth and development
Immunologic: Infections, sepsis (especially encapsulated organisms)
Cardiac: Congestive heart failure (due to chronic hypoxia, anemia, and hemochromatosis)
Pulmonary: Increased intrapulmonary shunting
Renal: Papillary necrosis (more in sickle trait), concentrating deficiency
Neurologic: Stroke and sequelae
Hematologic: Chronic anemia, aplastic anemia (parvovirus B19 associated)
Genital: Priapism
Gastrointestinal: Cholelithiasis
Splenic: Infarcts, asplenia, acute sequestration
Skeletal: Avascular necrosis, osteomyelitis
Skin: Ulcers (ankle)
Metabolic: Hemochromatosis

2. What are preoperative considerations for patients with homozygous SCD (HbSS)?

It is helpful to think about the perioperative management in terms of a **quartet of key factors: oxygenation, hydration, normothermia, and hematocrit**. Preoperative hydration is mandatory with some institutions admitting patients anywhere from 4 hours to 24 hours preceding the surgery in order for them to receive intravenous (IV) hydration. Preoperative transfusion is indicated for patients undergoing intermediate- and high-risk surgery with or without an underlying pulmonary disorder, with a target hemoglobin 10 g/dL or higher. Preoperative anxiolytics may be administered as necessary, with caution as respiratory suppression can result in oxygen desaturation, which can trigger sickling. Therefore, supplemental oxygen in patients receiving preoperative sedatives is reasonable. A forced-air warmer or similar device is helpful to maintain normal body temperature, and applying it prior to induction of anesthesia helps reduce the drop in temperature that results within the first hour of general anesthesia. Regarding packed red blood cell transfusions, data suggest that a conservative regimen targeting a total hemoglobin level of 10 g/dL offers the same efficacy in preventing perioperative complications as an aggressive regimen (target HbSS <30% total) but with half of the transfusion-related complications (Vichinsky et al., 1995). Patients with sickle cell trait do not require preoperative transfusion except before open heart surgery or extensive thoracic surgery.

3. How does hydroxyurea work in SCD?

The treatment of sickle cell anemia can be divided in two groups: prophylactic and symptomatic.

Hydroxyurea is used as part of **prophylactic treatment** to prevent crisis and complications related to the disease. **Hydroxyurea** stimulates hemoglobin F production. Higher levels of hemoglobin F diminish the severity of crises by preventing hemoglobin S polymerization (Charache et al., 1995). Other widely used prophylactic interventions include administration of pneumococcal vaccine and antibiotics in febrile illness/acute chest syndrome. Folic acid is prescribed to prevent megaloblastic anemia. Bone marrow transplantation is reserved for patients younger than 16 years of age who have had multiple serious complications related to sickle cell anemia and crises.

Symptomatic treatment of painful vaso-occlusive crises starts with rehydration. Pain management follows an ascending algorithm beginning with acetaminophen and nonsteroidal anti-inflammatory drugs (NSAIDs). Patients in crisis usually have moved beyond this step by the time they present to the hospital and often have begun oral opioids at home. Advancing the oral regimen or adding IV opioids, either intermittently or via patient-controlled analgesia pump, is appropriate, depending on previous history of chronic analgesic use, severity of pain, and symptoms. Regional and neuraxial analgesia are also good options. For long-term pain management, acetaminophen, NSAIDs, opioids, and adjuncts have been used (e.g., gabapentin for bone pain, the tricyclic antidepressant amitriptyline for abdominal pain and sleep disturbances).

4. What is acute chest syndrome, and how is it managed?

Acute chest syndrome is a medical emergency that is a feared complication in the postanesthetic phase, with significant morbidity and mortality (mortality up to 10%). Patients present with an acute pain crisis (lower chest), fever, cough, pleuritic **chest pain**, hypoxemia, pulmonary hypertension, and **lung infiltrates** of the lower bases on chest radiograph. Patients with acute chest syndrome may have concomitant rib infarcts. Recurrent episodes progress to pulmonary fibrosis and chronic respiratory insufficiency. The management involves mechanisms that will address the quartet of key factors: oxygenation, hydration, normothermia, and hemoglobin to maintain adequate hemoglobin level. Start **supplemental oxygen via nasal cannula** or face mask to maintain normal oxygen saturation. Hydrate the patient—replace deficits first, maintain hydration with close attention to losses (due to sweating, high fever, urine output, vomiting), and treat fever or hypothermia. **Transfusion** may be indicated, either simple or exchange, depending on the severity of symptoms. Inhaled bronchodilators may be indicated in patients with acute chest syndrome if there is a component of increased airway reactivity. There are few data regarding antibiotic administration in patients with acute chest syndrome; the treatment to date is empiric. An infectious etiology can be identified in only 30% of patients; 10% suffer an embolic event (fat embolism from necrotic marrow), but the majority of patients have an unclear etiology. Pain medications—preferably NSAIDs such as ketorolac or cautious use of opioids (avoid respiratory depression and worsening oxygenation)—and incentive spirometry are frequently indicated. Epidural analgesia may be helpful for patients whose analgesia is limited by opioid side effects. Patients may require **admission to the intensive care unit** or another unit where they can be more closely monitored, and their hematologist should be consulted. Hyder and colleagues (2013) found that the six most common inpatient surgeries in the pediatric SCD population include cholecystectomy, tonsillectomy/ adenoidectomy, splenectomy, umbilical hernia repair, appendectomy, and myringotomy. They also showed that the most common complication was acute chest syndrome after these elective procedures, and stroke and death were rare (Hyder et al. 2013).

5. What are the intra- and postoperative concerns for these patients?

If a patient with SCD has been adequately prepared preoperatively, then the outcome of the anesthetic should be favorable. Intraoperative management again follows the quartet of key factors—*oxygenation, hydration, normothermia, and hemoglobin*. There is no single best anesthetic for all SCD patients. The use of tourniquets during surgery is discouraged although not strictly contraindicated.

Regional anesthesia has been successfully used as the sole anesthetic but has also been used as an adjunct to general anesthesia. For cardiac surgery, cardiopulmonary bypass represents a unique challenge as it is a combination of hypothermia, acidosis, and low peripheral blood flow. However, SCD patients seem to tolerate it without increased risk (Yousafzai et al., 2010). Postoperatively, the homeostatic quartet should be maintained through the postanesthesia care unit (PACU) until the patient has fully emerged and is ready to be discharged from the PACU. Shivering in the PACU should be treated aggressively, as vigorous exertion can trigger sickling. Note that SCD patients may require larger quantities of opioids for analgesia when compared to other patients; this is due to chronic exposure-induced tolerance. Neri and colleagues (2013) showed a potential benefit from use of ketamine in sickle cell patients. When SCD patients appear to not receive relief from their vaso-occlusive crisis pain, it may be prudent to consider adding ketamine for better analgesia (Neri et al., 2013). A recent review by Hagedorn and Monico (2016) suggests that ketamine's analgesic and anesthetic properties may make it an ideal choice in the treatment of Sickle cell vaso-occlusive crises pain.

The hematology team should be contacted immediately in the postoperative phase in order to coordinate care for these patients, especially for those with a previous history of stroke, acute chest syndrome, or splenic sequestration.

SUMMARY

1. Consider early preoperative admission, from 4 to 24 hours prior to surgery, for hydration, and also for transfusion (the latter if hemoglobin is less than 10 g/dL).
2. Key intraoperative factors to maintain are oxygenation, hydration, body temperature, and hemoglobin over 10 g/dL.
3. Postoperatively, maintain oxygenation, hydration, and body temperature; start incentive spirometry early; and consider overnight observation.
4. For postoperative pain management, patients may be opioid-tolerant. The full range of analgesics should be used; regional analgesia can be used for either postoperative pain or pain from vaso-occlusive crises.
5. Additionally, ketamine should be considered when managing opioid-tolerant patients.

ACKNOWLEDGMENTS

The authors wish to thank the first edition authors, Alexandra Szabova and Kenneth Goldschneider.

ANNOTATED REFERENCES

Charache S, Terrin ML, Moore RD, et al. Effect of hydroxyurea on the frequency of painful crises in sickle cell anemia. Investigators of the Multicenter Study of Hydroxyurea in Sickle Cell Anemia. *N Engl J Med.* 1995;332(20):1317–1322.

This double-blind randomized controlled trial tested the efficacy of hydroxyurea versus placebo on the frequency and severity of crises in adult patients. The trial was terminated prematurely due to strong evidence for patient benefit.

Hagedorn JM, Monico EC. Ketamine infusion for pain control in acute pediatric sickle cell painful crises. *Pediatr Emerg Care.* 2016 Nov 29. [Epub ahead of print]

This is a literature review that discusses the benefit of ketamine use when treating pain in sickle cell patients.

Hyder O, Yaster M, Bateman BT, et al. Surgical procedures and outcomes among children with sickle cell disease. *Anesth Analg.* 2013;117(5):1192–1196.

This study is a retrospective analysis of the billing data from the National Inpatient Sample database over an 11-year period that shows 3.6% of all hospital discharges of pediatric SCD patients involved surgery. By looking at these surgeries, it was discovered that acute chest syndrome was the most common complication and stroke and death were rare.

Neri CM, Pestieau SR, Darbari ES. Low-dose ketamine as a potential adjuvant therapy for painful vaso-occlusive crises I sickle cell disease. *Paediatr Anaesth.* 2013;23(8):684–689.

This review article discusses the potential benefit of low-dose ketamine boluses and infusions as adjuvants in managing pain in pediatric sickle cell patients.

Vichinsky EP, Haberkern CM, Neumayr L, et al. A comparison of conservative and aggressive transfusion regimens in the perioperative management of sickle cell disease. Preoperative Transfusion in Sickle Cell Disease Study Group. *N Engl J Med.* 1995;333(4):206–213.

The landmark randomized controlled trial that showed that an aggressive transfusion regimen (hemoglobin S <30%) was comparable to a conservative regimen (to achieve a hemoglobin level of 10 g/dL) in preventing perioperative complications in patients with HbSS. The conservative approach reduced transfusion-associated complications by 50%.

Yaster M, Tobin JR, Billett C, Casella JF, Dover G. Epidural analgesia in the management of severe vaso-occlusive sickle cell crisis. *Pediatrics.* 1994;93(2):310–315.

An early retrospective study of 9 patients admitted with vaso-occlusive crisis who failed to respond to conventional analgesia. Epidural analgesia was effective in treating vaso-occlusive pain without causing sedation, respiratory depression, or limitation on ambulation.

BIBLIOGRAPHY

Alhashimi D, Fedorowicz A, Alhashimi F, Dastgiri S. Blood transfusion for treating acute chest syndrome in people with sickle cell disease. *Cochrane Database Syst Rev.* 2010;1:CD007843. doi:10.1002/14651858.CD007843.pub2

de Montalembert M. Management of sickle cell disease. *BMJ.* 2008;337:a1397.

Frietsch T, Ewen I, Waschke KF. Anaesthetic care for sickle cell disease. *Eur J Anaesth.* 2001;18(3):137–150.

Marchant WA, Walker I. Anaesthetic management of the child with sickle cell disease. *Paediatr Anaesth.* 2003;13(6):473–489.

Wethers D. Sickle cell disease in childhood: part I. Laboratory diagnosis, pathophysiology and health maintenance. *Am Fam Physician.* 2000;62:1013–1028.

Wethers D. Sickle cell disease in childhood: part II. Diagnosis and treatment of major complications and recent advances in treatment. *Am Fam Physician.* 2000;62:1309–1314.

Yousafzai SM, Ugurlucan M, Al Radhwan OA, Al Otaibi AL, Canver CC. Open heart surgery in patients with sickle cell hemoglobinopathy. *Circulation.* 2010;121(1):14–19.

34

Hemophilia

REBECCA MCINTYRE

INTRODUCTION

Recent advances in the management of patients with hemophilia have led to significantly improved outcomes. Transmission of infectious diseases through blood product administration and severe arthropathies from recurrent joint bleeds are now rare. In the past, hemophilia was considered a contraindication to having some elective surgeries, such as adenotonsillectomy, due to the risk of life-threatening bleeding complications. Now, management of elective surgery in these patients can be straightforward and safe, provided adequate planning and consultation with a hematologist occur.

LEARNING OBJECTIVES

1. Understand the pathophysiology and classification of hemophilia.
2. Be familiar with the methods of diagnosis of hemophilia and other bleeding disorders.
3. Know the principles of management of patients with hemophilia undergoing elective surgery.
4. Understand the complications of therapy for hemophilia.

CASE PRESENTATION

A 12-year-old boy is booked to have elective adenotonsillectomy and insertion of myringotomy tubes. He has severe ***hemophilia A*** *(factor VIII 0%). He weighs 36 kg.*

Anesthesiology and hematology were notified of the planned surgery date by the otolaryngologist. ***Hematology formulated a plan for factor replacement*** *that was written in the patient notes for reference on the day of surgery. Otherwise his preoperative assessment was unremarkable. The patient does not have difficult veins and is not anxious about having a peripheral intravenous line placed preoperatively.*

Just prior to induction, 2,000 units (50 units/kg) of recombinant factor VIII (rFVIII) are given via a peripheral intravenous line. After induction, a second intravenous cannula is placed in case of rapid bleeding. Ultrasound guidance is used to minimize unsuccessful attempts at venous cannulation. Surgery proceeds uneventfully. At the conclusion of surgery, laryngoscopy reveals a dry surgical field, with minimal blood suctioned from the oropharynx. The patient is transferred to the bed and placed in the lateral position. He is extubated when he opens his eyes to command and coughs. He is transferred to recovery, where a further bolus dose of 1,000 units (30 units/kg) of rFVIII is given intravenously. On the ward, the team runs a continuous infusion of 108 units/hr (3 units/kg/hr) for 72 hours. The team also prescribes tranexamic acid 750 mg orally three times a day, to be continued for 14 days. For analgesia, he receives acetaminophen (paracetamol) and oxycodone as required. ***Nonsteroidal anti-inflammatory drugs are avoided.*** *At 72 hours his status is reviewed on the ward by hematology. As there are no bleeding problems, he is given a further intravenous bolus dose of 1,000 units rFVIII and discharged home. At home, he self-administers 1,000 units of rFVIII intravenously every second day until 10 days after surgery.*

DISCUSSION

1. How does hemophilia affect coagulation?

The current model of coagulation describes a complex network of various elements that are activated by tissue injury. This model describes interactions that occur on two cell types: tissue factor-bearing cells and platelets. In this model, coagulation can be divided into an initiation phase, an amplification phase, and a propagation phase. Coagulation is initially triggered by low levels of circulating activated factor VII (fVIIa) binding to tissue factor, which is exposed following vessel injury. fVIIa then activates factor X, which then generates small amounts of thrombin. This reaction is inhibited by tissue factor pathway inhibitor and antithrombin until high enough levels of tissue factor generate enough thrombin to overcome this inhibition (amplification). When this occurs, thrombin activates platelets, factor V, factor VIII, and factor XI, which further increases thrombin generation in a positive feedback mechanism (propagation). Propagation occurs effectively only on the surface of platelets and requires sufficient levels of circulating coagulation factors in the blood (Hoffman, 2003; Tanaka et al., 2009).

In hemophilia A (factor VIII deficiency) and hemophilia B (factor IX deficiency), the initiation of coagulation is normal, but the propagation phase at the platelet level, which is dependent on VIIIa and IXa, is severely impaired. This leads to the clinical picture of uncontrolled bleeding.

Hemophilia is classified as mild, moderate, or severe, according to the concentration of plasma factor level measured. A factor level below 1% of normal is classified as severe, 1% to 5% of normal is moderate, and 5% to 40% of normal is mild.

Patients with severe hemophilia are susceptible to frequent and often spontaneous bleeding. This bleeding may be into joints, soft tissues, the central nervous system, the airway, or the retroperitoneum or around major organs. Patients with mild disease will usually not have spontaneous hemorrhage but will bleed following surgery or trauma. The child in this scenario has severe hemophilia A. Therefore, without treatment he is prone to spontaneous bleeds and will bleed uncontrollably after trauma or surgery. He is dependent on factor VIII injections to prevent and treat bleeding episodes.

Von Willebrand disease is an inherited bleeding disorder which occurs in 1% to 3% of the population. In von Willebrand disease there is a deficiency of the amount or efficacy of von Willebrand factor (vWF). vWF is a peptide which acts both as an adhesive link between platelets and injured endothelium and as a stabilizer of circulating factor VIII. Patients with von Willebrand disease may present with spontaneous bleeding episodes or abnormal bleeding following trauma.

2. How is hemophilia diagnosed?

The clinical features of hemophilia A and hemophilia B are identical, and, as discussed, the clinical picture depends on the degree of factor deficiency. In severe disease, bleeding episodes begin at an early age, are frequent, and occur spontaneously or with only minor trauma. In mild disease, bleeding occurs only with major trauma and may not present until later in life. A history of excessive bleeding following minor trauma, bleeding following dental procedures, or a family history of hemophilia can raise suspicion. As hemophilia A and B are X-linked inherited disorders, males inherit the gene from female carriers (Table 34.1). Carriers may have a mild form of the disease and can also be at risk of bleeding during surgery.

A coagulation screen will show a prolonged activated prothrombin time (aPTT) and normal prothrombin time (PT). Specific factor-level assays confirm the diagnosis and the severity of disease.

In von Willebrand disease, PT and aPTT may be normal. There are more than 20 types of von Willebrand disease, and interpretation of laboratory tests in suspected patients is complex. Further evaluation includes measuring ristocetin cofactor activity, vWF antigen levels, factor VIII coagulant activity, and platelet count.

Other less common inherited bleeding disorders include deficiencies of factor II, factor V, factor VII, factor X, factor XI, and factor XIII (Lee, 2004).

TABLE 34.1. INHERITANCE OF MAJOR BLEEDING DISORDERS

	Deficiency	Inheritance	Incidence
Hemophilia A	Factor VIII	X-linked recessive	1 in 10,000 live male births
Hemophilia B	Factor IX	X-linked recessive	1 in 25,000 live male births
Von Willebrand disease	Von Willebrand factor	Autosomal dominant (common forms)	1–3 in 100

3. How should a patient with hemophilia for elective surgery be managed?

If surgery is indicated in a patient with hemophilia, careful planning is important to ensure that the surgery can proceed safely (Table 34.2). The procedure should always be undertaken at a specialist center with hemophilia expertise.

The first step in the preoperative evaluation is to ascertain the type and severity of the hemophilia, as this will guide therapy. The aim is to restore factor levels to normal during the time that bleeding may occur. This is primarily achieved by factor replacement (either plasma-derived or recombinant), which can be given as an infusion or as a bolus. In this case, the patient has severe hemophilia A, so he requires factor VIII replacement to bring his factor VIII level to 100% during and immediately after surgery. In adenotonsillectomy, bleeding may occur up to 14 days after surgery. This patient was therefore given additional factor replacement for 10 days after surgery. As he was able to administer factor VIII at home, and was considered relatively low risk for postoperative bleeding after day 2 with suitable factor replacement, he was discharged home on day 3. This may not always be possible, and other issues must be considered in making this decision. For instance, the patient must be able to access emergency hospital services promptly in case of a problem at home. Distance from the hospital, social factors, and willingness to comply with treatment at home must all be taken into account.

TABLE 34.2. LOGISTICAL EFFECTS OF HEMOPHILIA IN THE OPERATING ROOM

Venous Access
Difficult peripheral access due to scarring
Fear/anxiety about cannulation
Central line infection and clotting risks
Factor Administration
Antibody-mediated inhibitors affect achieving therapeutic levels of factor
Potential allergic response to administration of factor
Positioning and General Management
Arthropathy: contractures may affect positioning
Acquired brain injury from intracerebral bleeding may lead to seizure, behavioral and spasticity considerations
Minor Procedures
Bleeding risk from minor trauma requires judicious placement of nasogastric tubes, regional anesthesia blocks, arterial lines, intramuscular injections
Infection Control
Precautions are advisable (as for all patients) against HIV, hepatitis C and B, and Creutzfeld-Jacob disease; all can be acquired via repeated transfusions

In some cases of mild hemophilia A, normal factor levels may be achieved using desmopressin (DDAVP) alone. This acts by releasing stored factor VIII (and vWF) into the circulation. If a patient has been shown to have an adequate response to a DDAVP challenge, this may be the first line of therapy. The dose is 0.3 mcg/kg intravenously.

Antifibrinolytics (such as tranexamic acid and ε-aminocaproic acid) can be useful in preventing and treating mucous membrane hemorrhage (Association of Hemophilia Clinic Directors of Canada, 1995). The patient in this case was treated with tranexamic acid for 14 days to help prevent bleeding from the oral and nasal mucosa postoperatively.

Intraoperatively the anesthetist should be vigilant for abnormal bleeding. Should bleeding occur despite factor replacement, factor assays should be checked and hematology consulted. If bleeding occurs despite adequate factor replacement, the likely problem is surgical, though the development of inhibitors should be considered and tested for.

Other considerations in managing a child with hemophilia include assessment of any long-term complications of the disease. The life-limiting complications of hemophilia in the past were related to the transmission of infectious diseases such as HIV and hepatitis C and debilitating arthropathy due to recurrent hemarthroses. Fortunately, with the advent of better blood screening and recombinant factors, blood transfusion-related infections are almost nonexistent (although the potential for prion disease transmission is still unknown). With prophylactic factor replacement used to prevent recurrent hemarthroses, joints are now well preserved. Boys with hemophilia now have a normal life expectancy without severe disability. Treatment costs are high, but the outcomes are excellent.

Children with hemophilia can have difficult problems related to venous access. Those with difficult access who require regular treatments may have a long-term surgically placed central venous catheter in place. These catheters are prone to complications, particularly infection, and must be treated with care when used. Strict asepsis must be adhered to when accessing and using these long-term lines. Patients who do not have a central line may have an established and effective way of managing intravenous access to help make a potentially painful and stressful procedure acceptable to them. Local anesthetic cream, premedication, parental presence, play therapy, and distraction techniques may be used. The patient or parent may also know which veins are the easiest to cannulate. Discussing how the patient prefers to have his or her veins accessed is the best way to ensure the patient's cooperation and the anesthetist's success. Use of ultrasound can improve the success rate of venous cannulation for patients with veins which are difficult to see or palpate.

In general, regional blocks, intramuscular injections, and arterial punctures should be avoided in patients with hemophilia. Aspirin and nonsteroidal anti-inflammatory drugs should be avoided. Intravenous cannulas should be treated with care and checked frequently to ensure correct placement. If venipunctures are required, firm pressure should be applied for 3 minutes to the site afterwards.

4. What are potential adverse effects of therapy in hemophilia?

DDAVP is useful in patients with mild hemophilia A and some types of von Willebrand disease. DDAVP can increase factor VIII levels two- to three-fold within 30 to 60 minutes of infusion. However, there have been case reports of severe hyponatremia and seizures related to its use (Dunn & Gill, 2010.). Close monitoring of electrolytes and avoidance of hypotonic fluids with the use of DDAVP is prudent.

Replacement of factors in patients with hemophilia with plasma-derived products carries the risk of transmission of viruses, such as HIV and hepatitis C. The development of recombinant factor concentrates as well as improved screening of blood donors has reduced the incidence of virus transmission in this group.

Development of inhibitors is the most challenging complication of hemophilia today. An inhibitor is an antibody directed against exogenously administered factor VIII or IX, which renders factor replacement ineffective. It occurs in about 20% of cases of severe hemophilia A and in 3% of patients with severe hemophilia B (Lee, 2004). Inhibitors to factor IX can be associated with anaphylaxis.

Treatment of patients with inhibitors can be challenging, but there has been some success in inducing immune tolerance in these patients by exposing them to frequent high doses of factor replacement over a period of time. In acute bleeding episodes in patients with inhibitors, treatment options include activated recombinant factor VII or prothrombin complex concentrates. Perioperative management of patients with inhibitors should be guided by a hematologist, with careful planning and monitoring of the efficacy of chosen treatment with thrombin generation assays and clinical observation.

SUMMARY

1. Hemophilia A and B (deficiencies of factor VIII and IX) pose severe hemorrhagic risk for boys.
2. Cooperative management with hematology and aggressive replacement of the appropriate factor are important.
3. Preoperative evaluation of these patients should include looking for vascular access difficulties, infectious sequelae of repeated transfusions, and joint and neurologic sequelae of prior bleeding episodes.
4. Development of inhibitors to factors is a complication which makes management of surgical procedures very challenging. Multidisciplinary planning for these patients is imperative.

ANNOTATED REFERENCES

Hoffman M. Remodeling the blood coagulation cascade. *J Thrombosis Thrombolysis*. 2003;16(1–2):17–20.

This paper describes a cell-based model of coagulation that, unlike older biochemical models, is better able to explain why hemophiliacs have a bleeding tendency.

Lee J-W. Von Willebrand disease, hemophilia A and B, and other factor deficiencies. *Int Anesth Clin*. 2004;42(3):59–76.

Aimed at anesthesiologists, this practical review of the pathophysiology of the common inherited bleeding disorders outlines recommended perioperative management strategies.

Tanaka, KA, Key NS, Levy JH. Blood coagulation: hemostasis and thrombin regulation. *Anesth Analg*. 2009;108:1433–1446.

This review comprehensively describes the current concepts of coagulation, its regulation, and responses to surgery and bleeding. It also outlines drugs used to modulate the coagulation system to control bleeding and thrombotic complications.

BIBLIOGRAPHY

Association of Hemophilia Clinic Directors of Canada. Hemophilia and von Willebrand's disease: 2. Management. *Can Med Assoc J.* 1995;153(2):147–157.

Conlon B, Daly N, Temperely I, McShane D. ENT surgery in children with inherited bleeding disorders. *J Laryng Otol.* 1996;110:947–949.

Dargaud Y, Pavlova A, Lacroix-Desmazes S, et al. Achievements, challenges and unmet needs for haemophilia patients with inhibitors. *Haemophilia.* 2016;22(Supp 1):1–24.

Dunn AL, Cox Gill J. Adenotonsillectomy in patients with desmopressin responsive mild bleeding disorders: a review of the literature. *Haemophilia.* 2010;16:711–716.

Roberts HR, Monahan PE. Pediatric hemophilia: diagnosis, classification, and management. Medscape CME Pediatrics; 2010. http://cme.medscape.com/viewprogram/30887

35

The Oncology Patient

ANN NG AND ERIN S. WILLIAMS

INTRODUCTION

The pediatric cancer, or oncology, population presents many challenges to the pediatric anesthesiologist. Many of these patients undergo multiple procedures for their treatment protocol such as lumbar punctures and bone marrow aspirations. Radiation therapy is another treatment modality that requires children to lie still on a small treatment table away from all personnel and thus can often require the assistance of an anesthesiologist. Echocardiograms, line placements, hearing screens, and magnetic resonance imaging are other potential procedures requiring anesthesia for these patients. While seemingly minor, these procedures are a source of anxiety for patients and parents. Furthermore, patients can present with a number of physiological derangements such as anemia, coagulopathies, and toxicities from chemotherapeutic agents. Finally, these patients vary in age from infant to teen, making attention to their specific developmental level and anxiety a requirement for an effective anesthetic plan.

LEARNING OBJECTIVES

1. Understand the advantages of general anesthesia for common painful procedures for the pediatric oncology patient.
2. Review the medical problems of oncology patients important to the preanesthetic evaluation, including toxicities of chemotherapies, anemia, and thrombocytopenia.
3. Discuss the advantages of various anesthetic techniques for the pediatric oncology patient undergoing lumbar puncture.
4. Promote the importance of combining procedures in order to minimize potential complications including anesthetic neurotoxicity.
5. Outline the challenges of providing anesthesia for the radiation oncology patient.

CASE PRESENTATION

A 3-year-old boy with a recent diagnosis of acute lymphoblastic leukemia presents for lumbar puncture and administration of intrathecal chemotherapy. The patient was diagnosed a few weeks ago after presenting with lethargy, pallor, and lower extremity pain. After a 1-week hospital stay where the patient had an initial bone marrow biopsy, lumbar puncture with intrathecal chemotherapy, and a blood transfusion, he was discharged home on oral chemotherapy and now arrives to continue his induction regimen. His bone pain has improved and radiation treatment is currently deferred. His labs have been drawn in clinic and are significant for mild anemia. ***His platelet count is 35,000 mL-1. Echocardiography*** *reveals normal anatomy and biventricular function. On initial evaluation in the preoperative holding area, the patient appears fearful. His vital signs are normal and his examination is remarkable only for signs of a recent* ***upper respiratory tract infection*** *with nasal congestion 3 days ago.*

DISCUSSION

1. What are common hematologic derangements in oncology patients? To what extent are they a concern?

Patients with leukemia and solid malignancies present with bone marrow involvement or have poor marrow production from chemotherapy. The resulting myelosuppression can cause pancytopenia, and the anesthesiologist often encounters patients who are thrombocytopenic, anemic, and leukopenic. In patients with leukemia, thrombocytopenia is common at diagnosis and throughout early treatment (Latham & Greenberg, 2010b). However, data recommending perioperative transfusion of platelets prior to procedures in children with cancer is limited. One retrospective review in children with acute lymphoblastic leukemia found few complications of lumbar puncture in children with platelet counts of greater than **10,000 mL^{-1}** (Howard et al., 2000). However, spinal epidural hematomas have occurred at various platelet counts, suggesting that other factors besides thrombocytopenia are important to consider (Latham & Greenberg, 2010b). At our institution, in the absence of coagulopathy and liver dysfunction, **platelet counts above 50,000 mL^{-1} for newly diagnosed patients presenting for their first lumbar puncture and 30,000 mL^{-1} for all other patients** are acceptable to proceed with lumbar puncture and administration of intrathecal chemotherapy. Platelet transfusion is considered for those below that level to reduce the risk of epidural hematoma formation. For major invasive procedures, the American Society of Clinical Oncology guidelines suggest that platelets of 40,000 to 50,000 mL^{-1} is sufficient, while platelets >100,000 mL^{-1} are required prior to neurosurgical procedures (Latham & Greenberg, 2010b).

For bone marrow aspiration, the coagulation status of the patient is less important. Oozing stops with pressure whether an anterior or posterior approach is chosen. Though a hematoma may form, these tend to be small and limited and will not compress key structures.

Anemia is a concern, and most patients are transfused based upon their clinical status. Most otherwise healthy patients can tolerate hematocrits in the mid-20s under general anesthesia. For patients who are physiologically stressed or have concurrent cardiac or pulmonary disease, a higher hematocrit may be necessary.

Leukopenia commonly occurs due to toxicity from chemotherapy treatment. Neutropenia <1000 cells per mm^3 can lead to increased infections, and, in a patient with neutropenia and fever, further evaluation for sepsis is warranted. Anesthesiologists taking care of immunocompromised patients should use standard precautions to prevent further infection including aseptic techniques for invasive procedures, avoidance of medications per rectum, and appropriate perioperative isolation of the patient (Latham & Greenberg, 2010a).

2. What cardiotoxic effects are seen with chemotherapy?

Leukemia and lymphoma protocols call for the use of anthracyclines (ACs), such as doxorubicin, that are known to be cardiotoxic. Toxicity can be seen early within days or weeks of initiation of treatment or late after months to years after treatment. Acute AC-induced cardiomyopathy can present as hypotension, congestive heart failure, and arrhythmias. Late AC-induced cardiomyopathy is dose-dependent, and most protocols in children keep cumulative doses <250 to 300 mg/m^2 (Latham & Greenberg, 2010a). In late AC-induced cardiomyopathy, chronic effects can be persistent and progressive and cardiac dysfunction including heart failure and arrhythmias can occur even at small dosages. Children who have received ACs usually have echocardiograms prior to treatment, at various time intervals or dosages during therapy, at the end of therapy, and at times during remission. In the absence of a documented cardiac evaluation, a patient history evaluating exercise tolerance, dyspnea on exertion, and orthopnea should be performed. Other comorbidities as well as the nature of the surgery should also be part of the assessment to determine if the patient should have additional cardiac studies prior to an anesthetic. Other chemotherapeutic agents such as mitoxantrone, cyclophosphamide, mitomycin, fluorouracil, cytarabine, and cisplatin have been associated with cardiotoxicity (Latham & Greenberg, 2010a).

3. What are the advantages of general anesthesia for this patient population?

When compared to conscious sedation, general anesthesia offers several benefits to all concerned: patients and their families, the nursing staff, and the oncologist. While children can tolerate these painful procedures with distraction, topical anesthesia, and conscious sedation, the potential psychological stress from these techniques can inflict considerable distress to all those involved. There is evidence that considerable anxiety and behavioral distress occurs as a result of repeated painful procedures.

Children undergoing painful procedures with conscious sedation may find them difficult to tolerate.

Considerable physical restraint may be necessary, causing further anxiety and fear. A failed sedation can lead to significant **anticipatory anxiety**, which has to be addressed at future procedures. Furthermore, in busy, high-acuity centers, failure to complete the procedure results in delayed diagnosis, delayed treatment, and disrupted clinical roadmaps. One study found that when conscious sedation was used compared to general anesthesia, physical restraint was required in 94% of the sedation group, 66% required firm restrain and there was a 10% failure to perform the procedure in the conscious sedation group. Hospital nursing staff are more satisfied with general anesthesia, since restraining a resisting child causes them considerable distress as well. Therefore, general anesthesia offers fewer procedural failures and greater satisfaction for the patient, family, and staff (Crock et al., 2003). In addition, despite significant pain that children report during the treatment for cancer, the single most painful episode was during a painful medical procedure or surgery. Zernikow et al. (2005) found that the only variable that led to a reduction in pain scores from medical procedures, such as lumbar puncture and bone marrow aspirate, was general anesthesia.

4. Which anesthetic techniques have been demonstrated to be the safest and most effective?

The ideal general anesthetic technique minimizes anxiety on induction, has few side effects, is readily titratable, and permits a rapid wake-up. Most oncology patients have established central venous access, providing an easy route for rapid intravenous induction. Maintenance can be achieved with inhalational agents or propofol as an intermittent bolus or infusion technique. Intravenous maintenance with propofol results in fewer airway complications such as laryngospasm and lowers the risk of emergence delirium compared to sevoflurane. In patients with a history of postoperative nausea or vomiting, intravenous maintenance with propofol can be beneficial. If volatile anesthetic is used, an antiemetic such as ondansetron can be considered. A careful review of the patient's medication list is required as antiemetics may often already be taken. Dexamethasone, which is commonly used as an antiemetic in patients at moderate risk with general anesthesia, is avoided in oncology patients as administration has been associated with tumor lysis syndrome in a child with acute leukemia.

Additionally, if the patient has significant anxiety, the anesthesiologist must address the patient's and family's concerns and consider utilizing the child life services department, parental presence during induction, or even premedicating the patient with intravenous midazolam in order to have a pleasant patient experience. It is important to **involve the child and his or her parent in discussion of the anesthetic plan** as often the children may have developed a preferred routine for induction of anesthesia (Latham & Greenberg, 2010b).

5. What are the challenges that face the anesthesiologist during radiation therapy?

Safe and effective **radiation therapy** for children requires the patient to remain motionless so that the radiation beams focus only on the pathological tissue or field, minimizing radiation exposure to healthy tissues. Multiple treatments are often required over a period of weeks, each requiring exactly the same position of the patient. Treatments may last from 5 to 60 minutes, and regimens may include 1 to 35 treatments, with each treatment occurring on successive days. During the radiation treatment, no one can be present in the treatment room with the child. Many children ages 7 and above can do this awake with proper instruction and encouragement from family and staff, but younger children and older children with developmental delays are not able to hold still without sedation or general anesthesia.

There are many challenges to the anesthesiologist. The radiation oncology environment is hostile for the anesthesiologist. During the treatment, the patient is isolated in the lead-lined treatment room, and the anesthesiologist, who sits outside the treatment room, can only observe the patient via a video monitor (Fig. 35.1). If the patient requires immediate care from the anesthesiologist, the radiation treatment must be interrupted. Therefore, preanesthetic planning should include learning the location of the emergency stop button and door releases. One should plan these emergency interventions with the radiation technologist.

In addition, many patient-related factors are problematic. Patients undergoing craniospinal radiation therapy are placed in a rigid mask that covers the his or her face and attaches to the treatment table. This mask ensures exactly the same position of the patient for each of the treatments, but it limits access to the patient's airway. Use of an endotracheal

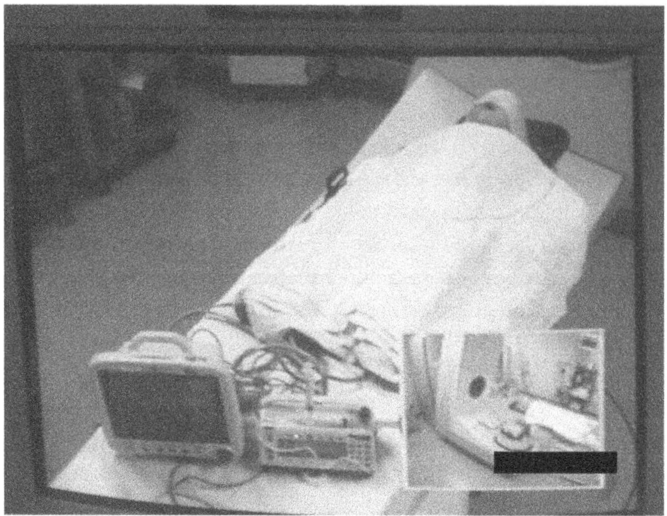

FIGURE 35.1: Patient having radiation therapy. Note head-positioning mask and need for remote video monitoring.

tube or laryngeal mask airway is only occasionally needed, but it can be awkward to place and maintain it when the positioning mask is in place. In some cases, a poorly fitted mask can contribute to airway obstruction and cause pain. Although seeing a patient daily can make the process seem routine, the patient's airway needs to be reassessed daily. As treatment progresses, mucositis and airway edema can occur, and adjustments to airway management may be needed at any time in the series of treatments.

Anesthetic technique for nonemergent treatment involves an intravenous induction with propofol. The airway can be maintained with an oropharyngeal airway or nasopharyngeal airway using a spontaneous respiration technique. The eyes are taped closed and the patient is monitored with pulse oximetry, electrocardiography, noninvasive blood pressure cuff, and capnography. Maintenance can be accomplished with boluses of propofol for brief treatments and with infusions of propofol for longer treatments. The treatments are not stimulating to the patient, so lower doses can often be used.

For common elective cases, such as hernia repair, cancellation of the procedure may be prudent; generally, there are few medical consequences. In contrast, diagnostic and therapeutic procedures for oncology patients are not elective in nature, and delaying procedures may have serious consequences. Therefore, the decision to proceed with or cancel the anesthetic must be made with careful consideration and discussion with the oncology team.

6. What are some considerations for potential neurotoxicity due to anesthetics?

In December 2016, the Food and Drug Administration (FDA) released a statement that stated all currently used general anesthetics pose an increased risk of neurologic complication of varying degree in animal studies. These studies showed **increased neurologic derangement in animals younger that the age of 3 years** as well as animals exposed to more than 3 general anesthetics. Given this information, the FDA promoted public awareness of the potential neurologic risks for humans. Even though the exact implication of animal data to humans is not clear, it is prudent to be cautious and to heavily consider any potential increase in harm to patients. Some potential changes that can be made include considering rescheduling surgeries in patients younger than 3 years old that pose no urgency or complication potential if delayed. This is certainly not possible for the pediatric oncologic patient given the urgent need for diagnosis and treatment of the oncologic process. However, one major change that can be instituted is **combining the many procedures that these patients require**. At our institution, we combine as many procedures as possible with the goal of minimizing the number of visits to the hospital, nil per os occurrences, and potential complications such as neurotoxicity. Parents and patients overall appreciate the combined anesthetic technique.

SUMMARY

1. Pediatric oncology patients often present with serious medical problems related to their cancer as well as to complications of their cancer treatment (e.g., chemotherapy-induced cardiac toxicity, anemia, and coagulopathy).
2. General anesthesia has advantages over conscious sedation for lumbar puncture. It offers fewer procedural failures and greater patient, family, and staff satisfaction.
3. Poorly conducted sedation can result in considerable longstanding harm to children undergoing repeat procedures.
4. Combining multiple procedures in one anesthetic may limit exposure to the potential complications of anesthesia.

BIBLIOGRAPHY

Crock C, Olsson C, Phillips R, et al. General anaesthesia or conscious sedation for painful procedures in childhood cancer: the family's perspective. *Arch Dis Child.* 2003;88:253–257.

Food and Drug Administration Drug Safety Communication. FDA review results in new warnings about using general anesthetics and sedation drugs in young children and pregnant women. 2016 Dec 14. https://www.fda.gov/Drugs/DrugSafety/ucm532356.htm

Howard SC, Gajjar A, Ribeiro RC, et al. Safety of lumbar puncture for children with acute lymphoblastic leukemia and thrombocytopenia. *JAMA.* 2000;284:2222–2224.

Latham GJ, Greenberg RS. Anesthetic considerations for the pediatric oncology patient—part 2: systems-based approach to anesthesia. *Pediatr Anesth.* 2010a;20:396–420.

Latham GJ, Greenberg RS. Anesthetic considerations for the pediatric oncology patient—part 3: pain, cognitive dysfunction, and preoperative evaluation. *Pediatr Anesth.* 2010b;20:479–489.

Zernikow B, Meyerhoff U, Michel E, et al. Pain in pediatric oncology—children's and parents' perspectives. *Eur J Pain.* 2005;9:395–406.

36

The Opioid-Tolerant Patient

MICHAEL BLAINE ZELISKO

INTRODUCTION

Caring for patients taking chronic opioids may present several challenges in the perioperative period. Opioid-tolerant patients tend to have a higher incidence of anxiety, pain, and unanticipated hospital admissions. The goal of the anesthesiologist is to provide sufficient analgesia to blunt the adverse emotional and physiologic effects of painful stimuli, while preventing withdrawal symptoms. Acute pain from surgical procedures and the patient's baseline chronic pain must be addressed simultaneously. Pain control in the chronic pain patient should be multimodal in nature. Pharmacologic and nonpharmacologic coping mechanisms need to be considered. Pharmacologic treatment should include opioids, non-opioid adjuncts, and regional and neuraxial analgesia, when applicable. Adequate pain control increases patient satisfaction, improves surgical outcomes, prevents unnecessary hospital admissions, and decreases length of hospital stay (Deer, 2013). Factors such as addiction, tolerance, opioid-induced hyperalgesia, and withdrawal can complicate perioperative management. This chapter addresses special considerations for the opioid-tolerant patient throughout the perioperative process.

LEARNING OBJECTIVES

1. Understand how to manage opioid-tolerant patients throughout the perioperative process.
2. Know the difference between tolerance, addiction, and pseudo-addiction.
3. Understand mechanisms of opioid-induced hyperalgesia.
4. Understand mechanisms of opioid tolerance.
5. Review basic principles of opioid rotation (switch).
6. Describe alternatives to treat the opioid-tolerant patient with acute or chronic pain.

CASE PRESENTATION

A 17-year-old, 50-kg girl with a history of tibial osteosarcoma presents for thoracoscopic biopsy of a new lung nodule. She underwent a limb salvage procedure about 10 months ago during which the sciatic nerve was injured. She has had significant neuropathic pain, which is being treated with gabapentin 900 mg 3 times a day, ***MS Contin 30 mg twice a day,*** *and oxycodone 15 mg as needed. Her average pain score with this regimen has been 4 to 5 out of 10 on a numeric rating scale. She has no other medical problems, and has suffered no apparent long-term effects from her chemotherapy. The anesthetic is uneventful, although the resident remarks that the patient requires 4.5% end-tidal sevoflurane concentration through the case. Fifteen minutes after the patient arrives in the recovery room, the nurse calls to report that the patient has extreme pain and needs more rescue pain medications.*

The patient received 10 mg intravenous (IV) morphine in the operating room and an additional 9 mg of IV morphine in the recovery room over the past 30 minutes. She says that she took her gabapentin and methadone with dinner, and a last dose of oxycodone before bed, but did not take her medications this morning because she was told not to eat or drink before surgery. She reports that her abdomen hurts her but not because she is hungry. She feels "weird," cold but sweaty, almost shaking. A ***titration*** *scheme is established, and the nurse is made aware that the patient is opioid-****tolerant*** *and* ***will require high doses of opioids*** *to become comfortable.*

DISCUSSION

1. How should a patient on chronic opioids be approached preoperatively?

Adequate pain control in the perioperative period begins with preoperative assessment and planning. It is imperative to recognize patients taking chronic opioids preoperatively. When caring for these patients, it is easy to overlook, or underestimate, their chronic opioid use. Recognition allows for coordination between medical teams, and collaboration with the patient, to create a pain management plan and ensure proper patient education.

Patients, and their families, should be informed that daily maintenance opioid regimen should be taken preoperatively. All oral regimens should be given the morning of surgery. Sustained-release opioid regimens provide 12 or more hours of analagesic effect, and supply patients with their basal opioid requirement. Transdermal fentanyl patches and epidural/intrathecal infusions should be continued. In the event the patient does not receive his or her scheduled regimen preoperatively, an equivalent dose of IV medication should be given. It is important to provide equianalgesic doses of oral or IV opioid that match the patient's daily dose, in 1:1 substitution. If the patient's dose in the perioperative period does not match his or her daily needs, the patient may face withdrawal.

Patient education is vital before surgery to improve perioperative pain control. When applicable, these patients should meet with the Pain Service preoperatively. The patient's baseline level of pain should be determined, and goals for acceptable and realistic pain levels should be established (Brooks & Golianu, 2016). Patients and their families should be aware that opioid requirements will increase after the procedure. Furthermore, inclusion of patients in the creation of a treatment plan, increases patient satisfaction in the postoperative period. Once established, perioperative pain plans should be well documented and communicated between all services involved in the patient's care.

2. What are some considerations for managing these patients intraoperatively?

Opioid requirements during surgery consist of the patient's daily regimen plus the additional pain medications needed to cover surgical stimulation. Individual patient opioid requirements in response to surgical stimulation can be difficult to determine due to variability in patient responsiveness. The total dose required by opioid-tolerant patients may exceed the "usual" dose anywhere from **30% to 100%** (Geary et al., 2011). Patients who were unable to take their daily home regimen prior to surgery should receive an equianalgesic 1:1 substitution of IV medication. Additional IV medication can then be given to cover surgical pain. When applicable, most authors recommend titrating pain medication based on spontaneous ventilation. Opioids are titrated to a ventilation rate slightly lower than the normal rate for the patient's age range. The degree of miosis, heart rate, and blood pressure are other parameters clinicians can consider when titrating meds (Geary et al., 2011).

A multimodal approach is the most effective method for managing pain in this subset of patients. Non-opioid adjuncts, regional nerve blockade, and neuraxial analgesia, should be considered when formulating a pain management plan for opioid-tolerant patients.

Peripheral nerve blocks should be considered in patients undergoing procedures involving the extremities. Common blocks of the upper extremities, include: interscalene, supraclavicular, infraclavicular, and axillary blocks. Femoral and sciatic blocks are common for procedures involving the lower extremities. Peripheral nerve blocks reduce oral and parenteral opioid requirements both intraoperatively and postoperatively. However, patients still require their basal regimen in order to prevent withdrawal symptoms. Single-injection blocks wear off variably in the postoperative period. A pain regimen with either oral or parenteral opioids must be in place to alleviate painful stimuli before regional anesthesia begins to subside. Continuous peripheral nerve block catheters should be considered in patients with chronic pain.

If indicated, neuraxial analgesia is an excellent way to decrease opioid requirements. As with peripheral nerve blocks, the patient's basal regimen is still needed to prevent withdrawal. Continuous epidural catheters are very effective for procedures involving the thoracic cavity, abdominal cavity, pelvis, and lower extremities. Opioid requirements are reduced both intraoperatively and postoperatively when epidurals are placed before surgical stimulation. Epidurals also reduce postoperative nausea, vomiting, ileus, pulmonary complications, and the incidence of thromboembolism (Deer, 2013). An oral or parenteral pain plan should be in place prior to the decision to remove the epidural catheter.

3. How should pain in opioid-tolerant patients be approached postsurgically?

Acute pain in the immediate postoperative setting is best managed by titration. Titration to effect is key, whether for IV rescue medications, patient-controlled analgesia (PCA), or as-needed analgesics. If one opioid is not sufficient for rescue analgesia, clinicians tend to give small doses of several different opioids. They may think the patient is failing to respond to treatment when, in fact, the treatment has not been optimized and maximized. It is better to stick to one drug, repeating loading doses as needed, and titrating to effect. Furthermore, multimodal analgesia should be continued.

Opioid management postoperatively depends on the surgical setting. After ambulatory surgery, patients can be restarted on their oral home regimen. Depending on the extent of surgical stimulus, the patient may require a higher dose of oral opioid. Presurgical regimens may need to be increased 20% to 50% above baseline, to cover acute pain from surgical procedures (Saberski, 1992). Patients requiring admission after surgery may benefit from the use of IV pain medication until they can be transitioned back to their oral home regimen. PCA or nurse-controlled analgesia is useful in this patient population.

PCA can be used to manage acute and underlying chronic pain simultaneously. Baseline opioid requirements can be calculated and converted in a 1:1 equianalgesic substitution to the medication chosen for the PCA. Morphine, hydromorphone, and fentanyl are the most commonly used PCA opioids. The calculated baseline conversion can be started as a continuous infusion on the PCA. Acute pain is then managed by adding intermittent bolus dosing on the PCA. While using a PCA, patients should be monitored closely for poor pain control, side effects, and withdrawal symptoms. The Anesthesia Patient Safety Foundation recommends vigilant monitoring of patients receiving PCA opioids. Specifically, pulse oximetry and respiratory rate should be monitored continuously (Coté et al., 2008). The primary advantage of PCA is that it gives patients the autonomy to titrate opioids to meet their pain requirements. Patients receiving PCAs report improved, analgesia and demonstrate lower pain scores when compared to patients receiving nurse-dependent rescue medications.

Non-opioid adjuncts play a key role in improving pain management in the opioid-tolerant patient postoperatively. Neuraxial and peripheral nerve catheters should be continued postsurgically when applicable. Clinicians must be prudent to continue equianalgesic doses of presurgical opioid to prevent withdrawal symptoms after surgery.

4. What adjuncts can improve the pain management of the opioid-habituated patient?

Opioids bind to four major types of opioid receptors: *mu, kappa, delta,* and *sigma*. Once bound, opioid receptor agonists inhibit the presynaptic release of acetylcholine and substance P. This inhibits the postsynaptic response in nociceptive neurons thus interrupting the transmission of pain impulses. In opioid-tolerant patients, these receptors are downregulated and desensitized. Furthermore, opioids themselves are metabolized more quickly. For these reasons, non-opioid adjuvants play a vital role in the management of pain in these patients. Adjunct medications relieve pain via mechanisms of action outside of the opioid receptor family. When used appropriately, these adjuncts can significantly reduce total opioid requirements.

Benzodiazepines

Benzodiazepines act by facilitating GABA-receptor binding, thus enhancing the inhibitory effects of GABA on various neurotransmitters. These medications serve as anxiolytics, reducing stress and fear. This improves patient cooperation in the preoperative period. Benzodiazepines also reduce intraoperative anesthesia and postoperative opioid requirements. In the postoperative period, benzodiazepines aid in the relief and treatment of muscle spasms.

Nonsteroidal Anti-inflammatory Drugs

Nonsteroidal anti-inflammatory drugs (NSAIDs) have been shown to reduce postoperative opioid consumption by inhibiting cyclooxygenase, resulting in decreased prostaglandin synthesis. NSAIDs are weak analgesics and are best utilized in multimodal pain regimens. Ketorolac can be given intramuscularly or intravenously. Ketorolac pediatric dosing is 0.5 mg/kg up to a maximum of 30 mg every 6 hours. IV ibuprofen (Caldolorâ) is also now available. Pediatric dosing is 10 mg/kg up to a maximum dose of 400 mg every 4 to 6 hours. Chronic NSAID use can be associated with gastric ulcers and kidney disease. Precautions should be taken in patients when platelet dysfunction and concern for postoperative bleeding.

Acetaminophen

Acetaminophen is useful in the treatment of mild to moderate pain. When used as a multimodal adjunct, it reduces overall opioid requirements. Acetaminophen acts as a COX-2 and COX-3 inhibitor, thus reducing inflammation. IV acetaminophen (Ofirmevâ) is available and has been shown to be more effective and faster acting than oral regimens. Pediatric dosing is 10 to 15 mg/kg every 6 hours. The maximum daily dose should not exceed 75 mg/kg.

Tramadol

Tramadol is a weak opioid mu agonist used to treat mild to moderate pain. Tramadol also inhibits the reuptake of norepinephrine and serotonin. Tramadol, like codeine, is ineffective in patients deficient in the CYP2D6 enzyme and thus has a variable response throughout the patient population. Tramadol should be avoided in patients taking tricyclic antidepressants (TCAs), selective serotonin reuptake inhibitors (SSRIs), and selective norepinephrine reuptake inhibitors (SNRIs) in order to prevent serotonin syndrome.

Alpha-2 Agonists

Clonidine and dexmedetomidine are alpha-2 agonists that act on muscarinic and nicotinic receptors in the substantia gelatinosa to inhibit pain pathways. Alpha-2 agonists potentiate the effects of opioids, resulting in the reduction of opioid consumption. Alpha-2 agonists have also proven vital in preventing withdrawal symptoms during opioid weaning. Side effects, include: sedation, bradycardia, and hypotension. Respiratory depression is not seen with these medications.

Ketamine

Ketamine works as a noncompetitive antagonist at the NMDA receptor resulting in the inhibition of monoaminergic pain pathways. Ketamine also acts directly on the kappa opioid receptor to provide analgesia. Ketamine potentiates opioid effects, decreases opioid consumption, and reduces the risk of developing opioid-induced hyperalgesia in the postoperative period (De Kock & Lavand'homme, 2007; Joly et al., 2005). Side effects include: increased salivation, hallucinations, delirium, tachycardia, and hypertension from increased sympathetic stimulation. Unlike opioids, ketamine does not cause respiratory depression.

Gabapentinoids

Gabapentin and pregablin are classified in a group of medications known as gabapentinoids. Gabapentinoids act on calcium channels centrally to reduce the release of glutamate. Neurontin was originally used as an anticonvulsant drug but has become a valuable resource in the management of chronic pain. It is well documented that gabapentinoids are beneficial in the treatment of neuropathic pain. Some studies have shown that gabapentin reduces total opioid consumption in pediatric patients undergoing spinal fusion for idiopathic scoliosis (Rusy et al., 2010). Similar studies have not yielded the same results (Bailey, 2004). Therefore, based on current literature, it is uncertain how much of a role gabapentin plays in reducing opioid consumption in the postoperative period. Side effects include: edema, dizziness, and drowsiness.

Antidepressants

TCAs, SSRIs, and SNRIs are used in chronic pain patients to treat both depression and neuropathic pain. These medications should be continued perioperatively. If discontinued, patients have increased symptoms of pain and depression in the postoperative period. Anesthesiologists should be aware that patients taking these medications may have an exaggerated sympathetic response when given pressors.

5. What is opioid-induced hyperalgesia (OIH)?

OIH is a state of heightened pain perception caused by exposure to opioids. This is a paradoxical effect in which patients taking narcotics for the treatment of pain become less tolerant to painful stimuli. OIH presents as increased pain without the evidence of disease progression. Moreover, the patient's pain increases as opioid dose is increased. The type of discomfort experienced may mimic the original underlying pain, or present as hyperesthesia and allodynia of the affected area. Treatment of OIH involves opioid rotation, reduction of opioids, and NMDA receptor antagonists, such as, ketamine. Ketamine appears to reduce central sensitization, which seems to be a component of OIH. It can be useful in reducing the incidence of OIH in patients who are taking large doses of opioids.

6. What is incomplete opioid cross-tolerance?

As defined in Table 36.1, opioid tolerance is a physiologic response that manifests as the need for an increased drug dose to achieve the same clinical effect. Opioid cross-tolerance is tolerance to all other opioids caused by short- or long-term use of one opioid. Recent research shows that different opioids bind to different sites on the mu opioid receptor—or, as newly termed, the mu opioid peptide (MOP) receptor. One explanation could be multiple MOP receptor subtypes. Different binding sites then determine slightly different analgesic effects. This leads to the incomplete opioid cross-tolerance observed clinically. Practically, it translates into the need for lower doses (up to 50% reduction) of the newly initiated opioid compared to the discontinued opioid.

TABLE 36.1. KEY TERMS

Tolerance: Physiologic response to opioid analgesics resulting in a decrease in pharmacologic response following repeated or prolonged drug administration. Can be of two types:

- *Innate:* Predisposition to exhibit drug sensitivity or insensitivity due to pharmacogenetic makeup
- *Acquired*: Three subtypes:
  - *Pharmacokinetic:* Occurs when drug disposition or metabolism is altered as a function of time, frequently a consequence of the drug being an inducer or inhibitor of a specific metabolic enzyme or transporter system
  - *Pharmacodynamic:* Occurs when the intrinsic responsiveness of the receptor system diminishes over time
  - *Learned:* Occurs when an individual learns to function despite repeated exposure to a drug

Opioid-Induced Hyperalgesia: A paradoxical effect of opioids leading to heightened pain perception

Pseudo-addiction: A term describing a patient with legitimate but undertreated pain who demands more pain medication to achieve relief and comfort

Addiction: A psychophysical condition in which a patient's focus becomes acquisition and use of a drug regardless of physical, psychological, or social harm caused by the use. *Tolerance* is one component of addiction.

Withdrawal: Occurs in the setting of tolerance, with sudden cessation of a medication, leading to a combination of physical symptoms, including abdominal pain/cramping, diarrhea, tachycardia, tremors, sweating, piloerection, anxiety, and/or generalized body achiness

7. How does the use of methadone differ from that of other opioids?

Unlike other opioids, where slow-release forms need to be manufactured, methadone possesses innate features as a long-acting pain medication. Methadone has regained popularity recently as a drug for opioid rotation (see later discussion). It is a complex drug, and every clinician prescribing it must be aware of its specific issues, especially its unpredictable pharmacokinetics. It has a long terminal half-life of 7 to 65 hours, causing the potential for sedation with rapid titration. Reaching a steady state may take 35 to 325 hours (1.5–13.5 days). Methadone's potential for significant drug interactions (either an increase in free methadone plasma levels or an increase/decrease in the effectiveness of coadministered drugs [e.g., SSRIs, TCAs, fluconazole, ciprofloxacin, doxorubicin, vinblastine] and risk of torsades de pointes via QT-interval prolongation; it structurally mimics the calcium channel blocker verapamil) cannot be emphasized enough. It also carries a stigma due to its use for opioid addiction management. The main advantage of methadone is its high oral bioavailability (almost 90%). It is a drug with not only mu opioid receptor agonistic effect, but also NMDA antagonistic properties that provide slower development of tolerance and beneficial effects on neuropathic pain.

8. How does one execute opioid rotation?

Over time, opioid-tolerant patients experience a reduction in the efficacy of an opioid. Patients require higher doses in order to manage their baseline pain. Furthermore, patients may develop side effects that are as bothersome as their pain. Opioid rotation is a potential solution to these problems.

Opioid rotation (or switching) is a change in opioid drug, or route of administration, with the goal of improving outcomes: analgesia, reduced side effects, and better functioning or quality of life. It is a complex process, and several factors that influence the new drug and dose selection must be taken into consideration: age, race, disease state, disease treatment, comorbidities, and concomitant pharmacotherapy (see Fig. 36.1). The provider executing an opioid rotation must be prepared to deal with

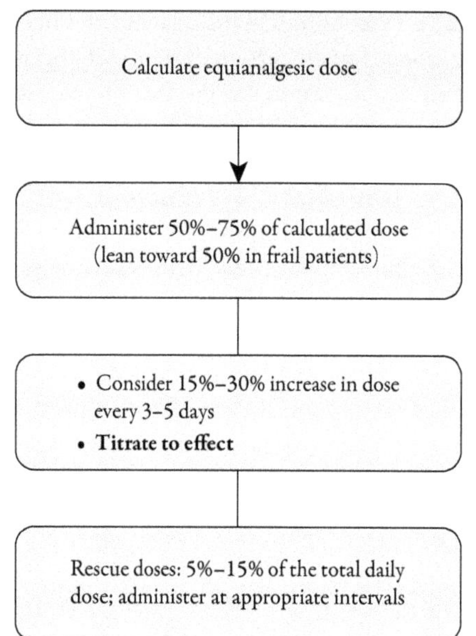

FIGURE 36.1: Guidelines for opioid rotation. (Note that methadone conversion is beyond the scope of this chapter, so these suggestions pertain to other opioids only.)

withdrawal, both acute and protracted (manifesting as dysphoria, fatigue, sleep disturbance).

SUMMARY

1. Patients on long-term opioids can have very high opioid requirements in the perioperative period.
2. Multimodal pain regimens are necessary to properly manage pain in opioid-tolerant patients.
3. Tolerance and addiction are not the same, and confusing the two can have adverse effects on patient care.
4. Patients who are not responding well to one medication or in whom side effects limit dose escalation may benefit from opioid rotation.
5. Use of adjunct analgesics is important in limiting side effects of opioids such as sedation and OIH.

ACKNOWLEDGMENTS

The author would like to thank Alexandra Szabova and Kenneth R. Goldschneider for their contributions to the first edition.

ANNOTATED REFERENCES

Chu LF, Angst MS, Clark D. Opioid induced hyperalgesia in humans: molecular mechanisms and clinical considerations. *Clin J Pain.* 2008;24(6):479–496.

This review highlights the important mechanistic underpinnings and clinical ramifications of opioid-induced hyperalgesia and discusses future research directions and the latest clinical evidence for modulation of this potentially troublesome clinical phenomenon.

Dumas EO, Pollack GM. Opioid tolerance development: a pharmacokinetic/pharmacodynamic perspective. *AAPS J.* 2008;10(4):537–551.

This review article explains some pharmacokinetic and pharmacodynamic aspects of opioid-tolerance development. It presents several pharmacodynamic modeling strategies that have been used to characterize time-dependent attenuation of opioid analgesia.

Fine PG, Portenoy R. Establishing "best practices" for opioid rotation: conclusions of an expert panel. *J Pain Symptom Manage.* 2009;38(3):418–425.

This is a very practical article, easy to read and understand. It will be helpful for clinicians who do not deal with opioid rotation on a daily basis. It provides helpful and simple rules to follow and factors to consider when attempting opioid rotation.

Fredheim OMS, Moksnes K, Borchgrevink PC, Kaasa S, Dale O. Clinical pharmacology of methadone for pain. *Acta Anaesthesiol Scan.* 2008;52:879–889.

A useful literature review with a focus on methadone's properties, pharmacokinetics, interactions, pharmacogenetics, and use in cancer and chronic non-cancer pain. It offers switching strategies, equianalgesic dosing, and detailed information on QT-prolongation side effects.

BIBLIOGRAPHY

Anand KJS, Willson DF, Berger J, et al. Tolerance and withdrawal from prolonged opioid use in critically ill children. *Pediatrics.* 2010;125(5):e1208–e1225. doi:10.1542/peds.2009-0489

Bailey CR. Analgesic effects of gabapentin after spinal surgery. *Surv Anesthesiol.* 2004;48(6):312. doi:10.1097/01.sa.0000144252.13625.02

Brooks MR, Golianu B. Perioperative management in children with chronic pain. *Pediatr Anesth.* 2016;26(8):794–806. doi:10.1111/pan.12948

Coté CJ, Lerman J, Todres DI, eds. *A Practice of Anesthesia for Infants and Children:* 4th ed. Philadelphia: Saunders/Elsevier; 2008.

De Kock MF, Lavand'homme PM. The clinical role of NMDA receptor antagonists for the treatment of postoperative pain. *Best Pract Res Clin Anaesthesiol.* 2007;21(1):85–98. doi:10.1016/j.bpa.2006.12.006

Deer TR. Acute management of opioid-dependent patient. In: Leong MS, ed. *Comprehensive Treatment of Chronic Pain by Medical, Interventional, and Integrative Approaches: The American Academy of Pain Medicine Textbook on Patient Management*. New York: Springer; 2013:119–133.

Geary T, Negus A, Anderson BJ, Zernikow B. Perioperative management of the child on long-term opioids. *Pediatr Anesth*. 2011;22(3):189–202. doi:10.1111/j.1460-9592.2011.03737.x

Joly V, Richebe P, Guignard B, et al. Remifentanil-induced postoperative hyperalgesia and its prevention with small-dose ketamine. *Anesthesiology*. 2005;103(1):147–155. doi:10.1097/00000542-200507000-00022

Rusy LM, Hainsworth KR, Nelson TJ, et al. Gabapentin use in pediatric spinal fusion patients. *Anesth Analg*. 2010;110(5):1393–1398. doi:10.1213/ane.0b013e3181d41dc2

Saberski L. Postoperative pain management for the patient with chronic pain. In: Sinatra RS, ed. *Acute Pain: Mechanisms and Management*. St. Louis, MO: Mosby Yearbook; 1992:422–431.

Zempsky WT. Postoperative pain management. In: McGrath PJ, Stevens BJ, Walker SM, eds. *Oxford Textbook of Paediatric Pain*. Oxford: Oxford University Press; 2013:269–279.

37

Mediastinal Mass Biopsy

LISA CAPLAN

INTRODUCTION

Anterior mediastinal masses (AMMs) comprise a heterogeneous collection of neoplasms that have an estimated prevalence of 0.4% (Nishino et al., 2014). The anterior mediastinum contains many vital structures to the cardiopulmonary system. Consequently, the mass effect of these neoplasms can compress the trachea/mainstem bronchi, heart, or large vessels, such as, the superior vena cava (SVC) (Ng et al., 2007). Formulating a safe perioperative anesthetic plan becomes challenging in this population, as the rate of life threatening cardiopulmonary complications is estimated to be 7-20%. (Azizkhan et al., 1985; Ng et al., 2007). Preoperative anesthetic plans should consider presenting signs, symptoms, and the extent of cardiopulmonary involvement ,to help risk stratify and select the proper airway technique and sedation plan.

LEARNING OBJECTIVES

1. Identify signs and symptoms that contribute to the pathophysiology of children who present with AMMs.
2. Perform a risk assessment of patient symptomatology and design a perioperative care plan.
3. Risk stratify patients and procedures to determine appropriate anesthetic and airway techniques.

CASE PRESENTATION

The anesthesiologist on-call is notified that a 3-year-old girl requires an emergent pericardial window. She presented with cough, congestion, and fatigue and has most recently developed "panic episodes" while lying flat. The chest X-ray obtained in the emergency department demonstrated a wide mediastinum and bilateral pleural effusions. This prompted a chest computed tomography (CT) scan which revealed a large 7 cm × 5 cm × 6 cm mass diffusely narrowing the trachea and posteriorly displacing the great vessels which included partial occlusion of the SVC. She was unable to lie flat for the unsedated scan and required her head raised 30 degrees. Transthoracic echocardiography (TTE) revealed a pericardial effusion with tamponade physiology. On physical exam, she is tachycardic, tachypneic, and orthopneic and has diminished peripheral pulses.

Prior to proceeding to the operating room (OR), a multidisciplinary team meeting was briefly held. Due to the diffuse tracheal involvement and concurrent tamponade physiology, the decision was made to have extracorporeal membrane oxygenation (ECMO) specialists and otolaryngology with rigid bronchoscopy on standby in the OR. The patient was brought to the OR with the plan to maintain spontaneous ventilation via a simple facemask, in her position of comfort (head of bed at 45 degrees). Intravenous (IV) sedation was administered using ketamine, glycopyrrolate, and a field block utilizing local anesthetic. The surgeon created a pericardial window, which drained 200 mL of fluid.

DISCUSSION

1. What types of tumors typically present as AMMs?

Not all mediastinal masses are neoplastic, and some can be infectious or cystic in origin. The incidence of mediastinal malignancy in adults is approximately 25%, and in children, this incidence doubles. The most common mediastinal masses in order of prevalence, are: lymphomas, neurogenic tumors, and germ cell tumors. Roughly half of all mediastinal masses occur in the anterior mediastinum, and of those 80% are malignant (Ricketts, 2001).

When considering solely anterior mediastinal tumors, the most common types are lymphomas, germ cell tumors, and thymic masses (Cheung & Lerman, 1998; Ricketts, 2001). Lymphomas have a 60:40 prevalence of non-Hodgkin's to Hodgkin's type. Children diagnosed with mediastinal masses due to non-Hodgkin's lymphoma tend to be younger and more severely symptomatic due to the faster-growing tumors. These children are also more likely to have more ominous symptoms, such as, SVC syndrome, pleural effusions, and airway compression.

2. What are signs and symptoms of an AMM?

The presenting signs and symptoms of AMMs depend on the type, clinical evolution, size and relationship to adjacent structures (i.e., carina, pulmonary artery, and SVC). Table 37.1 lists possible signs and symptoms of an AMM. Respiratory symptoms are due to the tumor extrinsically compressing the respiratory tree. Factors such as the weight of the tumor, position of the child, and duration of compression will influence the degree of airway narrowing, bronchomalacia, and laryngomalacia. Lying supine can be particularly treacherous as the weight of the mass, combined with decreased lung volumes, may completely occlude the airway (Cheung & Lerman, 1998). Furthermore, central blood volume increases when supine, which can augment the size of a well-vascularized mass.

Cardiovascular symptoms associated with AMMs occur less frequently than respiratory dysfunction and as a result are less commonly considered the etiology of acute decompensation during anesthesia (Cheung & Lerman, 1998). AMMs may invade structures, such as, the pericardium and myocardium, thus compressing the pulmonary artery and SVC. The aorta is usually not affected by the AMM due to its location and the high intraluminal pressure countering that of the mass. On the other hand, AMM compression may potentially reduce pulmonary artery diameters. The physiologic consequence of this is impaired pulmonary perfusion resulting in hypoxemia, acute right ventricular failure, and cardiac arrest. Other cardiac manifestations, although rare, may occur due to direct compression of the heart. Large tumors, such as lymphomas and thymomas, can cause arrhythmias or low cardiac output from pericardial tamponade and tumor-related pericardial effusion.

In contrast to the pulmonary arteries, the SVC is susceptible to mechanical compression with its low intravascular pressure, thin vascular wall, and adjacent firm structures. SVC obstruction can limit cardiac preload and filling, which may lead to reduced cardiac output. The obstruction can ultimately lead to syncope when the patient must lie flat, such as for most surgical procedures. SVC syndrome is a particularly ominous symptom of AMMs and can present with varied symptomatology: headache, ear fullness, nausea, chest pain, or distortion of vision. Physical exam may reveal vein dilatation of the face, neck or

TABLE 37.1. POSSBLE SIGNS AND SYMPTOMS OF AN ANTERIOR MEDIASTINAL MASS

Body System	Signs	Symptoms
Respiratory	• Acute respiratory distress • Carinal, bronchial, or tracheal compression • Pleural effusion • Reduction in airway luminal diameter	• Dyspnea at rest • Dysphagia • Cough • Hoarseness • Orthopnea • (Pleuritic) pain • Stridor • Wheezing • Shortness of breath
Cardiovascular	• Constrictive pericarditis • Impaired left ventricular function • Pericardial effusion • Pulmonary artery compression • Tamponade	• Chest pain or fullness • Syncope • Superior vena cava syndrome
Gastrointestinal	Vomiting	Nausea
Hematologic	Lymphadenopathy	Night sweats

upper body, edema, flushed or violet hue, proptosis, or conjunctival edema

3. What is the pathophysiology behind airway compromise during anesthesia in these patients?

Cardiopulmonary collapse following induction of anesthesia is associated with a high risk of morbidity and mortality (Hammer, 2004). Acute decompensation is not just limited to induction and may occur during intubation, positioning, or extubation. Forty to 60% of patients will exhibit some sort of respiratory symptom at presentation, but no single symptom is predictive of anesthetic risk (Shamberger, 1999).

Respiratory decompensation in children with AMMs is due to mechanical compression of the trachea or main bronchi and is exacerbated by awake postural changes or induction of general anesthesia. This causes an acute critical increase in airway pressure that significantly impairs ventilation and oxygenation. Having the patient assume a supine position for any procedure can decrease the lung's functional residual capacity, reduce the transverse diameter of the thorax, and cause cephalad displacement of the diaphragm, leading to external compression of the mass on the trachea or main bronchi. Additionally, lung compliance becomes decreased especially due to the tumor burden, and the lung retractive force is increased.

The child's precarious clinical situation can be further worsened by the institution of positive pressure ventilation and muscle relaxation during induction. These physiologic changes may cause the airway lumen to collapse as negative airway pressure is lost, causing the chest wall to collapse inward on the airway and abdominal contents to shift cephalad. Thus, if a patient already has an airway diameter narrowed by the tumor, the shift from spontaneous to positive pressure ventilation may potentially reduce the diameter to a critical level.

How do anesthesiologists differentiate a "critical" and thus high-risk airway under anesthesia from those that are not? Shamberger et al. (1991) conducted a retrospective chart review of pediatric patients undergoing general anesthesia and found that the complication rate increased for those patients whose tracheal cross-sectional diameter was reduced more than 50% of expected. Spiral CT has become an established practice to evaluate the airway in the context of AMMs, especially to categorize airway involvement. In addition to detailing the airway diameter, CT also reports information on the size and location of the mass; further benefits include brief scan time and the ability for the upper body to be elevated without affecting scan quality.

4. What type of preprocedural labs and imaging are important before proceeding with anesthesia?

Labs and imaging can reveal critical information characterizing the extent and systemic impact of the mass. A chest radiograph will often alert providers to the presence of an AMM due to the presence of a widened mediastinum, and will provide additional useful information as to the presence of pleural or pericardial effusions. A CT scan provides the care team with information such as extent and compression of the airway, compression of cardiac structures and vessels, and presence of pleural/pericardial effusions. A CT is ideal in that it can be performed rapidly, does not require supine position unlike magnetic resonance imaging, and may not require sedation to accomplish. Other useful imaging in pediatric patients may include TTE to delineate the presence of tamponade physiology in the case of pericardial effusions, function, and compression of the SVC, pulmonary arteries, or right ventricular outflow tract. Pulmonary function tests have been used in adult or older pediatric patients to delineate disease severity. In this instance, a critical airway compression is noted when there is a 50% reduction in peak expiratory flow rate.

Despite the various means of preprocedure imaging, no one modality can provide the tumor tissue diagnosis. Optimum treatment protocols for mediastinal tumors depend on obtaining a tissue diagnosis, by the least invasive means possible, to tailor treatment. This may be accomplished by less invasive methods, such as, venous blood sampling; and more invasive methods requiring a procedure (and perhaps requiring anesthesia), such as, pleural and pericardial fluid aspiration, lymph node biopsy, or tumor biopsy.

5. How does one assess risk for GA in these patients?

Although there are many case reports of perioperative morbidity and mortality for children with AMMs, there are only a few retrospective observational studies attempting to risk stratify patients based upon tumor burden and symptoms (Anghelescu et al., 2007; Hack et al., 2008).

In one such study, Hack et al. (2008) reviewed 56 anesthetic records over a 7-year period to identify cases with a high risk of anesthesia-related complications. Complications, which were graded as mild, moderate, or severe, were noted in 11/55 patients (19.6%). No perioperative deaths were observed in this retrospective study. The presence of the following preoperative clinical signs was associated with an increased risk of anesthesia-related complications: cough, dyspnea, orthopnea, stridor, wheezing, and SVC obstruction. In those patients where a CT scan was available for analysis, respiratory complications occurred almost exclusively in 6 patients (7 general anesthetics) with tracheal cross-sectional area (%CSA) ≤70%. If patients with significant carinal or bronchial compression are excluded, anesthetic respiratory complications were confined to 3 patients (4 general anesthetics) with a %CSA ≤30%.

Preoperative administration of steroids, which is often controversial in this patient population, as it may preclude tissue diagnosis, was given to 33% of patients (n = 18) at the discretion of the attending hematologist (Hack et al., 2008). All 18 patients demonstrated clear evidence of severe airway compromise with statistically significant smaller tracheal cross-sectional area and/or tumor encasing the great vessels. Despite the use of preoperative steroids, a clear cancer diagnosis was made in 17/18 (95%) of the subgroup.

Based upon this and other available retrospective studies, patients with an AMM and at least one of the following symptoms should have additional precautions taken in the perioperative period due to an increased risk of anesthetic complications (Anghelescu et al., 2007; Hack et al., 2008):

- Three or more symptoms of respiratory distress
- Upper body edema
- Inability to lie flat
- Orthopnea
- Tracheal involvement with cross-sectional area <50%
- Mediastinal mass ratio >0.45%
- Great artery involvement
- Evidence of pericardial tamponade or ventricular dysfunction
- Evidence of pneumonia

6. What is the perioperative management of these patients?

Prior to administering anesthesia, a good history and physical should be performed by either querying the patient or caretaker. The anesthesiologist should check for respiratory symptoms, such as, wheezing, shortness of breath, and inability to lie flat. Identifying the patient's position of comfort is especially important, as is identifying which positions exacerbate symptoms. This is especially important when coordinating potential positioning for the procedure. Other physical exam findings, such as, edema, especially when it concerns the upper body, neck, or face, may indicate SVC syndrome along with distended nonpulsatile neck veins. In this instance, the location of peripheral vascular access should be considered, as a lower body peripheral IV may be desired preoperatively.

There is no standardized diagnostic algorithm accepted for children with AMM, since resources such as cardiopulmonary bypass, ECMO, and specialized cardiac anesthesiologists will vary by institution. However, multidisciplinary planning and good communication among pediatric anesthesiology, pediatric surgery, pediatric cardiovascular surgery, hematology/oncology, critical care, and radiology is necessary to manage these patients perioperatively. The patient or patient's family should be counseled on anesthetic concerns, such as, the greater risk of acute cardiopulmonary collapse, anesthetic recall or awareness if a monitored anesthetic care will be used, and even death.

Figure 37.1 is a proposed perioperative anesthetic plan for children with AMMs utilized at our institution based upon an evidenced-based review of the literature. The following precautions are taken for anesthetic management for patients with AMMs:

- Use additional personnel present in the operating room in case of complications.
- Maintain the patient's spontaneous ventilation.
- Avoid positive pressure ventilation and muscle relaxants if possible.
- Maintain the patient's position of comfort.
- If impending respiratory collapse, intubate past the obstruction and stent the airway with a rigid bronchoscope.
- Initiate ECMO if impending cardiovascular collapse (if institutionally available).
- If the patient has an ejection fraction <35% or pericardial effusion, contact an otolaryngologist to be present in the operating room with rigid bronchoscopy equipment.

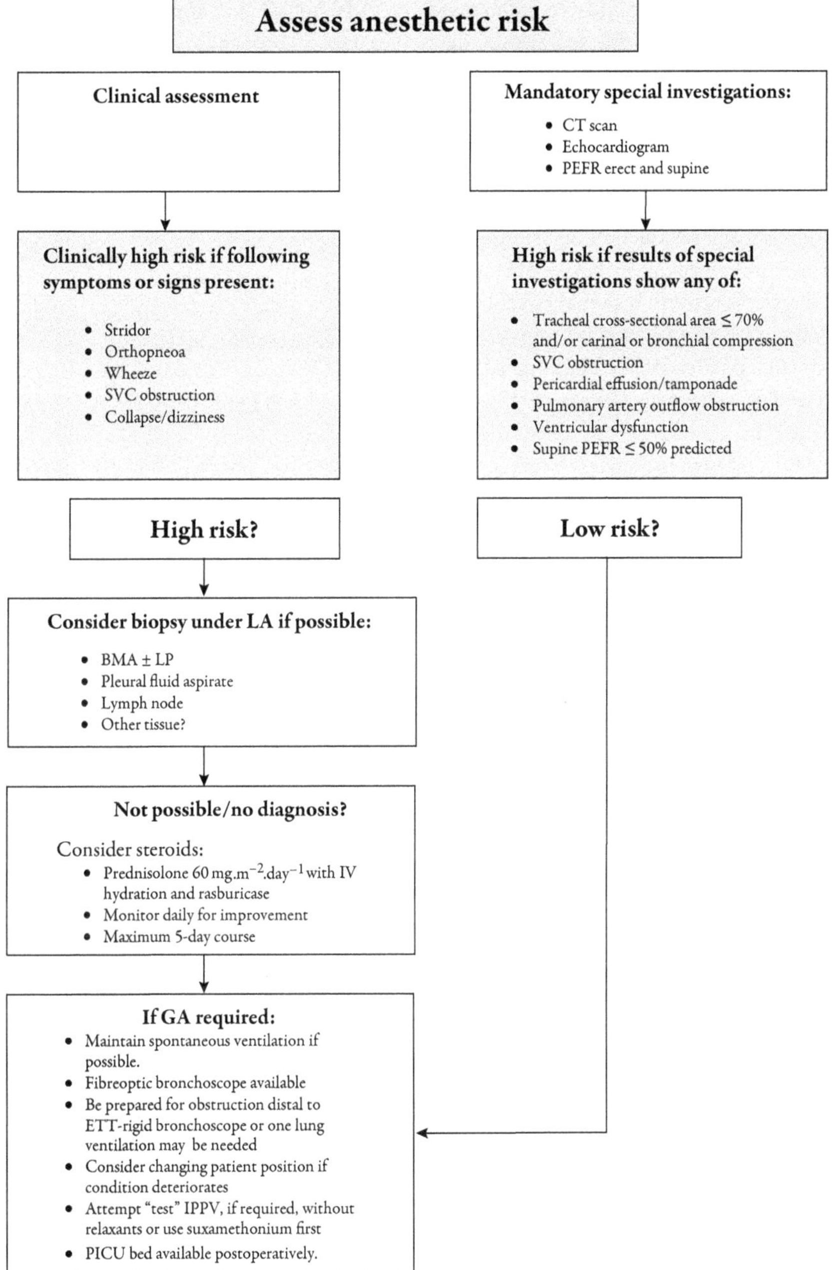

FIGURE 37.1: Proposed perioperative anesthetic plan for children with anterior mediastinal mass Anterior Mediastinal Masses, Evidence Based Outcomes Center, Texas Children's Hospital. Anterior Mediastinal Mass and Perioperative Care. 2015 http://connect2depts.texaschildrens.org/depts/1/nursing/Evidence%20Based%20Outcomes%20Center/Documents/DEPARTMENT%20SPECIFIC%20Evidence%20Based%20Summaries/Periop%20Mgt%20Anterior%20Mediastinal%20Mass/Anterior%20Mediastinal%20Mass%20algorithm%20final%20031915.pdf

7. What is the approach to acute decompensation in these patients?

There are numerous case reports of patients with AMMs undergoing general anesthesia who have had a perioperative demise due to airway complications (Slinger & Karsli, 2007). As stated, collapse of a "critical airway," which many agree is >50% reduction in tracheal airway diameter, may occur at any point during the procedure or thereafter. Acute decompensation is the consequence of the mass affecting the respiratory or cardiovascular system. Should acute changes in peak ventilatory airway pressure, loss of end-tidal carbon dioxide, or cardiovascular collapse occur, mass effect of the AMM should be suspected, with immediate maneuvers taken to relieve this obstruction. Repositioning the child should occur rapidly, especially if he or she is supine, by changing to the lateral decubitus or prone position ventilation is improved. Other maneuvers may include intubating the patient past the point of airway obstruction under direct vision, especially with a ridged bronchoscope if an otolaryngology surgeon is present. It should be cautioned that blindly advancing an endotracheal tube past the point of obstruction may lead to further complications with airway bleeding (Cheung & Lerman, 1998).

If cardiovascular collapse is imminent despite performing the aforementioned interventions, other considerations (albeit controversial) include instituting ECMO or cardiopulmonary bypass. It should be noted that even with "cardiopulmonary bypass standby," femoral cannulation will take at least 5 to 10 minutes under the best of circumstances. This would require perfusionists, a primed pump, and a surgeon to place the cannulas in the procedure area in anticipation of the event. There is no guarantee in this scenario that ECMO or cardiopulmonary bypass will prevent profound neurologic injury, in the case of cardiopulmonary collapse (Slinger & Karsli, 2007). That is why some authors argue that children with AMMs do not need to have their procedures performed in centers with ECMO capabilities but in places that have good perioperative planning before embarking on the procedure (Hack et al., 2008).

SUMMARY

1. The presenting signs and symptoms of AMMs depend on the type, clinical evolution, size, and relationship to adjacent structures.
2. Multidisciplinary teamwork with anesthesiology, oncology, otolaryngology, surgery, and interventional radiology is crucial to ensure a safe and effective outcome.
3. For high-risk patients, consider performing the biopsy under local anesthesia. Also, consider whether preoperative cancer management with radiation or steroid therapy is necessary prior to biopsy.

ACKNOWLEDGMENTS

The author would like to thank Jon Tomasson, Mohamed A. Mahmoud, and James P. Spaeth for their contributions to the first edition.

ANNOTATED REFERENCES

Cheung S, Lerman J. Mediastinal masses and anesthesia in children. *Anesthesiol Clin North America*. 1998;16(4):893–910.

An excellent review of anesthetic considerations of AMMs in children. Covers anatomy pathophysiology and presentation.

Hack H, Wright B, Wynn RF. The anaesthetic management of children with anterior mediastinal masses. *Anaesthesia*. 2008;63(8):837–846.

Case series describing a single institution's 7-year experience with AMMs.

BIBLIOGRAPHY

Anghelescu D, Burgoyne L, Liu T, et al. Clinical and diagnostic imaging findings predict anesthetic complications in children presenting with malignant mediastinal masses. *Pediatr Anesthesiol*. 2007;17(11):1090–1098.

Azizkhan RG, Dudgeon DL, Buck JR, et al. Life-threatening airway obstruction as a complication to the management of mediastinal masses in children. *J Pediatr Surg*. 1985;20(6):816–822.

Ferrari LR, Bedford RF. General anesthesia prior to treatment of anterior mediastinal masses in pediatric cancer patients. *Anesthesiology*. 1990;72:991–995.

Goh MH, Liu XY, Goh YS. Anterior mediastinal masses: an anaesthetic challenge. *Anaesthesia*. 1999;54:670–682.

Hammer GB. Anaesthetic management for the child with a mediastinal mass. *Pediatr Anesth*. 2004;14:95–97.

Ng A, Bennett J, Bromley P, Davies P, Morland B. Anaesthetic outcome and predictive risk factors in children with mediastinal tumors. *Pediatr Blood Cancer*. 2007;48(2):160–164.

Nishino M, Araki T, Dupuis J, Washko GR, Hunninghake GM, Hatabu H. Anterior mediastinal masses in the Framingham Heart Study: prevalence and CT image characteristics. *Eur J Radiol Open*. 2014;2:26–31.

Ricketts R. Clinical management of anterior mediastinal tumors in children. *Semin Pediatr Surg*. 2001;10(3):161–168.

Shamberger R. Preanesthetic evaluation of children with anterior mediastinal masses. *Semin Pediatr Surg*. 1999;8(2):61–68.

Shamberger R, Holzman RS, Griscom NT, Tarbell NJ, Weinstein J. CT quantitation of tracheal cross-sectional area as a guide to the surgical and anesthetic management of children with anterior mediastinal masses. *J Pediatr Surg*. 1991;26(2):138–142.

Slinger P, Karsli C. Management of the patient with a large anterior mediastinal mass: recurring myths. *Curr Opin Anesthesiol*. 2007;20:1–3.

Stricker P, Gurnaney H, Litman RS. Anesthetic management of children with an anterior mediastinal mass. *J Clin Anesthesiol*. 2010;22(3):159–163.

38

Neuroblastoma Resection

STEFANO SABATO

INTRODUCTION

Neuroblastoma is the most common extracranial solid tumor of childhood, and limited or complete surgical resection is performed in most cases. Anesthesia for these children can be challenging because of the size and location of the tumor, the secretion of vasoactive metabolites from the tumor, and because it involves major surgery in a potentially immunocompromised patient. Adequate preparation for these procedures can prevent intraoperative instability.

LEARNING OBJECTIVES

1. Know how to assess and optimize a child with neuroblastoma for surgery.
2. Appreciate some of the difficulties of anesthesia for the child with cancer.
3. Understand the principles of management of major blood loss during pediatric surgery.

CASE PRESENTATION

*A previously healthy, 20-month-old, 13-kg boy with a **stage M abdominal neuroblastoma** is scheduled for surgical resection of the tumor. The diagnosis of neuroblastoma was made using histology with tissue obtained via a needle biopsy, and **elevated urinary catecholamine concentrations**. Staging was based on magnetic resonance imaging (MRI), metaiodobenzyl guanidine scanning, analysis of bone marrow, and biopsy data. The patient received induction **chemotherapy** consisting of four cycles of carboplatin, etoposide, cyclophosphamide, and doxorubicin over 12 weeks. Repeat MRI scanning demonstrated residual disease in the left suprarenal region extending across the midline and encasing the origin of the superior mesenteric artery and the celiac trunk. Post-chemotherapy, echocardiography, chest x-ray, and serum biochemistry were all normal. On examination, his vital signs are a blood pressure of 75/40 mm/Hg, a heart rate of 95, and a respiratory rate of 30, and he is afebrile.*

*In the operating room an intravenous (IV) induction is followed by maintenance anesthesia of 3% sevoflurane in oxygen and air (FiO_2 = 0.3). **Intravenous access** is obtained for rapid fluid volume replacement with two 18-gauge intravenous cannulas. A 22-gauge radial arterial line and a 4 Fr left internal jugular double-lumen central line are placed using ultrasound guidance. A urinary catheter is placed to allow further indirect **assessment of intravascular volume** and organ perfusion.*

*A transverse upper abdominal incision is made and the tumor is exposed. The 7-hour surgery is notable for a prolonged, slow ooze of blood and serous fluid throughout the case. Crystalloids and 5% albumin are initially used to maintain mean arterial pressure, central venous pressure, and urine output targets. A full blood count, arterial blood gas, and coagulation profile are checked every 2 hours to monitor ventilation, blood sugar, serum electrolytes, and hemoglobin (Hb). Red blood cell transfusions are administered to maintain an Hb of approximately 9 g/dL. When two-thirds of the **estimated blood volume** has been replaced, fresh frozen plasma is administered in 10-mL/kg increments to maintain intravascular volume and a normal coagulation profile.*

*The surgeon applies vascular ligatures to the renal and splenic arteries, intermittently obstructing blood flow during the resection of the tumor. This results in decreased urine output and the development of a metabolic acidosis. Postoperatively, the patient is transferred to the intensive care unit, where the metabolic acidosis improves. Urine output improves with further fluid boluses, and **IV analgesics** are used to provide pain relief.*

DISCUSSION

1. What is the staging system for neuroblastoma? How are patients classified according to their risk of disease progression? How does this affect anesthesia?

Peripheral neuroblastic tumors are derived from neuroectodermal embryonic cells and include neuroblastoma, ganglioneuroblastoma, and ganglioneuroma. The diagnosis of neuroblastoma is made with histology from a tissue biopsy. The International Neuroblastoma Risk Group (INRG) has developed a widely used staging system based on clinical criteria and pre-surgical imaging (Monclair et al., 2009). Analysis of the bone marrow and 20 image-defined risk factors are used to stage the tumor (Table 38.1). The INRG classifies each malignancy into very low, low, intermediate, and high risk groups; based on the INRG stage, age at diagnosis, histologic category, grade of tumor differentiation, presence of MYCN oncogene amplification, presence or absence of chromosome 11q aberration, and tumor cell ploidy. In children with neuroblastoma, the **stage of disease** is the most important prognostic indicator. Age at diagnosis is the only other independent risk factor, with an age of less than 18 months associated with higher survival rates (Weinstein et al., 2003).

Very low-risk patients (localized ganglioneuromas/ganglioneuroblastomas) and low-risk L1 patients are treated with surgery alone. This surgery can be performed by a minimally invasive laparoscopic approach. MS stage patients are often observed, as the tumor resolves without intervention for reasons yet to be discovered. However, the majority of patients require chemotherapy, followed by open surgical resection to prevent primary recurrence. Some will also have additional postresection radiotherapy.

TABLE 38.1. THE INRG STAGING SYSTEM

Stage	Description
L1	Localized tumor not involving vital structures as defined by the list of image-defined risk factors and confined to one body compartment
L2	Locoregional tumor with presence of one or more image-defined risk factors
M	Distant metastatic disease (except stage MS).
MS	Metastatic disease in children younger than 18 months with metastases confined to skin, liver, and/or bone marrow

It is important to understand the aim of the surgical procedure, in order to provide the appropriate anesthetic. The initial surgery aims to establish or confirm the diagnosis by obtaining tissue and potentially resecting as much tumor as is safely possible. If the tumor is thought to be unresectable, or if it is easily accessible by percutaneous needle biopsy, then adequate tissue for diagnosis and stratification may be obtained by minimally invasive techniques. After chemotherapy has reduced the disease burden, a second surgical procedure is undertaken. This second operation may be a near-total resection that leaves tumor that is too dangerous to remove, or a complete resection of all remaining disease, including stripping the adventitia off the large arteries to which the cancer is adherent (Kiely, 2007). The role of complete resection of the tumor in Stage M disease is still controversial as it decreases the risk of local recurrence but does not improve overall survival (von Allmen et al., 2017).

2. Who is at risk of hemodynamic instability from circulating catecholamines?

Like pheochromocytomas, neuroblastomas are tumors derived from neural crest cells and can synthesize catecholamines. Most patients with neuroblastoma have **elevated urinary catecholamines** and catecholamine metabolites at diagnosis. Dopamine is the most common catecholamine produced by neuroblastomas, and levels can be assessed quickly from a random urine sample by the ratio of homovanilic acid (its major metabolite) to creatinine to aid the initial diagnosis. However, in contrast to patients with pheochromocytoma, there are usually no signs or symptoms of excessive circulating catecholamines. Although many case reports of hemodynamic instability during anesthesia for children with neuroblastoma exist (Kako et al., 2013), fortunately it is relatively rare (Haberkern et al., 1992). Those at risk of hemodynamic instability may exhibit signs and symptoms of excessive catecholamine production, such as, sweating, palpitations, diarrhea, tachycardia, hypertension, pallor, diaphoresis, and cardiomegaly on radiographs. Isolated hypertension without other signs of excessive catecholamines may be due to renal artery compression. If the child is exhibiting clinical signs of excessive catecholamine production, it is important to test for epinephrine (adrenaline) and norepinephrine (noradrenaline) from a 24-hour urine collection. These findings warrant preoperative consultation with the endocrinology and cardiology departments to guide **preoperative alpha and beta blockade**.

Chemotherapy may decrease the likelihood of encountering hemodynamic instability due to reduced tumor bulk and endocrinologic activity (Creagh-Barry & Sumner, 1992). Thus, the likelihood of catecholamine-induced instability is greater in a primary resection or biopsy prior to chemotherapy than during second operations after chemotherapy. However, there are reports of intraoperative hemodynamic instability during resection of tumors already treated with chemotherapy (Kain et al., 1993). Therefore, IV alpha and beta blockers need to be readily available during all surgeries. Finally, the presence of elevated levels of endogenous catecholamines preoperatively does not necessarily predict the need for inotrope or vasopressor administration in the postoperative period, as this is more dependent on the extent and duration of surgery (Ross et al., 2009).

3. What are the practical issues concerning IV access and fluid administration in major abdominal surgery?

The patient described had a tunneled cuffed central venous catheter already in situ. This line was used for the administration of chemotherapy, but its use in the perioperative setting has limitations. The long, thin lumen is not suitable for rapid infusion of IV fluids. Also, if the line has been in situ for an extended period of time, it may not aspirate freely, rendering measurement of central venous pressure unreliable and making it unsuitable for postoperative venous blood sampling. Finally, the tunneled line was placed for long-term access, and therefore all attempts to avoid colonization of bacteria and subsequent line infection should be made. Intraoperatively, many drugs and blood products are given, and they often need to be given rapidly. This makes it difficult to maintain strict asepsis when handling IV access devices. Therefore, in this case, **large-bore peripheral IV access** was obtained, and a second central venous catheter was inserted. A fluid warmer is necessary to warm blood products, as this patient is prone to hypothermia due to the large degree of exposure from the surgical wound and the anticipated large volume of fluid resuscitation.

In this case, as in most, there was no catastrophic hemorrhage during the operation, but the anesthesiologist still needs to **be prepared for extensive blood loss**, as abdominal neuroblastomas will often surround major vessels. It is important to have all blood products readily available for urgent rapid transfusion. It is helpful to have calculated the patient's **estimated blood volume** (EBV) prior to surgery (in toddlers EBV = 70 mL/kg). The intraoperative Hb (and hence the point at which transfusion may be needed) may be very roughly estimated by considering the observed blood loss. However, observed blood loss is very difficult to accurately quantify, so using serial intraoperative Hb measurements is a better method to guide the need for transfusion. When total fluid replacement approaches one blood volume, consider transfusing clotting factors. With slow, continuous bleeding, as opposed to rapid exsanguination, platelet administration is often unnecessary due to recruitment of platelets from splenic and endothelial reserves (Barcelona et al., 2005). However, if total fluid replacement approaches two blood volumes, platelet transfusion is likely to be required. In the event of a massive transfusion, it is important to avoid hypocalcemia and hypofibrinogenemia (see Chapter 20).

The anesthesiologist maintained a Hb concentration of 9 g/dL, even though a lower concentration would otherwise be acceptable. This was to provide a margin of safety given the possibility of sudden bleeding. Even without sudden hemorrhage, there is still often a need for transfusion and fluid replacement over the course of the operation.

Large losses of extracellular fluid occur as well. An exposed abdomen will lose up to 7 mL/kg/hr in evaporative losses alone, and aggressive tumor resection disrupts abdominal lymphatics, resulting in loss of lymphatic fluid. In summary, **large volumes of fluid administration may be required**, and replacement should be guided by the available clinical, laboratory, and invasive and noninvasive measurements. Hypovolemia is not the only cause for poor urine output; ligation of the renal vessels, pressure on the ureters, and even renal infarction should also be considered. Urine output is not always a reliable guide to intravascular volume and end organ perfusion pressure.

4. What are the anesthetic implications of chemotherapy?

Intense multi-agent chemotherapy reduces disease burden and facilitates resection. There are many different chemotherapeutic regimens, and which agents are selected depend on the institution. Many of the toxic effects of an individual drug are common across its class (Table 38.2). Anorexia, nausea, and vomiting are universal adverse effects throughout the duration of treatment. **All patients will be immunosuppressed**, and the utmost precautions against introducing infection must be taken. Thorough assessment by history, examination, and investigation of the cardiac, respiratory, renal, and hematologic systems is necessary prior to anesthesia. Anthracycline-induced cardiomyopathy may occur over a year after completion of therapy. A consultation by cardiology may be helpful in assessing the cardiac effects of the anthracyclines. Recently, immunotherapy has been introduced into the medical management of neuroblastomas. Monoclonal antibodies against the glycolipid disialoganglioside GD2 (anti-GD2 antibody) are used in high-risk patients after radiotherapy, when in a minimal residual disease state. It is also used in patients who have relapsed. Adverse effects of the anti-GD2 antibody, include: severe pain, hypotension, increased capillary permeability, visual disturbance, fever, and a high incidence of severe allergic reactions including anaphylaxis.

5. Are there specific needs for postoperative analgesia?

There is no single preferred approach to treating postoperative pain in this population. This child had extensive elective surgery with an anticipated long duration and the potential for coagulopathy. The anesthesiologist planned to ventilate the child for the first 12 to 24 hours postoperatively, and therefore

TABLE 38.2. COMMON TOXICITIES FROM CHEMOTHERAPY

Drug/Class	Toxicities
Cyclophosphamide/Alkylating agent	**Immediate**: metallic taste⁺, inappropriate ADH, blurred vision, arrhythmias*, myocardial necrosis* **Prompt**: myelosuppression⁺, alopecia⁺, hemorrhagic cystitis⁺ **Delayed**: immunosuppression, gonadal dysfunction, pulmonary fibrosis⁺* **Late**: secondary malignancy*, bladder fibrosis*
Etoposide/Podophyllotoxin derivative	**Immediate**: hypotension*, anaphylaxis* **Prompt**: myelosuppression, alopecia, peripheral neuropathy*, stomatitis* **Late**: secondary malignancy*
Carboplatin/Heavy metal antineoplastic agent	**Immediate**: metallic taste* **Prompt**: myelosuppression, electrolyte disturbance⁺, peripheral neuropathy*, hepatotoxicity*, renal toxicity⁺*, ototoxicity⁺*
Doxorubicin/Anthracycline antibiotic	**Immediate**: arrhythmias, local ulceration if extravasated, pink urine, anaphylaxis* **Prompt**: myelosuppression⁺, alopecia⁺, stomatitis⁺, mucositis⁺, hepatotoxicity⁺ **Delayed**: immunosuppression, cardiomyopathy (cumulative dose-dependent) **Late**: secondary malignancy*

Immediate: Within 1–2 days. Prompt: Within 2–3 weeks. Delayed: Anytime later during therapy. Late: Any time after the completion of treatment. ⁺ indicates that toxicity may occur later. * indicates a rare toxicity.

Source: Baker DL, Schmidt ML, Cohn SL, et al. Outcome after reduced chemotherapy for intermediate-risk neuroblastoma. *N Engl J Med.* 2010;363:1313–1323.

an epidural catheter would not have avoided postoperative ventilation. Neither of these two reasons are absolute contraindications to an epidural catheter, and individual/institutional preference varies. Most of the systemic analgesics can be used effectively. Neuroblastoma patients are often too young to directly use patient-controlled analgesia (PCA). Use of PCA by proxy can allow parents to help control their child's pain. Monitoring and family and nursing education are critical if this modality is used. Nonsteroidal anti-inflammatory drugs are generally avoided due to their antiplatelet effect and potential nephrotoxicity.

SUMMARY

1. Staging of neuroblastomas has prognostic value and guides therapy and intervention; therapy may include extensive surgery and chemotherapy.
2. Several of the chemotherapeutic agents have significant physiologic effects, which have both immediate and long-term implications for anesthetic management.
3. It is important to recognize the minority of patients who are at risk of catecholamine-induced hemodynamic instability and formulate a plan for their preoperative and intraoperative care.
4. Intraoperative fluid management is challenging, and adequate venous access is important.

ANNOTATED REFERENCES

Creagh-Barry P, Sumner E. Neuroblastoma and anesthesia. *Pediatr Anesth.* 1992;2:147–152.

A case series that discusses patients at risk of hemodynamic instability.

Weinstein JL, Katzenstein HM, Cohn SL. Advances in the diagnosis and treatment of neuroblastoma. *Oncologist.* 2003;8:278–292.

An excellent review of neuroblastoma from an oncology perspective. Details staging, prognostic indicators, and conventional and novel treatments.

BIBLIOGRAPHY

Barcelona SL, Thompson AA, Coté CJ. Intraoperative pediatric blood transfusion therapy: a review of common issues. Part II: transfusion therapy, special considerations, and reduction of allogenic blood transfusions. *Pediatr Aneseth.* 2005;15:814–830.

Gupta A, Kumar A, Walters S, Chait P, Irwin MS, Gerstle JT. Analysis of needle versus open biopsy for the diagnosis of advanced stage pediatric neuroblastoma. *Pediatr Blood Cancer.* 2006;47:875–879.

Haberkern CM, Coles PG, Morray JP, Kennard SC, Sawin RS. Intraoperative hypertension during surgical excision of neuroblastoma: case report and review of 20 years' experience. *Anesth Analg.* 1992;75:854–858.

Kain ZN, Shamberger RS, Holzman RS. Anesthetic management of children with neuroblastoma. *J Clin Anesth.* 1993;5:486–491.

Kako H, Taghon T, Veneziano G, Aldrink JH, Ayoob R, Tobias JD. Severe intraoperative hypertension after induction of anesthesia in a child with neuroblastoma. *J Anesth.* 2013;27:464–467.

Kiely E. A technique for excision of abdominal and pelvic neuroblastomas. *Ann R Coll Surg Eng.* 2007;89:342–348.

Monclair T, Brodeur GM, Ambros PF, et al. The International Neuroblastoma Risk Group (INRG) staging system: an INRG task force report. *J Clin Oncol.* 2009;27(2):298–303.

Ross SL, Greenwald BM, Howell JD, et al. Outcomes following thoracoabdominal resection of neuroblastoma. *Pediatr Crit Care Med.* 2009;6:681–686.

Sendo D, Katsuura M, Akiba K, et al. Severe hypertension and cardiac failure associated with neuroblastoma: a case report. *J Pediatr Surg.* 1996;12:1688–1690.

von Allmen D, Davidoff AM, London WB, et al. Impact of extent of resection on local control and survival in patients from the COG A3973 study with high-risk neuroblastoma. *J Clin Oncol.* 2017;35(2):208–216.

Wagner LM, Danks MK. New therapeutic targets for the treatment of high-risk neuroblastoma. *J Cell Biochem.* 2009;107:46–57.

PART 10

Challenges in Metabolic and Endocrinologic Conditions

39

The Diabetic Patient

MARIO PATINO AND ANNA M. VARUGHESE

INTRODUCTION

Diabetes is the most common metabolic disorder in children. Its incidence is increasing at a rate of 2% to 3% per year, with 70,000 new cases diagnosed every year worldwide. Its peak incidence occurs between the ages of 11 and 14 years old. Perioperative management of diabetic patients demands knowledge of pathophysiology, current treatment, degree of control and compliance with therapy, previous complications, complexity and duration of the surgical procedure, and expected postoperative course. The rapid development of new, complex regimens for treatment and the availability of many forms of insulin make the management of these patients complex, and best conducted using a multidisciplinary approach, that involves optimal communication among the various teams involved in the care of these patients and, in particular, in conjunction with a pediatric endocrinologist.

LEARNING OBJECTIVES

1. Differentiate appropriate preoperative metabolic control from nonoptimal control in a diabetic child.
2. Define the perioperative risks and complications for diabetic patients.
3. Describe perioperative goals in the management of children with diabetes and conceptualize a perioperative plan to meet these goals.
4. Know how to effectively manage life-threatening complications, such as, severe hypoglycemia.

CASE PRESENTATION

A 7-year-old, 20-kg girl with a past history of bladder exstrophy is undergoing a bladder augmentation procedure for intractable urinary incontinence. A year ago, she was diagnosed with ***type 1 diabetes mellitus*** *after being admitted with urosepsis and diabetic ketoacidosis. Over the past 9 months, she has been managed with a* ***continuous subcutaneous insulin infusion (CSII)*** *of insulin lispro (Humalog®) at a* ***basal rate*** *of 0.3 units/hr, with* ***prandial boluses*** *of 2 to 3 units of insulin lispro. On average, she receives 15 units of insulin lispro per day. Her blood glucose level is checked three or four times a day, and is usually below 250 mg/dL (13.9 mmol/L). The patient is scheduled as the first case of the day and is to be admitted after surgery. Complete blood count and electrolytes are normal. There is no evidence of ketonuria, and her hemoglobin A1C (***HbA1C***) is 8.5%. A preoperative blood sugar is 275 mg/dL (15.3 mmol/L). Using a* ***correction formula*** *calculation, an additional 0.6 units of insulin lispro (Humalog®) is administered subcutaneously. The CSII is discontinued, and maintenance fluids are administered with dextrose 5% with half-normal saline. A continuous infusion of* ***intravenous*** *(IV) regular* ***insulin*** *is started at 0.05 units/kg/hr. Intraoperative blood glucose levels are measured every hour. Blood glucose levels are between 90 and 180 mg/dL (5.0–10 mmol/L) during the first 2 hours of the procedure, after which they increase to 350 mg/dL (19.4 mmol/L). Two units of rapid-acting insulin (insulin lispro) are administered subcutaneously, and the continuous infusion of insulin is increased by 25% to 0.06 units/kg/hr; over the next hour the blood glucose level drops to 110 mg/dL (6.1 mmol/L). At the end of the procedure, the patient is* *breathing spontaneously and ready to be extubated; but she is unable to follow commands. There are no residual effects of muscle relaxants or inhalation agents present. The patient is clammy to the touch and has an elevated heart rate. Her blood glucose level is 35 mg/dL (1.9 mmol/L).* ***The IV insulin infusion*** *is immediately stopped and* ***20 mL of 50% dextrose*** *is rapidly administered through* ***the central line****. Shortly after, the patient wakes up and is extubated and transferred to the intensive care unit (ICU). In the ICU, maintenance fluids of 5% dextrose with half-normal saline are restarted with a continuous infusion of regular insulin at a rate of 0.05 units/kg/hr. On the second postoperative day, the patient is placed on a liquid and soft diet, the* ***CSII*** *is restarted with her regular settings, and the patient is transferred to a regular ward.*

DISCUSSION

1. How can one determine if a diabetic child is in optimal condition prior to undergoing an elective operation?

Initial assessment should include determining current regimen and stability, previous complications, and recent evaluation by a pediatric endocrinologist. Evaluation by pediatric endocrinology must be performed several days before surgery to allow for assessment and optimization of glycemic control. It is important to identify patients who are at risk for episodes of hyperglycemia or hypoglycemia, such as, those with a prolonged fasting time, bowel preparation prior to surgery, steroid therapy, or continuous total parenteral nutrition infusion.

If the patient presents with an acute disease process and uncontrolled blood glucose levels, the presence of acidosis and ketonuria must be evaluated to rule out ketoacidosis. A preoperative blood sugar is mandatory, and recent electrolytes should be evaluated. **Glycosylated hemoglobin levels (HbA$_{1C}$)** provide information about the degree of glycemic control in the past 2 to 3 months. The American Diabetes Association (2016) currently recommends an **HbA$_{1C}$** below 7.5% across all pediatric age-groups.

If the patient has uncontrolled diabetes with a *persistent blood glucose level above 250 mg/dL* (13.9 mmol/L), *electrolyte imbalances*, and/or *ketonuria*, an elective procedure should be postponed and preoperative optimization by a pediatric endocrinologist is recommended. If surgery cannot be postponed, diabetic ketoacidosis must be ruled out, given the accentuated stress response and higher insulin requirements. It is important to note that diabetic ketoacidosis may present as an "acute abdomen" and that acute illness may precipitate diabetic ketoacidosis.

2. What are the risks and complications of diabetic patients undergoing major and prolonged procedures?

The response to surgical stress is characterized by an increase in the counterregulatory hormones (glucagon, cortisol, catecholamines, and growth hormone) that enhance gluconeogenesis, glycogenolysis, and protein and fat catabolism and make control of blood glucose levels more challenging. Also, surgical stress can increase inflammatory cytokines (interleukin-6 and tumor necrosis factor alpha) that impair insulin secretion. Therefore, the perioperative period can be marked by episodes of hyperglycemia due to this increase in counterregulatory hormones, and the insulin deficiency of type 1 diabetes mellitus (or the relative insulin deficiency and insulin resistance of type 2 diabetes mellitus). Patients are also susceptible to episodes of hypoglycemia due to preoperative fasting and the exogenous administration of insulin. Uncontrolled hyperglycemia compromises immune function; this increases the risk of surgical site infection and alters the wound healing process. Also, diabetic patients are at greater risk of developing autonomic dysregulation, with poor compensatory effects for episodes of hypotension. They may have gastroparesis, with a resultant increased risk for aspiration. Insulin overdose can lead to a life-threatening episode of hypoglycemia. Given the susceptibility to fluctuating blood glucose levels during the perioperative period, frequent measurement of blood glucose (every 30 to 60 minutes) is strongly suggested.

3. What are the goals of perioperative management of pediatric diabetic patients undergoing major procedures? How is insulin therapy optimally managed?

From the metabolic standpoint, the goal is to maintain a blood glucose concentration between 90 and 180 mg/dL (5.0–10 mmol/L). Intensive and tight glycemic control must be balanced with the associated risk of hypoglycemia. Ideally, diabetic children would be scheduled as the first case of the day to avoid prolongation of the fasting time, and to facilitate the implementation of an insulin/carbohydrate regimen.

Knowing the following terms will aid better understanding of perioperative insulin therapy:

- ***Total daily dose (TDD) of insulin***: Number of units given in 24 hours
- ***Basal insulin***: Physiological insulin levels produced by the pancreas when not stimulated by glucose. Basal insulin prevents gluconeogenesis and ketogenesis. To provide the needs of basal insulin in diabetic children, long-acting insulin (peakless), intermediate-acting insulin (neutral protamine Hagedorn [NPH] insulin) or continuous subcutaneous (SC) insulin infusion is administered.
- ***CSII*: Continuous subcutaneous insulin infusion** administered via a portable pump
- ***Insulin-to-carbohydrate ratio* (I:C ratio)**: Number of units of insulin administered per gram of carbohydrate. During the perioperative period, the I:C ratio is usually 1:5 to 1:8 for the administration of continuous IV insulin. The I:C ratio may be modified according to the patient's response. Postpubertal children are more resistant to insulin and may need an I:C ratio of 1:3 to 1:5.
- ***Insulin correction factor or insulin sensitivity factor***: This is a determination of the expected decrease in blood sugar concentration (in mg/dL) after the administration of 1 unit of insulin. It is calculated by dividing 1,500 by the TDD ("the 1,500 rule").
- ***Correction formula***: Knowing the insulin sensitivity factor, this formula is used to estimate the dose of insulin needed to bring a patient's blood glucose level to a target or goal level:

CF = (patient's blood glucose level – goal blood glucose) / insulin sensitivity factor

4. How does the correction formula factor into perioperative insulin dosing?

Perioperative insulin management is based on providing the usual pattern of physiological secretion of insulin. However, insulin requirements during the perioperative period increase. Insulin therapy consists of three different elements: **basal, prandial,** and **supplemental** administration.

Basal administration of insulin is given by either long-acting insulin, intermediate-acting insulin (NPH), or by continuous SC administration of rapid-acting insulin with the use of a portable pump (CSII). Patients receiving NPH have a less predictable response to its administration with larger variability of peak and duration of action than patients on newer forms of insulin. Basal administration is equivalent to the physiological insulin levels that avoid gluconeogenesis and ketogenesis. Basal insulin therapy is approximately 50% of the total daily dose and is necessary in type I diabetics, independent of the patient's fasting status.

Prandial administration uses rapid-acting insulin, which is determined by the amount of carbohydrates to be consumed (insulin-to-carbohydrate ratio).

Supplemental administration is determined by the level of glucose above the goal. Supplemental administration of insulin is calculated using a **correction formula**. Knowing the insulin sensitivity factor, a correction formula is used to calculate the insulin dose to be administered to maintain a blood glucose level at 150 mg/dL (8.3 mmol/L). Usually 100% of the correction factor is administered, but in prepubertal children and in patients with history of hypoglycemia, 50% or 75% of the correction factor may be administered since prepubertal children are more sensitive to the effects of insulin and have a higher risk of hypoglycemia.

Current perioperative management of insulin with the administration of the basal requirements, prandial dose (if allowed to eat), and the administration of correction factor, when needed, has shown better glycemic control and lower rate of perioperative complications than the traditional use of a sliding scale which is now discouraged.

Considering the higher risk of metabolic decompensation in patients undergoing longer procedures, guidelines for management are divided by the duration of the procedure (see Tables 39.1 and 39.2).

The insulin daily dose for the patient in this case is 15 units. The insulin *correction factor* or *insulin sensitivity factor* is 1,500/15 = 100. Theoretically, 1 unit of insulin administered subcutaneously to this patient would decrease the blood glucose level by 100 mg/dL (5.5 mmol/L). If this patient's preoperative blood glucose level is 275 mg/dL (15.3 mmol/L) and the perioperative blood glucose goal is 150 mg/dL (8.3mmol/L), then: **CF** = (275 – 150)/

TABLE 39.1. MANAGING DIABETIC PEDIATRIC PATIENTS FOR SHORTER PROCEDURES (<2 HOURS)

- Administer the usual evening dose of basal/ long acting insulin
- On the morning of surgery, if the patient is on the conventional therapy (NPH), administer 50% of the NPH insulin (basal insulin requirements) and check preoperative blood glucose level and electrolytes. Check ketones (blood or urine) if BG > 250 mg/Dl. If the BG level is <100 mg/dL (5.5 mmol/L), start fluids at maintenance rate with 5% to 10% dextrose. If the BG level is >250 mg/dL (13.9 mmol/L), administer a supplemental dose of rapid-acting insulin SC with the calculation of a correction factor (administer 50% of the correction factor to titrate response). Given the lower predictability of response and peak effect of NPH insulin with higher risk of hypoglycemia in fasting patients, maintenance fluids with dextrose fluids must be considered even in normoglycemic patients undergoing short procedures receiving NPH insulin.
- If the patient is receiving continuous SC administration of rapid-acting insulin, continue the same basal rate. If the BG level is >250 mg/dL (13.9 mmol/L), administer an additional bolus of SC rapid-acting insulin with 50% of the correction factor.
- If the patient is receiving long-acting insulin (i.e., insulin glargine [Lantus®]) once every 24 hours administered at night, there is no requirement for additional doses on the day of surgery. If a patient is on long-acting insulin every 12 hours, give the full morning dose, since there is no associated peak effect and this will provide the basal insulin needs. For a BG level of >250 mg/dL (13.9 mmol/L), an additional bolus of SC rapid-acting insulin is given according to the correction factor.
- Intraoperative fluid management during short procedures for patients receiving continuous SC administration of rapid-acting insulin, or for patients receiving long-acting insulin with supplementation of bolus short-acting insulin, usually does not require dextrose-containing fluids unless hypoglycemia is an issue.

Note. NPH = neutral protamine Hagedorn (intermediate-acting insulin); BG = blood glucose; SC = subcutaneous.

TABLE 39.2. MANAGING DIABETIC PEDIATRIC PATIENTS FOR LONGER PROCEDURES (>2 HOURS)

- Administer the usual evening dose of basal/ long acting insulin.
- All morning doses of insulin are held. Start maintenance fluids with 5% dextrose with half-normal saline and continuous insulin intravenous infusion. Insulin infusion doses depend of the BG levels and are as follows: for BG (6–7 mmol/L /110–140 mg/dL) 0.03 units/kg/hour, BG (8–12 mmol/L / 140–220 mg/dL) 0.05 units/kg/hour, BG (>12 mmol/L / 220 mg/dL) 0.075 units/kg/hour. Insulin is diluted in normal saline to a concentration of 1 unit/mL (or 0.5 unit/mL for younger children). Both insulin and glucose are administered through the same intravenous line. For a BG level >250 mg/dL (13.9 mmol/L), administer a correction factor dose with the administration of SC insulin.
- Intraoperatively, insulin is administered by continuous intravenous infusion at the doses recommended here according to the BG levels with a goal to maintain BG levels between 90 and 180 mg/dL (5.0–10 mmol/L).
- Continue maintenance fluids with 5% dextrose with half-normal saline. Administer isotonic fluids to replace the deficit and third-space losses. Monitoring of electrolytes is critical given the risk of hyponatremia with the administration of hypotonic fluids. Replace half normal saline with isotonic fluids if hyponatremia is detected.
- Check BG hourly. After any adjustment to the therapy, check BG every 30 minutes.
- If the BG level is >180 mg/dL (10 mmol/L), administer a correction factor dose (calculated with the 1,500 rule with an ideal BG level of 150 mg/dL [8.3 mmol/L]) with the administration of SC rapid-acting insulin. Considering the biological effect of the rapid-acting insulin given SC, do not administer a correction factor more frequently than every 3 hours.
- For a persistent BG level >180 mg/dL (10 mmol/L), consider increasing the continuous intravenous insulin infusion (20%–25%).
- For BG levels >60 mg/dL (3.3 mmol/L) and <110 mg/dL (6.1 mmol/L), decrease the insulin infusion and increase the dextrose infusion. Follow BG levels every 30 minutes.
- For a BG level <60 mg/dL (3.3 mmol/L), discontinue the insulin infusion and administer 0.5 to 1 g/kg of intravenous dextrose.
- Important consideration must be given to patients scheduled for surgery in the afternoon (not ideal). If allowed to eat breakfast, the patient must receive a dose of short-acting insulin based on the I:C ratio (prandial dose) and the full usual dose of basal/long-acting insulin (basal requirements). If receiving NPH, administer 50% of the morning dose. Dextrose fluids and insulin infusion must be started 2 hours before surgery and not later than noon.

Note. NPH = neutral protamine Hagedorn (intermediate-acting insulin); BG = blood glucose; SC = subcutaneous.

100 = 1.25 units. Theoretically 1.25 units of insulin would decrease the blood glucose level to the target level. However, 0.6 units of insulin were administered instead of 1.25 units (50% of the correction formula) to avoid the risk of hypoglycemia in this prepubertal patient. When administering a dose of correction factor, it is important to avoid the IV route. The administration of IV regular insulin peaks in 4 to 5 minutes and has a biological half-life of 15 to 20 minutes, leading to rapid and transient changes in blood glucose levels.

5. What are other issues in the perioperative management of the diabetic patient?

Other important considerations are the risks of hypokalemia and hyponatremia. Frequent monitoring is required. The risks of surgical site infection should also be considered; appropriate antibiotic prophylaxis must be given prior to the surgical incision, and adequate antibiotic redosing is required. Given the alterations in wound healing, appropriate positioning and padding in these patients is important to avoid any skin breakdown and/or pressure on the skin.

Postoperative care requires adequate pain control to blunt the increase in counterregulatory hormones, and to facilitate the control of blood glucose levels. Maintenance fluids with 5% to 10% dextrose and the administration of IV or SC insulin are continued at the previously titrated insulin dose. Blood glucose should be measured hourly as long as the patient continues on **continuous IV insulin infusion**. Transition to the previous insulin therapy based on the child's usual I:C ratio and correction factor must be established as soon as the patient is tolerating oral intake. It is expected that diabetic patients during the first 48 hours after surgery will have an increase in insulin requirements due to the stress response. Well-defined written protocols for postoperative management must be available on the units where postoperative care of diabetic patients occur.

6. What are the preoperative recommendations for patients with type 2 diabetes on oral hypoglycemic agents? How does the insulin management of patients with type 2 diabetes differ from patients with type 1 diabetes?

Lactic acidosis secondary to the use of metformin has been well recognized, with risk increased by renal insufficiency. For major surgery lasting for more than 2 hours, and concomitant risk factors, such as, tissue hypoperfusion or renal insufficiency, metformin should ideally be discontinued 24 hours before the procedure. In situations such as emergency surgery with <24 hours since the last oral dose of metformin, precaution should be taken to maintain adequate hydration with IV fluids throughout the perioperative period. Metformin may be discontinued on the day of surgery for minor, short surgical procedures lasting less than 2 hours. In all types of surgical cases, it is recommended that metformin be withheld for at least 48 hours after surgery and restarted once normal renal function has been confirmed. Other oral hypoglycemic agents can be discontinued the day of surgery. Preoperative and postoperative recommendations for insulin infusions in patients with type 2 diabetes treated with insulin are similar to those for patients with type 1 diabetes in which consideration must be given to the duration of the procedure. Importantly, greater rates of insulin infusion are commonly required in type 2 diabetes.

7. How should hypoglycemia be treated?

The patient in this case developed a serious episode of hypoglycemia at the end of the procedure. Hypoglycemia is a life-threatening situation and requires immediate treatment to avoid a neurologic injury: **25% or 50% dextrose** is recommended, and continuous infusion of insulin must be *immediately discontinued*. Although concentrations of dextrose above 10% are considered hypertonic and carry the risk of causing phlebitis and venous thrombosis, in an emergency situation 25% dextrose can be administered through a peripheral vein. However, **50% dextrose** must always be administered through a **central line**. The recommended dose is 0.5 to 1 g/kg of dextrose. This is equivalent to 1 to 2 mL/kg 50% dextrose, 2 to 4 mL/kg 25% dextrose, 4 to 8 mL/kg 12.5% dextrose, or 5 to 10 mL/kg 10% dextrose. Another option is the intramuscular administration of glucagon in a dose of 0.25 mg (<5 years of age), 0.5 mg (5–12 years), and 1 mg (>12 years). Important consideration must be given to the risk of rebound hyperglycemia in patients who were receiving a continuous infusion of insulin and develop hypoglycemia. The insulin infusion is discontinued if the blood glucose level is below 60 mg/dL (3.3 mmol/L). For patients on a continuous insulin infusion with blood glucose between 60 mg/Dl (3.3 mmol/L) and 90 mg/dL (5.0 mmol/L), the rate of infusion is decreased but not stopped abruptly due to the risk of rebound hyperglycemia.

SUMMARY

1. Preoperative evaluation includes blood glucose, HbA_{1C}, and electrolytes. For blood glucose levels >250 mg/dL (13.8 mmol/L), blood or urine ketones must be checked. Basal insulin requirements and duration of fasting should also be considered.
2. Perioperative fluxes in blood glucose levels are to be expected; the patient requires close monitoring and manipulation of the insulin and glucose regimen.
3. Hypoglycemia is more dangerous than hyperglycemia and requires rapid intervention.

ANNOTATED REFERENCES

Rhodes ET, Gong C, Edge JA, Wolfsdorf JI, Hanas R. Management of children and adolescents with diabetes requiring surgery. *Pediatr Diabetes.* 2014;15(Suppl. 20):224–231.

Clinical practice consensus guidelines with evidence grading system developed by the International Society for Pediatric and Adolescent Diabetes.

Sperling M, Tamborlane W, Battelino T, Weinzimer S, Philip M. Diabetes Mellitus. In: Sperling M, ed. *Pediatric Endocrinology*. Cambridge, MA: Saunders; 2014: 839–900.

In-depth chapter about diabetes mellitus and its management.

Rhodes ET, Ferrari LR, Wolfsdorf JI. Perioperative management of pediatric surgical patients with diabetes mellitus. *Anesth Analg.* 2005;101:986–999.

A hallmark article in the perioperative management of diabetic children.

BIBLIOGRAPHY

American Diabetes Association. Standards of medical care in diabetes—2016. *Diabetes Care.* 2016;39 (Suppl 1):S86–S104.

Atkinson, M. Type 1 diabetes mellitus. In: Melmed S, Polonsky KS, Larsen PR, Kronenberg H, eds. *Williams Textbook of Endocrinology,* 16th ed. Cambridge, MA: Elsevier; 2016:1451–1483.

Betts P, Brink S, Silink M, Swift P, Wolfsdor J, Hanas R. Management of children and adolescents with diabetes requiring surgery. *Pediatr Diabetes.* 2009;10:169–174.

Delli A, Lernmark A. Type 1 (insulin-dependent) diabetes mellitus: etiology, pathogenesis, prediction, and prevention. In: Jameson JL, ed. *Endocrinology Adult and Pediatric.* Cambridge, MA: Saunders; 2016:672–690.

Rodbard HW, Blonde L, Braithwaite SS, et al. Medical guidelines for clinical practice for the management of diabetes mellitus. *Endocrine Practice.* 2007;13:1–68.

Shamsuddin A, Barash P, Inzucchi S. Scientific principles and clinical implications of perioperative glucose regulation and control. *Anesth Analg.* 2010;110:478–497.

40

Diabetic Ketoacidosis in a Child with Acute Surgical Abdomen

RAHUL BAIJAL AND CARLOS J. CAMPOS

INTRODUCTION

Diabetic ketoacidosis (DKA) is a complication of insulin deficiency, leading to hyperglycemia, glucosuria, dehydration, ketogenesis, and acidosis. DKA is a complication of type I diabetes mellitus (DM) with potentially significant morbidity.

LEARNING OBJECTIVES

1. Identify children at risk for DKA.
2. Understand the clinical presentation and pathophysiology of DKA.
3. Identify children at risk for cerebral edema (CE) and manage CE in children with DKA.
4. Discuss the management of DKA.
5. Describe the anesthetic implications in children with DKA.

CASE PRESENTATION

A 9-year-old boy with ***type 1 DM*** *presents to the emergency department with fever and intermittent* ***abdominal pain*** *for 10 days, and vomiting for the past 3 days. His home insulin regimen consists of insulin Lantus 10 U at night, and regular insulin for carbohydrate correction. He has no other past medical history.*

Physical examination reveals an alert, thin, ill-appearing patient. His vital signs are: weight 30 kg, height 150 cm, blood pressure 90/52, respiratory rate 50, heart rate 144, and oxygen saturation 98%. He has reduced skin turgor, dry mucous membranes, sunken eyes, and a distended abdomen with rebound tenderness in the right lower abdomen.

Laboratory analysis reveals serum glucose of 420 mg/dL, Na 134 mmol/L, K 5.0 mmol/L, HCO_3 *14 mEq/L, and BUN 27 mg/dL. Subsequent arterial blood gas analysis shows a* ***pH 7.21****,* pCO_2 *30 mmHg,* pO_2 *102 mmHg,*HCO_3^- *12 mEq/L, and* ***BE -9****. His urine analysis shows a* ***glucose >1,000 mg/dL*** *with* ***elevated ketones****. Complete blood count reveals elevated white blood cells at* 16.3×10^9*/L with 74% neutrophils and an* $HbA1_c$ *of 12. His abdominal computed tomography (CT) scan demonstrates a* ***perforated appendix*** *with a* ***periappendiceal abscess.***

The ***consulting endocrinology service*** *initiates management with a 10-mL/kg bolus of lactated Ringer's (LR). Body surface area (BSA,* m^2*) is calculated to start maintenance intravenous (IV) fluids. A continuous IV* ***insulin infusion*** *is started to treat the ketonuria and metabolic acidosis. A* ***D10LR*** *infusion is started when blood glucose falls below 300 mg/dL. The insulin infusion is continued until the anion gap resolves and the bicarbonate levels reach 18 mEq/L at which point the child is transitioned to Lantus and regular insulin therapy. The perforated appendicitis is initially medically managed with IV antibiotics and the patient is scheduled for a periappendiceal drain when the laboratory values and hypovolemia are corrected. The anesthesiologist, in consultation with the endocrinologist, continues the* ***fluids and insulin therapy in the operating room.*** *Eight weeks later, the serum glucose is normal, the ketonuria has resolved, and the HbA1c has improved. The patient returns for an uneventful laparoscopic appendectomy.*

DISCUSSION

1. Which patient is at risk for DKA?

Type 1 DM is the most common metabolic disease of childhood, with a yearly incidence of 15 to 21 cases per 100,000 people younger than 18 years. Approximately one-third of children with type I DM present with DKA at the time of initial diagnosis. The severity at presentation is inversely related to age. Ethnic minority status, lack of health insurance, lower body mass index, missed diagnosis at previous health care visits, and preceding infection, increase the risk of DKA at initial diagnosis. The incidence of DKA is 25% in children with a known diagnosis of DM, with absence of insulin therapy as the most common etiology.

2. What is the definition and pathophysiology of DKA?

DKA is characterized by the metabolic triad of hyperglycemia, anion gap metabolic acidosis, and ketonemia. Biochemically, DKA is defined as **hyperglycemia** above 200 mg/dL (11.1 mmol/L), arterial pH below 7.3, or bicarbonate below 15 mEq/L (15 mmol/L) with **ketonemia** or **ketonuria**. The severity of DKA is categorized by the degree of **acidosis** as either mild (venous pH <7.3 or bicarbonate <15 mEq/L), moderate (pH <7.2 or bicarbonate <10 mEq/L), or severe (pH <7.1 or bicarbonate <5 mEq/L).

Insulin is the primary hormone for blood glucose regulation, promoting peripheral glucose uptake and stopping gluconeogenesis. DKA results from absolute or relative insulin deficiency, either from pancreatic β-cell failure or insulin deficiency. The imbalance of counterregulatory hormones (glucagon, catecholamines, cortisol, and growth hormone) promotes glycogenolyis, gluconeogenesis, and lipolysis. Lipolysis produces two primary ketone bodies, acetoacetate and β-hydroxybutyrate, contributing to ketonemia and an anion gap metabolic acidosis by overwhelming the body's buffering capacity. Acetone, a minor by-product of lipolysis metabolized through the lungs, is responsible for the fruity odor in DKA. Gluconeogenesis and glycogenolyis produce hyperglycemia and an osmotic diuresis. Stress situations, such as, infection, trauma, and dehydration may precipitate DKA.

3. What is the clinical presentation of DKA?

Classic symptoms of DKA, are: polyuria, polydipsia, and weight loss. Dehydration and electrolyte abnormalities may produce muscle cramps and abdominal pain that may mimic an acute surgical abdomen. Dehydration may result not only from a hyperglycemia-induced osmotic diuresis, but also ketonemia-induced emesis. Assessing the degree of dehydration is imprecise, but abnormal skin turgor, dry mucous membranes, a prolonged capillary refill >3 seconds, and sunken eyes are the most useful signs for predicting degree of dehydration in young children. Respiratory compensation for metabolic acidosis results in Kussmaul respirations, with shallow-rapid breathing and subsequent respiratory alkalosis. Sodium, potassium, chloride, phosphorus, calcium, and magnesium electrolyte abnormalities occur in DKA, with hypokalemia being the most life-threatening. Phosphate loss occurs secondary to the osmotic diuresis, with subsequent phosphate depletion exacerbated by insulin therapy, which promotes phosphate entry into cells. Although potassium shifts out of cells from insulin-deficiency and metabolic acidosis, total body potassium is depleted from renal (osmotic diuresis) and gastrointestinal losses (emesis). Potassium depletion is also exacerbated by insulin administration promoting potassium entry into cells, with hypokalemia predisposing to cardiac arrhythmias. Potassium replacement therapy is indicated regardless of serum potassium concentration, unless renal failure is present.

The major morbidity and mortality associated with DKA is **cerebral edema (CE),** occurring in approximately 0.5% to 1% of all cases of DKA. Headache, mental status changes, focal neurologic deficits, and age-inappropriate incontinence, are signs of CE. Most episodes occur 4 to 12 hours after treatment, and mortality can be as high as 23%. CE accounts for 70% to 80% of diabetic-related deaths in children under 12 years.

4. What are the risk factors for DKA-induced cerebral edema (DKA CE)? What is the treatment?

Important predictors of DKA CE are younger age, new-onset DM, longer duration of symptoms, degree of acidosis (pH <7.1) at presentation, greater hypocapnia (PaCO2 <20 mmHg) at presentation, greater initial rate of fluid resuscitation (>50 mL/kg in first 4 hours) at presentation, insulin administration within the first hour of fluid resuscitation, high blood urea concentration at presentation, slow increase of sodium concentration with treatment, and bicarbonate therapy. Treatment of DKA CE involves elevation of the head of the bed, decrease in fluid administration, and mannitol (0.5–1 g/kg) or 3% NaCl (2.5–5mL/kg). If the patient is intubated, hyperventilation may help temporarily. A CT scan should be obtained to rule out other potential causes of neurological deterioration, but treatment should not be delayed to obtain imaging.

5. What is the clinical management of DKA in pediatric patients?

After obtaining an **endocrinology consult**, DKA management should use standardized pediatric-specific treatment protocols (an example is shown in Table 40.1) and flow sheets to ensure safe correction of metabolic abnormalities while minimizing the high risk of developing CE. The International Society for Pediatric and Adolescent Diabetes published its Clinical Practice Consensus Guidelines for DKA in 2009. The primary goals are fluid resuscitation, correction of ketoacidosis and hyperglycemia with inhibition of lipolysis and ketogenesis with insulin administration, correction of acid–base and electrolyte imbalances, and avoidance of complications, particularly DKA CE. The mainstay of therapy is fluid replacement and insulin therapy.

Fluid resuscitation should begin with an isotonic solution, typically 10 to 20 mL/kg over 1 to 2 hours. Repeat boluses may be administered for children who are hemodynamically unstable. Resuscitation volumes should not exceed 40 to 60 ml/kg during the first 4 hours of treatment to avoid increasing the risk of DKA CE, unless the child is hemodynamically unstable. The remaining rehydration should be administered evenly over 48 hours. If the patient is hemodynamically unstable, the resuscitation volume can be infused as quickly as necessary; urinary losses should not be added to the calculation of replacement fluid. Normal saline (NS) is the most commonly used replacement fluid, but recent evidence suggests that a hyperchloremic metabolic acidosis from excessive NS administration may mask treatment effect in DKA with base deficit as an endpoint. LR and Plasma-Lyte have shown similar resolution of acid-base and electrolyte abnormalities, hyperglycemia, duration and total dose of insulin, and intensive care unit length of stay. Institutional preference guides choice of isotonic crystalloid.

A two-bag system is recommended for fluid therapy, with one bag containing identical electrolyte contents as the second bag but different dextrose concentrations (0% to 10%) that are administered simultaneously. The first bag rate is determined by the degree of dehydration, and the second bag rate and concentration of the dextrose-containing solution depends on the serum glucose and the rate of decline with insulin treatment.

Low-dose insulin therapy is now the standard of care, which should be started 1 to 2 hours after intravascular volume expansion has begun and an initial potassium level has been obtained, since insulin shifts potassium intracellularly. Insulin therapy restores normal cellular metabolism and suppresses lipolysis and ketogenesis. Insulin should be continued until resolution of the ketoacidosis (pH >7.3, bicarbonate >18 mmol/L, β-hydroxybutyrate <1 mmol/L, and closure of the anion gap) with a serum glucose target of 200 mg/dL. A dextrose-containing fluid is started when the serum glucose reaches 250 to 300 mg/dL, or when the rate of decline is more than 100 mg/dL. IV insulin boluses may increase the risk of CE and should ***not*** be used. Intravenous sodium bicarbonate has not been shown to be beneficial with DKA, except for treatment of life-threatening hyperkalemia.

6. What are the anesthetic implications of DKA?

The decision to proceed with surgery in a child with DKA is a multidisciplinary decision, between the surgeon, endocrinologist, and anesthesiologist. Surgery should be ideally delayed until after appropriate fluid resuscitation and correction of glycemic, acid-base, and electrolyte abnormalities. If surgery is emergent, fluid resuscitation and insulin therapy should be continued intraoperatively similar to a prescribed DKA management protocol. Additional isotonic crystalloid may be necessary for hemodynamic instability and insensible losses from the surgical procedure. Invasive monitoring, including arterial line and central venous pressure, may be necessary to assess volume and hemodynamic status, from not only hypovolemia but also myocardial dysfunction from electrolyte and acid-base abnormalities. Invasive monitoring additionally allows rapid assessment of glycemic, acid-base, and electrolyte abnormalities. Vasopressors may be necessary for systemic vascular resistance

TABLE 40.1 DKA MANAGEMENT

Initial Assessment

- Assess airway, breathing, circulation, and mental status
- Vital signs hourly
- Neurologic assessment hourly (to assess for DKA CE)
- Obtain current height and weight for body surface area (BSA m^2) calculation: $\sqrt{\text{weight(kg)} * \text{height(cm)}/3600}$
- Record last known meal, blood glucose, and home urine ketone measurement, if available.
- Establish IV access and obtain **initial diagnostic workup:**
  - Arterial or venous blood gas
  - Serum glucose
  - Serum electrolytes with calcium, phosphorus, and magnesium
- Calculate corrected serum Na: Corrected Na = serum Na+([(serum glucose−100)/100] × 1.6)
  - Blood urea nitrogen, creatinine
  - Complete blood count
  - HgA1c (to evaluate duration of hyperglycemia)
  - β-hydroxybutyrate
  - Urinalysis to assess for urine ketones
  - Electrocardiogram (specifically to assess for arrhythmias from hyper/hypokalaemia

Fluid and Electrolyte Therapy

- Begin fluid replacement therapy before insulin therapy.
- LR 10–20 ml/kg over 1–2 hours. If hemodynamically unstable, consider additional boluses of LR until hemodynamically stable prior to initiation of maintenance fluid therapy.
- Start maintenance therapy following initial rehydration therapy with LR at 2.5L/ m^2/24 hour for 48 hours.
- **<u>Phosphate</u>: Phosphate bolus not recommended.**
- **<u>Bicarbonate</u>: Bicarbonate therapy not recommended (may cause paradoxical central nervous system acidosis as well as hypokalemia).**

• **<u>Potassium</u>**: If serum K^+<5.5 mEq/L, begin with 40mEq/L with half as KCl, half as KPhosphate.

Note: If initial serum K^+<4.0 mEq/L, begin with 60 mEq/L with half as KCl, half as KPhosphate. With severe hypokalemia (<3.5 mEq/L), higher concentration of K^+ may be necessary.

- **Two-Bag System**
  - o **If K^+<5.5mEq/L**
- Bag A: LR + KCl 20mEq/L + KPhosphate 20mEq/L
- Bag B: D10LR + KCl 20mEq/L + KPhosphate 20mEq/L
  - o **If K^+>5.5mEq/L**
- Bag A: LR
- Bag B: D10LR + KCl 20mEq/L + KPhosphate 20mEq/L
  - o Total IVF mL/hr= Bag A mL/hr +Bag B mL/hr

Blood Glucose	A (%)	B %)
>300	100	0
251–300	75	25
201–250	50	50
151–200	25	75
<150	0	100
If <100	De	

Insulin Therapy

• If ketone positive and bicarbonate < 15 mEq/L: Begin continuous IV infusion of 0.1 units/kg/hr of regular insulin. **Insulin bolus not recommended.**

• If isolated hyperglycemia or ketone positive with bicarbonate >15 mEq/L: May forego insulin infusion and start subcutaneous rapid-acting insulin according to home regimen, with the following supplemental doses added to each home baseline dose.

TABLE 40.1 CONTINUED

Monitoring

- Bedside glucoses: Q1 hr while on insulin drip
- Chemistry panel: Q2 hrs until bicarbonate >15 mEq/L, then Q6 hrs until bicarbonate >20 mEq/L. Consider additional renal panels as needed.
- Ca, Mag, Phos: Q4 hrs while on insulin drip.
- β-hydroxybutyrate: Q6 hrs
- Urine ketones: Dip all urine for ketones until negative × 3
- Strict inputs and outputs

Introduction of Oral Fluid Therapy and Transition to Subcutaneous Insulin Injection

- Stop insulin infusion therapy when: patient is hungry and able to take adequate oral intake by mouth **and**
  - anion gap resolved, or
  - Bicarbonate >18 mEq/L
  - Absence of ketonuria should **not** be used as an endpoint for determining resolution of DKA (may persist several hours after β-hydroxybutyrate levels have returned to normal).
  - Total fluid therapy is sum of IV and oral fluids: fluid restriction should be applied for 48 hours from admission.
- For patients who have not yet received Lantus or Levemir: Give the basal insulin dose 1 hour before discontinuing insulin drip.
- Initial subcutaneous rapid-acting insulin dose: Give first rapid-acting insulin dose 15–30 minutes before discontinuing insulin drip.

Consider PICU management if:	Patient has altered mental status, pH < 7.0, age less than 5, altered mental status, >40 mL/kg of volume resuscitation (given risk of cerebral edema), treatment with bicarbonate, associated with sepsis/systemic inflammatory response
Consider giving IV $NaHCO_3$ if:	Significant metabolic acidosis (pH < 7.0) and hemodynamically unstable following initial infusion of LR. Administer 1–2 mEq/kg slowly over 2–4 hours to prevent paradoxical central nervous system acidosis.
Worry about cerebral edema if:	Headache, mental status changes, neurologic deficits Elevate the head of the bed. Empirically treat with Mannitol 0.5–1mg/kg/dose over 20–30 minutes or 3% NS 2.5–5 ml/kg/dose; intubate for severe neurologic deterioration or impending respiratory failure.

Note. DKA = diabetic ketoacidosis; DKA CE = DKA-induced cerebral edema; IV = intravenous; Na = sodium; LR = lactated Ringer's; PICU = pediatric intensive care unit; NS = normal saline.

support in the setting of limited fluid resuscitation prior to the emergent surgery. A baseline head CT is also recommended in children at high risk of CE, as those signs may be masked under general anesthesia. Nonemergent surgery should be delayed until appropriate fluid resuscitation with correction of hemodynamic instability and improvement of glycemic, acid-base, and electrolyte abnormalities. Acidosis may directly depress myocardial function, and hypocalcemia, hypomagnesemia, and hypokalemia may predispose to arrhythmias. Furthermore, hypophosphatemia and hypomagnesemia may exacerbate neuromuscular weakness.

Perioperative insulin therapy should be dictated by the institutional DKA protocol and in close consultation with the endocrinology service. Patients with DKA whose glycemic, acid-base, and electrolyte abnormalities have corrected are transitioned to subcutaneous (SC) insulin therapy; those patients may be managed by SC insulin therapy perioperatively.

SUMMARY

1. Risk factors for DKA, include: new-onset type 1 DM, younger age, ethnic minority status, lack of health insurance, lower body mass index, missed diagnosis at previous health care visits, preceding infection, and noncompliance of insulin therapy.
2. DKA is characterized by hypovolemia, hyperglycemia, acidosis, and ketonemia or ketonuria.
3. Cerebral edema is a severe complication of DKA.
4. The mainstay of DKA management is fluid resuscitation and insulin therapy, with

correction of hypovolemia, glucose, acid-base, and electrolyte abnormalities.
5. The decision to proceed with surgery in a child with DKA should occur following a multidisciplinary discussion between the surgeon, endocrinologist, and anesthesiologist.

ACKNOWLEDGMENTS

The authors wish to thank the first edition editors, Ximena Soler and Lori A. Aronson.

ANNOTATED REFERENCES

Glaser N. Cerebral injury and cerebral edema in children with diabetic ketoacidosis: could cerebral ischemia and reperfusion injury be involved? *Pediatr Diabetes.* 2009;10:534–541.

This article reviews cerebral injury and cerebral edema caused by DKA.

Wolfsdorf J, Craig ME, Daneman D, et al. International Society for Pediatric and Adolescent Diabetes (ISPAD). Clinical practice consensus guidelines 2009 compendium: diabetic ketoacidosis. *Pediatr Diabetes.* 2009;10(Supp 12):118–133.

This article provides clinical guidelines in the management of DKA.

FURTHER READING

Grimberg A, Cerri RW, Satin-Smith M, Cohen P. The "two bag system" for variable intravenous dextrose and fluid administration: benefits in diabetic ketoacidosis management. *J Pediatr.* 1999;134(3):376–378.

Olivieri L, Chasm R. Diabetic ketoacidosis in the pediatric emergency department. *Emerg Med Clin North America.* 2013;31(3):755–773.

Orlowski JP, Cramer CL, Fiallos MR. Diabetic ketoacidosis in the pediatric ICU. *Pediatr Clin North America.* 2008;55(3):577–587.

Rhodes ET, Ferrari LR, Wolfsdorf JI. Perioperative management of pediatric surgical patients with diabetes mellitus. *Anesth Analg.* 2005;101:986–999.

Wolfsdorf J, Glaser N, Sperling MA, American Diabetes Association. Diabetic ketoacidosis in infants, children, and adolescents: a consensus statement from the American Diabetes Association. *Diabetes Care.* 2006;29(5):1150–1159.

41

Hypopituitarism

MATTHEW D. SJOBLOM, DIANE GORDON, AND LORI A. ARONSON

INTRODUCTION

Hypopituitarism refers to the decreased secretion of pituitary hormones, which can result from diseases of the pituitary gland or hypothalamus. Surgery in the presence of untreated panhypopituitarism is rare. It is important to recognize the presence of hypopituitarism, and most importantly, adrenal insufficiency, a condition that can result in mortality from adrenal crisis without stress-dose corticosteroid treatment.

LEARNING OBJECTIVES

1. Understand the pathophysiology of hypopituitarism.
2. Recognize the clinical features of hypopituitarism.
3. Discuss the optimal perioperative management of patients with hypopituitarism.

CASE PRESENTATION

A 9-year-old boy presents for bilateral removal of tibial orthopedic hardware. The hardware was placed 18 months earlier at the time of a severe bicycling collision. His injuries at the time included multiple fractures and head trauma (initial Glasgow Coma Scale 11), with a moderate traumatic brain injury (TBI). In the interim, the patient's recovery has gone smoothly although his pediatrician has recently noted that his growth has begun to lag behind his growth curve prior to the accident.

After a smooth induction and intubation, the patient becomes hypotensive. A fluid bolus is given with minimal improvement in his blood pressure. A dose of hydrocortisone is administered due to concern for ***hypocortisolism****. During the operation, he is noted to have an increased output of dilute urine. Intraoperative labs show significant hypernatremia (Na 154 mEq/L) and increased serum osmolality (326 mEq/L). In consultation with the endocrine service, the decision is made to administer* ***desmopressin****. Vasopressin infusion is considered for further management. Based on estimation of water deficit and the level of hypernatremia, a fluid management plan is discussed to correct the hypernatremia slowly and to manage the polyuria. Postoperatively, the patient is admitted to the intensive care unit for further management of his* ***diabetes insipidus****.*

DISCUSSION

1. What are the hormones of the pituitary gland?

The pituitary gland, situated in the sella turcica at the base of the brain, is divided into anterior and posterior components. The anterior pituitary secretes six hormones, which act on target organs and modulate hypothalamic and anterior pituitary activity: corticotropin, thyrotropin, prolactin, follicle-stimulating hormone, luteinizing hormone, and growth hormone. The posterior pituitary stores vasopressin, or antidiuretic hormone (ADH), and oxytocin.

2. What is the clinical relevance of hypopituitarism?

Hypopituitarism may be either partial or complete, and results from either pituitary or hypothalamic disease. Cortisol and thyroxine are regulated by corticotropin and thyrotropin, respectively. Cortisol secretion varies with the circadian rhythm; it is highest in the morning and traditionally rises with stress, fever, hypoglycemia, and surgery. Surgery is one of the most potent activators of the *hypothalamic–pituitary–adrenal (HPA) axis.* Adrenocorticotropic hormone (ACTH) concentrations increase with incision and during surgery, with greatest secretion during emergence from anesthesia, extubation, and in the immediate postoperative period. *Adrenal insufficiency* may result from destruction of the pituitary or adrenal glands, or from long-term administration of exogenous glucocorticoid. Under anesthesia, this may manifest as refractory hypotension. In children, supraphysiological doses of oral corticosteroids (>8–12 mg/m^2/day—hydrocortisone equivalent) for greater than 2 weeks likely suppresses the HPA axis. Children taking inhaled corticosteroids for 3 to 6 months with ≥500 mcg/day of fluticasone or ≥1000 mcg/day of budesonide/beclomethasone are also at risk (Ahmet et al., 2011). For adults, prednisone or its equivalent in doses of greater than 20 mg/day for longer than 3 weeks suppresses the HPA axis for up to 1 year after cessation of steroids. The HPA axis is not suppressed with doses of less than 5 mg/day of prednisone or its equivalent. Despite the risk of HPA suppression, the role for supraphysiologic corticosteroid dosing has come into question in more recent literature (Kelly & Domanjnko, 2013).

Pituitary or hypothalamic insufficiency can cause secondary hypothyroidism. Patients who are euthyroid on replacement therapy are not at increased risk of perioperative morbidity. However, patients with myxedema coma, those with severe clinical symptoms of chronic hypothyroidism, or those with markedly decreased T3 and T4 levels are at increased risk of having complications during the perioperative period. Clinical manifestations include cardiovascular depression refractory to catecholamine administration, hypothermia, airway difficulties due to generalized edema, and aspiration due to delayed gastric emptying. Elective surgery in symptomatic hypothyroid patients should be postponed until the euthyroid state is achieved.

Diabetes insipidus (DI) reflects the absence of ADH due to destruction of posterior pituitary (neurogenic DI) or failure of renal tubules to respond to ADH (nephrogenic DI). DI is differentiated based on the response to desmopressin, concentrating urine in the presence of neurogenic but not nephrogenic DI. DI that develops during or immediately after pituitary gland surgery is generally transient and due to trauma to the posterior pituitary.

3. What are the risk factors for hypopituitarism?

The prevalence of hypopituitarism is 46 cases per 100,000 individuals, with an incidence of 4 cases per 100,000 per year (Schneider et al., 2007). Most cases are due to pituitary tumors or their treatment. The mechanisms by which pituitary tumors cause hypopituitarism include, mechanical compression of normal pituitary tissue, impaired blood flow to the normal tissue, and interference with the delivery of hypothalamic-regulating hormones through the hypothalamic-hypophyseal portal system. Reducing the size of the mass may relieve the pressure and restore pituitary function. Patients with brain, head, or neck tumors treated with radiation may have damage to the hypothalamus or pituitary gland resulting in partial or complete hypopituitarism. Since loss of pituitary function can be delayed several years after radiation, hormonal evaluation should be performed every 6 months.

Risk factors for postoperative pituitary deficiency, are: the size of the tumor, the degree of destruction of adjacent normal tissue, and the ability of the neurosurgeon to remove the tumor without disturbing the normal pituitary tissue. If a total hypophysectomy is performed, panhypopituitarism, including DI, results.

Table 41.1 lists causes of hypopituitarism in children. *Empty sella syndrome* refers to an enlarged pituitary fossa resulting from arachnoid herniation through an incomplete sellar diaphragm. Forty-eight percent of children with either an isolated growth hormone deficiency or a combination of pituitary hormone deficiencies may have empty sella syndrome. Other causes of hypopituitarism include a tumor or cyst in the hypothalamus or infundibulum, infiltrative and vascular disorders, infection, hemochromatosis, granulomatous disease, and trauma (Geffner, 2002; Vance, 1994).

TABLE 41.1. CAUSES OF HYPOPITUITARISM IN CHILDREN

Pituitary adenoma and treatment
Empty sella syndrome
Head trauma
Radiation therapy
Infiltrative diseases (e.g., eosinophilic granuloma)
Sheehan's syndrome (pituitary necrosis after postpartum hemorrhage)
Genetic: congenital and syndrome-associated hypopituitarism

Pituitary dysfunction occurs in 23% to 69% of adults following head trauma, and the limited studies looking at children suggest a similar incidence (Rose & Auble, 2012). Endocrine abnormalities after TBI can improve, resolve, or worsen; therefore, serial screening is recommended with surveillance 6 to 12 months after injury and then annually (Reifschneider et al., 2015). Delayed presentation of growth hormone deficiency followed by gonadotropin-releasing hormone deficiency are most common in children, and should raise a high index of suspicion for other endocrinopathies, given ACTH deficiency, hypothyroidism, and DI are the most challenging to manage perioperatively.

4. What are the clinical signs of hypopituitarism?

The clinical manifestations of hypopituitarism vary depending on the extent and severity of the pituitary hormone deficiency. Damage to the anterior pituitary can occur suddenly or slowly; can be mild or severe; and can affect the secretion of one, several, or all of its hormones. Some diseases, such as pituitary apoplexy (abrupt destruction of the pituitary gland by infarction or bleeding into the gland, usually in the context of an undiagnosed tumor), develop rapidly; causing sudden impairment of ACTH secretion and consequently sudden onset of symptoms of cortisol deficiency. Other insults, such as radiation therapy to the pituitary or hypothalamus, usually act slowly, causing symptoms many months or years later. The presentation of patients with deficiencies of those hormones that control target glands is often similar to the presentation of patients with primary deficiencies of the target gland hormones they control. Patients in whom the hypopituitarism is due to a pituitary or sellar mass may also have symptoms related to the mass: headache, visual loss, or diplopia.

The symptoms of corticotropin deficiency, include: fatigue, weakness, headache, anorexia, weight loss, nausea, vomiting, abdominal pain, and altered mental status. In its most severe form, cortisol deficiency leads to death due to vascular collapse. Physical examination is notable for lack of the hyperpigmentation that occurs in patients with primary adrenal insufficiency. Orthostatic hypotension is common. Women with longstanding adrenal insufficiency often have loss of axillary and pubic hair. Hyponatremia may occur as a result of increased ADH secretion, but the serum potassium concentration is usually normal, since adrenal production of aldosterone is not dependent on corticotropin. In contrast, both hyponatremia and hyperkalemia are common in patients with primary adrenal insufficiency. Normochromic, normocytic anemia, and eosinophilia may also occur with corticotropin deficiency. Orthopedic manifestations have been seen, and slipped capital femoral epiphysis is associated with endocrinopathies, including panhypopituitarism, in a little over 5% of cases (Bowden & Klingele, 2009).

The clinical presentation of thyroid-stimulating hormone deficiency is exclusively that of thyroxine deficiency, and includes fatigue, weakness, cold intolerance, constipation, facial puffiness, bradycardia, and dry skin. Impaired memory or altered mental activity is characteristic of severe hypothyroidism. Physical examination may reveal bradycardia, periorbital puffiness, and delayed relaxation of tendon reflexes.

Growth hormone deficiency in children typically presents as short stature. Deficient secretion of the gonadotropins, follicle-stimulating hormone and luteinizing hormone, causes infertility and sexual dysfunction in both men and premenopausal women. Pubic and axillary hair is present, unless there is concomitant adrenal failure. Children may have hypogonadism or delayed puberty. Prolactin deficiency manifests as inability to lactate after delivery.

Classic manifestations of DI, are: polydipsia and a high output of poorly concentrated urine despite increased serum osmolarity, volume contraction, and dehydration. A simple calculation of serum osmolality may be helpful (normal 285–295 mOsm/kg or mmol/L).

Serum osmolality (mmol/L) = $2\,[Na^+] + 2\,[K^+]$ + Glucose + Urea (all in mmol/L) or

Serum osmolality = $2[Na^+]$ + [Glucose]/18 + [BUN]/2.8 (where [Glucose] and [BUN] are measured in mg/dL).

Without treatment, intravascular volume depletion occurs, cardiac stroke volume decreases, and heart rate increases in an effort to maintain cardiac output. These patients may have weak peripheral pulses, orthostatic hypotension, cold, clammy skin, shallow and rapid breathing, and a reduced level of consciousness. Hypernatremia may manifest as seizures and hyperreflexia.

5. What studies can be performed to confirm hypopituitarism?

Pituitary insufficiency can be confirmed by using endocrine laboratory and imaging studies. Although basal serum hormone measurements may be all that is needed to confirm hypopituitarism, dynamic tests are used for equivocal results or partial deficiencies. Both the target hormone concentration and the pituitary hormone concentration should be measured to assess the appropriateness of both values. After clinical and biochemical diagnosis of hypopituitarism has been made, an imaging study of the hypothalamic–pituitary region should be performed to determine whether a mass is present. The most informative image is a magnetic resonance imaging scan. A high-resolution computed tomography scan with contrast administration is an adequate alternative.

6. What is the best way to manage patients with hypopituitarism postoperatively?

Management of anesthesia for patients with hypocortisolism may include, administration of exogenous corticosteroid supplementation and a high index of suspicion for primary adrenal failure if unexplained intraoperative hypotension occurs. Selection of anesthetic drugs and muscle relaxants is not influenced by the presence of treated hypocortisolism, with the possible exception of etomidate. Etomidate has been shown to transiently inhibit synthesis of cortisol in normal patients. If surgery becomes necessary, perioperative management must include administration of supplemental corticosteroids and intravenous infusion of sodium-containing fluids. Minimal doses of anesthetic drugs should be administered as these patients may be exquisitely sensitive to drug-induced myocardial depression. Invasive monitoring of systemic blood pressure and cardiac filling pressures may be indicated. Plasma concentrations of glucose and electrolytes should be measured frequently during the perioperative period. In view of skeletal muscle weakness, the initial dose of muscle relaxant may need to be decreased, and the response monitored using a peripheral nerve stimulator.

Elective surgery should be deferred in patients with symptomatic hypothyroidism, although controlled clinical studies have not confirmed an increased risk when patients with mild to moderate hypothyroidism undergo elective surgery. Complications from hypothyroidism and anesthesia may include increased sensitivity to depressant drugs, a hypodynamic cardiovascular system with bradycardia and decreased cardiac output, slow metabolism of drugs, impaired ventilatory responses to arterial hypoxemia or hypercarbia, hypovolemia, hyponatremia, hypoglycemia, and delayed gastric emptying time (Bennett-Guerrero et al., 1997).

Fluid management must be closely followed in patients with DI. Exogenous replacement of ADH is with either **desmopressin** or aqueous vasopressin. Desmopressin lacks the vasoconstrictor effects of vasopressin and thus is less likely to cause hypertension or abdominal cramping. Those on baseline therapy may require some degree of fluid restriction, while those manifesting DI acutely intraoperatively will need adequate resuscitation and possible treatment. In the conscious patient with intact thirst mechanism, desmopressin may be administered intranasally on a daily basis and fluid intake monitored closely. Management through fluid restriction and volume contraction alone is also possible (Laxton & Petrozza, 2007).

Management of the unconscious surgical patient is more difficult. For the patient with pre-existing DI, desmopressin may be either withheld several days before surgery or continued until the evening before surgery. Expert consensus only specifies hypotonic fluids intraoperatively for insensible losses and/or urine output replacement, with varying strategies using 0.45 normal saline (NS) to D5 water to D5 + 0.45 NS with 20 mEq/L KCl (Dabrowski, 2016). DI is seen most frequently in neurosurgical patients; and osmotic diuresis with mannitol is avoided and urine output monitored closely. If urine output rises abruptly and simultaneously obtained urine and serum osmolalities suggest DI, intravenous vasopressin administration should begin. Postoperative DI most commonly begins the evening following surgery and may resolve in 3 to 5 days if osmoregulatory structures have not been permanently injured. Perioperative glucocorticoid administration may facilitate development of polyuria.

SUMMARY

1. The pituitary gland is instrumental in regulating many hormonal systems. Patients with adrenal insufficiency, hypothyroidism, and diabetes insipidus are at greatest risk in the perioperative period.

2. The primary risk factor for hypopituitarism is a tumor and its subsequent treatment. In children, one may also see empty sella syndrome or TBI as a cause.
3. Pituitary endocrinopathy should be identified and treatment initiated prior to elective and nonemergent surgery.
4. It is important to recognize those at risk for adrenal suppression and treat with stress-dose corticosteroids prior to or during surgery, especially if refractory hypotension is present. Close attention should also be paid to intraoperative manifestations of DI.

ACKNOWLEDGMENT

The authors wish to acknowledge the first edition author, Liana G. Hosu.

ANNOTATED REFERENCES

Ahmet A, Kim H, Sper S. Adrenal suppression: a practical guide to the screening and management of this under-recognized complication of inhaled corticosteroid therapy. *Allergy Asthma Clin Immunol.* 2011;7:13.

This article presents information to serve as a guide for physicians in the management of adrenal suppression.

Geffner ME. Hypopituitarism in childhood. *Cancer Control.* 2002;9(3):212–222.

This article is a thorough overview of the etiology, clinical features, diagnosis, and treatment of hypopituitarism.

Reifschneider K, Auble BA, Rose SR. Update of endocrine dysfunction following pediatric traumatic brain injury. *J Clin Med.* 2015;4(8):1536–1560.

This article discusses the pathophysiology and reviews the latest literature regarding endocrine aberrations after TBI.

BIBLIOGRAPHY

Bennett-Guerrero E, Kramer DC, Schwinn DA. Effect of chronic and acute thyroid hormone reduction on perioperative outcome. *Anesth Analg.* 1997;85:30–36.

Bowden SA, Klingele KE. Chronic bilateral slipped capital femoral epiphysis as an unusual presentation of congenital panhypopituitarism due to pituitary hypoplasia in a 17-year-old female. *Int J Pediatr Endocrin.* 2009;609131.

Dabrowski E, Kadakia R, Zimmerman D. Diabetes insipidus in infants and children. *Best Pract Res Clin Endocrinol Metab.* 2016;30(2):317–328.

Kelly KN, Domanjnko B. Perioperative stress-dose steroids. *Clin Colon Rectal Surg.* 2013;26:163–167.

Laxton MA, Petrozza PH. Pituitary tumors: diabetes insipidus. In: Atlee J, ed. *Complications in Anesthesia*, 2nd ed. Philadelphia: Saunders; 2007:712–713.

Rose SR, Auble BA. Endocrine changes after pediatric traumatic brain injury. *Pituitary.* 2012;15:267–275.

Schneider HJ, Aimaretti G, Kreitschmann-Andermahr I, Stalla GK, Ghigo E. Hypopituitarism. *Lancet.* 2007;369(9571):1461–1470.

Vance ML. Hypopituitarism. *N Engl J Med.* 1994; 330:1651–1662.

42

Mitochondrial Disease and Anesthesia

MARY A. FELBERG

INTRODUCTION

Mitochondrial disease is a genetically, biochemically, and clinically heterogeneous group of disorders that arise from defects in cellular oxidative phosphorylation, most commonly within the electron transport chain involved in energy metabolism. Patients with mitochondrial disease have an increased risk for cardiac, respiratory, neurologic, and metabolic complications from anesthesia. Awareness of the anesthetic considerations for patients with mitochondrial disease is necessary for the development of an anesthesia plan to minimize adverse events.

LEARNING OBJECTIVES

1. Recognize the complexities of mitochondrial defects resulting in variable expression of the disease.
2. Identify common clinical presentations of a patient with mitochondrial disease.
3. Discuss anesthetic management for patients with mitochondrial disease.

CASE PRESENTATION

*A 7-year-old girl with intractable seizures is scheduled for vagal nerve stimulator implantation. She presents for a preanesthesia consultation. The patient's medical history is significant for **complex I mitochondrial disease**, intractable seizures despite maximal antiepileptic medications and a **ketogenic diet**, gastroesophageal reflux disease (**GERD**), aspiration pneumonia, and developmental delays. Her symptoms include muscle weakness, 4 to 5 generalized **seizures**/month, and a chronic "wet" cough. Her developmental age is 3 to 4 years old. She had a normal echocardiogram and normal sleep study 9 months ago. Her parents have surfed the Internet and state that she should not be given **propofol,** and they are concerned that their daughter might be at risk for **malignant hyperthermia (MH)**.*

DISCUSSION

1. What is a mitochondrial disease? How does it present?

Mitochondrial disease is a heterogeneous group of disorders that arise from defects in cellular oxidative phosphorylation (OXPHOS), most commonly in the electron transport chain (ETC) involved in energy metabolism. The prevalence of mitochondrial disease at birth is 1:5,000. Over 1,400 proteins are involved in mitochondrial energy metabolism, making identification and classification of the disorders challenging.

Mitochondrial disorders may be classified into two broad categories: primary or secondary. Primary disorders involve defects in the actual OXPHOS machinery caused by either inherited or spontaneous mutations or deletions of nuclear DNA or mitochondrial DNA. Secondary disorders may be caused by a broad spectrum of entities ranging from drugs or disease processes to environmental factors, all of which result in abnormal mitochondrial function. Systems most often involved are those with high energy demands: neurologic, cardiac, and musculoskeletal.

A confounding feature of mitochondrial disease is that identical genetic mutations may not produce identical clinical symptoms *and* different genetic mutations can lead to the same clinical expression. This is due in part to inconsistent distribution of dysfunctional mitochondria within cells (heteroplasmy) and throughout tissues. Due to a large overlap, there is no clear correlation between clinical findings and

TABLE 42.1. COMMON CLINICAL PRESENTATIONS OF MITOCHONDRIAL DISEASE

System	Presentation
Respiratory	Frequent pulmonary infections due to pulmonary aspiration, respiratory muscle weakness, central alveolar hypoventilation syndrome, obstructive sleep apnea, stridor, choking episodes
Cardiac	Exercise intolerance, conduction defects (heart blocks which may require a pacemaker), preexcitation syndromes (Wolff-Parkinson-White), cardiomyopathy (dilated or hypertrophic)
Neurology	Encephalopathy, seizure disorder, developmental delay, ataxia, stroke-like episodes, myoclonus, dysphagia, ophthalmoplegia, hearing loss, neuropathy
Renal	Renal tubular dysfunction, interstitial nephritis, glomerular pathology
Fluid/Electrolytes/Nutrition	Intolerance to fasting, failure to thrive, altered glucose levels, elevated lactate level, altered renal function
Gastrointestinal	Swallowing difficulties, gastroesophageal reflux disease (GERD), GI dysmotility, altered hepatic function, cholestasis
Hematology	Anemia, neutropenia
Musculoskeletal	Hypotonia, weakness, myopathy, muscle wasting

the site of biochemical defect. Table 42.1 summarizes common presentations of mitochondrial disorders.

2. What preoperative testing is necessary?

A thorough history, physical exam, baseline vital signs, and consultation with the patient's primary physician and specialists should guide additional testing for the planned surgery. Considerations include: obtaining a complete blood count, basic metabolic panel, liver function test, urine analysis, blood gases, chest x-ray, sleep study, electrocardiogram, and echocardiography.

3. What is the risk of MH in a patient with mitochondrial disease?

There are currently only two neuromuscular disorders for which a clear link to MH has been established: central core disease and King-Denborough syndrome. Although susceptibility to **MH** was previously thought to have an association with mitochondrial myopathies, the risk of MH does not seem to be increased in these patients. The Mitochondrial Medicine Society 2015 Consensus Statement supports this conclusion as well as work done by Footitt et al. (2007).

The dilemma for the anesthesiologist comes when anesthetizing a patient with neuromuscular deficits of unknown etiology. Evidence-based guidelines, including those for patients with mitochondrial disorders, are lacking. Flick et al. (2007) found no MH occurred in a diverse population of children undergoing muscle biopsy for suspected neuromuscular disorder with a range of anesthetics but went on to estimate the "risk of MH (or rhabdomyolysis) in the setting of no observed events" to be 1% or less. Each clinician must decide whether this risk justifies the use of a nontriggering anesthetic.

4. What is the best anesthetic plan for a patient with mitochondrial disease?

Given the heterogeneity of the disease, patients with mitochondrial disease will have diverse responses to anesthetics depending on their unique expression of the disease, and thus the plan must be individualized. Lacking guidance in the literature as to the "best" anesthetic technique; a reasonable anesthesia plan reflects the overall goals to *maintain normoglycemia* and *normovolemia* and to *avoid metabolic stresses* that may provoke metabolic decompensation, commonly lactic acidosis. In addition, the anesthesiologist is also concerned with the potential for respiratory failure, cardiac decompensation, conduction defects, and dysphagia. Despite in vitro evidence that almost every anesthetic agent studied has been shown to decrease mitochondrial function, all anesthesia agents have been used safely. Patients with mitochondrial disease often are predisposed to hypoglycemia and lactic acidosis, which may be exacerbated by perioperative stressors (i.e., fasting, surgical procedure, postoperative pain, or postoperative nausea and vomiting (PONV). Fasting shifts metabolism toward fat utilization as an energy source. As beta-oxidation of fatty acids occurs in the mitochondria, patients with mitochondrial disease may be limited in their ability to metabolize fat, thus leading to the depletion of carbohydrate stores. Anaerobic metabolism of glucose can cause serum lactate levels to rise acutely in these patients. Strategies to avoid hypoglycemia or lactic acidosis include allowing liberal clear sugar-containing liquids until 2 hours prior to surgery, scheduling the procedure as first case, providing adequate dextrose-containing *lactate-free intravenous (IV) fluids* at maintenance rates when the patient is nil per os, and continuing the fluids throughout the perioperative period. Of note, patients on a **ketogenic diet** for seizure management or who have demonstrated an adverse reaction to a higher glucose intake *should not* receive dextrose-containing fluids.

Monitoring of blood glucose should be considered regardless of choice of fluids. Administering insulin to treat hyperglycemia is recommended over decreasing the glucose infusion (if dextrose is used). In addition to controlling hyperglycemia, insulin serves as a potent anabolic hormone, promoting protein and lipid synthesis, removing plasma free fatty acids, and decreasing fatty acid beta-oxidation.

Although providing dextrose-containing fluids throughout the perioperative period is recommended, non-dextrose, non-lactate containing balanced salt solutions should be used for large volume replacement. Minimize perioperative stressors, this includes smooth separation from parents. Sedative premedication should be given judiciously to avoid respiratory depression. Impaired respiratory responses to hypoxemia and hypercarbia have been reported in these patients, along with prolonged somnolence following barbiturates.

Impaired upper airway and lower esophageal sphincter tone may predispose mitochondrial disease patients to reflux and aspiration. In patients with overt signs of **GERD** and/or bulbar muscle dysfunction, the use of pharmacologic prophylaxis with histamine-2 receptor antagonists, proton pump inhibitors, and nonparticulate antacids may be indicated. Rapid sequence intubation, avoiding succinylcholine if possible, should be considered. Succinylcholine-induced rhabdomyolysis in this population remains a concern. Induction and maintenance of anesthesia should be titrated carefully. Sensitivity to IV anesthetic agents has been described, although thiopental, propofol (discussed more fully later), etomidate, ketamine, and dexmedetomidine have all been used safely. Volatile inhalational anesthetic agents appear to be safe in the majority of mitochondrial disease patients, but those with **complex I dysfunction** appear more sensitive. In vitro studies (Hanley et al., 2002) demonstrated reduction in complex 1 activity by 20% (2 MAC halothane or isoflurane) and by 10% (sevoflurane). Though these inhibitory effects are unlikely to compromise cardiac performance, careful titration of volatile agents is advisable.

Thermoregulation may be impaired, as patients with mitochondrial disease may not adapt well to hypothermia or hyperthermia. Attention to heat conservation perioperatively is important.

5. Should muscle relaxants be avoided?

Response to nondepolarizing muscle relaxants in children with mitochondrial disorders is variable depending on organ involvement. Because the main complications of mitochondrial myopathies range from respiratory failure to cardiac depression to conduction defects, muscle relaxants and cardiac depressants must be used cautiously (Niezgoda & Morgan, 2013). Renal or hepatic involvement may decrease clearance. Sensitivity may be increased due to myopathy or decreased due to concurrent antiepileptic medications. Nondepolarizing muscle relaxants have been safely used; judicious dosing and close monitoring with a nerve stimulator are recommended. The use of succinylcholine does not have the same safety profile. While patients with mitochondrial disease may not be susceptible to MH, risks for rhabdomyolysis with hyperkalemia still exist. Succinylcholine has the potential to cause unexpected cardiac arrest from hyperkalemia due to rhabdomyolysis in children with myopathies. Avoidance of succinylcholine in these patients is recommended, given the availability of alternative relaxants.

6. Is propofol safe for these patients?

Propofol has high plasma clearance and rapid metabolism, making it an ideal agent for total IV anesthesia. Although propofol has been safely used in patients with mitochondrial diseases, propofol use in patients with mitochondrial disorders has been questioned.

Propofol has been shown in vitro to interfere with mitochondrial processes at several points: inhibition of OXPHOS complexes I and IV, uncoupling the ETC, and inhibition of long-chain fatty acid transport into the mitochondria. Given the lipid-based formulation for propofol, there is concern over adding to the fatty acid load in a patient with possible impaired fatty acid oxidation. Mtaweh et al. (2013) reported a case of an acutely ill child with mitochondrial encephalomyopathy, lactic acidosis, and stroke-like episodes (MELAS) who received propofol for emergent magnetic resonance imaging without concomitant dextrose-containing IV fluids. MELAS is characterized by encephalopathy presenting as dementia or seizures, stroke-like episodes before 40 years of age, and evidence of mitochondrial dysfunction, such as lactic acidosis and/or ragged red fibers. These patients have a high glycolytic rate, increased lactate production, reduced glucose oxidation, and markedly reduced adenosine triphosphate production. The case report described an ensuing severe, nonfatal metabolic crisis in the postoperative period. Administration of propofol without a concurrent dextrose-containing solution in the setting of a pre-existing catabolic state due to illness was postulated to trigger the crisis.

Even in children without mitochondrial disease, there have been cases in which propofol infusions have resulted in metabolic crisis, known as the propofol-related infusion syndrome (PRIS). Clinical features of PRIS, include: acute refractory bradycardia leading to asystole, metabolic acidosis, rhabdomyolysis, hyperlipidemia, and enlarged or fatty liver. Risk factors for PRIS, include: young age, acute illness, dose of propofol >4 mg/kg/hr and duration of infusion >48 hours, and administration of catecholamine or steroids. Avoidance of propofol is recommended in more symptomatic mitochondrial disease patients; its use in these patients has been associated with an increased incidence of metabolic acidosis, prolonged anesthesia recovery, and intensive care unit admission. If propofol infusions are necessary, the anesthetic plan should include monitoring lactate and glucose levels, ensuring adequate dextrose infusion rate to suppress fat metabolism, and minimizing propofol dose by using it in combination with other anesthetics (e.g., ketamine, opioids, dexmedetomidine, regional or local anesthetics).

7. What are the options for postoperative analgesia?

Pain management in patients with mitochondrial disorders is critical because the stress response to pain may worsen their risk of metabolic decompensation. Whenever possible a multimodal analgesic approach should be used including, if indicated, local or regional anesthesia. Although opioids have been used without adverse event, cautious titration is still advised. Decreased ventilatory response to both hypoxia and hypercarbia (unrelated to muscle weakness) has been described. Renal function should be reviewed if using nonsteroidal anti-inflammatory medications. Regional techniques enable reduction of other anesthetic agents, thus reducing risk of mitochondrial depression with subsequent sequelae. Assessment of coagulation function should precede any neuraxial technique, due to the possibility of hepatic dysfunction in patients with mitochondrial disease. Long-acting local anesthetics (bupivacaine, levobupivacaine, ropivacaine) have been shown in vitro to inhibit complex I and uncouple OXPHOS, causing mitochondrial membrane depolarization and Ca^{2+} dysregulation (Nouette-Gaulain et al., 2007); the clinical significance is unknown. Maslow et al. (1993) observed that in patients with mitochondrial disease demyelination of the spinal cord or peripheral nerves may occur. While it is possible that patients without clinically evident neuropathy are not at increased risk of sequelae from regional anesthesia or interactions with local anesthetics, it may be prudent to avoid regional anesthetic techniques if the patient demonstrates evidence of peripheral nerve or spinal cord abnormalities.

8. Is prophylactic antiemetic therapy indicated?

In addition to being an unpleasant experience, PONV may contribute to metabolic decompensation for patients with mitochondrial disorders. Unless contraindicated, consider prophylactic antiemetic therapy for these patients. Ondansetron has been linked to postoperative headaches when administered to patients with a history of migraines (Sharma & Panda, 2010).

9. What complications are likely?

Postoperative complications are related to the clinical condition of the patient prior to surgery, and the complexity of the surgical procedure. Adverse events reported, include: respiratory difficulties, cardiac arrhythmias, metabolic decompensation, new neurologic problems, such as, stroke, worsening of the overall neurologic status, seizures, prolonged coma, and death. Continuation of medications preoperatively, and promptly resuming therapy postoperatively, combined with close postoperative monitoring for respiratory compromise, cardiovascular instability, or metabolic dysfunction, is important to help prevent complications.

SUMMARY

1. Patients with mitochondrial disorders display wide variation in their clinical presentation and disease severity. Multiple organ systems are often affected.
2. Mitochondrial disorders have not been linked to an increased incidence of MH.
3. Despite in vitro evidence that almost every anesthetic agent studied has been shown to decrease mitochondrial function, all anesthesia agents have been used safely.
4. Anesthetic goals are to maintain normoglycemia and normovolemia and to avoid metabolic stresses.
5. Adequate dextrose-containing, lactate-free IV fluids should be administered in the perioperative period *unless* the patient is on a ketogenic diet or has a history of an adverse reaction to a higher glucose intake.
6. Succinylcholine is probably best avoided. Use nondepolarizing muscle relaxants cautiously with nerve stimulator monitoring.
7. Although propofol has been used safely, consider avoiding propofol in the more symptomatic patient with mitochondrial disease.
8. Meticulous preoperative assessment, a thoughtful anesthetic plan, and close monitoring of the patient allows for the safe administration of general anesthesia to patients with mitochondrial diseases.

ACKNOWLEDGMENTS

The author would like to acknowledge J. Fay Jou, Lori A. Aronson, and Jacqueline W. Morillo-Delerme for their contributions to the first edition.

ANNOTATED REFERENCES

Driessen J, Willems S, Dercksen S, Giele J, van der Staak F, Smeitink J. Anesthesia-related morbidity and mortality after surgery for muscle biopsy in children with mitochondrial defects. *Pediatr Anesth.* 2007;17:16–21.

This is a retrospective case review study of 155 children who underwent diagnostic muscle biopsy for suspected mitochondrial and muscle disorders. With standard preoperative assessment, monitoring, and anesthesia management, there were no serious adverse events attributed to anesthesia in the 122 children who were later diagnosed with mitochondrial disease.

Niezgoda J, Morgan P. Anesthetic considerations in patients with mitochondrial defects. *Pediatric Anesthesia.* 2013;23(9):785–793.

A detailed review of mitochondrial disease for the anesthesiologist concentrating on normal mitochondrial physiology, genetics, pathophysiology, and anesthetic management of this heterogeneous disorder.

Parikh S, Goldstein A, Koenig MK, et al. Diagnosis and management of mitochondrial disease: a consensus statement from the Mitochondrial Medicine Society. *Genet Med.* 2015;17(9):689–701.

Consensus-based recommendations for the diagnosis and treatment of mitochondrial disease with a section on anesthesia (p. 696) by the Mitochondrial Medicine Society. The group consisted of 19 mitochondrial medicine experts including anesthesiologist Phil Morgan, MD, who coauthored a review article for *Pediatric Anesthesia* in 2013.

BIBLIOGRAPHY

Flick RP, Gleich SJ, Herr MMH, Wedel, DJ. The risk of malignant hyperthermia in children undergoing muscle biopsy for suspected neuromuscular disorder. *Pediatr Anesth.* 2007;17:22–27.

Footitt EJ, Sinha MD, Raiman JA, Dhawan A, Moganasundram S, Champion MP. Mitochondrial disorders and general anaesthesia: a case series and review. *Br J Anaesth.* 2008;100:436–441.

Hanley PJ, Ray J, Brandt U, Daut J. Halothane, isoflurane, and sevoflurane inhibit NADH: ubiquinone oxidoreductase (complex I) of cardiac mitochondria. *J Physiol.* 2002;544(3):687–693.

Maslow A, Lisbon A. Anesthetic considerations in patients with mitochondrial dysfunction. *Anesth Analg.* 1993;76:884–886.

Mtaweh H, Bayır H, Kochanek PM, Bell MJ. Effect of a single dose of propofol and lack of dextrose administration in a child with mitochondrial disease: a case report. *J Child Neurol.* 2013;29(8):NP40–NP46.

Nouette-Gaulain K, Sirvent P, Canal-Raffin M, et al. Effects of intermittent femoral nerve injections of bupivacaine, levobupivacaine, and ropivacaine on mitochondrial energy metabolism and intracellular calcium homeostasis in rat psoas muscle. *Anesthesiology.* 2007;106:1026–1034.

Sharma R, Panda A. Ondansetron induced headache in a parturient mimicking postdural puncture headache. *Can J Anesth.* 2010;57:187–188.

43

Obesity

KIM-PHUONG NGUYEN AND CHRIS D. GLOVER

INTRODUCTION

The rising prevalence of childhood obesity in the United States has become a major public health concern with rates increasing from 7% to 18% in children ages 6 to 11 years, and 5% to 21% in adolescents from 1980 to 2012. Similarly, the rates of obesity are increasing in European countries with almost 20% of children and adolescents considered overweight, and 7% of them considered obese. Previously believed to be a high-income country problem, this epidemic is now on the rise in low- and middle-income countries. According to the World Health Organization, 43 million children under age 5 were considered overweight or obese in 2014 with nearly half living in Asia. Worldwide, the percentage of obese and overweight children increased from 4.7% in 1990 to 6.7% in 2010 (Kendrick et al., 2015). The cardiopulmonary and metabolic comorbidities associated with obesity can result in a higher number of anesthesia-related complications; therefore, anesthesiologists must have a comprehensive knowledge of the pathophysiology of obesity in order to prevent morbidity and mortality.

LEARNING OBJECTIVES

1. Understand the anesthetic implications of obesity and its effects on various body systems.
2. Discuss the principles of perioperative management of obese children.
3. Gain a working knowledge of pharmacokinetics of common anesthetic drugs in obese children and dosage implications.

CASE PRESENTATION

A 13-year-old boy who weighs 120 kg and is 160 cm tall (body mass index [BMI] 47) with late-onset Blount disease, or tibia vara, presents for proximal tibial osteotomy with internal fixation. He has a history of ***sleep and behavioral disturbances****, and a sleep study showed a Respiratory Disturbance Index of 36. Though he has been fitted with* ***nasal continuous positive airway pressure (CPAP)*** *of 8 cmH_2O, he has not tolerated it well and is noncompliant. His parent reports that he is* ***not very active*** *due to significant* ***knee pain*** *and has recently gained another 5 pounds in the last 2 months. His pediatrician has diagnosed him with* ***non-insulin-dependent diabetes mellitus*** *for which he takes metformin 500 mg/day. An echocardiogram showed left ventricular dilation but adequate cardiac function. He has properly fasted for surgery. His physical examination is significant for blood pressure of 130/82, obesity with excess adipose tissue deposits behind his neck and under his chin, and a pear-shaped appearance. He is noted to have* ***acanthosis nigricans*** *in the folds of his neck and axilla. He appears anxious and reports being "nervous" about surgery. On* ***airway*** *examination, he has adequate mouth opening, restricted neck extension, and a Mallampati class 2 airway. A peripheral intravenous (IV) line is placed in the holding area using a portable vein finder device. He is given* ***midazolam*** *2 mg preoperatively, which makes him very sleepy. On arrival to the operating room (OR), his room air oxygen saturation is 94%. Standard monitors are placed, and he is positioned in a sniffing position with sheets stacked under his head and shoulders. After preoxygenation for 3 minutes,* ***rapid sequence induction*** *is done with propofol and succinylcholine (suxamethonium).*

*The patient **desaturates** to 78% before the airway is intubated and secured. Despite clear bilateral breath sounds, **high airway pressures** are needed to ventilate the patient with a tidal volume of 8 mL/kg. After a few breaths with airway pressures of 35 cmH_2O and positive end-expiratory pressure (PEEP) of 5 cmH_2O, his saturation normalizes. An orogastric tube is placed and **300 mL of gastric fluid** is suctioned. Anesthesia is maintained with oxygen/air, desflurane, cisatracurium, fentanyl, and then morphine towards the end of the operation.*

*At the end of surgery, he is given **ketorolac** for pain relief and prophylactic ondansetron to prevent nausea/vomiting. The surgeon injects bupivacaine 0.25% locally into the wound. Neuromuscular relaxation is reversed and the patient is **extubated awake** in the OR. The patient complains of knee pain and is given 0.5 mcg/kg of fentanyl. As the patient is being transported to the recovery room, his airway becomes obstructed, requiring a vigorous jaw thrust and positive pressure by mask. In the recovery room, a lubricated nasal airway is inserted, but he continues to snore and remain sleepy with an oxygen saturation oxygen of 92%. CPAP is initiated and his saturations improve to 96%. Due to his need for pain medication and his sleep apnea, he is admitted for overnight observation and monitoring and is discharged uneventfully the next day.*

DISCUSSION

1. How is obesity defined in children?

Obesity refers to an individual who has excess adiposity. Adolphe Quetelet originally proposed the mathematical formula to measure excess adiposity called the Quetelet index, which is now known as body mass index, or BMI. The formula does not differentiate between age, gender, or types of tissues being weighed and can be skewed in the upper or lower ranges of height. In comparison to other indexes used to estimate excess fat, BMI is preferable due to its ease of calculation and applicability to all populations at all times. Adult obesity is defined as a BMI (weight in kilograms/height in meters^2) greater than 30 kg/m^2. Due to dynamic changes in height and weight in growing children with resultant changes in BMI with age, a different criteria has been used to describe obesity in children. In 2000, the Centers for Disease Control and Prevention published sex-specific BMI for age growth charts. Children whose BMI for age percentile measurements are between the 85th and 95th percentile are "overweight," and those above the 95th percentile are "obese" (Ogden & Flegal, 2010). Other terms used for calculation of drug doses are: ideal body weight (IBW) = BMI at the 50th percentile for the child's age × (height in m)^2 and lean body mass (LBM); which comprises all nonfatty tissues and accounts for 99% of the body's metabolic activity. Obesity is associated with a 20% to 40% increase in LBM compared to normal-weight children, due to an increase in muscles, bones, and other lean body tissues.

2. What are the effects of obesity on various organ systems? What are the anesthetic implications?

Airway: Studies (Nafiu et al., 2007; Tait et al., 2008) demonstrated that obese children compared to normal-weight children had a greater incidence of difficult mask ventilation, postoperative airway obstruction, bronchospasm, major oxygen desaturation, and overall critical respiratory events. In adults, morbid obesity and neck thickness are risk factors for difficult intubation. However, few studies predict difficult laryngoscopy in children. Nafiu et al. reported an increased difficulty in laryngoscopy (1.3% vs. 0.4%), while Tait et al. did not. Others report equivalent rates of difficulty in intubation (10%) in obese and nonobese children. Factors that can contribute to a difficult airway in obese children include diminished mandibular and atlanto-occipital joint mobility, narrowed upper airway and small mouth, short distance from mandible to sternal fat, and redundant oral tissue. Positioning the patient with the head and shoulders elevated, so that the ears and the sternum are at the same level, can improve the laryngoscopic view dramatically in obese patients (Collins et al., 2004). It is important to have help and emergency airway backup available.

Childhood obesity is highly associated with *obstructive sleep apnea* (OSA), with reported incidence between 13% and 59%. Unlike adults, OSA in children is associated more with hyperactivity and learning difficulties than daytime somnolence. Disordered sleep breathing (as in the case scenario) occurs up to 6 times more frequently in obese children, than their normal-weight counterparts. Polysomnography can be used to quantify sleep apnea and to assess the need for **CPAP** or bilevel positive airway pressure (BiPAP) during sleep, to improve OSA symptoms.

Respiratory: Obese children have reduced lung volumes and forced expiratory volume/forced vital capacity ratios; in addition to lower functional residual capacity (FRC), they have reduced diffusion capacity and higher oxygen consumption. Rapid oxygen **desaturation** occurs on induction and during periods of apnea, as a result of high closing volume causing atelectasis, air trapping, and intrapulmonary right to left shunting. Obese children have reduced chest compliance due to the weight of adipose tissue on the neck and chest. They are at an increased risk of bronchial hyperreactivity and asthma, for which the severity is related to increasing BMI (Lang et al., 2009). Practically, preoxygenation in the upright position helps reduce desaturation episodes, and alveolar recruitment strategies, such as, elevated peak inspiratory pressures and optimal PEEP may be required for successful ventilation intraoperatively.

Cardiac: Obesity is associated with *hypertension* due to increased cardiac output and increased hemodynamic load. Echocardiogram findings show increased ventricular dimensions and early subclinical findings of ventricular dysfunction, though cardiac reserves are preserved. In patients with OSA, increased oxygen demand, hypoxia, hypercapnia, increased pulmonary blood flow, and polycythemia are common physiologic changes. The extreme example is the patient with Pickwickian syndrome, who is hypercapnic and has right ventricular strain/failure and somnolence (obesity hypoventilation syndrome). It is important to assess cardiac function with an echocardiogram in inactive children who fit this picture or who are coming in for a major operation.

Gastrointestinal: Traditionally, obesity has been associated with an increased incidence of gastroesophageal reflux, hiatal hernia, attenuated gastric emptying, and lower gastric pH, with a predisposition to aspiration during bag-mask ventilation and intubation. Gastric acid pretreatment with proton pump inhibitors, histamine receptor-2 blockers, and sodium bicitrate has been advised preoperatively. Recent evidence refutes this increased risk for aspiration in obese children. The gastric fluid volume in obese children (1 mL/kg IBW) was found to be no different from nonobese children (Cook-Sather et al., 2009), and they may be allowed clear liquids up to 2 hours before surgery. Other gastrointestinal comorbidities, include: nonalcoholic fatty liver disease, nonalcoholic steatohepatitis, cirrhosis, and cholelithiasis.

Endocrine: Obese children are at increased risk for type 2 diabetes mellitus, which may require treatment, and metabolic syndrome (abdominal obesity, dyslipidemia, hypertension, and hyperglycemia). Thyroid function abnormalities, such as, elevated thyroid stimulating hormone levels are frequently seen in obese children with associated hypothyroidism. Polycystic ovarian syndrome and hyperandrogenism may be present in adolescent girls with obesity resulting in hirsutism, irregular menses, and acne.

Mental health: The social stigma associated with childhood obesity can be profound. Psychosocial complications may include: symptoms of depression, body dissatisfaction, impaired social relationships, and decreased quality of life (Gungor, 2014). Overall, 35% of obese children have a psychiatric diagnosis.

Thromboembolic: Longer hospital stays with immobilization increase the risk of **deep vein thrombosis and pulmonary embolism.** Therefore, compression stockings and other preventive measures are indicated.

3. What are other perioperative considerations in caring for an obese patient?

Preoperative: Preoperative laboratory studies may be indicated based on the planned operation and the patient's medical condition. Arterial blood gas determination may be indicated in patients with obesity hypoventilation syndrome (Pickwickian syndrome), and preoperative glucose measurement is important for diabetic patients. Premedication must be individualized and given judiciously, especially in the face of OSA, when the patient must be monitored closely with pulse oximetry and direct observation. For individuals with suspected cardiac disease, an electrocardiogram and echocardiography should be obtained. Pulmonary function tests should be considered for respiratory comorbidity.

Intraoperative: IV access may be difficult due to obesity. Routine noninvasive monitors are acceptable. However, if an appropriate-size blood pressure cuff fails to read due to the thickness or conical shape of the arm or forearm, an arterial line may be necessary for monitoring blood pressure. Adequate preoxygenation is imperative, as obese children may develop hypoxemia faster due to higher oxygen consumption and decreased FRC. Current literature does not support the routine use of rapid sequence induction for obese patients, as they are not at increased risk of pulmonary aspiration compared to normal-weight children. A ventilation strategy incorporating a PEEP of 10 cm H_2O during ventilation resulted in better oxygenation intraoperatively and postoperatively with lower atelectasis and fewer pulmonary complications when compared to a PEEP of 0 or 5 cm H_2O in bariatric patients (Talab et al., 2009). Careful padding of pressure points is important as these patients are at increased risk for neuropathies. As in adults, regional anesthesia techniques may be more challenging in obese children due to difficult positioning, increased fatty tissue, and increased lordosis. Despite these difficulties, regional anesthesia may significantly decrease the opioid doses needed for postoperative analgesia. Though most data regarding neuraxial blocks and obesity come from obstetrics, it would be prudent to assume that reduced epidural local anesthetic volume is needed for similar levels of anesthesia compared to nonobese patients. Awake extubation combined with elevation of the head of the bed are methods to decrease the risk of airway collapse and postoperative atelectasis.

Postoperative: It is important to watch for airway obstruction, apnea, and respiratory failure. Preoperative CPAP should be resumed postoperatively. Caution is warranted while using positive airway pressure by mask after gastric bypass surgery, due to the risk for gastric insufflation and anastomotic leak. It is important to remember that patients with sleep apnea are very sensitive to respiratory depressants and opioids. Pain control can be achieved by patient-controlled analgesia, or carefully titrated doses of analgesics. Use of regional techniques and nonopioid analgesics, like ketorolac, are important adjuncts that decrease the risk of respiratory depression. Patients with severe sleep apnea should be **admitted for observation and monitoring** after general anesthesia.

4. How is medication dosing altered in an obese child like this one?

With a paucity of information specifically on the pharmacokinetics and pharmacodynamics of many common drugs, including anesthetic agents, in obese children, conclusions are largely drawn from adult literature. Typically, volume of distribution (V_d) determines the loading dose for a drug and clearance determines the maintenance dose. Dosing drugs in obese patients may be difficult to predict. In general, *highly lipophilic* drugs, such as, propofol, fentanyl, dexmedetomidine, cisatracurium, and benzodiazepines, have increased V_d and are dosed to total body weight (TBW). Sodium thiopental (thiopentone) is an exception and is dosed to IBW, as obese patients have increased sensitivity to its effects. Remifentanil has a lower than expected V_d for lipid-soluble drugs and, due to its rapid extrahepatic metabolism, is dosed based on IBW, not TBW.

Weakly lipophilic drugs, such as ketamine, vecuronium, rocuronium, and morphine, are dosed by LBW because their limited volume of distribution is not influenced by fat stores. The V_d of muscle relaxants and other *hydrophilic* drugs is not affected by increased fat stores, and hence they are dosed based on IBW. Although succinylcholine is hydrophilic, it is dosed according to TBW because of an increased pseudocholinesterase activity in this population. IBW can be calculated using the formula IBW = (BMI at the 50th percentile for child's age) × Height $(m)^2$. For the patient in the case presentation (TBW 120 kg), IBW $18 \times 1.6^2 = 46.1$ kg, LBW = IBW + 0.3x(TBW − IBW) = 68.3 kg), the following doses are used:

- Midazolam: 0.05 to 0.1 mg/kg (IBW) = 2 to 4 mg. For patients with OSA, medication administration should be in a monitored area due to concern for airway obstruction and respiratory depression.
- **Propofol:** 1 to 2 mg/kg (TBW) = 2 × 120 ~ 200 mg. Clearance and V_d have been found to correlate with TBW. Rates for infusion have been successfully calculated using an empirical formula: Corrected weight = IBW + [0.4 × excess weight]. Caution needs to be exercised in administering boluses based on TBW, especially for drugs that cause hemodynamic changes; it is best to administer these drugs by *titration to clinical effect.*
- **Fentanyl:** 1 to 2 mcg/kg (TBW) = 100 to 200 mcg, followed by morphine at the end of the case (0.1–0.2 mg/kg) (LBW) = 5 to 10 mg.
- **Succinylcholine:** 1 to 2 mg/kg at TBW = 120 to 240 mg. A dose of 120 to 200 mg is usually adequate.
- **Local anesthetics** should be dosed based on IBW. Doses should be reduced by 25% for epidural and spinal techniques due to engorged epidural veins and reduced volume of the spaces.

TABLE 43.1. GENERAL PHARMACOKINETIC IMPLICATIONS OF OBESITY

Physiological Factors	Volume of Distribution		Clearance		Dosing Recommendations, Based on Weight	
	LD	HD	LD	HD	LD	HD
Body Composition *						
Increased adipose tissue ↑ ↑	↑	↔	↔	↔	Loading dose—total body weight Maintenance dose—lean body weight	Dose based on ideal body weight
Increased lean body mass ↑	↑	↔	↑	↑		
Organ Function and Blood Flow						
Increased renal blood flow, increased GFR, increased tubular secretion	↔	↔	↑	↑	Insufficient data for dose recommendations	
Altered hepatic metabolism (fatty degeneration of the liver)	↔	↔	↓	↓	Insufficient data for dose recommendations	
Protein binding changes	**Effect**				**Recommendations**	
Increased concentrations of free fatty acids, cholesterol, triglycerides, and lipoproteins inhibit protein binding	Increased free drug levels				No dosage changes recommended	
Plasma albumin unchanged, increased α_1-acid glycoprotein	Decreased free drug levels					

Note. LD = lipophilic drugs; HD = hydrophilic drugs; GFR = glomerular filtration rate.
* 75% excess weight is fat mass generally, but there is high variability in fatness for same BMI.
Sources: (1) Casati A, Putzu M. Anesthesia in the obese patient: Pharmacokinetic considerations. *J Clin Anesth* 2005; 17(2): 134–145 and (2) Mulla H, Johnson TN. Dosing dilemmas in obese children. *Arch Dis Childhood Education Practice* 2010; 95(4): 112–117.

With the steady increase in the epidemic of obesity, the pediatric anesthesiologist must remain knowledgeable about the systemic effects of obesity, as well as, the alterations in drug dosing in this patient population in order to minimize and prevent perioperative complications. See Table 43.1.

SUMMARY

1. Careful preoperative airway evaluation is fundamental, and IV induction may be preferred in an obese child with severe OSA, due to prolonged second stage during inhalational induction, and risk for airway obstruction. Rapid sequence intubation may still be advisable for morbidly obese children.
2. Obese children with OSA may be extremely sensitive to narcotics and respiratory depressants.
3. Preoxygenation in the upright position helps reduce desaturation episodes.
4. Alveolar recruitment strategies, such as, elevated peak inspiratory pressures to ventilate, and optimal PEEP to prevent atelectasis, are important for successful ventilation intraoperatively.
5. Opioid-sparing analgesics and regional analgesia are important for quicker postoperative recuperation. Use lower incremental doses of local anesthetic when dosing an epidural block in obese patients.

ACKNOWLEDGMENTS

The authors would like to thank Vidya Chidambaran and Senthilkumar Sadhasivam for their contributions to the first edition.

ANNOTATED REFERENCES

Gungor NK. Overwieght and obesity in children and adolescents. *J Clin Res Pediatr Endocrinol.* 2014 Sep;6(3)129–143.

This article discusses the overall systemic and psychological effects of childhood obesity.

Kendrick JG, Carr RR, Ensom MH. Pediatric obesity: pharmacokinetics and implications for drug dosing. *Clin Therap.* 2015;37:1924–1932.

This is a review article about the epidemiology and the effect pediatric obesity has on pharmacokinetic common drug dosing.

Mulla H, Johnson TN. Dosing dilemmas in obese children. *Arch Dis Child Educ Pract Ed.* 2010;95 (4):112–117.

A guide to optimal dosing in children, with discussion of factors affecting pharmacokinetics.

Nafiu OO, Reynolds PI, Bamgbade OA, Tremper KK, Welch K, Kasa-Vubu JZ. Childhood body mass index and perioperative complications. *Pediatr Anesth.* 2007;17(5):426–430.

In this retrospective review of 6,094 children who underwent general anesthesia, difficult airway, upper airway obstruction in the postanesthesia care unit (PACU), PACU stay longer than 3 hours, and the need for 2 or more antiemetics were more common in overweight and obese than normal-weight children.

Samuels PJ. Anesthesia for adolescent bariatric surgery. *Int Anesthesiol Clin.* 2006;44(1):17–31.

A comprehensive review of anesthetic considerations for morbidly obese children undergoing bariatric surgery.

Talab HF, Zabani IA, Adbelrahman HS, et al. Intraoperative ventilatory strategies for prevention of pulmonary atelectasis in obese patients undergoing laparoscopic bariatric surgery. *Anesth Analg.* 2009;109(5): 1511–1516.

BIBLIOGRAPHY

Almarakbi WA, Fawzi HM, Alhashemi JA. Effects of four intraoperative ventilatory strategies on respiratory compliance and gas exchange during laparoscopic gastric banding in obese patients. *Br J Anaesth.* 2009;102(6):862–868.

Casati A, Putzu M. Anesthesia in the obese patient: pharmacokinetic considerations. *J Clin Anesth.* 2005;17:134–135.

Collins JS, Lemmens HJ, Brodsky JB, Brock-Utne JG, Levitan RM. Laryngoscopy and morbid obesity: a comparison of the "sniff" and "ramped" positions. *Obes Surg.* 2004;14(9):1171–1175.

Chidambaran V, Tewari A, Mahmoud M. Anesthetic and pharmacologic conciderations in obese children. *J Clin Anesth.* 2018 Mar;45:39–50.

Cook-Sather SD, Gallagher PR, Kruge LE, et al. Overweight/obesity and gastric fluid characteristics in pediatric day surgery: implications for fasting guidelines and pulmonary aspiration risk. *Anesth Analg.* 2009;109(3):727–736.

Lang JE, Feng H, Lima JJ. Body mass index-percentile and diagnostic accuracy of childhood asthma. *J Asthma.* 2009;46:291–299.

Mortensen A, Lenz K, Abidstrom H, Laurisen TLB. Anesthetizing the obese child. *Pediatr Anesth.* 2011;21:623–629.

Ogden CL, Flegal KM. Changes in terminology for childhood overweight and obesity. *National Health Statistics Reports.* June 25, 2010. http://cdc.gov/nchs/data/nhsr/nhsr025.pdf

Rowland TW. Effect of obesity on cardiac function in children and adolescents: a review. *J Sports Sci Med.* 2007;6:319–326.

Tait AR, Voepel-Lewis T, Burke C, Kostrzewa A, Lewis I. Incidence and risk factors for perioperative adverse respiratory events in children who are obese. *Anesthesiology.* 2008;108(3):375–380.

44

Perioperative Management of Pheochromocytoma

YANG LIU

INTRODUCTION

Pheochromocytomas (PCC) are rare neuroendocrine tumors arising from catecholamine-producing chromaffin cells in the medulla of the adrenal glands. Extra-adrenal paragangliomas are closely related tumors of extra-adrenal sympathetic or parasympathetic paraganglia. Both tumors can secrete high amounts of catecholamines, may have similar presentations, and may be cured completely by surgical removal. If left untreated, PCC can result in resistant arterial hypertension or a life-threatening hypertensive emergency, which is not well controlled with standard blood pressure (BP) medications. PCC most commonly appears between the ages of 20 and 50, but it can present at any age. In the pediatric population, catecholamine-secreting tumors typically present around ages 11 to 12, and occur in 0.8% to 1.7% of hypertensive children. Thirty to 40% of children diagnosed with PCC/paraganglioma have an associated familial disorder, such as von Hippel-Lindau (VHL) syndrome, multiple endocrine neoplasia type 2 (MEN2), and neurofibromatosis type 1 (NF1).

PCC represent significant management challenges to the anesthesiologist, particularly when undiagnosed. Preoperative evaluation and appropriate preparation to optimize the patient's condition are keys to successful perioperative management.

LEARNING OBJECTIVES

1. Review the preoperative evaluation and management of a patient presenting for resection of PCC.
2. Evaluate the options for the anesthetic management of a patient coming for resection of PCC.
3. Develop a postoperative management plan for the resection of PCC.

CASE PRESENTATION

A 12-year-old, 25-kg male presents for a scheduled laparoscopic cortical sparing adrenalectomy for unilateral PCC. He presents with 6 months of episodes of ***headaches, palpitations, sweating, and high blood pressure*** *of more than 156/100 mmHg. The cardiologists previously performed an initial evaluation and referred to an endocrinologist. Total urine metanephrines were 1500 mcg/24 hours, and a following* ***computed tomography (CT) of the abdomen revealed a right adrenal mass*** *(3.6 cm × 4.6 cm × 3.7 cm).*

The patient has no other medical history and his family history is negative for familial neuroendocrine syndromes.

His BP is currently managed with a regimen of doxazosin 2 mg daily, metoprolol 40 mg daily, and amlodipine 5 mg daily, and is well controlled with systolic blood pressure (SBP) 110–130s and diastolic blood pressure 40–60s. He occasionally has mild orthostatic hypotension.

Physical examination reveals a healthy-appearing but nervous boy. Vital signs are BP 132/68 mmHg, heart rate 86 bpm, and respiratory rate 20 breaths/min with 98% oxygen saturation on room air. His airway, cardiac, pulmonary, and abdominal examinations are normal.

Complete blood count and comprehensive metabolic panel are within normal limits. Electrocardiogram shows a normal sinus rhythm, no preexcitation, and no hypertrophy. A previous transthoracic echocardiogram from 1 week prior revealed normal ventricular function and size.

The patient is premedicated with midazolam 1 mg intravenously. After standard monitors are applied, the child is preoxygenated and anesthesia is induced with propofol 2 mg/kg and fentanyl 2 ug/kg. Endotracheal intubation was facilitated with vecuronium 0.1 mg/kg. A right radial arterial line and second larger bore peripheral intravenous (IV) line are placed. A thoracic epidural is also placed and 0.2% ropivacaine 12 mg is bolused and maintained at a rate of 12 mg/hr during surgery.

The patient is positioned in the left lateral decubitus position. Anesthesia is maintained throughout the case with sevoflurane 1.8% to 2.5% in 50% oxygen/50% air without further major complications. Ventilation is adjusted to maintain end-tidal carbon dioxide between 35 and 40 mmHg. The nicardipine infusion is titrated to maintain SBP <130 mmHg. Esmolol infusion is used intermittently for heart rate >130 bpm. There are significant fluctuations in BP and heart rate during the surgery, especially with tumor manipulation. The tumor is successfully removed without complications. After tumor removal, nicardipine and esmolol infusion are stopped immediately. The BP normalizes. Total IV fluid administered is 55 mL/kg and estimated blood loss approximately 100 ml. After surgery, the patient is extubated immediately in the operating room and admitted to the pediatric intensive care unit for overnight monitoring. Postoperative analgesia is managed with an epidural infusion of 0.1% ropivacaine with 2 mcg/mL of fentanyl at 5 ml/hr and supplemental doses of IV morphine. The remainder of his hospital course is uneventful and he is discharged to home. At his 2-week postoperative follow-up, his BP and heart rate were normal.

DISCUSSION

1. What are the common symptoms of patient with PCC?

A PCC is usually suspected because of signs and symptoms of excessive catecholamines (norepinephrine, epinephrine, and dopamine) produced by a tumor. The most common symptoms of PCC and paraganglioma in children are: hypertension (64%), palpitations (53%), headaches (47%), and mass-related effects (30%), similar to the presentation in adults. Other signs and symptoms that may be associated with PCC and paraganglioma, include: pallor, visual blurring, orthostatic hypotension, weight loss, polyuria/polydipsia, hyperglycemia, and cardiomyopathy. However, in some patients with PCC, the tumor may not produce any signs or symptoms. The lack of symptoms leaves the patient undiagnosed, and may cause a sudden hypertensive crisis which can have an 80% mortality rate (Ramakrishna, 2015). Additionally, the tumor may be discovered serendipitously by abdominal CT.

2. What labs or imaging would be diagnostically useful?

Laboratory tests: Diagnostic options for PCC and paraganglioma have changed considerably in the past two decades. Catecholamines are metabolized within chromaffin cells to metanephrines (epinephrine to metanephrine and norepinephrine to normetanephrine); studies have confirmed that measurements of fractionated metanephrines in urine (24-hour collection) or plasma provide superior diagnostic sensitivity over measurements of parent catecholamines. There is no consensus on whether plasma or urine measurements are superior. In the young pediatric patient in whom a 24-hour collection is not possible, measurement of plasma fractionated metanephrines is a reasonable initial test. This is a relatively newer test that is becoming increasingly available. Measurement of plasma or urine catecholamines and metabolites are highly sensitive and specific in pediatric patients with symptoms. Other tests that have been described in adult patients with PCC, such as, the clonidine suppression test and glucagon stimulation test, have not been validated in studies of children with suspected PCC.

Imaging tests: Localization of a PCC or paraganglioma should be considered if the clinical evidence for the presence of a tumor is reasonably compelling. Either CT or magnetic resonance imaging (MRI) is recommended for initial tumor localization. The higher specificity of functional imaging such as 123-I-metaiodobenzylguanidine (MIBG) imaging may be useful to detect tumors not detected by CT or MRI. Also, MIBG imaging may be useful to further evaluate disease extent and presence of multiple tumors or metastases. Positive emission tomography (PET) scanning with 18F-flourodeoxyglucose or 11C-hydroxyephedrine or 6-[18F] fluorodopamine is a newer radionuclide localization technique which in recent studies demonstrates superiority to MIBG in detection of metastases. OctreoScan is another functional imaging modality that, like PET scanning, should be reserved for patients with negative MIBG imaging or rapidly growing tumors.

Genetic tests: Genetic testing should be considered if a patient has bilateral adrenal PCC, paraganglioma, presentation at a young age, family history of PCC/paraganglioma, or clinical findings suggestive of an associated familial disorder. Mutation testing is routinely available for the genes associated with VHL, MEN2, NF1, and familial paraganglioma.

3. What is the typical medical management of hypertension secondary to PCC?

Once a PCC or paraganglioma is diagnosed, a patient should undergo surgical resection after appropriate medical preparation as it is the primary treatment (Chen et al., 2010). Although proper and adequate preoperative preparation is essential for the anesthetic management of PCC, no universally accepted method of preparation for surgery in children with PCC has been established. Perioperative management of PCC requires a multidisciplinary approach for optimal care and successful outcome.

The major goals of preoperative management, include: the overall goals of normalization of BP and heart rate, control of secondary symptoms, expansion of the contracted blood volume, and decreasing tumor catecholamine synthesis. Administration of α-adrenergic blockers has been the cornerstone of management. The most commonly used drugs, include: phenoxybenzamine, prazosin, and a phentolamine infusion. Phenoxybenzamine, an irreversible noncompetitive α-adrenoceptor blocker, is the most widely used because of its longer duration of action. The starting dose of phenoxybenzamine in children is 0.25 to 1 mg/kg per day; the dose is increased every few days until the patient's symptoms and BP are controlled and mild orthostasis has been induced. Phenoxybenzamine can cause significant orthostatic hypotension, and is often accompanied by a β-blocker to control reflex tachycardia. β-blockers should never be used in isolation and should only be initiated in the presence of established α-adrenergic blockade due to the catastrophic hypertensive crisis. Blockade of vasodilatory peripheral β-adrenergic receptors with unopposed α-adrenergic receptor stimulation can lead to further increases in BP. Magnesium sulfate, angiotensin-converting enzyme inhibitors, and calcium channels blockers have also been used with α-blockers to achieve hemodynamic stability.

Another approach in the preoperative preparation of children undergoing PCC or paraganglioma resection is the administration of metyrosine, a catecholamine synthesis inhibitor. Metyrosine competitively inhibits tyrosine hydroxylase, the rate-limiting step in catecholamine synthesis, decreasing tumor catecholamine stores. In conjunction with α-blockade, the use of metyrosine may facilitate better perioperative hemodynamic control.

Adequate preoperative α-blockade may be gauged by: (a) no in-hospital BP readings of >160/90 mmHg for 24 hours prior to surgery; (b) no orthostatic hypotension with BP <80/45 mmHg; (c) no ST or T wave changes for 1 week prior to surgery; and (d) no more than 5 premature ventricular contractions per minute.

4. What is the anesthetic plan?

Complete surgical resection remains the only curative therapy for PCC. Although open surgical approaches to treat PCC have been used since the 1920s, the laparoscopic approach is a relative safe procedure for PCC resection and has been successfully used since 1992. An adrenal cortex-sparing approach has been advocated in some patients with hereditary forms of primary or recurrent PCC, thereby avoiding or postponing permanent adrenal insufficiency; the risk of this approach is recurrent PCC.

Various anesthetic techniques have been used in the resection of PCC and paraganglioma in pediatric patients. Anesthesiologists should choose an anesthetic plan with which they are most experienced. Close communication with the surgical team throughout the procedure is crucial.

Because anxiety can predispose to catecholamine surges, preoperative sedation is a key component and may obviate the need for antihypertensive medications preoperatively. Adequate dosing of anxiolytics, such as, midazolam prior to entry to the operating room will help prevent hypertensive crises (Ramakrishna, 2015).

Agents commonly used for induction, include: propofol and etomidate. Etomidate has the advantage of conferring cardiovascular stability, especially in hypovolemic patients. Ketamine is usually avoided due to its sympathomimetic effects. All agents that cause histamine release should also be avoided.

If bilaterally adrenalectomy is performed, the patient should receive glucocorticoid stress coverage perioperatively.

5. What are the main anesthetic concerns for intraoperative management of PCC resections?

Hemodynamic changes and wide fluctuations in BP are common during PCC resection. Blood-circulating volume is decreased in patients with a PCC secondary to chronic peripheral vasoconstriction. Therefore, euvolemia and liberal nil per os status should be maintained preoperatively. Volume resuscitation should be judicious in those patients with decreased myocardial function. Euvolemia is often restored in those patients who have been taking α-blockers for 2 weeks or more.

6. What monitors should be used?

In addition to standard monitoring, an intra-arterial catheter for pressure monitoring is essential for immediate identification of hemodynamic fluctuations during the tumor resection. A central venous catheter is commonly used to monitor central venous pressure, administer medication infusions, and provide fluid resuscitation. The use of pulmonary artery catheters and transesophageal echocardiography is uncommon in pediatric patients undergoing PCC resection.

7. Should a thoracic epidural be placed in this patient?

The use of epidural analgesia has been described in pediatric patients with satisfactory results. Epidural analgesia may blunt the sympathetic response from surgical incision and the creation of pneumoperitoneum in laparoscopic procedures. However, it does not protect against catecholamine release during tumor manipulation. The epidural can be placed either awake or after induction depending on the level of anxiety and cooperation of the patient.

8. What vasopressors and antihypertensives should be used to control the fluctuations in BP?

Depending on the stage of the procedure, acute variation in serum catecholamine levels may cause hypertensive or hypotensive crises. Intubation, induction of pneumoperitoneum, and tumor manipulation can cause catecholamine release; which may cause significant heart rate or BP changes without appropriate anesthesia management. Many different anesthetic techniques and various antihypertensive agents have been used to attenuate intraoperative BP variations. Drugs used to control intraoperative hypertension include:

- α-blockers, such as phentolamine and hydralazine. Phentolamine is a reversible nonselective α-blocker that can be given as an IV bolus or as an infusion to control intraoperative hypertension.
- β-blockers, such as esmolol and labetalol. Esmolol, a short-acting β1-blocker has hemodynamic effects that may be uniquely suited for the intraoperative management of PCC, and it has been used with good effect in pediatric patients.
- Calcium channel blockers, such as nicardipine. Using nicardipine as an IV bolus or as an infusion may quickly control BP variations. Advantages of nicardipine, over sodium nitroprusside, include: little reduction in preload, less potential for overshoot hypotension, less increase in heart rate, and absence of cyanide toxicity.
- Venodilators, such as nitroprusside and nitroglycerin. Sodium nitroprusside is a short-acting direct vasodilator that is frequently used to control intraoperative hypertension.
- Magnesium sulfate. Magnesium sulfate inhibits catecholamine release from both the adrenal medulla and peripheral adrenergic nerve terminals, directly blocks catecholamine receptors, and is also a direct vasodilator. It has been shown to be effective in controlling intraoperative hypertension in both adult and pediatric patients during PCC resection.

In contrast, a patient may also experience a significant BP decrease due to hypovolemia, residual effects of preoperative α-adrenergic blockade, abrupt decrease in catecholamine levels, and/or hemorrhage after adrenal vein ligation. Blood pressure may be maintained with direct-acting vasopressors, such as phenylephrine or norepinephrine, along with fluid administration. In patients with catecholamine-resistant hypotension after resection of PCC, aggressive exogenous catecholamine replacement may not effectively restore vascular tone. Vasopressin can be used as an adjunctive agent for vascular rescue and provides an alternative pharmacologic route to reverse catecholamine-resistant vasoplegia.

9. What is the postoperative management of these patients?

Postoperatively, the patient should be transferred to a suitable postoperative care unit. Most patients will likely experience persistent hypotension related to pre-existing hypovolemia, alteration of vascular compliance, fluid losses from bleeding or third spacing, adrenal insufficiency, or residual effects of preoperative adrenergic blockade. Some patients may remain temporarily hypertensive postoperatively due to fluid excess, presence of residual tumor, or inadvertent ligation of a renal artery. In patients who undergo bilateral adrenalectomies, long-term steroid replacement therapy is required and endocrinology should be consulted. Decrease in circulating catecholamine levels following tumor resection will increase insulin secretion. Postoperative glucose monitoring is recommended in patients following PCC resection, due to concerns related to hypoglycemia. Effects of β-adrenergic blockade may also contribute to postoperative hypoglycemia.

Long-term periodic follow-up is highly recommended for all patients with PCC because of the high incidence of recurrence and malignancy.

SUMMARY

1. PCC and extra-adrenal paragangliomas are rare neoplasms that have similar clinical presentations and approaches of treatment. However, it is important to distinguish between them because of implications for associated neoplasms, risk of malignancy, and genetic testing.
2. Anesthesia management for PCC surgery is challenging. The anesthesiologist should have an understanding of the pathophysiological impact of the oversecreted catecholamines and a thorough knowledge of its pharmacology, to avoid or minimize the hemodynamic changes that may occur during surgery.
3. Prior to the operation, it is imperative that an α-adrenoceptor blocker be used to optimize hemodynamics and protect the patient against potential significant release of catecholamines due to anesthesia and surgical manipulation of the tumor.

ANNOTATED REFERENCES

Chen H, Sippel RS, O'Dorisio MS, Vinik AI, Lloyd RV, Pacak K. The North American Neuroendocrine Tumor Society consensus guideline for the diagnosis and management of neuroendocrine tumors: pheochromocytoma, paraganglioma, and medullary thyroid cancer. *Pancreas.* 2010;39(6):775–783.

An excellent overview of the pathophysiology and management of PCC.

Ramakrishna H. Pheochromocytoma resection: current concepts in anesthetic management. *J Anaesthesiol Clin Pharmacol.* 2015;31(3):317–323.

An updated review of current anesthetic management of PCC.

FURTHER READING

Augoustides JG, Abrams M, Berkowitz D, Fraker D. Vasopressin for hemodynamic rescue in catecholamine-resistant vasoplegic shock after resection of massive pheochromocytoma. *Anesthesiology.* 2004;101(4):1022–1024.

Deutsch E, Tobias JD. Vasopressin to treat hypotension after pheochromocytoma resection in an eleven-year-old boy. *J Cardiothorac Vasc Anesth.* 2006;20(3):394–396.

Gagner M, Lacroix A, Bolte E. Laparoscopic adrenalectomy in Cushing's syndrome and pheochromocytoma. *N Engl J Med.* 1992;327(14):1033.

Gagner M, Pomp A, Heniford BT, Pharand D, Lacroix A. Laparoscopic adrenalectomy: lessons learned from 100 consecutive procedures. *Ann Surg.* 1997;226(3):238–246.

Hack HA. The perioperative management of children with phaeochromocytoma. *Pediatr Anesth.* 2000;10(5):463–476.

Kenady DE, McGrath PC, Sloan DA, Schwartz RW. Diagnosis and management of pheochromocytoma. *Curr Opin Oncol.* 1997;9(1):61–67.

Mannelli M. Management and treatment of pheochromocytomas and paragangliomas. *Ann N Y Acad Sci.* 2006;1073:405–416.

Pham TH, Moir C, Thompson GB, et al. Pheochromocytoma and paraganglioma in children: a review of medical and surgical management at a tertiary care center. *Pediatrics.* 2006;118(3):1109–1117.

Pretorius M, Rasmussen GE, Holcomb GW. Hemodynamic and catecholamine responses to a laparoscopic adrenalectomy for pheochromocytoma in a pediatric patient. *Anesth Analg.* 1998;87(6):1268–1270.

Pullerits J, Ein S, Balfe JW. Anaesthesia for phaeochromocytoma. *Can J Anaesth.* 1988;35(5):526–534.

Tobias JD. Preoperative blood pressure management of children with catecholamine-secreting tumors: time for a change. *Pediatr Anesth.* 2005;15(7):537–540.

45

Thyroid Mass Resection

KALYANI GOVINDAN

INTRODUCTION

Thyroid nodules are uncommon in children. However, there is a greater risk of malignancy in nodules diagnosed in children compared with adults (Divarci et al., 2017). Estimates from ultrasound and postmortem examination suggest that 1% to 1.5% of children, and up to 13% of older adolescents or young adults have thyroid nodules. It also remains unclear how many of these nodules would reach a clinical threshold during childhood. Several risk factors are associated with the development of thyroid nodules in children, including: iodine deficiency, prior radiation exposure, a history of antecedent thyroid disease, and several genetic syndromes. One high-risk population is childhood cancer survivors who were treated for their primary malignancy with radiation therapy, especially survivors of Hodgkin's lymphoma, leukemia, and central nervous system tumors.

LEARNING OBJECTIVES

1. Recognize the clinical manifestations of hypo- and hyperthyroidism.
2. Identify the main preoperative considerations in thyroid surgeries.
3. Develop a plan for the optimal perioperative management of patients undergoing thyroid surgeries.

CASE PRESENTATION

A 13-year-old girl is scheduled for near-total thyroidectomy under general anesthesia. She presented to the pediatrician's office 12 months previously with history of diffuse swelling in her neck, palpitations, excessive sweating, and weight loss. Upon examination, she was found to have diffuse goiter with no difficulty in swallowing or breathing, mild exophthalmos, tremors, a heart rate of 126, and blood pressure of 132/78. Lab tests were consistent with a diagnosis of hyperthyroidism, with elevated triiodothyronine (T3), thyroxine (T4) levels, and undetectable thyroid-stimulating hormone (TSH) levels; she was started on antithyroid drugs (ATDs) and beta-blockers. After being on medications for 12 months, she was deemed euthyroid. However, with antithyroid drug withdrawal she relapsed and it has now been decided that she undergo a near-total thyroidectomy. She restarts ATD and presents for her preoperative assessment visit. Two days later, she undergoes an uneventful near-total thyroidectomy. Routine blood work on the first postoperative day shows that she has mild hypocalcemia. She has no other acute changes or abnormal lab work and she is discharged home on oral calcium supplements on postoperative day 2.

DISCUSSION

1. What are the causes of hyperthyroidism in children?

The most common causes are: congenital hyperthyroidism and Graves' disease (toxic goiter). Acute suppurative thyroiditis, thyroid carcinoma, and toxic uninodular goiter may also produce this syndrome. Congenital hyperthyroidism results from transplacental transfer of thyroid antibody from a mother with a history of Graves' disease. These infants have goiter, appear irritable, and may have hypermetabolic signs; like tachycardia, tachypnea, and elevated temperature progressing to high output cardiac failure with hepatomegaly in the severely affected infant. Since maternal immunoglobulins have a short half-life in infants, the hyperthyroid state resolves in a few weeks.

2. What are the signs and symptoms of hyperthyroidism and how is it evaluated?

Graves' disease is the most common cause of hyperthyroidism in children. It occurs during adolescence and is more common in girls. Early signs include motor hyperactivity, emotional disturbances, and irritability. They may also have sweating, loss of weight, increased appetite, palpitations, tremors, exophthalmos, and palpable thyroid gland. The cardiopulmonary symptoms, include: systolic hypertension, tachycardia, dyspnea, and cardiac enlargement progressing to cardiac failure, atrial fibrillation, or mitral regurgitation. Serum levels of T4 and T3 are usually elevated with decreased TSH levels. The TSH levels are suppressed due to the negative feedback by high T4 and T3 levels (Krane et al., 2009). Radionuclide scans are also useful in diagnosis. If x-ray reveals a large goiter, computed tomography or magnetic resonance imaging may be used to evaluate the extent of tracheal compression/deviation.

3. What are the treatment options for hyperthyroidism?

Beta-blockers are used to control the cardiovascular effects; propranolol (1–2 mg/kg/day) is titrated to effect. The antithyroid medications, propylthiouracil and methimazole, inhibit the incorporation of inorganic iodide; propylthiouracil also inhibits the conversion of T4 to T3. Oral potassium iodide suppresses the hormone secretion but is usually avoided in children due to side effects like thyroid cancer, damage to germ cells, and hypothyroidism.

Once a patient has started therapy, a clinical response may be evident in 1 to 3 weeks, but it can take up to 2 months. Efficacy of treatment is determined with normal levels of T3, T4, and TSH. Additionally, the patient returns to a euthyroid state which is manifested by normal heart rate, blood pressure, and reflexes. After a period of time on ATD a relapse may occur, and is a negative aspect of ATD. Such a recurrence of hyperthyroidism makes other treatment modalities, such as, long-term ATD versus radioactive iodine versus surgery a point of consideration and discussion (Laurberg et al., 2014).

4. What is thyroid storm and how is it managed?

Thyroid storm is a state of an acute onset of *hyperthermia, severe tachycardia*, and *restlessness* resulting from uncompensated thyrotoxicosis. If untreated, thyroid storm may deteriorate to delirium, coma, and death. Treatment consists of cooling blankets to treat hyperthermia, balanced salt solutions to maintain intravascular volume, and beta-blockers to ameliorate the cardiovascular response. Thyroid suppression therapy with propylthiouracil should be started. The clinical presentation of thyroid storm intraoperatively may be mistaken for malignant hyperthermia. Perioperative surgical stress can trigger thyroid storm in a patient with previously unrecognized thyrotoxicosis. The patients with signs and symptoms of hyperthyroidism should be rendered euthyroid prior to any elective surgery.

5. What are the causes, signs, symptoms, and treatment modalities for hypothyroidism?

Hypothyroidism may be caused by primary thyroid dysfunction or by decreased production of TSH from pituitary failure. Primary thyroid dysfunction may be congenital or acquired. Congenital hypothyroidism appears in infancy, and features, include: large tongue, decreased tendon reflexes, large fontanelle with wide sutures, and umbilical hernia. Older child may have growth failure, hypothermia with cold intolerance, and bradycardia with narrow pulse pressure. Severe hypothyroidism is associated with cardiovascular collapse, hyponatremia, respiratory failure, and coma. It is very important to correct hypothyroidism gradually, over a period of 2 to 4 weeks, before subjecting patients to surgery. It is suggested that these children receive one-fourth of the maintenance dose of thyroid hormone (6–8 mcg/kg/ day) and gradually increase over a period of 2 to 4 weeks to the required dose, monitoring the thyroid hormone and TSH levels. Patients with incompletely restored hormone levels may have hemodynamic instabilities. Severe hypothyroidism is also associated with adrenal insufficiency and should receive a stress dose of steroids.

6. What are the anesthetic considerations in the management of patients with hypothyroidism?

Considerations in management of symptomatic hypothyroid patients, include: prolonged drug effect from decreased metabolism, and minimizing heat loss since the patient is at risk for hypothermia. Depending on the surgery, or amount of blood loss or fluid shifts, invasive hemodynamic monitoring may be warranted since hypothyroidism can cause decreased cardia output, heart rate, and stroke volume. Additionally, postoperative ventilatory support may be required.

7. What are preoperative and intraoperative concerns in a patient undergoing thyroid surgery?

Patients should be pharmacologically euthyroid preoperatively. Beta-blockers are used to control the cardiovascular effects, and esmolol can be used intraoperatively. All medications should be continued until the morning of surgery. Possible airway compression and tracheal deviation should be evaluated by preoperative neck x-rays.

In children with no airway compromise, inhaled or intravenous (IV) induction can be done keeping in mind that inhaled induction may be prolonged in hyperthyroid patients because of increased cardiac output. In children with large goiters and tracheal compression, spontaneous ventilation should be maintained until the airway is secured. Drugs with fewer cardiovascular side effects are chosen, avoiding ketamine, pancuronium, and other drugs that may cause tachycardia. Ventilation should be controlled to avoid hypercapnia, which can cause sympathetic stimulation in an already hypermetabolic child.

At the conclusion of surgery, the child should be evaluated for vocal cord paralysis, which can be a result of trauma to recurrent laryngeal nerves. This can be done by doing direct or video laryngoscopy after deep extubation or through a fiberoptic bronchoscope placed via a laryngeal mask airway after extubation. Postoperatively, airway obstruction may occur due to residual tracheomalacia or hematoma.

8. What are the postoperative complications of thyroid surgery?

Postextubation croup, airway obstruction secondary to vocal cord paralysis, tracheomalacia, tetany, or a hematoma causing tracheal compression, are potential concerns in the immediate postoperative period after thyroidectomy. Unilateral vocal cord paralysis may result in a mild stridor, whereas a bilateral vocal cord paralysis may lead to complete airway obstruction requiring reintubation. Postextubation croup is treated with humidified oxygen, racemic epinephrine, and rarely continuous positive airway pressure. Tracheal compression from a hematoma is a potential complication in the postoperative period necessitating reintubation and surgical evacuation. Surgical manipulation of the neck tissues can also lead to subcutaneous emphysema, pneumomediastinum, or pneumothorax.

Accidental resection of parathyroid glands during surgery may result in acute hypoparathyroidism, as shown by low levels of serum-ionized calcium and parathyroid hormone. This is clinically manifested as tetany in the first 24 to 72 hours after surgery and is treated with IV calcium. One study looked at over 1,000 pediatric thyroidectomies from a national database and found 20% of the patients had hypocalcemia postoperatively, which may indicate the need for algorithms to prevent and or subsequently treat this finding (Hanba et al., 2017).

SUMMARY

1. There are several causes of childhood hyperthyroidism; Graves' disease is the most common etiology.
2. Antithyroid medications are the first line of treatment for hyperthyroidism.
3. Hypothyroidism may be caused by the primary failure of the thyroid gland or secondarily to the dysfunction of the pituitary gland leading to decreased levels of TSH.
4. Any patient who is hyperthyroid must be in an euthyroid state prior to surgery in order to minimize or prevent significant morbidity and mortality.
5. There are numerous potential complications that can occur after thyroid surgery, and the anesthesiologist must look for and be ready to treat complications, such as, vocal cord paralysis and neck hematoma.

ANNOTATED REFERENCES

Divarci E, Celtik U, Documcu C, et al. Management of childhood thyroid nodules: surgical and endocrinological findings in a large group of cases. *J Clin Res Pediatr Endocrinol*. 2017;9 (3):222–228.

This article discusses the management of the pediatric patient with thyroid nodules.

Hanba C, Svider PF, Siegel B. Pediatric thyroidectomy: hospital course and perioperative complications. *Pediatr Otolaryngol*. 2017;156(2):360–367.

This article reviews the hospital course of the pediatric thyroidectomy patient.

Krane EJ, Rhodes ET, Neely EK, et al. Essentials of endocrinology. In: Cote CJ, Lerman J, Todres ID, eds. *A Practice of Anesthesia for Infants and Children*, 4th ed. Philadelphia: Elsevier/Saunders; 2009:535–555.

This chapter provides a thorough overview of the endocrine and pediatric anesthesia.

Laurberg P, Krejbjerg A, Anderson SL. Relapse following antithyroid drug therapy for Graves' hyperthyroidism. *Curr Opin Endocrinol Diabetes Obesity*. 2014;21(5):415–421.

This article discusses the relapse that can occur with antithyroid drugs.

BIBLIOGRAPHY

Davis P, Cladis FP, eds. *Smith's Anesthesia for Infants and Children*, 9th ed. Philadelphia: Elsevier; 2017.

Diogini G, DelBosco A, Cantone G, et al. Anaesthesia for thyroid surgery: perioperative management. *Int J Surg*. 2008;6(Suppl 1):S82–S85.

Wood JH, Patrick DA, Barham HP, et al. Pediatric thyroidectomy: a collaborative surgical approach. *J Pediatr Surg*. 2011;46(5):823–828.

PART 11

Challenges in the Perinatal Period

46

Exploratory Laparotomy for Necrotizing Enterocolitis

KARLA E. K. WYATT AND OLUTOYIN A. OLUTOYE

INTRODUCTION

The survival rates of very low birth weight (birth weight <1500 g) and extremely low birth weight (birth weight <1000 g) infants have increased with improvements in antenatal and postnatal care. These include the use of antenatal steroids, artificial surfactant, and ventilation strategies that have reduced injury to the neonatal lung. As a result, the pediatric anesthesiologist is now more often faced with the task of safely caring for these infants, often in unfamiliar environments, and sometimes during episodes of life-threatening illness. One such life-threatening condition is necrotizing enterocolitis (NEC), which commonly requires surgical management.

> **LEARNING OBJECTIVES**
>
> 1. Identify comorbidities of the population commonly presenting with NEC.
> 2. Review the medical and anesthetic management strategies for NEC.
> 3. Compare the challenges and issues related to provision of anesthetic care in the neonatal intensive care unit (NICU) versus the operating room (OR).
> 4. Develop a plan for managing neonatal resuscitation.

CASE PRESENTATION

A 17-day-old, former 24-week premature female infant weighing 920 g is scheduled for an urgent laparotomy. She was intubated and ventilated at birth for poor respiratory effort. At day 13 she was extubated to nasal continuous positive airway pressure, but was reintubated for signs of ***sepsis*** *(shock, tachypnea, and increased work of breathing) on day 17. During fluid resuscitation, a radial arterial line, a urinary catheter, and a 4Fr triple-lumen internal jugular central line (central venous catheter) are inserted. X-ray reveals* ***free intraperitoneal gas.*** *She is scheduled for an urgent laparotomy. Due to escalating ventilator requirements, she is placed on a* ***high-frequency oscillating ventilator*** *(HFOV), with ΔP 30 mmHg, mean airway pressure of 14 cmH$_2$O, frequency of 8 Hz, and fraction of inspired oxygen (FiO$_2$) of 0.8. Preoperatively her vital signs are pulse 190/min, blood pressure 42/20 mmHg, oxygen saturation (SpO$_2$) 89%, and esophageal T 36.3° C. Her abdomen is tense and distended. She appears mottled with some generalized edema, and urine output is 1 mL/hour. The chest x-ray shows no focal changes; the endotracheal and nasogastric tubes are in good position. Her medications are dobutamine and dopamine (both 20 mcg/kg/min), morphine (40 mcg/kg/hour), midazolam (1 mcg/kg/min), antibiotics, and maintenance fluids 1 mL/hr (10% dextrose, 0.225% saline, 20 mmol/L KCl). Cranial and renal ultrasounds are normal. An echocardiogram shows a moderate-sized patent foramen ovale, a large* ***patent ductus arteriosus (PDA)*** *with left-to-right shunt and some evidence of* ***pulmonary hypertension.*** *Arterial blood gas results are pH 7.13, pCO$_2$ 64 mmHg, pO$_2$ 51 mmHg, Hb 10.6 g/dL, and lactate 5.3 mmol/L.*

During surgery in the NICU, the anesthetic includes fentanyl (5 mcg initially, then 2.5-mcg boluses dependent on hemodynamics) and vecuronium 2 mg. Surgery reveals free intraperitoneal fluid and a 50-cm segment of necrotic distal small bowel; it is managed with bowel resection, peritoneal lavage, and an ileostomy with distal mucus fistula. Hepatic bleeding is noted; the MAP drops to 18 mmHg. There is no response to a bolus of 15 mL/kg of ***fresh packed red blood cells*** *(PRBCs), 15 mL/kg of fresh frozen plasma (FFP), and 0.4 mL 10%* ***calcium gluconate****. Norepinephrine (noradrenaline) 0.4 mcg/kg/min is started with an increase in MAP to 31 mmHg. During wound closure, continued* ***hepatic bleeding occurs****; she is given 20 mL/kg fresh PRBCs, 10 mL/kg cryoprecipitate, 15 mL/kg platelets, and 3 doses of 0.4 mL 10%* ***calcium gluconate****. The bleeding persists. The abdomen is packed and a bolus of 180 mcg* ***recombinant factor VIIa*** *is given; hemostasis is subsequently achieved allowing for abdominal wall closure. She is discharged from the NICU 4 months later.*

DISCUSSION

1. What is NEC, and which babies are predisposed to developing this?

NEC is a severe *inflammatory disorder* of the intestine most commonly affecting premature infants. The incidence is 5% to 15% for infants weighing less than 1500 grams at birth, and the incidence decreases with increasing gestational age. A diagnosis of NEC is associated with significant morbidity, and a mortality rate of 10% to 30% (Coté et al., 2013). The inflammatory process of NEC is initially managed with fluid resuscitation, antibiotics, and ventilatory and inotropic support (Henry & Ross, 2008), but may rapidly progress to full-thickness necrosis and bowel perforation. It may involve a localized segment of bowel or be more generalized. Despite extensive research, the pathogenesis is not fully understood; however, it is thought to be multifactorial. This multifactorial pathogenesis includes an inciting insult related to enteral feeding, milk exposure, bacterial colonizations, or alterations in intestinal blood flow, which then cascades a sequence of bowel mucosal injury. The most common sites of injury are the terminal ileum, ascending colon and cecum. Typical clinical features, include: poor feeding, abdominal distention, bile-stained vomiting, lethargy, electrolyte disturbances, and occult or gross blood in the stool. In addition, apneic spells, respiratory insufficiency, and poor perfusion may be early nonspecific signs. Sepsis may be suspected before the diagnosis of NEC is made. Radiologic data can show evidence of distended, edematous bowel and gas within the intestinal wall (pneumatosis intestinalis; see Fig. 46.1), and, when perforation is present, free air in the abdomen is visualized. Deterioration can be rapid with circulatory compromise, acidosis, coagulopathy, and multiorgan failure.

2. What are the preoperative cardiorespiratory issues for consideration?

As more preterm neonates are surviving despite younger ages at delivery, a lot of patients with NEC have accompanying bronchopulmonary dysplasia and chronic lung disease. The use of predelivery maternal steroids, administration of surfactant, and use of early noninvasive ventilation in the preterm

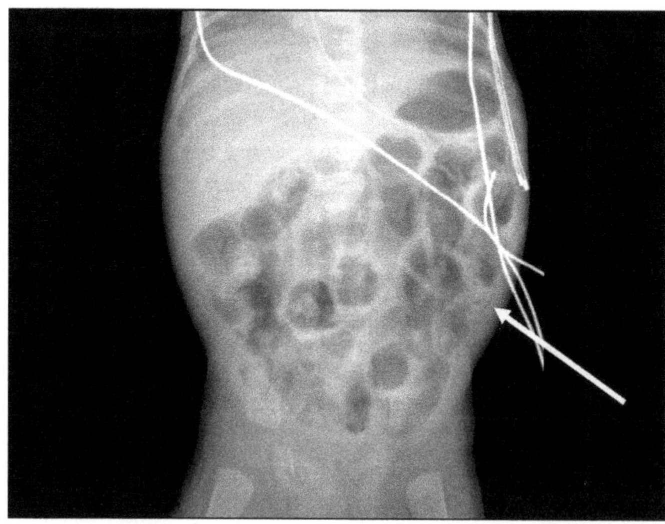

FIGURE 46.1 Abdominal x-ray depicting distended bowel. Arrow points to air within the wall of the bowel.

neonate, have reduced morbidity and mortality from lung disease in this population. However, the presence of a tense, distended abdomen in a baby with NEC, further compromises respiratory function and may necessitate conventional mechanical ventilation or mechanical ventilation requiring significant amount of positive end-expiratory pressure (PEEP). In extreme cases, **HFOV** may be necessary. The use of this specialized mode of ventilation during surgery requires perioperative cooperation between the neonatologist and anesthesiologist.

The cardiovascular system in the ex-premature neonate is also affected, as the myocardium is less compliant and more reliant on heart rate, as well as extracellular **calcium,** to preserve cardiac output when compared to older children. The immature cardiovascular system poorly tolerates deviations from homeostasis, has limited functional reserve, and copes poorly with acute increases in afterload (Lönnqvist, 2004) or significant changes in preload. NEC is also more prevalent in former premature infants with concomitant congenital heart disease, with an estimated incidence of 3% to 7% (Giannone et al., 2008); this subset of infants has an earlier age of onset of NEC, as well as, increased morbidity and mortality. Furthermore, on clinical review, those patients born with left-sided cardiac obstructive lesions demonstrate evidence of intestinal hypoperfusion, predisposing them to NEC. The most common lesion is a **PDA**, with an incidence of up to 80% in infants weighing less than 1200 g. The shunt is usually left to right through the PDA, causing excessive pulmonary circulation at the expense of systemic oxygen delivery. This shunt may be reversed when **pulmonary hypertension** is present (precipitated in part by systemic acidosis and hypoxia in the sick neonate). A laparotomy with significant fluid shifts can worsen this marginal cardiopulmonary function. A preoperative cardiology consultation, including echocardiography, is important as the presence of congenital heart disease can be evaluated with quantification of cardiac function and ventricular filling.

3. What are the other essential features of the preoperative visit?

After investigating comorbidities, cardiorespiratory status, pharmacologic and ventilatory support, it is imperative to review the arterial blood gas analysis, complete blood count, glucose, coagulation studies, and electrolytes (including Ca^{2+}). In addition, any radiographic and/or ultrasonography data should be assessed, including a "babygram" x-ray to confirm the position of lines and the endotracheal tube. Intra-arterial blood pressure monitoring is highly desirable (if not essential) for this surgery, both for continuous pressure measurement and for blood sampling. Evaluation for adequate venous access is also important. Good peripheral access (multiple venous access sites) is mandatory in the absence of a central venous catheter. Central venous access is ideal for anticipated inotrope delivery and fluid balance monitoring; however, if central venous access and invasive monitoring are not in place preoperatively, time taken to establish these needs to be weighed against surgical delay. For surgery undertaken in the OR, in a relatively stable patient, placement of central venous access by the surgical team prior to commencing surgery should be considered or discussed. Finally, parents need to be counseled about the high perioperative risk and high likelihood of transfusion.

4. Is NEC a surgical emergency?

The diagnosis of NEC does not equate with emergency surgery. The decision to perform surgery on a patient with NEC should be based on a collaborative team-based clinical discussion. Certain findings in the setting of a diagnosis of NEC will prompt an emergent exploratory laparotomy, including evidence of free air in the abdomen (or a suspected perforation), clinical decompensation with worsening cardiopulmonary function, severe metabolic acidosis with evidence of global systemic hypoperfusion, and evidence of bowel necrosis (Frost et al., 2016).

5. Should this procedure be performed in the OR or the NICU?

Advantages of the OR, include: familiarity with equipment for all staff, the ability to deliver volatile anesthesia, and better surgical lighting conditions. Disadvantages of surgery in the OR, include: the need to disrupt any complex ventilator strategy the baby may be on for transport (OR ventilators may also differ in compliance from what the neonate has been stable on in NICU), and the development of hypothermia in transit (Frawley et al., 1999). Consequences of changing to manual ventilation for transport, include: loss of PEEP, atelectasis, hypoxemia, and the risks of barotrauma or volutrauma. It is more difficult to manage critical incidents during transport; in addition, movement of the baby carries the risk of inadvertent extubation, venous line removal, or endobronchial tube migration.

While the NICU offers the advantage of not disturbing the neonate in its critically sick milieu, the operating environment provides optimal surgical access and lighting. The size of the baby could also influence location of surgery, as micro-preemies may be operated on in the NICU for some of the aforementioned reasons.

6. How should the NICU environment be prepared for surgery?

Having assistance while providing anesthesia care for these patients is essential. This could be in the form of a trained assistant or a second anesthesiologist. The overhead heater built into the baby's NICU bed may need to be turned off while surgery is ongoing. Therefore, in order to avoid hypothermia, a warming pad may be placed under the baby or a U-shaped blanket can be placed around the baby and heated with a forced-air warmer. The use of waterproof drapes prevents irrigation and preparation fluid from spilling and coming into contact with the rest of the baby. *All fluids administered to the baby during surgery should be warmed.* A fluid warmer, with access ports on either side of the warming device, can be connected to the patient using a short, minimum-volume (0.5 mL) extension tube. This allows for aspiration of fluids through the warming device, with minimal dead space prior to administration to the patient. In addition to standard monitoring, a pre- and postductal oxygen saturation probe, a transcutaneous CO_2 monitor or in-line expiratory CO_2 monitor, and an esophageal temperature probe are useful. Before surgical draping, all intravenous and arterial lines should be reviewed for access points and potential sites of kinking. It is imperative to have *rapid access to the endotracheal tube and an alternate ventilatory source* (e.g., a Neopuff™ T-piece resuscitator [Fisher & Paykel Healthcare, Auckland, New Zealand]). Appropriately small-sized suction catheters (6Fr, 8Fr) should also be readily available. *Emergency drugs, inotropes, and neonatal airway* equipment should be checked. **Bleeding** should be anticipated; blood products need to be available in the room, checked, and ready to administer to the patient. PBRCs should be requested in 20 cc/kg aliquots in order to prevent wastage, decrease exposure of the baby to multiple blood donors, and prevent overtransfusion. This blood should also be irradiated prior to transfusion in order to prevent graft-versus-host disease. In addition, a thawed unit of FFP, as well as calcium, and albumin should be available at the bedside.

7. What are the major intraoperative risks?

Fluid shifts, potential massive **bleeding**, hypothermia, and glucose instability, on the background of significant comorbidities, are the major challenges (Table 46.1). The neonates' estimated blood volume

TABLE 46.1 CHECKLIST TO PREVENT AND MANAGE COMMON INTRAOPERATIVE RISKS

Intraoperative Risk	Action
Airway disconnection, tube kinking	Prevention: Check airway and connections before draping. During the case: Always have easy access to the tube and alternative ventilator source.
Changing ventilatory requirement with opening abdomen, closure, worsening sepsis	Monitor arterial blood gas, CO_2, SpO_2 closely and be prepared to change ventilation.
Worsening cardiovascular function due to sepsis, bleeding, coagulopathy, or hypocalcemia	Have inotropes ready, measure IABP. Have a plan and blood products ready (see text). Predict hypocalcemia after blood products; measure and treat.
Hyperkalemic dysrhythmias	Prevent: Use fresh blood (irradiated, washed)
Hypothermia	Measure temperature, use plastic drapes, light warmers, and a forced-air warmer.
Loss of IV access (kinking, disconnection, blockage)	Prevention: Check that lines are secure and not kinked before draping. Obtain large-bore peripheral and/or central venous access. During the case: Check the IV line and connections if the patient is not responding to fluid bolus or medication administration.
Hypoglycemia	Monitor glucose hourly. Administer dextrose containing maintenance solutions throughout the case.

Note: IV = intravenous; IABP = invasive arterial blood pressure.

should be calculated and adjusted for gestational age. A preoperative *massive blood loss plan* should be discussed. Communication with the surgical team is both visual and verbal, with constant surveillance of the operative field, monitors, and surgical suction. The maximal allowable blood loss should be calculated, as well as, the replacement requirements necessary to maintain an appropriate hematocrit. In order to prevent falling behind blood replacement, it is helpful to start transfusion of blood products as soon as bleeding is identified on the operating field. Warmed PRBCs should be administered, guided by arterial blood pressure, central venous pressure, and hemoglobin levels. Pulse pressure variation, often associated with hypotension, will not be evident with respirations if the neonate is on **HFOV**. Extrapolating from studies of blood transfusion in preterm neonates not acutely bleeding (Bell, 2008), a reasonable hemoglobin target is probably 10 g/dL. This target should be reconciled with any underlying cardiopulmonary conditions for which a higher oxygen-carrying capacity and hence hematocrit is ideal.

Babies with NEC are at risk for coagulopathy due to **sepsis**, hypothermia, and dilution of coagulation factors and platelets. Once blood loss exceeds one blood volume, it is expected that clotting factor deficiency would be demonstrated clinically in the surgical field with oozing from mucosal surfaces (Barcelona et al., 2005). To prevent impending coagulopathy, it is reasonable to begin FFP when transfused blood volume reaches 40 mL/kg (or sooner if there is diffuse microvascular bleeding and/or abnormal international normalized ratio/activated partial prothrombin time). Platelet numbers have been shown to be reduced to 60%, 40%, and 30% of their initial value after one, two, and three blood volumes have been lost, respectively. The lowest acceptable platelet count during neonatal surgery is unknown. In the setting of ongoing bleeding and a worsening coagulation profile, a platelet count of above 100×10^9/L is an acceptable target, but recommendations vary (Chang, 2008). Platelet transfusion is usually not required until when one to two blood volumes have been lost, depending on the initial platelet count. Fibrinogen, in the form of cryoprecipitate, should be replaced when the fibrinogen level is less than 1 g/L, or when hemorrhage is uncontrolled and one blood volume replacement is being approached.

Of particular importance to the neonate during blood transfusion, is the risk of hyperkalemic arrest; the [K^+] is high in stored PRBCs due to prolonged storage and irradiation. Thus, neonates should be given **fresh PRBCs;** the time between irradiation and administration should also be minimized. Methods to prevent hyperkalemic arrhythmias, include: washing and warming of packed cells prior to transfusion. Infusing via a peripheral vein will reduce the concentration of potassium being presented to the atria and thus the risk of nodal dysfunction (Sloan, 2011). Citrate is used as an anticoagulant in stored blood products; it binds calcium and magnesium and therefore results in hypocalcemia. **Hypocalcemia** not only worsens hypokalemia but also has an especially strong negative effect on inotropy in neonates. The highest amount of citrate is found in FFP and platelets.

8. In addition to coagulopathy, what are other etiologies for bleeding?

Fluid overload in the setting of NEC is a significant problem. Preoperative aggressive filling of the heart may be associated with liver congestion; obtaining surgical access into a tense abdomen may release any tamponade effect on the liver. Rapid hepatic expansion can follow, eventually leading to capsular rupture and **spontaneous hepatic bleeding** (Pumberger et al., 2002). If fluid therapy is too aggressive intraoperatively, spontaneous intraoperative liver hemorrhage may occur. It is vital to communicate closely with the surgical team about the potential hepatic congestion and enlargement during the operation. The combination of possible liver congestion and the fragile liver anatomy associated with prematurity poses an increased risk for retraction injury (Frost et al., 2016).

Other causes of bleeding, include: lysis of intestinal strictures and adhesions following bowel perforation, disseminated intravascular coagulopathy and iatrogenic vessel or organ injury secondary to surgical trauma (Frost et al., 2016). Cardiovascular instability in children with NEC needs to be treated with the ongoing liberal transfusion of blood products. Low systemic vascular resistance and increased capillary leak seen in these patients may continue to cause unacceptable hypotension and third spacing despite adequate volume resuscitation. Increasing doses of inotropes in such cases may be protective against hepatic hemorrhage. There are many reports of **recombinant factor VIIa** being used successfully for liver hemorrhage in this situation (Mathew & Young, 2006), and this could be considered for resuscitation of a baby *in extremis from hemorrhage*. The clinical utility and benefit of this modality in neonates and infants is ongoing, alongside the potential deleterious effects.

SUMMARY

1. NEC most commonly affects the small, preterm neonate with coexistent conditions of prematurity.
2. Communication and planning between the neonatologist, surgeon, and anesthesiologist is vital. This will help facilitate decisions, such as, location of surgery, ventilation strategies, and early management of blood loss.
3. Coagulopathy and/or massive transfusion in the neonate with NEC should be anticipated, and appropriate blood products should be ordered from the blood bank prior to the start of the case.
4. Use of intraoperative inotropes, with increasing doses as required, as well as, intraoperative blood transfusion should be considered to support the patient's hemodynamics, especially in the septic patient.

ACKNOWLEDGMENT

The authors wish to thank the first edition author, Dugald McAdam.

ANNOTATED REFERENCES

Caplan MS, Fanaroff A. Necrotizing: A historical perspective. *Semin Perionatol.* 2017;41(1):2–6.

Royal Children's Hospital. Massive transfusion clinical practice guidelines, 2005. http://www.rch.org.au/clinicalguide/cpg.cfm?doc_id=11225

BIBLIOGRAPHY

Barcelona SL, Thompson AA, Cote CJ. Intraoperative pediatric blood transfusion therapy: a review of common issues. Part II: transfusion therapy, special considerations, and reduction of allogenic blood transfusions. *Pediatr Anesth.* 2005;15:814–830.

Bell EF. When to transfuse premature babies. *Arch Dis Child Fetal Neonatal.* 2008;93:F469–F473.

Chang T-T. Transfusion therapy in critically ill children. *Pediatr Neonatol.* 2008;49(2):5–12.

Emergency surgery: necrotizing enterocolitis. In Coté CJ, Lerman J, Todres ID, eds. *A Practice of Anesthesia for Infants and Children,* 5th ed. Philadelphia: Elsevier; 2013.

Frawley G, Bayley G, Chondros P. Laparotomy for necrotizing enterocolitis: intensive care nursery compared with operating theatre. *J Paediatr Child Health.* 1999;35:291–295.

Frost BL, Modi BP, Jaksic T, et al. New medical and surgical insights into neonatal necrotizing enterocolitis: a review. *JAMA.* 2016;171(1):83–88.

Giannone PJ, Luce WA, Nankervis CA, et al. Necrotizing enterocolitis in neonates with congenital heart disease. Minireview. *Life Sci.* 2008,82:341–347.

Henry MC, Ross RL. Neonatal necrotizing enterocolitis *Semin Pediatr Surg.* 2008;17:98–109.

Lönnqvist PA. Major abdominal surgery of the neonate: anaesthetic considerations. *Best Pract Res Clin Anaesth.* 2004;18(2):321–342.

Mathew P, Young G. Recombinant factor VIIa in paediatric bleeding disorders: a 2006 review. *Haemophilia.* 2006;12:457–472.

Moss RL, Dimmitt RA, Barnhart DC. Laparotomy versus peritoneal drainage for necrotizing enterocolitis and perforation. *N Engl J Med.* 2006;354:2225–2234.

Pumberger W, Kohlhauser C, Mayr M, Pomberger G. Severe liver hemorrhage during laparotomy in very low birthweight infants. *Acta Pædiatr.* 2002;91:1260–1262.

Sloan RS. Neonatal transfusion review. *Pediatr Anesth.* 2011;21:25–30.

47

Former Premature Infant for Hernia Repair

GEOFF FRAWLEY

INTRODUCTION

Hernia repair is the most common surgery in ex-premature infants, with the incidence of inguinal hernias being inversely proportional to gestational age at birth (13% incidence in infants born <32 weeks' gestation, and 30% in those born with a birth weight <1000 g; Coté et al., 1995). Postoperative apnea is a significant complication in this age group. Both awake regional and general anesthetic techniques are widely used for infant hernia repair, with recent concerns about the impact of anesthesia in the neonatal period on neurocognitive outcome influencing anesthetic management.

> **LEARNING OBJECTIVES**
>
> 1. Describe the risk of apnea and/or bradycardia in the postoperative period and contributing factors that increase the risk.
> 2. Understand the risks and benefits of different anesthetic techniques for infant hernia repair.
> 3. Discuss the potential implications of anesthetic exposure in the neonatal period on subsequent neurodevelopment.
> 4. Understand the basic principles in avoiding and managing apnea in this group.

CASE PRESENTATION

A 5-month-old, former 28-week estimated gestational age premature infant, presents with an incarcerated inguinal hernia that needs urgent repair. The infant has a history of respiratory distress syndrome requiring intubation at birth, ventilation for 2 weeks, and a further 3 weeks of nasopharyngeal continuous positive airway pressure. Episodes of apnea were treated with intravenous, and then oral, caffeine. Echocardiography had revealed a patent ductus arteriosus, which closed with indomethacin treatment. The child went home about 1 month ago with an apnea and bradycardia monitor. The current medications are iron and vitamin supplements, and he weighs 5 kg. The parents are concerned about the effects of general anesthesia (GA) on their baby's brain and raise the possibility of avoiding GA, or delaying surgery for hernia repair until the baby is older.

An awake spinal anesthetic is given with 1 mL of 0.5% bupivacaine without epinephrine (adrenaline). The block is rapidly effective. The surgery starts well but the inguinal hernia is larger than expected and surgical repair is long and difficult. After taking 60 minutes to repair the first side, the surgeon starts the contralateral side. Twenty minutes later the infant becomes unsettled and his leg movement becomes troublesome to the surgeon. A general anesthetic is given. Induction is with sevoflurane, and a size 1 laryngeal mask (LMA) is used for the airway. Upon removal of the LMA in the operating room there is occasional apnea with oxygen desaturation to 88%. The infant requires intermittent stimulation and positive-pressure ventilation via an anesthetic circuit. The infant is transferred to the postanesthesia care unit (PACU) once respiration is regular.

In the PACU, the infant again has bradycardia to 80 bpm with apneas requiring intermittent stimulation to maintain saturations above 85%. Caffeine (10 mg/kg) is given. The surgeon asks if the baby can be discharged to home.

DISCUSSION

1. What factors increase the risk of postoperative apnea?

Ex-premature infants have been identified as a group at risk of postoperative apnea and oxygen desaturation. In an early comprehensive review, Coté et al. (1995) combined data from eight prospective studies (255 patients) where halothane and enflurane were the main anesthetic agents used, found that gestational age at birth, postmenstrual age (PMA), and anemia were independent risk factors for postoperative apnea. PMA is the time elapsed between the first day of the last menstrual period and birth (gestational age) plus the time elapsed after birth (chronological age). Coté et al. concluded that the risk of apnea in an infant born at 35 weeks is at least 5% until a PMA of 48 weeks with gestational age being a significant influence. The General Anesthesia Spinal (GAS) study has demonstrated a much lower rate of apnea with sevoflurane anesthesia and awake regional techniques (Davidson et al., 2015). Significant postoperative apnea occurred in 4% of ex-premature infants, with no difference between regional anesthesia (RA; 2.8%) and GA (4.2%). Early apneic episodes in the first 60 minutes in the recovery room were more common with GA (3.4% vs. 0.9%) whilst late apnea (30 minutes to 12 hours postoperatively) was similar with RA (2.2%) and GA (2%). The most significant predictor of postoperative apnea was low gestational age. Although it is difficult to exactly identify those at risk, extreme prematurity and low PMA are still generally regarded as the most significant risk factors for postoperative apnea.

2. What is the risk of anesthetic-induced neuroapoptosis?

A relationship between the administration of general anesthetics and sedatives during periods of rapid brain growth, and an increase in neuronal apoptosis and subsequent long-term behavioral impairment, was first reported in 2003 (Jevtovic-Todorovic et al., 2003). Non-human research has established that fetal and neonatal exposure to N-methyl-D-aspartate antagonists (ketamine and nitrous oxide) and gamma-aminobutyric acid agonist drugs (benzodiazepines, barbiturates, propofol, and all volatile anesthetics) leads to accelerated neuroapoptosis, albeit at doses not consistent with human exposure. Local anesthetics and narcotics seem to be free of concerns. Translation of these observations to humans has proven much more difficult, and the clinical relevance remains uncertain. A number of retrospective human clinical trials have suggested there may be an association between multiple episodes of anesthesia and surgery and the subsequent development of learning disabilities. In December 2016, the US Food and Drug Administration issued a "Drug Safety Communication" and mandated warnings to be added to the labels of drugs commonly used for anesthesia and sedation in children. The safety communication warns over the use of drugs for GA and sedation for prolonged (over 3 hours) or repeated procedures in children under 3 years old and pregnant women in their third trimester.

In contrast, there are a number of prospective human studies which have reassuringly suggested that a single exposure of around an hour or less is not associated with any lasting neurodevelopmental changes. The GAS study compared awake RA with sevoflurane anesthesia (GA) in infants undergoing inguinal hernia repair (Davidson et al., 2016). Interim analyses using a standardized international test to evaluate the psychomotor development (Bayley-III) have been reported in *The Lancet* and is the strongest indication yet that a 1-hour sevoflurane-based anesthesia does not increase the risk of an adverse neurological outcome at the age of 2 years. Sun et al. (2016) recently published another landmark trial, the Pediatric Anesthesia Neurodevelopment Assessment (PANDA) study. This study compared neurocognitive and behavior outcomes in children exposed to a single general anesthetic for inguinal hernia surgery prior to age 3 and their unexposed sibling. There was no statistically significant difference in full-scale IQ score at 10 years of age between the exposed and unexposed siblings. There were also no statistically significant differences between groups in scores of memory, executive function, motor and processing speed, language, attention, visuospatial function, or behavior. The sibling-matched controls effectively reduced confounders, such as, genetics, socioeconomic status, and parental educational level. In both series, however, the duration of anesthesia was just under one hour, which means that the effects of longer and repeated anesthesia exposure still needs to be investigated.

3. Which anesthetic is best?

The goal of anesthesia for the ex-premature infant having hernia repair is to provide acceptable operating conditions, a safe anesthetic, and an anesthetic that will minimize intra- and postoperative cardiorespiratory complications. The 10-N principle for safe conduct of neonatal anesthesia has been promoted by the SAFETOTS network (Weiss et al., 2016). **The principles of maintaining homeostasis are emphasized** such that quality conduct of anesthesia in children includes avoidance of fear and pain, as well as, maintenance of normotension, normal heart rate, normovolemia, normoxemia, normocarbia, normal electrolytes, normoglycemia, and normothermia. GA with regional nerve blockade, awake spinal anesthesia (SA), and awake caudal anesthesia (CA) are options well described in the anesthesia literature. A recent Cochrane database meta-analysis has reported that there is moderate-quality evidence to suggest that the administration of SA, in preference to GA, without pre- or intraoperative sedative administration may reduce the risk of postoperative apnea by up to 47% in preterm infants undergoing inguinal herniorrhaphy at a postmature age (Jones et al., 2015). For every 4 infants treated with SA, 1 infant may be prevented from having an episode of postoperative apnea (number needed to treat in order to benefit = 4). In those infants without preoperative apnea, there is low-quality evidence that SA rather than GA may reduce the risk of postoperative apnea by up to 66% (Jones et al., 2015).

GA: The incidence of postoperative apnea with newer anesthetic agents (sevoflurane or desflurane) is significantly lower (5%) than reported with older volatile agents, such as, halothane and enflurane (up to 30%). The incidence of postoperative apnea is most prominent in infants with a history of preoperative apnea. Apart from increased risk of apnea, there are several other reasons that make GA a less appealing option. GA with tracheal intubation has the potential for further airway trauma in infants who have been previously intubated and are at risk for subglottic stenosis or cysts. In addition, a number of series have reported a 20% to 25% incidence of moderate hypotension (MAP <35 mmHg) in infants undergoing GA (McCann & Schouten, 2014). The prevalence of hypotension is paradoxically higher in GA than infants receiving regional techniques, and a number of authors have suggested that hypotension may be a more significant contributing factor to neurodevelopmental delays than anesthetic agents (Weber et al., 2016; Weiss et al., 2013). Ex-premature infants have normative blood pressure data that are generally higher than that of term infants, so a MAP of 35 in an ex-preemie may represent relative hypotension compared to term infants. Only by 4 weeks of age do full-term infants attain comparable blood pressure values. The reason for this difference in cardiovascular development is unclear, but the extrauterine stress may lead to a higher systemic vascular resistance in ex-premature infants. Neonatal blood pressure may not be an accurate predictor of neurocognitive outcomes in preterm infants if the duration is brief.

Awake SA: While RA has been demonstrated to reduce the risk of postoperative apnea in at-risk neonates, its greatest drawback is the failure rate even in experienced hands (Frawley et al., 2015; Williams et al., 2006). The largest awake neonatal RA series published (the Vermont Infant Spinal Registry's 1,554 infants) reports a 97.4% success rate, but with some sedation required in 20% (Williams et al., 2006). The GAS series have reported a significantly higher incidence of failure, mainly because sedation for partial blocks was not allowed. SA was more effective (87% success) than combined spinal CA (76%) or awake CA (55%). Unfortunately, risk factors for failure of RA could not be identified; gestational age, age at surgery, weight at surgery, drugs used, anesthetic technique, and experience of the anesthetist were not predictive for success of RA. In the event of block failure, the question of whether to delay surgery or continue with volatile anesthesia has not been resolved. It is worth noting that supplemental sedation or converting to GA significantly increases the risk of postoperative apnea (Frawley et al., 2015).

Table 47.1 lists cases where SA could have significant advantages over GA.

Awake CA: Successful CA in awake infants has been reported with bupivacaine 0.25% at doses ranging from 0.8 to 1.2 mL/kg (2.0–3.0 mg/kg). The Pediatric Regional Anesthesia Network group report significant variability in local anesthetic dosing with 24.7% (4,406 of 17,867) receiving doses of bupivacaine over 2 mg/kg (Suresh et al., 2015). Awake caudal blocks often demonstrate slow onset, inconsistent motor block, and an increased risk of local anesthetic toxicity if the larger doses are used (Breschan et al., 1988). Marhofer et al. (2015) recommended that awake caudal and epidural anesthesia be used more frequently in infants but did not specifically study ex-premature infants. Their protocol is to perform neuraxial regional blocks with initial sevoflurane or propofol sedation to establish a vascular access, and to keep the children immobile

TABLE 47.1 RELATIVE RISK-BENEFIT OF ANESTHETIC TECHNIQUES APPROPRIATE FOR INFANT INGUINAL HERNIA REPAIR

Anesthetic Technique	Patient Cohort	Pros	Cons
Awake regional anesthesia[a]	Ex-premature infants born at <35 weeks' gestational age	Profound muscle relaxation	Significant failure rate (2%–10%)
	Currently <45 weeks PMA	Hemodynamic stability	Limited duration of block (70–80 min with spinal)
	Past or current apnea of prematurity requiring caffeine or methylxanthines		
	Significant neonatal history, including IVH, NEC, retinopathy of prematurity	Avoidance of volatile anesthetic induced neurotoxicity	May be challenging with laparoscopic hernia repair
	Chronic lung disease requiring home oxygen	No airway instrumentation	Team may be uncomfortable with technique
General anesthesia	Term infants currently >45 weeks PMA	Facilitates laparoscopy or prolonged surgery	Postoperative apnea, laryngospasm, desaturations
	Extremely large hernias	Greater familiarity with caudal or ilio-inguinal blocks	Hypotension more common; longer induction and emergence time
	Parental refusal for spinal anesthesia	Sevoflurane anesthesia of less than 1 hour considered low risk	Ill-defined risk of anesthetic induced neurodevelopmental delays

Note: PMA = postmenstrual age (gestational age + postnatal age); IVH = intraventricular hemorrhage; NEC = necrotizing enterocolitis.

[a]Awake regional anesthesia includes spinal anesthesia, caudal anesthesia, or combined caudal spinal anesthesia.

during the performance of the neuraxial block. A recent study comparing awake SA to awake CA in premature and ex-premature infants failed to demonstrate any advantage to awake CA over SA. The rate of postoperative apneas in the CA group was 8.9% compared to 5.6% in the SA group (Henderson-Smart et al., 2001).

4. What is the role of perioperative caffeine?

There is limited evidence that prophylactic caffeine and theophylline can reduce the rate of postoperative apnea after GA. A Cochrane review stated that caffeine can be used for this indication but emphasized the small number of patients studied. It is not clear whether there is a benefit in giving caffeine prophylactically to all patients receiving GA with newer insoluble agents, such as, sevoflurane or desflurane. In the event of apnea or bradypnea after GA, caffeine or aminophylline should be given without delay. Of the methylxanthines, theophylline is the most extensively used, but caffeine is at least as effective as theophylline, has a longer half-life, is associated with fewer adverse events, and is easier to administer (Henderson-Smart & Steer, 2010). Any postoperative bradycardia or apnea is predictive of both early and late cardiorespiratory events, and mandates admission until a 12-hour event-free interval has elapsed.

5. Is there a role for day-stay hernia repair?

The best time to discharge these patients is controversial. The most widely practiced and conservative measure is to admit all ex-premature infants less than 60 weeks PMA for overnight apnea monitoring, regardless of the anesthetic. Factors which predict postoperative complications usually occur more frequently in the complicated ex-premature infant. Silins et al. (2012) found prematurity, low gestational age, postconceptual age <45 weeks, GA, and perioperative opioids, predicted prolonged postanesthesia care unit stay or admission; whereas SA was protective. Babies at risk for sudden infant death syndrome (e.g., parental smoking, single-parent families, low socioeconomic status) should be considered for admission as well. Some units consider "early" discharge

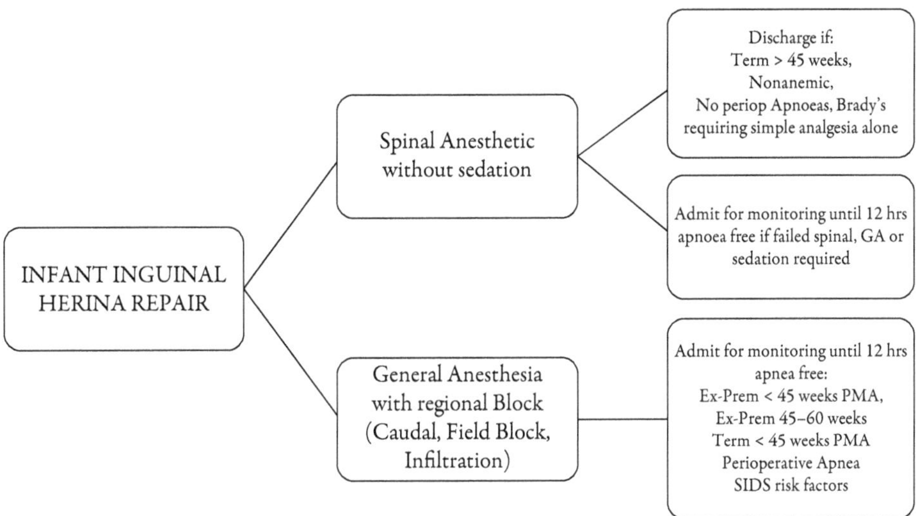

FIGURE 47.1 Algorithm for postoperative management. General anesthesia with sevoflurane or desflurane. Perioperative sedation (with propofol or volatile anesthetics) and/or perioperative opioids (including codeine) increases the apnea risk to that consistent with general anesthesia. GA, general anesthesia; PMA, postmenstrual age (gestational age + postnatal age); SIDS, sudden infant death syndrome.

for uncomplicated term infants who do not have any risk factors, and who have demonstrated no apnea, bradycardia, or desaturations during the surgery and for 8 hours postoperatively. Figure 47.1 summarizes an algorithm to consider for the management of the former premature infant.

6. What do we tell parents about the risks of neonatal anesthesia?

First, we should emphasize to parents that very few neonatal procedures are elective and delaying the procedure introduces more significant risks. Second, we believe it is not ethical to withhold anesthesia for procedures in infants and children. Third, the evidence for an association between anesthetic exposure and neurodevelopmental issues in humans is far from clear-cut. It is worth emphasizing that recent well-designed, prospective large-scale studies reassuringly show minimal or no impairment in neurocognitive development in children who received GA. Lastly, there is no evidence suggesting that any one anesthetic technique is risk-free.

Up-to-date information and consensus statements are readily available to parents from the "Strategies for Mitigating Anesthesia Related neuro-Toxicity in Tots" (SmartTots) website (Weiss et al., 2015). SmartTots is a public-private partnership between the US Food and Drug Administration and the International Anesthesia Research Society which promotes prospective investigation of anesthesia effects on neurodevelopment, and investigates agents which may protect the neonatal brain.

SUMMARY

1. Ex-premature infants less than 60 weeks PMA are at increased risk for postoperative apnea, especially those with a complicated neonatal history and previous apneas.
2. The ideal anesthetic for hernia repair in these infants is not clear-cut, with significant drawbacks associated with both GA and RA. Whatever the approach taken, the maintenance of neonatal homeostasis, especially normotension and normocarbia, should be adhered to.
3. Neonatologists, pediatric surgeons, and anesthetists should all be aware of the immediate and long-term effects of GA and should book cases appropriately.

BIBLIOGRAPHY

Breschan C, Hellstrand E, Likar R, Lonnqvist PA. Bupivacaine plasma concentrations associated with clinical and electroencephalographic signs of early central nervous system toxicity in infants during awake caudal anaesthesia. *Anaesthesist.* 1988;47:290–294.

Coté CJ, Zaslavsky A, Downes JJ, et al. Postoperative apnea in former preterm infants after inguinal herniorrhaphy: a combined analysis. *Anesthesiology.* 1995;82:809–822.

Davidson AJ, Disma N, de Graaff JC, et al. Neurodevelopmental outcome at 2 years of age after general anaesthesia and awake-regional anaesthesia in infancy (GAS): an international multicentre, randomized controlled trial. *Lancet.* 2016 Jan 16;387(10015):239–250.

Davidson AJ, Morton NS, Arnup SJ, et al. Apnea after awake regional and general anesthesia in infants: the General Anesthesia Compared to Spinal Anesthesia Study—comparing apnea and neurodevelopmental outcomes, a randomized controlled trial. *Anesthesiology.* 2015;123(1):38–54.

Frawley G, Bell G, Disma N, et al. Predictors of failure of awake regional anesthesia for neonatal hernia repair: data from the General Anesthesia Compared to Spinal Anesthesia Study comparing apnea and neurodevelopmental outcomes. *Anesthesiology.* 2015;123(1):55–65.

Henderson-Smart DJ, Steer PA. Prophylactic caffeine to prevent postoperative apnea following general anaesthesia in preterm infants. *Cochrane Database Syst Rev.* 2001;4: CD000048.

Henderson-Smart DJ, Steer PA. Caffeine versus theophylline for apnea in preterm infants. *Cochrane Database Syst Rev.* 2010;1:CD000273.

Hoelzle M, Weiss M, Dillier C, Gerber A. Comparison of awake spinal with awake caudal anesthesia in preterm and ex-preterm infants for herniotomy. *Paediatr Anaesth.* 2010;20(7):620–624.

Jevtovic-Todorovic V, Hartman RE, Izumi Y, Benshoff ND, Dikranian K, Zorumski CF, . . . Wozniak DF. Early exposure to common anesthetic agents causes widespread neurodegeneration in the developing rat brain and persistent learning deficits. *J Neurosci.* 2003;23:876–882.

Jones LJ, Craven PD, Lakkundi A, Foster JP, Badawi N. Regional (spinal, epidural, caudal) versus general anaesthesia in preterm infants undergoing inguinal herniorrhaphy in early infancy. *Cochrane Database Syst Rev.* 2015 Jun 9;6:CD003669.

Marhofer P, Keplinger M, Klug W, et al. Awake caudals and epidurals should be used more frequently in neonates and infants. *Pediatr Anesth.* 2015;25:93–99.

McCann ME, Schouten AN. Beyond survival: influences of blood pressure, cerebral perfusion and anesthesia on neurodevelopment. *Pediatr Anesth.* 2014;24:68–73.

Silins V, Julien F, Brasher C, Nivoche Y, Mantz J, Dahmani S. Predictive factors of PACU stay after herniorraphy in infants: a classification and regression tree analysis. *Pediatr Anesth.* 2012;22(3):230–238.

Sun LS, Li G, Miller TL, et al. Association between a single general anesthesia exposure before age 36 months and neurocognitive outcomes in later childhood. *JAMA.* 2016 Jun 7;315(21):2312–2320.

Suresh S, Long J, Birmingham P, De Oliveira G. Are caudal blocks for pain control safe in children? An analysis of 18,650 caudal blocks from the pediatric regional Anesthesia Network (PRAN) database. *Anesth Analg.* 2015;120(1):151–156.

Weber F, Honing GH, Scoones GP. Arterial blood pressure in anesthetized neonates and infants: a retrospective analysis of 1091 cases. *Pediatr Anesth.* 2016;26(8):815–822.

Weiss M, Bissonnette B, Engelhardt T, Soriano S. Anesthetists rather than anesthetics are the threat to baby brains. *Pediatr Anesth.* 2013;23:881–882.

Weiss M, Hansen TG, Engelhardt T. Ensuring safe anaesthesia for neonates, infants and young children: what really matters. *Arch Dis Child.* 2016;101:650–652.

Weiss M, Vutskits L, Hansen TG, Engelhardt T. Safe anesthesia for every tot—The SAFETOTS initiative. *Curr Opin in Anaesthesiol.* 2015;28:302–307.

Williams RK, Adams DC, Aladjem EV, Kreutz JM, Sartorelli KH, Abajian JC. The safety and efficacy of spinal anesthesia for surgery in infants: the Vermont Infant Spinal Registry. *Anesth Analg.* 2006;102(1):67–71.

48

Tracheoesophageal Fistula Repair

CATHERINE P. SEIPEL AND TITILOPEMI A. O. AINA

INTRODUCTION

Tracheoesophageal fistula (TEF) and esophageal atresia (EA) is a congenital malformation occurring in 1:3,000 to 4,500 births. The condition presents specific challenges to the anesthesiologist in the perioperative period. The presence of a fistula means that infants born with TEF/EA are at risk of pulmonary aspiration, and positive-pressure ventilation may be hazardous. These babies often have coexistent problems associated with prematurity and/or low birth weight; additionally, 50% have associated abnormalities, most commonly congenital cardiac malformations.

LEARNING OBJECTIVES

1. Explain the anatomy of the various abnormalities of the trachea and esophagus and the commonly associated conditions.
2. Identify how TEF/EA presents and what investigations are required during the preoperative assessment.
3. Assess the potential problems associated with anesthetizing an infant with TEF/EA.
4. Construct an appropriate postoperative management plan.

CASE PRESENTATION

A 2.5-kg boy is born at 35 weeks' gestation after his mother went into preterm labor secondary to polyhydramnios. No other antenatal problems were present. APGAR scores were 8 at 1 minute and 10 at 5 minutes. He is now spontaneously ventilating with normal saturations on room air, with no increased work of breathing. The baby is transferred to the neonatal intensive care unit (NICU) for feeding. On arrival, placement of a nasogastric tube (NGT) is unsuccessful; the whole-body x-ray ("babygram") demonstrates the ***NGT*** *is* ***coiled in the upper esophagus,*** *and* ***gas is noted in the stomach.*** *Based on this, a diagnosis of TEF/EA is made with surgical consultation placed. On examination, he is well-perfused with no dysmorphic features. Cardiorespiratory examination reveals a II/VI systolic murmur. He has passed urine and meconium. Maintenance intravenous (IV) fluid of 10% dextrose is continued at 60 mL/kg/day. The baby is kept 30 degrees head up to prevent aspiration and the NG tube is suctioned regularly. An* ***echocardiogram*** *diagnoses a small ventricular septal defect and confirms a left-sided aortic arch. Complete blood count, urea, electrolytes, and renal and cranial ultrasounds are normal. A type and screen is taken, and he is booked on the emergency surgical list.*

In the warmed operating room, the baby is placed on a blanket connected to a forced-air warmer. IV dextrose is continued. Anesthesia is induced using sevoflurane/oxygen. ***Gentle positive-pressure ventilation*** *is applied with no significant expansion of the stomach. He is intubated with a size 3 uncuffed endotracheal tube (ETT) after muscle relaxation; the tube is passed into the bronchus and gently pulled back until bilateral air entry is heard. Hand ventilation is possible without stomach expansion, so fentanyl 2 mcg/kg and antibiotics are given. A 24G radial arterial line and nasopharyngeal temperature probe are inserted. Anesthesia is maintained with sevoflurane at an end-tidal concentration of 2.8% in an oxygen/air mix with FiO_2 0.4. Rigid esophagoscopy shows a blind-ended upper esophageal pouch; no upper pouch fistula is seen. He is positioned in the left lateral position and endotracheal tube position and ventilation are* *rechecked. A right thoracotomy and extrapleural dissection allows the fistula to be ligated. The FiO_2 is increased to 0.8 to compensate for the SpO_2 fall due to lung retraction. There is a short gap, so the upper and lower esophageal segments are anastomosed over a size 10 nasogastric feeding tube; during this, the mean blood pressure (MAP) drops 20 mmHg. This is instantly corrected with release of the surgical traction.* ***Hand ventilation*** *is required throughout the procedure; this allows instant recognition of two episodes of* ***large airway obstruction*** *due to surgical retractors. A total of 30 mL/kg of albumin is given for the 150-minute procedure. A* ***morphine infusion*** *is started at 10 mcg/kg/hr. The baby is transferred ventilated to the NICU to allow controlled extubation the following morning.*

DISCUSSION

1. What are the anatomical variants of TEF/EA, and what are the common associated abnormalities?

In the majority of patients (80% to 85%), the lesion consists of an EA, with a distal esophageal pouch and a proximal TEF (Holder et al., 1987). The remaining 15% to 20% of patients have variations on this (Fig. 48.1).

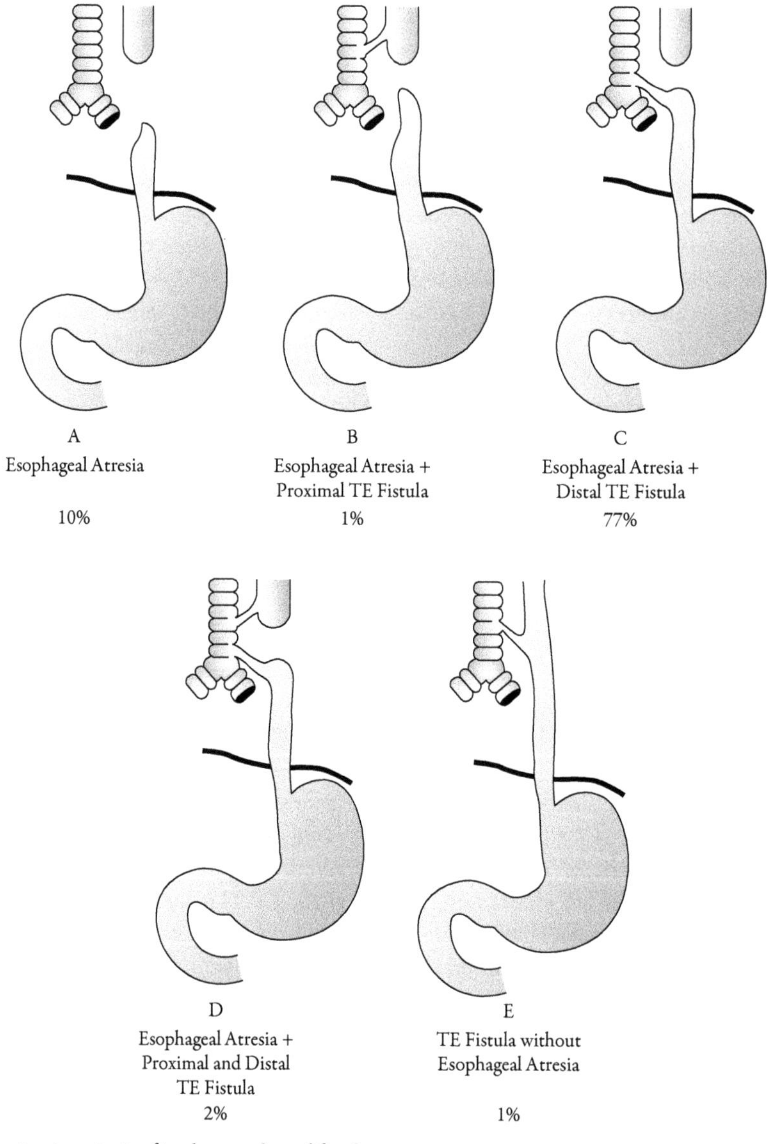

FIGURE 48.1 Anatomic variants of tracheoesophageal fistula.

Urgent diagnosis and treatment is important to avoid aspiration of saliva, feeds, and possibly gastric contents. TEF/EA is linked with other clinical defects in more than 50% of babies; the most common is cardiac (30%). The most frequent cardiac anomalies, are: ventriculoseptal defects and tetralogy of Fallot (Greenwood & Rosenthal, 1976). **Echocardiogram** is also used to exclude a right-sided aortic arch, which would influence the surgical approach. This anomaly occurs in 2.5% of cases. There is a link with associations, such as vertebral, anorectal, cardiac, tracheoesophageal, renal, and limb defects (VACTERL); coloboma, heart defects, anal atresia, retarded growth, genital hypoplasia, ear anomalies (CHARGE); and trisomy 18. Isolated abnormalities also occur, such as renal abnormalities, imperforate anus, duodenal atresia, and cleft lip and palate.

2. How does TEF/EA present, and how is it diagnosed?

TEF/EA can present *in utero* with the absence of stomach bubble on ultrasound, or it may be suspected in the presence of polyhydramnios. Polyhydramnios, however, is a nonspecific finding, and the majority of TEF/EAs are diagnosed postnatally. The baby may be "mucousy"—with copious oral secretions—and EA is confirmed with the inability to pass a NG tube. However, it may be that TEF/EA is not discovered until the baby chokes or aspirates with his first feeding. An isolated TEF can present at an older age with recurrent pneumonia. A "babygram" x-ray is the initial investigation used to diagnose EA. Typically the **NG tube is coiled in the upper mediastinum** and **air in the stomach** confirms the presence of a TEF (Fig. 48.2). The x-rays are also useful to examine the vertebrae for bony abnormalities, to check the positions of umbilical lines (and ETT), and to look for signs of aspiration or congenital heart disease. Electrolytes should be checked, as they may become deranged, with large amounts of suctioned secretions and subsequent replacement.

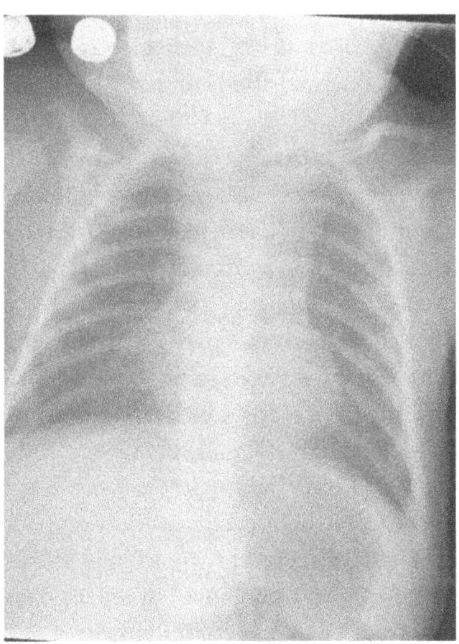

FIGURE 48.2 Typical radiograph of a baby with a TEF. Note nasogastric tube coiled in esophagus and air bubble in stomach.

3. What are the key problems associated with anesthetizing an infant with TEF/EA?

Comorbidities: Infants with extreme prematurity or severe lung disease can be difficult to ventilate; the ventilatory gases can easily flow down the low-resistance fistula, and this is worsened if lung compliance is poor. The result is inadequate ventilation and gastric distention; the latter can further impede ventilation or even cause gastric rupture and pneumoperitoneum. In the past, a gastrostomy would have been performed in these high-risk neonates and thoracotomy postponed until respiratory function improved (Ulma et al., 2001). However, in these cases it is now generally accepted that emergency transpleural ligation of the TEF is the procedure of choice, with the aim to reoperate in 8 to 10 days to divide the fistula and repair the atresia. Very low birth weight (<1500 g) premature infants have a higher rate of anastomotic complications and overall morbidity; a staged repair is often considered. This involves ligation and division of the TEF with gastrostomy placement followed by a delayed primary repair when the child is clinically stable or has reached a weight of 2000 g (Greenwood & Rosenthal, 1976). Premature or low birth weight babies can also have hypoglycemia and hypocalcemia, which need to be evaluated and treated perioperatively. Particular care needs to be taken with temperature control, and checking ETT placement with any position change.

Location and size of fistula: In an otherwise well infant, the majority of anesthetic problems are due to the location and size of the fistula. Carinal and multiple fistulas make it difficult to exclusively ventilate the lungs. Rigid bronchoscopy, performed before intubation and thoracotomy, has been used to assess the presence, type, size, and location of the fistula. It may also aid in the diagnosis of tracheomalacia or bronchial abnormalities, which can alter the surgical plan and influence the timing of extubation. Flexible bronchoscopy through the ETT could be used during initial intubation and following changes in the patient position, to confirm placement below the TEF and above the carina. However, in premature infants the airway may be too small to accommodate the bronchoscope. The main disadvantage to presurgical bronchoscopy is that preterm infants with severe respiratory compromise may not tolerate spontaneous ventilation. Complications, such as, desaturation, airway trauma, laryngospasm, or bronchospasm can occur. Controversy still exists as to the best way to induce and intubate while minimizing ventilatory difficulties. In theory, maintaining spontaneous ventilation seems to be the optimal technique, as the negative intrathoracic pressure causes the gas to preferentially enter the lungs, rather than the TEF. However, in an already compromised neonate with poor lung compliance, adequate gas exchange may not be possible without **positive-pressure ventilation**. Inadequate depth of anesthesia can lead to coughing, splinting, or inadequate ventilating conditions. Some authors choose to use succinylcholine (suxamethonium) before intubation (McEwan, 2004).

Surgical retraction: Lung retraction can be poorly tolerated, requiring higher FiO_2, and altered ventilation settings. Direct **large airway compression** can also occur; for these reasons, many anesthetists prefer to **hand ventilate** throughout these periods for immediate recognition of altered respiratory compliance. Surgical compression of the great vessels and right atrium can cause rapid loss in preload and hence a rapid fall in MAP. This is one reason an arterial line is useful (although some would argue not "absolutely essential") in these procedures. Continued open dialogue with the surgeon throughout the case is essential.

4. How can positive-pressure ventilation difficulties after intubation be managed?

After intubation, it is usually difficult to maintain spontaneous ventilation until the time of fistula ligation; the combination of lung retraction, opioids, and comorbid lung insufficiency requires positive-pressure ventilation. Ventilation problems occur due to gas preferentially flowing into the fistula rather than the lungs. Various anesthetic and surgical maneuvers are possible; the choice depends on the clinical urgency and the *predetermined plan* made between the anesthesiologist and the surgical team (Table 48.1).

5. What are the postoperative respiratory complications?

Generally, infants return to the NICU for postoperative management of pain and ventilation. The timing of extubation depends on many factors, including: preoperative lung disease, prematurity, congenital abnormalities, and surgical preference. Airway edema and postoperative stridor may occur. The most common early postoperative complication is pneumonitis or atelectasis from secretions in the bronchial tree. Severe tracheomalacia and bronchomalacia occur in 10% to 20% of infants. It can result in apnea, cyanotic spells, and reintubation. Rare life-threatening tracheomalacia may require urgent aortopexy.

6. What are the potential analgesic modalities?

IV opioid infusion, with adjunct nonopioid analgesics, regional techniques, epidural catheters, extrapleural catheters, or a combination, have all been used. The choice depends on several factors, including the timing of extubation, the type of ventilation being used, the anesthesiologist's familiarity with a technique, and ability of the NICU to care for the modality.

Continuous **infusions of morphine** or fentanyl have been used safely and with good effect. Some institutions prefer the use of fentanyl due to concerns over accumulation of morphine and its metabolites in neonates. Epidural catheters can be inserted via the caudal, lumbar, or thoracic spaces, and advanced to the mid-thoracic level; verification of the tip is recommended, and this can be achieved by electrical stimulation, ultrasound, or x-ray screening (see Chapter 54). Local anesthetic clearance is reduced in the neonate, so both maximum dose and duration should be reduced; most providers limit infusions to 48 hours. Regional techniques can reduce opioid requirement and ventilator days, though the evidence for improved outcome is lacking.

TABLE 48.1 ANESTHETIC AND SURGICAL TECHNIQUES TO MANAGE PROBLEMS WITH POSITIVE-PRESSURE VENTILATION

Anesthetic Technique	Advantage	Disadvantage
Maintain spontaneous ventilation	Avoid positive-pressure ventilation down fistula	Inadequate ventilation or apnea during thoracotomy
"Blind" placement of ETT below fistula	Simple if anatomy allows	May not be possible if fistula is at or below level of carina
Bronchoscopic ETT placement	Accuracy ensured	ETT may be too small for bronchoscope; time-consuming in an emergency
Occlusion of fistula with embolectomy balloon catheter via trachea (with or without bronchoscope)	Can be effective	Difficult in practice if unfamiliar with technique; time-consuming in emergency
Deliberately intubate the bronchus	Can be effective	Difficult to intubate the correct (left) bronchus; right bronchial intubation is not sustainable intraoperatively with right thoracotomy
Surgical Technique	Advantage	Disadvantage
Emergency ligation of fistula	Effective; probably ***most preferable technique*** unless the baby is in extremis. Surgeon familiar with technique.	Requires lateral positioning
Needle decompression of stomach	Rapid; used if gastric distention is causing cardiorespiratory depression or imminent gastric rupture	Temporary measure, invasive
Gastrostomy to decompress stomach	Can keep patient supine. An underwater seal may reduce ventilation "egress" into the decompressed stomach (Domajnko et al., 2007).	More time-consuming than needle decompression. Invasive. Inevitable gastropexy caused may make long-gap esophageal anastomosis more difficult. May reduce fistula resistance and worsen ventilation.
Occlude fistula with embolectomy catheter via gastroscopy	Effective	Can be difficult, time-consuming
Occlude gastroesophageal junction	Effective; performed supine; some may reserve this for those in extremis	Invasive, time-consuming

Note. ETT = endotracheal tube.

Reprinted from Knottenbelt G, Skinner A, Seefelder C. Tracheo-oesophageal fistula and oesophageal atresia. *Best Pract Res Clin Anaesthesiol.* 2010;24:387–401, with permission from Elsevier.

SUMMARY

1. TEF/EA represents a perioperative challenge, and up to 30% of patients are preterm.
2. Many patients have respiratory compromise, and up to 50% have other congenital comorbidities.
3. The surgery involves the lateral position and thoracotomy with the inherent potential hemodynamic, ventilatory, and analgesic problems.
4. Communication with cardiologists, surgeons, and neonatologists is essential to optimize the preoperative assessment, intraoperative emergency planning, and postoperative analgesia and ventilation.

ACKNOWLEDGMENTS

The authors would like to thank Lorna Rankin for her contributions to the first edition.

ANNOTATED REFERENCES

Knottenbelt G, Skinner A, Seefelder C. Tracheo-oesophageal fistula and oesophageal atresia. *Best Pract Res Clin Anaesthesiol.* 2010;24:387–401.

An excellent recent article. A good overview of anesthetic management of TEF/EA, including recent evidence for the use of preoperative bronchoscopy.

McEwan A. Anaesthesia for repair of oesophageal atresia and trachea-oesophageal fistula. In: Stoddart PA, Lauder GR, eds. *Problems in Anaesthesia: Paediatric Anaesthesia.* London: Taylor & Francis; 2004:7–11.

A nice summary chapter on the anesthetic management of TEF/EA.

BIBLIOGRAPHY

Domajnko B, Drugas GT, Pegoli W Jr. Temporary occlusion of the gastroesophageal junction: a modified technique for stabilisation of the neonate with esophageal atresia and tracheoesophageal fistula requiring mechanical ventilation. *Pediatr Surg Intern.* 2007;23:1127–1129.

Greenwood RD, Rosenthal A. Cardiovascular malformations associated with tracheoesophageal fistula and oesophageal atresia. *Pediatrics.* 1976;57: 87–91.

Holder TM, Ashcraft KW, Sharp RJ. Care of infants with oesophageal atresia, tracheoesophageal fistula and associated abnormalities. *J Thorac Cardiovasc Surg.* 1987;94:828–835.

Orenstein S, Peters J, Khan S Youssef N, Hussain SZ. The digestive system. Congenital abnormalities: esophageal atresia and trachesophageal fistula. In: Behrman RE, Kliegman RM, Jenson HB, Stanton BF, eds. *Nelson Textbook of Paediatrics.* 18th ed. Philadelphia: Saunders Elsevier; 2007:1219–1220.

Petrosyan M, Estrada J, Hunter C, Russell W, Stein J, Ford H, Anselmo DM. Esophageal atresia/tracheoesophageal fistula in very low birth-weight neonates: improved outcomes with staged repair. *J Pediatr Surg.* 2009;44:2278–2281.

Ulma G, Geiduschek J, Zimmerman A, Morray J. Esophageal atresia and tracheosophageal fistula: anesthesia for thoracic surgery. In: Gregory GA, ed. *Pediatric Anesthesia.* 4th ed. Philadelphia: Churchill Livingstone; 2001:440–443.

49

Omphalocele/Gastroschisis

KARLA E. K. WYATT AND OLUTOYIN A. OLUTOYE

INTRODUCTION

Gastroschisis and omphalocele comprise the majority of congenital abdominal wall defects (AWD). These conditions are not surgical emergencies but do require urgent intervention within a few hours of birth. The incidence of gastroschisis and omphalocele vary among different countries; however, the current global incidence of gastroschisis is 1 to 5 per 10,000 (~1 in 6,000 in the United States) and that of omphalocele is 1 to 3 per 10,000 (1 in 15,000 in the United States). For unclear reasons, gastroschisis rates have continued to increase over the past few decades. Nevertheless, improved management of these congenital defects has resulted in a fall in mortality to less than 5%. Infants born with AWDs are at risk of prolonged hospitalizations, infection, feeding intolerance, cardiopulmonary complications, and overall mortality. The approach to anesthetic management for both of these conditions reflect similar goals of care.

LEARNING OBJECTIVES

1. Compare and contrast clinical presentation and associated comorbidities of gastroschisis and omphalocele.
2. Develop a plan for the perioperative management of abdominal wall defects.
3. Review the complications and outcomes of gastroschisis and omphalocele.

CASE PRESENTATION

A 1.6-kg male infant is delivered vaginally at a district hospital at 34.1 weeks to a 19-year-old, former smoker, primigravid mother. The neonate was diagnosed with a gastroschisis via prenatal ultrasound at 32 weeks. Delivery was accompanied by meconium-stained amniotic fluid and the APGAR scores were 1 at 1 minute and 7 at 5 minutes. After resuscitation and intubation, he was transferred to the neonatal intensive care unit. Two doses of surfactant were administered via the endotracheal tube. An 8Fr ***orogastric*** *tube was inserted for stomach decompression, and he was started on 80 mL/kg/24 hr intravenous 10% dextrose.* ***Prophylactic antibiotics*** *and intramuscular vitamin K were also administered. A bowel bag was applied to contain the intraabdominal contents (Fig. 49.1).*

The pediatric surgeon decides to reduce the viscera in the operating room under general anesthesia. The operating room is ***warmed*** *to 26°C (humidity 50%), and the infant is laid on an air mattress attached to a forced-air warmer. An overhead heater is utilized while monitoring is applied (including pre- and post-ductal SpO_2). The baby is ventilated to normocapnia using pressure-controlled ventilation. The surgeons remove the plastic bowel wrap to visualize intraabdominal contents (Fig. 49.2), mainly distended bowel with possible malrotation, and portions of the colon. When the bowel is externally manipulated, the* ***tidal volumes decrease*** *despite an incremental increase in the ventilation pressures from 12/4 to 26/4 cmH_2O. The* ***end-tidal carbon dioxide ($ETCO_2$) drops*** *to 22 mmHg, heart rate rises from 130 to 166, and the* ***postductal saturations drop*** *compared to the measured SpO_2 in the right hand (preductal). The mean arterial pressure falls from 38 to 30 mmHg despite administration of 2 boluses of 20ml/kg of crystalloid. Further manipulation is abandoned, and a silastic pouch is placed (Fig. 49.3). Cardiovascular*

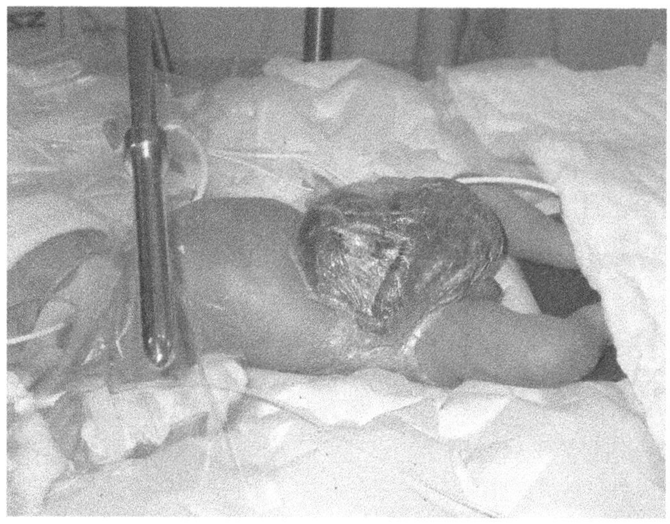

FIGURE 49.1 On arrival to the operating room, the baby's intestines were covered by plastic wrap to prevent evaporative losses.

stability returns with normalization of ventilation pressures. A peripherally inserted central catheter is placed for ***parenteral nutrition*** *before the baby is transferred back to the neonatal intensive care unit where he remains intubated for 1 week with the silo suspended above. Following 2 subsequent operating room silo reduction manipulations, the remaining bowel is returned to the abdominal cavity. The silo is removed and the abdomen closed by pulling the umbilical cord over the defect and suturing of the AWD. Over the ensuing days to weeks, the patient is extubated, parental nutrition weaned, and enteral feedings gradually implemented.*

DISCUSSION

1. What are the similarities and differences between gastroschisis and omphalocele?

Gastroschisis and omphalocele are the two most common congenital AWDs, resulting in the herniation of abdominal viscera through a defect in the upper or lower abdominal wall. These neonates present with herniated abdominal contents which may or may not have a covering sac, and, on occasion, intestinal obstruction is also present. The herniated viscera may have impaired blood supply, and major fluid deficits can occur due to exposed intestines. While the surgical and anesthetic management for both conditions is similar, gastroschisis and omphalocele

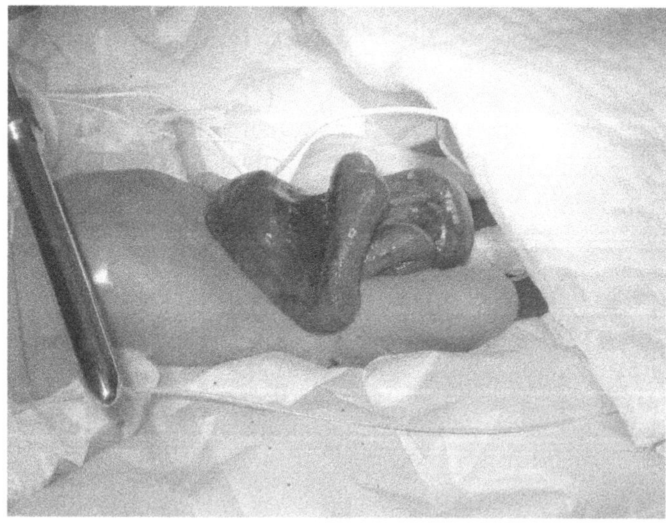

FIGURE 49.2 Gastroschisis unwrapped intraoperatively.

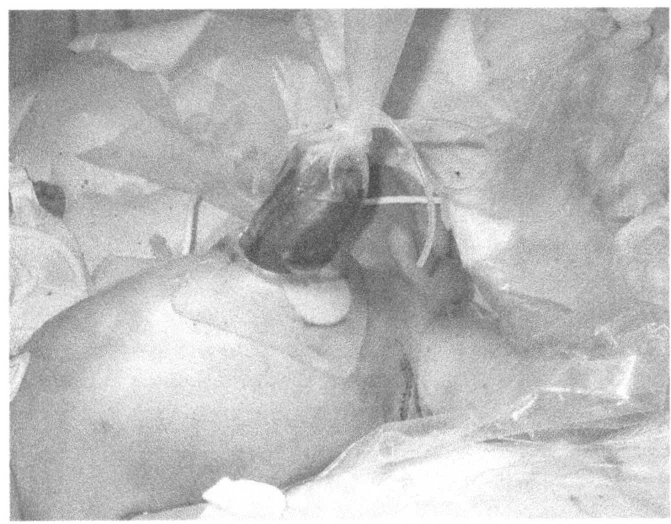

FIGURE 49.3 Silo reduction of gastroschisis.

have distinctly different etiologies, comorbidities, and prognoses (Table 49.1).

Gastroschisis can be classified into simple or complex; the latter is associated with bowel atresia (sometimes multiple) or other congenital abnormalities. Complex gastroschisis therefore has a poorer prognosis. Omphalocele is classified into minor (defects <5 cm) or major (defects >5 cm). The major defect may or may not include the liver in the sac. Omphalocele is associated with chromosomal abnormalities (e.g., trisomy 13, 18, 21, Turner, Klinefelter), syndromes including Beckwith-Wiedemann, cardiac defects (e.g., atrial septal defect/ventrical septal defect, tetralogy of Fallot, and transposition of the great vessels), and lung hypoplasia.

2. What are the management priorities for a neonate with an AWD?

The priorities for a neonate with exposed abdominal viscera is to maintain perfusion of the herniated viscera, and minimize evaporative fluid losses secondary to the exposed surface area. Babies with a prenatal diagnosis via ultrasound should be delivered in an obstetric unit that has a high-level neonatal intensive care unit within the same hospital. However, premature delivery may preclude this from happening. On examination of the baby, if there is no significant

TABLE 49.1 COMPARISON OF OMPHALOCELE WITH GASTROSCHISIS

Omphalocele	Gastroschisis
• Herniation of viscera into base of umbilical cord through a central defect; a membranous sac covers and protects the viscera, but this may rupture, especially at birth • Etiology: Failure of gut to migrate back into abdominal cavity between the 6th and 10th week post-conception • Lower risk of prematurity • 75% have associated congenital abnormalities, including chromosomal, cardiac, genito-urinary, and craniofacial	• Evisceration of gut and potentially other organs through 2- to 5-cm defect lateral to umbilicus (nearly always right-sided); no overlying sac: viscera exposed to chemical burn from amniotic fluid and environment • Etiology: Thought to be secondary to occlusion of the omphalomesenteric artery in utero. The lateral ventral wall folds fail to close during the 4th week post-conception • 60% associated with prematurity and intrauterine growth retardation • Associated with young maternal age (<20 years of age), low socioeconomic status, smoking, preterm labor, lower birth weights • Lower risk for congenital abnormalities, 10% to 30%

viscero-abdominal cavity disproportion, surgical closure of a simple gastroschisis may be accomplished at the bedside. However, in the case described, reduction was not immediately possible largely due to the size of the defect. In the case of ruptured abdominal contents in omphalocele, or exposed bowel as in gastroschisis, fluid and heat loss must be minimized by covering the bowel with a simple **plastic wrap** or placing the viscera and lower extremities in a "bowel bag." It is vital to maintain the vascular integrity of the bowel by *avoiding accidental volvulus* which may occur due to rotation of the bowel as it is being placed in the bag; therefore, the color and perfusion should be monitored frequently. Prior to definitive treatment, the baby should be positioned supine in a thermoneutral neonatal cot/incubator with *ongoing fluid resuscitation* with crystalloid and/or colloid solution, if indicated. To aid reduction of the viscera, an **orogastric tube** is required to decompress the bowel; this is preferred over a nasogastric tube in potentially obligate nasal-breathing premature infants. Some surgeons also use a Gastrografin lavage; however, there is no evidence that it increases primary closure rates, and it does carry a significant risk of an acute core temperature drop. Surgical repair of either of these conditions is not an emergency; many centers now keep the abdominal contents contained in a silo and gradually manually compress the silo to slowly reduce the contents back into the abdominal cavity. This approach decreases moderately long surgery with moderate to severe fluid losses when surgical closure eventually occurs.

Unruptured omphalocele sacs do not require additional cover but may need physical support to avoid rupture in major omphalocele defects. Associated abnormalities are common with omphalocele, so all affected infants routinely require an *echocardiogram* before surgery. Cardiac defects may also occur in 10% of infants with gastroschisis, so preoperative echocardiography should also be strongly considered for these infants as well.

Enteral **nutrition** is frequently delayed because of raised intra-abdominal pressure and/or additional gastrointestinal anomalies, such as, atresias, necrotizing enterocolitis (NEC), and intra-abdominal sepsis. Nutrition should therefore be initiated parenterally with early minimal enteral trophic feeding, if possible.

Prior to surgery, if the neonate is not intubated, gastric contents should be decompressed with an orogastric tube, followed by rapid-sequence induction. An appropriate-sized endotracheal tube should be placed. If necessary, a cuffed endotracheal tube with a low-pressure inflatable cuff should be used for intubation. These can safely be used in this population to reduce aspiration risk and promote adequate ventilation during bowel manipulation. Neuromuscular blockade is used to facilitate the reduction of abdominal contents. If complete reduction is not possible, surgeons will perform a staged reduction, as presented in this case. With this approach, the intestine is covered with a silastic pouch and the size of the pouch is subsequently reduced in stages, either in the operating room or intensive care unit. This staged procedure allows the abdominal cavity to gradually accommodate the increased mass without abruptly compromising ventilation or organ perfusion (Bachiller et al., 2013).

As wound infection and sepsis are particular risks following surgical reduction, **antibiotics** are started prior to surgery. This risk is particularly increased when a silo or a patch is used. Additionally, maintaining normothermia is also paramount in the anesthetic management of these patients. Hypothermia contributes to left shift in the oxygen-hemoglobin dissociation curve with decreased oxygen delivery to the tissues and platelet dysfunction leading to coagulopathy. Given the increased body surface area to weight ratio, minimal subcutaneous fat, and inability to shiver in the neonate, these babies are very prone to hypothermia. Various techniques should be utilized to warm the patient, including maintaining ambient temperature adjustments above 27°C, use of overhead radiant warmers, fluid warmers, forced-air warming devices and warming blankets, heat and moisture exchange filters, and occlusive surgical drapes to keep the rest of the baby dry.

3. What is the physiological effect of reducing the viscera, and what is abdominal compartment syndrome?

Returning the viscera into the abdominal cavity causes a rise in intra-abdominal pressure depending on the disparity between the volume of viscera reduced and the volume of the abdominal cavity. This can result in respiratory and cardiovascular compromise. Lung expansion may become limited by splinting of the diaphragm, which can cause a fall in tidal volume and atelectasis. Cardiac output may also fall (with concomitant rise in right atrial pressure) due to a reduction in venous return from the lower body and an increase in afterload. A rise in intra-abdominal pressure above 15 mmHg will reduce renal perfusion with disruption of fluid and salt homeostasis. Above 20 mmHg, abdominal compartment syndrome (ACS) can occur due to compromised splanchnic blood flow. Visceral ischemia (particularly bowel and liver) due to compromised blood supply results in prolonged ileus, metabolic acidosis, NEC, and sepsis (Marven & Owen, 2008). Increased intra-abdominal pressure can also decrease venous return from the lower body via compressive effects on the inferior vena cava, resulting in lower extremity congestion and cyanosis. Blood pressure and pulse oximetry determinations from a lower extremity may be different from those in the upper extremity, hence preductal and postductal pulse oximetry is recommended. Compartment syndrome must be avoided by individualizing the visceral reduction depending on the degree of abdominal cavity disproportion.

Intra-abdominal pressure may be measured via a nasogastric tube or bladder catheter. If the pressure does not rise above 20 mmHg during the reduction of a gastroschisis under general anesthesia, primary closure of the abdomen is likely to be achieved. Surrogate measures that suggest clinical decompensation secondary to ACS should be closely monitored, such as an acute **fall in ETCO$_2$** (reflecting falls in tidal volume or cardiac output), a significant **fall in measured tidal volume**, a rise in inspiratory plateau pressure above 25 cmH$_2$O, or a significant **fall in lower limb SpO$_2$** compared to postductal upper limb SpO$_2$. If any of these occur, primary closure and or manipulation should be abandoned, as in the scenario presented. In most neonatal intensive care units, a silo would be used to achieve a staged abdominal closure, or occasionally a prosthetic mesh patch may be used (particularly in large omphalocele defects).

4. What complications are associated with AWDs?

Preoperative and intraoperative fluid losses from exposed bowel and "third spacing" can be massive. Neonates can require up to 200 mL/kg/24 hr of crystalloid, with colloid supplement as indicated by heart rate, blood pressure, and capillary refill. Postoperatively these patients often become edematous and hyponatremic due to renal dysfunction and extravascular third-spacing; urine output, serum electrolytes, and fluid input need to be carefully monitored. Some infants may need inotropic support to improve renal and splanchnic perfusion pressure.

Postoperative intestinal dysfunction and failure is common due to a combination of inflammation, intestinal anomalies, atresias, dilatations, raised intra-abdominal pressure, and NEC. Considering that the majority of these infants are either premature or have low birth weight, in conjunction with prolonged gastrointestinal dysfunction, nutritional support is required. **Parenteral nutrition** should be instituted via a peripherally placed intravenous catheter or, if there is prolonged gut failure, a cuffed Hickmann/Broviac central line. Early trophic feeding with expressed human milk is of benefit to premature infants and potentially those with gastroschisis. Sepsis is a significant problem, particularly in very small neonates at high risk for NEC and wound and line infections. Sources of sepsis need to be actively sought if there is any deterioration in the baby's condition.

5. What are the long-term outcomes of infants born with AWDs?

The mortality of AWDs is dependent on coexisting genetic and/or congenital abnormalities, as well as, the gestational age and birth weight of the neonate. The majority of these affected neonates are premature, thus the associated comorbidities will play a pivotal role in short- and long-term outcomes. A recent retrospective review (Kong et al., 2016) demonstrated that infants with gastroschisis required significantly longer hospitalizations and parenteral nutrition with higher rates of infection compared to infants with omphalocele. In general, mortality rates have decreased for omphalocele, but mortality rates for infants with gastroschisis has continued to rise with unclear etiologies. A previous study on gastroschisis in low-risk neonates showed a mortality of 2.9%, compared with 24.4% in high-risk neonates (Chang et al., 2010). High risk was associated with NEC, complex cardiac anomalies, or lung hypoplasia/bronchopulmonary dysplasia. A rare but significant problem is intestinal failure secondary to short bowel syndrome caused by intrauterine or postdelivery volvulus, atresia, or NEC. This results in prolonged parenteral nutrition dependency and a need for small bowel transplantation +/– liver transplantation.

A good cosmetic result is typically achieved if multiple surgeries are not required, and if the umbilical cord is preserved in the correct position. Initially many neonates are growth-restricted, but following successful treatment most will attain a normal IQ and exercise tolerance.

SUMMARY

1. Gastroschisis and omphalocele are associated with different comorbidities and therefore different prognoses.
2. The aim of management is to reduce the eviscerated organs back into the abdominal cavity; primary closure of the abdomen is ideal, but abdominal compartment syndrome must be avoided.
3. Parenteral nutritional support is universally required, until full enteral feeding is established.
4. Long-term prognosis is good, except in the presence of significant prematurity, growth retardation, and/or associated genetic or congenital anomalies.

ACKNOWLEDGMENT

The authors wish to acknowledge the first edition author, Peter Stoddart.

ANNOTATED REFERENCES

Holland AJ, Walker K, Badawi N. Gastroschisis: an update. *Pediatr Surg Internat.* 2010;26:871–878.

A review of gastroschisis, including antenatal care and overall prognosis.

Kong JY, Yeo KT, Abdel-Latif ME, et al. Outcomes of infants with abdominal wall defects over 18 years. *J of Ped Surg.* 2016;51:1644–1649.

A contemporary large retrospective review of AWD outcomes in infants.

Marven S, Owen A. Contemporary postnatal surgical management strategies for congenital abdominal wall defects *Seminar Pediatr Surg.* 2008;17:222–235.

Review of the surgical management options for AWD.

BIBLIOGRAPHY

Bachiller P, Chou, J., Romanelli T, Roberts, J. Neonatal emergencies. In: Coté, CJ; Lerman, J; Anderson, B eds. *A Practice of Anesthesia for Infants and Children.* 6th ed. Philadelphia: Elsevier; 2013:746–765.

Bauman B, Stephens D, Gershone H, et al. Management of giant omphaloceles: a systematic review of methods of staged surgical vs. nonoperative delayed closure. *J of Ped Surg.* 2016;51:1725–1730.

Chang DC, Salazar-Osuna JH, Choo SS, Arnold MA, Colombani PM, Abdullah F. Benchmarking the quality of care of infants with low-risk gastroschisis using a novel risk stratification index. *Surgery.* 2010; 147:766–771.

Morton NS, Fairgrieve R, Moores A, Wallace E. Anesthesia for the full-term and ex-premature infant. In: Gregory G. Andropoulos D, eds. *Gregory's Pediatric Anesthesia.* 5th ed. Hoboken, NJ: Blackwell; 2012:479.

Ross AR, Hall NJ. Outcome reporting in randomized controlled trials and systematic reviews of gastroschisis treatment: a systematic review. *J of Ped Surg.* 2016;51:1385–1389.

Sadler T. Embryological origin of ventral body wall defects. *Sem Pediatr Surg.* 2010;19:209–214.

Vachharajani AJ, Rao R, Keswani S, Mathur AM. Outcomes of exomphalos: an institutional experience. *Pediatr Surg Int.* 2009;25:139–144.

50

Congenital Diaphragmatic Hernia Repair

JAGROOP MAVI, ANNE C. BOAT, SENTHILKUMAR SADHASIVAM, AND CATHERINE P. SEIPEL

INTRODUCTION

Congenital diaphragmatic hernia (CDH) affects approximately 1 in 2,500 live births. It results from an **embryologic defect** in diaphragm formation, allowing abdominal contents to enter into the fetal pleural cavity. Prognosis and treatment options vary depending on the extent and location of the diaphragmatic hernia. CDH remains a significant cause of neonatal morbidity and mortality.

LEARNING OBJECTIVES

1. Understand the pathogenesis of CDH.
2. Describe the prognostic indicators and treatment options for CDH.
3. Review the anesthetic considerations for CDH repair.

CASE PRESENTATION

An 11-day-old 3.5-kg boy was born at 38-weeks gestation, with a prenatal diagnosis of left-sided CDH, and is now scheduled for repair. The prenatal assessment of the severity of this neonates CDH on fetal magnetic resonance imaging MRI) include a ***lung-to-head ratio*** *(LHR) of 1.6 on prenatal ultrasound and 19% liver herniation. The patient was born via spontaneous vaginal delivery and intubated immediately after birth. Currently, the patient is ventilated with assist control/volume guarantee ventilation at a rate of 40 bpm, with tidal volumes of 4 ml/kg and a FiO_2 of 0.30. He is also on inhaled* ***nitric oxide*** *at 20 ppm for pulmonary hypertension estimated to be at systemic level.* ***Echocardiography*** *shows a small patent ductus arteriosus with bidirectional shunting, and normal right and left systolic ventricular function. Head ultrasound reveals a grade-1 intraventricular hemorrhage. He is currently sedated with both midazolam and morphine infusions.*

DISCUSSION

1. What is the embryologic defect responsible for CDH?

A common pleuroperitoneal cavity exists in the fetus during the first 4 weeks of human gestation. Subsequently, a pleuroperitoneal membrane forms and becomes the diaphragm at about 8 weeks of gestation, dividing this common cavity into the chest and abdomen. The left posterolateral section of this membrane is the last to develop. When the pleuroperitoneal membrane is not fully formed, abdominal contents, such as small and large intestine, stomach, spleen, and liver, can herniate and migrate into the chest cavity (Fig. 50.1). CDH can be classified by the location in the diaphragm, with a left posterolateral hernia (**foramen of Bochdalek**) occurring most frequently. Other possible sites for visceral herniation through the diaphragm include right posterolateral, anterior, (through the foramen of Morgagni), and through the esophageal hiatus.

2. What is the pathophysiology of CDH?

The presence of abdominal organs in the pleural cavity produces a mass effect, resulting in lung compression, pulmonary hypoplasia, pulmonary vascular changes, and cardiac malposition. **Pulmonary hypoplasia** is more pronounced in the ipsilateral lung, but lung development in the contralateral lung can also be affected. Visceral herniation occurs during a critical time in lung development, when the bronchi and pulmonary arteries are undergoing branching. Subsequently, CDH patients have **abnormal pulmonary vasculature** due to lung

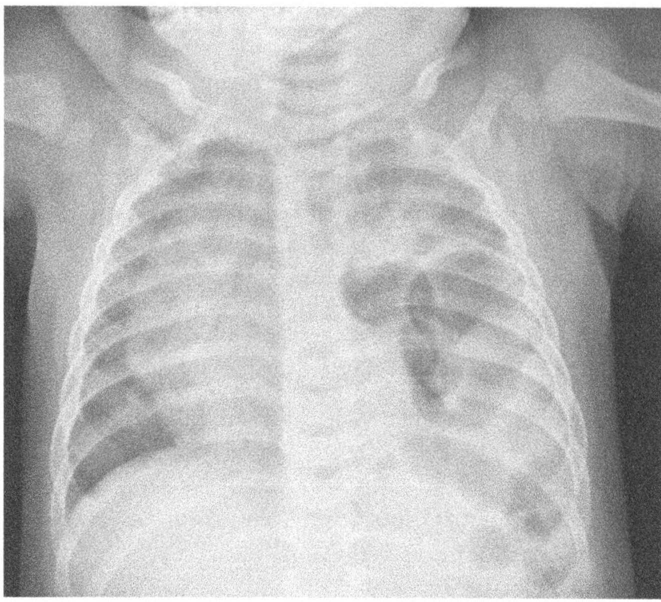

FIGURE 50.1 Typical radiograph of baby with CDH. Note bowel in left hemithorax with displacement of thoracic contents to the right.

hypoplasia-associated reduction in the vascular cross-sectional area, and abnormal thickening of the walls of the pulmonary arteries (Chinoy, 2002). The decreased functional lung volume and increased pulmonary vascular resistance lead to postnatal hypoxemia, acidosis, and, in severe cases, right heart failure. The hypoxemia and acidosis then further worsen the pulmonary vasoconstriction, which in turn exacerbates the cyanosis and respiratory distress. Cardiac malposition (mesocardia or dextroversion) is frequently found with left-sided CDH. Vascular compression of the inferior vena cava can occur and produce shock-like clinical conditions. Finally, **congenital heart anomalies** have been found in association with CDH in up to 23% of patients (Greenwood et al., 1976).

3. How is CDH diagnosed?

With the detailed level of prenatal care available today, CDH is often **diagnosed prenatally** with ultrasonography and fetal MRI. The diagnosis of CDH should be considered in any newborn with signs of **respiratory failure** shortly after birth. On physical examination of a patient with left-sided CDH, a scaphoid abdomen is often noted with a barrel-shaped chest and decreased or absent breath sounds over the left chest. A chest radiograph shows dilated loops of bowel in the chest and a shift of the mediastinum to the right (Fig. 50.1).

4. What prognostic indicators are used to determine the severity of CDH?

Multiple variables have been used to predict severity of CDH and subsequent mortality. The **observed-to-expected total fetal lung volumes (O/E-TFLV)** and **percentage of liver herniation** on fetal MRI have the highest accuracy in predicting survival and the need for extracorporeal membrane oxygenation (ECMO) (Akinkuotu et al., 2016). Liver herniation that is less than 20% on fetal MRI is associated with greater than 90% survival. Another acceptable prognostic predictor of CDH severity is the **lung-to-head ratio** (LHR) on fetal ultrasound (Zamora et al., 2014). An LHR of less than 1.0 is associated with severe CDH and increased mortality. A prenatal assessment of O/E-TFLV of <35% is a strong predictor of 6-month mortality in neonates with CDH.

Postnatally, the **Brindle clinical prediction score** is utilized in some institutions to educate families on mortality risk of CDH patients. It also stratifies high- and low-risk populations thereby allowing management strategies to be tailored according to severity. This score includes consideration of low birth weight, Apgar scores, and the presence of severe pulmonary hypertension, cardiac anomaly, and chromosomal anomaly (Brindle et al., 2014). Using this model, intermediate- and high-risk infants can be selected for transfer to high-volume centers for further care and those with severe disease can be considered for advanced medical therapy including ECMO. Severe or lethal anomalies, if present, may preclude aggressive CDH treatment.

5. What are the available treatment options?

The focus of treatment in patients with CDH is **medical management,** followed by **surgical repair** of the diaphragm. Respiratory and cardiovascular compromise are *primarily* due to pulmonary hypoplasia and pulmonary hypertension causing right-to-left cardiac shunting, hypoxemia, and right heart failure. With CDH patients, medical stabilization often means sedation and positive-pressure ventilation to manage hypoxemia, hypoventilation, acidosis, and prevent worsening of pulmonary hypertension. However, ventilator-associated lung injury, due to barotrauma caused by overdistention of the lungs, and oxygen toxicity can worsen pulmonary status. The ventilation strategy used should achieve preductal oxygen saturation of greater than 85%, while maintaining a $PaCO_2$ of 50 to 70 mmHg, and a pH greater than 7.2, with peak inspiratory pressures of 28 cmH_2O or less.

Other strategies for improving pulmonary blood flow include inhaled nitric oxide (iNO) and high-frequency oscillatory ventilation (HFOV). Nitric oxide is an endogenous regulator of vascular tone, and iNO can act as a selective vasodilator of the pulmonary vasculature. Although the use of iNO has shown benefit in other instances of neonatal pulmonary hypertension, the abnormal pulmonary vessels in some CDH patients with hypoplastic lungs may not respond appropriately to vasodilators (Finer & Barrington, 2006). In addition, the use of iNO in patients with CDH may be associated with increased mortality (Putnam et al., 2016); thus, the use of iNO in the treatment of CDH remains controversial.

Neonates who require more than 25 cmH_2O peak pressures for adequate oxygenation may benefit from HFOV which offers a decreased risk of barotrauma. HFOV uses an oscillator to produce high respiratory rates at low tidal volumes. This method is thought to evenly inflate the lungs and decrease overdistention and the subsequent release of inflammatory mediators from the lungs (Van den Hout et al., 2009). Though HFOV has been used in treatment of CDH patients, a recent multicenter analysis showed no difference in mortality between conventional ventilation and HFOV groups (Puligandla et al., 2015).

When medical stabilization fails, **extracorporeal membrane oxygenation (ECMO)** is often used to support cardiopulmonary status. ECMO will temporarily stabilize the patient's condition, allowing for time or medications to improve the pulmonary hypertension and respiratory failure. Exclusion criteria for ECMO, include: preterm birth before 34 weeks, weight less than 2 kg, presence of a grade II or greater intracranial hemorrhage, and presence of an irreversible disease process. An infant with CDH can undergo surgical repair of the diaphragm while on ECMO or after ECMO decannulation.

More recent modalities for CDH treatment involve **fetal interventions**. These include: fetal endoscopic tracheal occlusion (FETO) or ex-uterine intrapartum treatment (EXIT)-to-ECMO procedures. Fetal endoscopic tracheal occlusion is thought to promote fetal lung growth by preventing the outward movement of fluid from the lungs and increasing lung volumes. Between 26 and 30 weeks gestation, an endoscope is inserted in the mouth of the fetus and a balloon is deployed to sit just above the carina. The response of the fetal lungs is typically assessed biweekly until 34 weeks of gestation when the balloon is removed, also via a percutaneous endoscopic approach. While improvement in survival rates or morbidity with FETO were originally not proven (Harrison et al., 2003), it is believed to provide more rapid neonatal stabilization. Trials to determine the definitive role of FETO in CDH are ongoing. EXIT-to-ECMO procedures are performed in fetuses with severe CDH who require ECMO support at birth. In this scenario, to avoid the unstable period after delivery, but before ECMO initiation, the fetus undergoes ECMO cannulation while still on uteroplacental circulation. Once ECMO and invasive monitoring have been established, the umbilical cord is clamped and the fetus is delivered.

6. What are the anesthetic considerations for a neonate undergoing repair of CDH?

Depending on the clinical status of the patient, surgery may occur in the operating room, or in the intensive care unit (ICU) if the patient is on ECMO. In either situation, extensive knowledge of the patient's hospital course, medications, and ventilatory status is essential prior to providing an anesthetic for CDH repair. This includes an understanding of the coexisting congenital anomalies, results of echocardiograms, recent blood gases, the need for pulmonary vasodilators and inotropes, and sedation requirements. The patient is usually placed in the supine position for a transabdominal approach to the CDH repair. The diaphragmatic defect is typically closed primarily; however, if the defect is large, a prosthetic patch is often used. Vascular access for a CDH repair includes peripheral intravenous lines and an arterial line (preferably right radial to measure the preductal oxygenation). Central venous access may be necessary, but neck veins are usually preserved in case they may be required for ECMO cannulation.

In patients presenting for surgery who are not already on mechanical ventilation, a nasogastric tube should be placed to prevent gaseous distention of the bowel in the chest, which could further decrease functional lung volume. Similarly, prolonged mask ventilation and nitrous oxide should be avoided during induction of anesthesia as they may contribute to bowel distention. During the CDH repair, close attention must be paid to ventilatory parameters, such as, tidal volume, peak inspiratory pressure, and blood gas measurements. High ventilatory pressures should be avoided and "gentle ventilation" should be considered (Van den Hout et al., 2009). Sudden elevations in peak inspiratory pressures, a decrease in lung compliance, or sudden hypotension should alert the anesthetist to the possibility of pneumothorax. Pneumothorax usually occurs on the ipsilateral side but can also occur in the contralateral lung; immediate chest tube placement is required if this complication is suspected. Myocardial function and cardiac output must also be closely monitored. Treatment of hypotension and fluid management is paramount in maintaining adequate cardiac output. If hypotension and poor perfusion are not responsive to crystalloid and colloid administration, then the addition of inotropic support (such as dopamine, epinephrine, or dobutamine) may be necessary. Hypocalcemia may occur following transfusion of blood products and must be corrected to maintain optimal cardiac function. Although the use of iNO in CDH patients is controversial, if the patient is already on iNO, it may be prudent to continue this during the procedure as there is the potential for rebound pulmonary hypertension and right ventricular dysfunction if the iNO is discontinued abruptly.

As with all newborns undergoing surgery in the operating room, it is important to **avoid hypothermia**, which can increase oxygen consumption and alter platelet function. Warming the operating room and utilizing fluid warmers, warming blankets, and radiant warmers are important methods of maintaining normal body temperature in the neonate.

The type of anesthetic agent used during CDH repair depends on the cardiovascular status of the patient, mode of ventilation, and partially on the preference of the anesthesiologist. Halogenated inhalational anesthetics may be used, but can cause hemodynamic instability even at lower doses. The hemodynamic stability afforded by intravenous opioids, such as, fentanyl is often preferred. If the conventional ventilator on the anesthesia machine does not allow for adequate ventilation with the available varying modes of ventilation or for the use of iNO, it may be prudent to use the ICU ventilator. The addition of a neuromuscular blocking agent is recommended to decrease the amount of anesthetic required. Since CDH patients are sedated throughout the period of medical stabilization prior to surgical repair, they have often developed a tolerance to opioids and benzodiazepines and frequently require higher doses.

SUMMARY

1. CDH is a failure of the closure of the diaphragm during the early stages of fetal life, allowing abdominal contents to herniate into the chest cavity and causing lung hypoplasia and other morbidities. The most common site of a CDH is in the posterolateral aspect of the diaphragm.
2. The presence of abdominal viscera in the chest cavity results in pulmonary hypoplasia and an alteration in the structure of pulmonary vessels, leading to pulmonary hypertension. Pulmonary hypertension and right heart failure are a major source of morbidity and mortality in neonates with CDH.
3. Treatment of CDH now consists of delayed closure of the diaphragm after medical stabilization of the patient. Management options range from conventional ventilation to ECMO to fetal intervention.
4. Anesthesia for CDH repair requires close attention to the ventilatory status of the patient. Pneumothorax is a risk in both the ipsilateral and contralateral lungs and should be considered if there is a sudden increase in peak inspiratory pressure, decrease in lung compliance, or hypotension. A "gentle ventilation"

strategy may decrease the likelihood of pneumothorax and barotrauma to the hypoplastic lungs.
5. iNO therapy for pulmonary hypertension, instituted preoperatively, may need to be continued intraoperatively to avoid sudden rebound pulmonary hypertension.
6. Cardiovascular status must also be monitored closely with invasive arterial monitoring and aggressive treatment of hypotension.

ACKNOWLEDGMENTS

The author wishes to acknowledge the first edition authors, Anne Boat and Senthilkumar Sadhasivan.

ANNOTATED REFERENCES

Brindle M, Cook E, Tibboel D, Lally K. Congenital Diaphragmatic Hernia Study Group. A clinical prediction rule for the severity of congenital diaphragmatic hernias in newborns. *Pediatrics.* 2014;134(2):e413–e419.

Description of a generalizable scoring system that can be calculated at bedside; helps identify patients at high risk for mortality.

Finer N, Barrington KJ. Nitric oxide for respiratory failure in infant born at or near term. *Cochrane Database of Syst Rev.* 2006;4:CD000399.

A review of the use of iNO for respiratory failure in term or near-term infants. The review found the outcome of infants with CDH was not improved and may have been slightly worsened with iNO.

Van den Hout L, Sluiter I, Gischler S, et al. Can we improve outcome of congenital diaphragmatic hernia? *Pediatr Surg Internat.* 2009;25:733–743.

A nice review of CDH discussing etiology, prenatal predictors of survival, treatment strategies, and long-term outcomes.

BIBLIOGRAPHY

Akinkuotu A, Cruz S, Abbas P, et al. Risk stratification of severity for infants with CDH: prenatal versus postnatal predictors of outcome. *J Pediatr Surg.* 2016;51(1):44–48.

Chinoy MR. Pulmonary hypoplasia and congenital diaphragmatic hernia: advances in the pathogenetics and regulation of lung development. *J Surg Res.* 2002;106:209–223.

Greenwood RD, Rosenthal A, Nadas AS. Cardiovascular abnormalities associated with congenital diaphragmatic hernia. *Pediatrics.* 1976;57(1):92–97.

Grivell RM, Andersen C, Dodd JM. Prenatal interventions for congenital diaphragm hernia for improving outcomes. *Cochrane Database Syst Rev.* 2015(11): CD008925.

Harrison M, Keller R, Hawgood S, et al. A randomized trial of fetal endoscopic tracheal occlusion for severe fetal congenital diaphragmatic hernia. *N Engl J Med.* 2003;349:1916–1924.

Langham MR Jr, Kays DW, Ledbetter DJ, Frentzen B, Sanford LL, Richards DS. Congenital diaphragmatic hernias: epidemiology and outcome. *Clin Perinatol.* 1996;23:671–688.

Puligandla P, Grabowski J, Austin M, et al. Management of congenital diaphragmatic hernia: a systematic review from the APSA outcomes and evidence based practice committee. *J Pediatr Surg.* 2015;50(11):1958–1970.

Putnam L, Tsao K, Morini F, et al. Evaluation of variability in inhaled nitric oxide use and pulmonary hypertension in patients with congenital diaphragmatic hernia. *JAMA Pediatr.* 2016;170(12):1188–1194. doi:10.1001/jamapediatrics.2016.2023

Zamora I, Olutoye O, Cass D, et al. Prenatal MRI fetal lung volumes and percent liver herniation predict pulmonary morbidity in congenital diaphragmatic hernia (CDH). *J Pediatr Surg.* 2014;49(5):688–693.

51

Myelomeningocele Repair

JAGROOP MAVI, ANNE C. BOAT, AND SENTHILKUMAR SADHASIVAM

INTRODUCTION

Myelomeningocele (MMC) is a spinal birth defect that occurs due to failure in the closure of the embryologic neural tube. The meninges and/or neural structures are exposed, resulting in nerve damage. MMCs are associated with significant direct morbidity, as well as, Chiari II malformations and hydrocephalus. The degree of sensory and motor deficits depends on the level of the defect, with bowel and bladder function often affected. Due to the risk of infection with an exposed spinal cord, surgical repair is usually performed in the first 24 to 48 hours of life, although prenatal correction is now performed in select cases after clinical trials demonstrated improved neurological outcomes. Anesthesia for MMC repair presents a unique challenge since positioning of these patients must prevent direct pressure on the exposed neural tissue; and, when repaired prenatally, both maternal safety and fetal outcomes must be considered.

LEARNING OBJECTIVES

1. Understand the pathogenesis and potential causes of MMC.
2. Review the treatment options for MMC, including prenatal and postnatal repair.
3. Review the anesthetic considerations for MMC repair.

CASE PRESENTATION

*A full-term baby girl with known **MMC, Chiari II malformation,** and **hydrocephalus** is born via cesarean section. APGAR scores are 7 and 8 at 1 minute and 5 minutes respectively. Birth weight is 4,070 g. The MMC is noted to be ruptured at birth and covered with **saline-soaked gauze**. She is transferred to the neonatal intensive care unit. Prenatal studies include fetal magnetic resonance imaging (MRI) showing a low lumbar, upper sacral open neural tube defect, severe hydrocephalus, and a Chiari II malformation with **herniation of the posterior fossa and brain stem** contents into the low cervical spinal canal. Fetal echocardiography shows normal cardiac anatomy. On physical exam, the infant is pink and active with no apparent distress. Macrocephaly is noted, with a head circumference of 46 cm and full, bulging anterior and posterior fontanels. Examination of the back shows a 6 × 3cm sacral lesion covered by a thin membrane. Spontaneous movement is present in all four extremities. The patient is positioned prone, on room air, with a saline drip over the MMC to keep the membrane and neural tissue moist. The neurosurgeon wants to proceed to the operating room immediately for MMC repair and possible ventriculoperitoneal (VP) shunt placement.*

DISCUSSION

1. What is a MMC, and at what point in embryologic development does it occur?

MMC, a type of spina bifida, is a birth defect that occurs during the third to fourth week of embryologic development, causing an abnormality in the spinal column and spinal cord. Incomplete closure of the neural tube causes a cleft in the vertebral column through which meninges, neural tissue, and cerebrospinal fluid can herniate. When only meninges protrude through the defect, the term "meningocele" is used. However, when meninges and neural elements are involved, it is called a "**myelomeningocele**". The opening may occur anywhere along the spinal column, but low thoracic, lumbar, and sacral regions

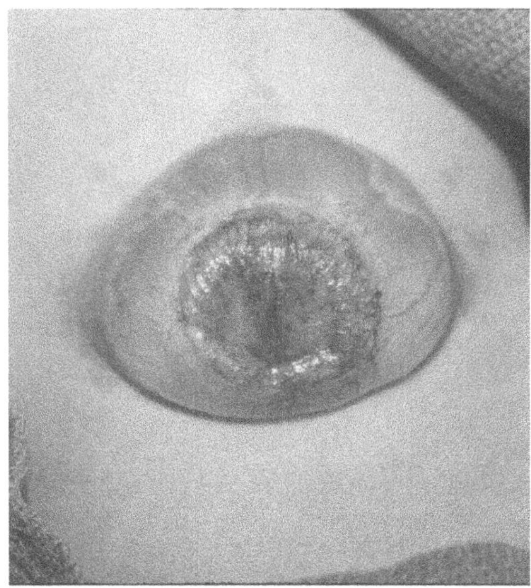

FIGURE 51.1 Lumbar myelomeningocele.

MMC is typically detected through routine ultrasound during the 18th to 22nd week of pregnancy. Preliminary diagnosis can be made as early as 16 weeks through a blood test that screens for maternal alpha-fetoprotein (AFP). Elevated AFP suggests the presence of a neural tube defect in which case an amniocentesis or ultrasound confirms the diagnosis.

are most commonly affected (Fig. 51.1). Typically, the exposed neural tissue develops abnormally, forming a flat neural placode. The neural placode is thought to be further damaged by *in utero* exposure to amniotic fluid. This is the "two-hit" hypothesis of the development of neurologic damage in MMC. The first insult occurs due to failure of primary neurulation in the embryonic period leading to myelodysplasia; and, due to the absence of skin and musculoskeletal coverage the second hit stems from chronic irritation of the exposed cord to amniotic fluid, leading to further damage (Walsh et al., 2001).

Although most patients with MMC are born alive and are relatively healthy, there are significant lifelong morbidities associated with this congenital defect. Depending on the location of the lesion, sensory and motor function and bowel, bladder, and sexual function are affected.

2. Why are hydrocephalus and Chari II malformations strongly associated with MMC?

Most infants with MMC develop **hydrocephalus**. Of the infants who develop hydrocephalus, 80% to 90% will require ventriculoperitoneal (VP) shunt placement. Evidence of hydrocephalus may occur within the first week of life, as repair of the MMC often worsens the degree of hydrocephalus. While some argue that placement of a VP shunt at the time of the MMC repair will decrease the hospital stay, others feel that MMC repair and shunt placement performed together will prolong surgery and increase the risk of shunt infection. Criteria for postnatal VP shunt placement include: the evidence of hydrocephalus, marked syringomyelia with ventriculomegaly, ventriculomegaly and symptoms of Chiari malformation, and persistent cerebrospinal fluid leakage from the MMC repair site (Pedreira et al., 2016).

Hydrocephalus is likely secondary to the **Chiari II malformation**, which is almost always present in patients with MMC. Chiari II malformations involve **herniation of the cerebellum and brain stem** tissue through the foramen magnum into the cervical spine. Symptoms associated with a Chiari II malformation, include: difficulty swallowing, inspiratory stridor, apnea, impaired cough/gag reflex, weakness or spasticity of the upper extremities, and difficulties with balance and coordination. One in 3 patients with MMC will be symptomatic from their Chiari II malformation, so anesthesiologists must handle airway management and neck positioning with care. It is important that the signs and symptoms of a Chiari II malformation are recognized early and followed with a decompressive procedure; otherwise, respiratory failure and loss of neurologic function can occur. Fifteen percent of MMC patients with a symptomatic Chiari II malformation will die by 3 years of age, and one-third will have permanent neurologic damage (Stevenson, 2004). Elevated intracranial pressure can mimic symptoms of Chiari II malformation. Therefore, it is important to rule out increased intracranial pressure as the cause of a patient's symptoms, often by radiologic or surgical evaluation of the ventriculoperitoneal shunt.

3. What are potential causes of MMC?

MMC affects approximately 1 in 2,000 live births and is thought to be caused by genetic as well as nongenetic factors (Mitchell et al., 2004). A family history of a sibling with MMC significantly increases the risk. MMC is a multifactorial polygenetic trait. Nongenetic factors associated with neural tube defects, include: folate deficiency; use of folate antagonists (for example, carbamazepine, valproic acid, and trimethoprim); and maternal pregestational diabetes mellitus. Since the 1960s, the incidence of spina bifida has been decreasing, largely due to enhanced prenatal diagnosis and early folate supplementation (Kshettry et al., 2014). Folate plays an important role in nucleic acid synthesis and methylation reactions, but the exact method by which low folate levels contribute to neural tube defects has yet to be fully understood.

4. What are the treatment options for MMC?

The treatment options for MMC include postnatal surgical repair in the first 24 to 48 hours of life or *in utero* repair of the lesion. Advances in prenatal diagnostic testing and ultrafast MRI imaging technology permit prenatal diagnosis of MMC (Maselli & Badillo, 2016). This allows for a planned cesarean section prior to the onset of labor, reducing the risk of rupture of membranes, and allows delivery in a medical center with pediatric neurosurgery services. Despite the success of postnatal neurosurgical repair and medical treatment of spina bifida, mortality remains approximately 10%, rising to 35% in children with brainstem dysfunction secondary to Chiari II malformation (Junior et al., 2015). A study showed that most infants with the most severe form of spina bifida had a surgical repair within the first 2 days of life and those born in a hospital with level I or II nursery care were less likely to have a timely surgical repair (Radcliff et al., 2016).

Open fetal surgery for MMC takes place between the 19th and 27th week of gestation. The neurosurgeon removes the MMC sac, if present, and repairs the spinal defect in layers, after which the skin is closed to protect the spinal cord from further exposure to amniotic fluid. The fetal team, includes: maternal-fetal medicine specialists, fetal surgeons, pediatric neurosurgeons, anesthesiologists, neonatologists, genetic counselors, developmental pediatricians, and social workers.

If postnatal repair is indicated, the infant is delivered, and after initial physical examination of the infant, the patient is placed prone or lateral to prevent pressure on the neural placode. The defect is covered with **sterile saline-soaked gauze** to prevent drying out of the neural tissue and further trauma. Postnatal MMC repair involves reconstruction of the neural placode, with care taken to prevent future tethering of the spinal cord with closure of the dura, the muscular layer, and the skin (Gaskill, 2004). The cerebrospinal fluid is cultured at the time of surgery, and the infant often remains on antibiotic therapy until cultures are negative.

Fetal surgery for MMC is undergoing investigation. The rationale behind *in utero* repair of MMC is the fact that additional trauma to the neural placode is believed to occur during the prolonged exposure to amniotic fluid and subsequent direct trauma or pressure on the neural tissue. This theory has been supported by both human and animal data (Bouchard et al., 2003; Meuli et al., 1996). With the routine use of ultrasonography for fetal screening and the ability to confirm the diagnosis of MMC with a fetal MRI, the diagnosis is often made by 18 weeks of gestation. This allows for fetal surgery to occur in the window of 19 to 25 weeks' gestation, when the integrity of the fetal tissue is amenable to repair but before extensive damage to the neural placode occurs.

A multicenter prospective randomized clinical trial, called the Management of Myelomeningocele Study (MOMS), was developed because of controversies between benefits versus risks of intrauterine MMC repair. The trial compared midgestation surgery with standard postpartum repair. The authors found much lower rates of demise (fetal or neonatal) and need for and placement (hydrocephalus needing VP shunt placement) of a VP shunt by 1 year of age. There was also significant improvement in the composite score for mental development and motor function at 30 months. Improvements were seen both in hindbrain herniation at 12 months and percentage of patients who were ambulatory at 30 months of age. Potential benefits of prenatal surgery must be balanced against associated higher rates of preterm birth, maternal morbidity, intraoperative complications, and uterine-scar defects apparent at delivery; along with a higher rate of maternal transfusion at delivery (Adzick et al., 2011).

Antenatal treatment of open spinal defects can also be performed using an entirely percutaneous endoscopic approach using a surgical technique that includes a bio-cellulose patch and a single layer closure. The technique used in the CECAM trial resulted in a watertight closure of the lesion, reversal of hindbrain herniation, and better level of neurologic function relative to anatomic level. In this trial, premature rupture of membranes and premature delivery remained significant complications (Pedreira et al., 2016). A recent case series described 10 fetuses with MMC who underwent completely percutaneous fetoscopic repair with 7 surviving long-term, and

6 demonstrating complete reversal of hindbrain herniation. (Maselli & Badillo, 2016).

5. What are the anesthetic considerations for MMC repair?

Ideal candidates for fetal surgery are: maternal age >18 years, 16 to 26 weeks of gestation, normal fetal echocardiogram, and singleton pregnancy. Preoperatively, it is important to establish if there is coexisting disease in the fetus. Many infants with MMC have been found to have a shortened trachea, and a chest x-ray may help assess that. The anesthesiologist should perform a thorough cardiac exam in the infant and review results of echocardiography. Screening echocardiograms have been suggested for all neonates with MMC, as over one-third of patients have congenital heart disease. Most commonly seen cardiac anomalies are secundum atrial septal defects and ventricular septal defects, with girls affected more than boys. Most patients with MMC develop hydrocephalus, and some may have an enlarged head, making airway management difficult. However, the increase in intracranial pressure often happens after the MMC defect is closed. Most neonates with MMC have a Chiari II malformation, but not all are symptomatic. Symptomatic patients may present with inspiratory stridor due to dysfunction of cranial nerve X (vagus nerve), apnea or disordered breathing due to disruption of the medullary respiratory center, or diminished gag reflex and dysphagia due to dysfunction of cranial nerve IX (glossopharyngeal nerve). Other signs and symptoms may include: hypotonia, opisthotonos, nystagmus, and a weak cry.

Infants for MMC repair should have peripheral intravenous (IV) access established prior to surgery. Volume status needs to be assessed preoperatively as there is the potential for significant fluid loss from the MMC. IV fluid replacement with crystalloid should cover maintenance requirements plus these losses. Glucose may be added to the IV fluids to prevent hypoglycemia, and glucose levels should be monitored at regular intervals. It is usually not necessary to establish central venous access or place an arterial line for postnatal MMC repair. Blood loss is not usually significant unless a large rotation flap is required to cover the defect. However, two well-functioning peripheral IVs are recommended.

Positioning of patients for induction of anesthesia and intubation can be a challenge. Care must be taken not to place pressure on or traumatize the MMC sac. This can be achieved by intubating the patient in the lateral position or placing the patient supine with the MMC sac supported in the hollowed portion of a cushioned ring. The approach to the airway should account for the fact that Chiari II malformations may cause significant cervical cord and brain stem compression, which is accentuated by cervical flexion during laryngoscopy and intubation. MRI images are helpful in understanding the extent of cord and brain stem compression.

After intubation, the patient is turned prone and supported on hip and chest rolls with the neck maintained in neutral position. It is important that the rolls are placed to minimize an increase in intra-abdominal pressure, which could compromise ventilation and cause increased surgical bleeding through engorged epidural veins. Anesthesia can be maintained with a combination of IV opioids and an inhalational anesthetic agent. Use of neuromuscular blocking agents should be discussed with the neurosurgeon prior to surgery; they may be undesirable if the surgeon plans to use nerve stimulation during surgery. Attention should be paid to maintaining the patient's body temperature. This may be achieved by preventing preoperative hypothermia, warming the operating room temperature, and using a forced-air warming blanket.

If comorbid conditions affect the airway or respiratory center, patients may need to remain intubated in the postoperative period to protect the airway and to ensure adequate ventilation. Otherwise, extubation can often be achieved with close monitoring for postoperative apnea. Some centers have used spinal anesthesia for MMC repair with direct injection of hyperbaric local anesthetic into the caudal aspect of the MMC sac (Viscomi et al., 1995). This approach prevents the need for intubation and general anesthesia but is limited by the duration of the block and the risk of a "high spinal." Currently, spinal anesthesia is not a widely accepted anesthetic technique for MMC repair.

Open fetal surgeries have unique anesthetic considerations which include performing a complete maternal history and physical exams, counseling on lumbar epidural placement, and arterial line placement intraoperatively. Rapid-sequence induction and intubation are performed and the mother is maintained in left uterine displacement. Maternal blood pressure is maintained with IV phenylephrine and ephedrine as high concentrations of volatile anesthetics are utilized for uterine relaxation. Fetal resuscitation drugs are available to the surgeon.

Intramuscular administration of fetal opioid and neuromuscular blocking agent are administered by the surgical team following hysterotomy and exposure to provide analgesia and better fetal surgical conditions. The epidural analgesia for mother is used for postoperative analgesia to minimize the risk of preterm labor. Tocolytic therapy is initiated at the termination of the procedure. Fetoscopic surgery avoids the maternal morbidity associated with a large hysterotomy which may reduce the incidence of preterm labor. Significantly less maternal morbidity in terms of length of stay, need for transfusion, and need for intensive care unit stay are the advantages of the fetoscopic approach compared to open fetal surgery (Ferschl et al., 2013).

It is unlikely that fetuses can experience pain before 24 weeks of gestation since the cortex must undergo significant development and establish highly complex neuronal networking prior to this point. Fetal anesthesia during open fetal surgery is provided primarily by the placental transfer of maternal volatile anesthetics, supplemented by intramuscular injection of opioids and neuromuscular blocking agents.

SUMMARY

1. MMC occurs due to a failure in the closure of the neural tube in the third to fourth week of gestation in 1:2,000 live births. Loss of sensory and motor function at and below the level of the lesion are often seen.
2. Chiari II malformation is seen in conjunction with MMC and contributes to the hydrocephalus seen in the majority of patients.
3. Prenatal surgical intervention options include both open and fetoscopic techniques, which have been shown to decrease the incidence of neurological complications in infants. Fetoscopic approach is likely to reduce maternal morbidity and preterm labor.
4. Anesthetic considerations for MMC repair (performed in the first 24–48 hours of life) include reviewing comorbidities (congenital heart disease and symptomatic Chiari II malformations), careful positioning, and evaluation and treatment of patient's volume status. MMC patients are at risk for hypoventilation in the postoperative period.

ANNOTATED REFERENCES

Gaskill A. Primary closure of open myelomeningocele. *Neurosug Focus.* 2004;16:1–4.

A nice review of the neurosurgical technique for postnatal MMC repair. It is helpful for anesthesia anesthesiologists to understand the phases of surgical care and the postoperative course.

Mitchell L, Adzick NS, Melchionne J, Pasquariello P, Sutton L, Whitehead A. Spina bifida. *Lancet.* 2004;364:1885–1895.

A thorough review of MMC, including epidemiology, diagnosis, treatment, and prevention. If the reader were to pick one review article to read on MMC, this should be it.

Stevenson KL. Chiari II malformation: past, present and future. *Neurosurg Focus.* 2004;16(2):E5.

This is an informative review of Chiari II malformations, including an extensive explanation of the clinical complexity of presenting signs and symptoms. Multiple images illustrate the anatomic derangement found with Chiari II malformations.

BIBLIOGRAPHY

Adzick NS, Thom EA, Spong CY, et al. MOMS Investigators. A randomized trial of prenatal versus postnatal repair of myelomeningocele. *N Engl J Med.* 2011;364:993–1004.

Bouchard S, Davey MG, Rintoul NE, Walsh DS, Rorke LB, Adzick NS. Correction of hindbrain herniation and anatomy of the vermis after in utero of myelomeningocele in sheep. *J Pediatr Surg.* 2003;38:451–458.

Ferschl M, Ball R, Lee H, Rollins M. Anesthesia for in utero repair of myelomeningocele. *Anesthesiology.* 2013;118:1211–1223.

Hirose S, Farmer D. Fetal surgery for myelomeningocele. *Clin Perinatol.* 2009;6(2):431–438.

Junior EA, Eggink AJ, Oepkes D. Fetal myelomeningocele repair: where are we and where can we go? *Rev Bras Ginecol Obstet.* 2015;37(11):495–497.

Kshettry V, Kelly M, Rosenbaum B, Seicean A, Hwang L, Weil R. Myelomeningocele: surgical trends and predictors of outcome in the United States, 1988–2010. *J Neurosurg Pediatr.* 2014;13:666–678.

Maselli K, Badillo A. Advances in fetal surgery. *Ann Transl Med.* 2016;4:394.

Meuli M, Meuli-Simmen C, Hutchins GM, et al. In utero repair of experimental myelomeningocele saves neurologic function at birth. *J Pediatr Surg.* 1996;31:397–402.

Pedreira D, Zanon N, Nishikuni K, et al. Endoscopic surgery for the antenatal treatment of myelomeningocele: the CECAM trial. *Am J Obstetr Gynecol.* 2016;214:e1–e11.

Radcliff E, Cassell C, Laditka S, Thibadeau J, Correia J, Grosse S, Kirby R. Factors associated with the timeliness of postnatal surgical repair of spinal bifida. *Child Nerv Syst.* 2016;32:1479–1487.

Rintoul NE, Sutton LN, Hubbard AM, et al. A new look at myelomeningoceles: functional level, shunting, and the implications for fetal intervention. *Pediatrics.* 2002;109(3):409–413.

Ritter S, Lloyd YT, Shaddy, RE, Minich LL. Are screening echocardiograms warranted for neonates with meningomyelocele? *Arch Pediatr Adolesc Med.* 1999;153:1264–1266.

Sival DA, Begeer JH, Staal-Schreinemachers AL, Vos-Niel JM, Beekhuis JR, Prechtl HF. Perinatal motor behavior and neurological outcome in spina bifida aperta. *Early Hum Dev.* 1997;50:27–37.

Viscomi CM, Abajian JC, Wald SL, Rathmell JP, Wilson JT. Spinal anesthesia for repair of meningomyelocele in neonates. *Anesth Analg.* 1995;81:492–495.

Walsh DS, Adzick NS, Sutton LN, Johnson MP. The Rationale for in utero Repair of Myelomeningocele. *Fetal Diag Ther.* 2001;16:312–322.

52

Anesthesia for Ex Utero Intrapartum Therapy

CAITLIN D. SUTTON AND OLUTOYIN A. OLUTOYE

INTRODUCTION

Advances in technology and imaging capabilities have resulted in an increasing number of procedures being performed on the fetus. These fetal procedures have lead to increased survival and decreased morbidity for fetuses that may have otherwise died *in utero* or at delivery or survived with significant impairment. The gamut of fetal interventions which are performed in established fetal centers may be categorized as minimally invasive fetal surgery, open mid-gestation fetal surgery, or *ex utero* intrapartum therapy (EXIT). Only the EXIT is performed at or near term. Fetal conditions warranting the EXIT procedure are likely to present at institutions that are not routinely involved with invasive or open *in utero* fetal procedures.

The care of patients undergoing an EXIT procedure involves a multidisciplinary approach, as well as one anesthesiologist dedicated to the mother and one for the baby. In addition to knowledge of maternal-fetal physiology, excellent communication skills and situational awareness are paramount to successful anesthetic management.

LEARNING OBJECTIVES

1. Identify the key maternal and fetal preoperative considerations for an EXIT procedure.
2. Develop an anesthetic plan for both mother and fetus undergoing the EXIT procedure.
3. Propose a plan for postoperative care that highlights considerations specific to EXIT procedures.
4. Review the team dynamics critical to successful management of these cases.

CASE PRESENTATION

A healthy 29-year-old female (gravida 3 para 1) was referred to the fetal center by her primary obstetrician after a 20-week ultrasound revealed severe retromicrognathia associated with possible Nager Syndrome. Magnetic resonance imaging (MRI) of the fetus confirmed a diagnosis of micrognathia versus agnathia, as well as bilateral upper extremity limb anomalies and no other apparent anomalies. The case was reviewed by physicians in pediatric surgery, pediatric otolaryngology, maternal-fetal medicine (MFM), anesthesiology, as well as labor and delivery nursing staff in their weekly multidisciplinary conference. All teams agreed that an EXIT-to-airway procedure was appropriate for this patient given the degree of anatomical compromise of the airway and the concern for failed intubation if a conventional delivery and airway management plan were pursued. Following a thorough consultation by physicians in surgery, maternal-fetal medicine, neonatology, and anesthesiology, as well as personnel in social work, informed consent was obtained and an EXIT-to-airway procedure with intubation versus tracheostomy was scheduled. The day prior to delivery, a meeting of all participating health care team members was held to confirm the plan for surgery including the step-by-step process of the procedure and to clarify any questions or concerns. The patient and her family were again counseled and their questions were answered.

On the morning of surgery, 16-gauge intravenous access was obtained in the preoperative holding area and aspiration prophylaxis was administered intravenously. An epidural was placed for postoperative analgesia. The patient was taken to the operating room and general anesthesia was induced smoothly. After obtaining additional venous and arterial access, surgery commenced. Uterine relaxation was achieved with 5% end-tidal sevoflurane concentration. Her blood pressure was maintained within 10% of baseline using a phenylephrine infusion at 0.5 mcg/kg/min.

After hysterotomy was performed with a stapling device, the fetal anesthesiologist placed a fetal pulse oximetry probe and administered a combination of intramuscular fentanyl 5 mcg/kg, vecuronium 0.3 mg/kg, and atropine 20 mcg/kg to the fetus. The otolaryngologist attempted direct laryngoscopy, but the fetal mandible was immobile and revealed a grade 4 view. During this time, pulse oximetry was lost but fetal echocardiography showed a fetal heart rate in the 120s throughout. A tracheostomy was successfully performed and confirmed with a colorimetric carbon dioxide detector. The umbilical cord was clamped and divided, and the baby was handed over to the neonatology team.

The volatile anesthetic was discontinued and oxytocin was administered via 2-unit bolus followed by an infusion of 7.5 units per hour. The uterine tone was found to be excellent, and surgical hemostasis was achieved. After loading the epidural with 0.25% bupivacaine and 3 mg preservative-free morphine, the patient was extubated awake. Estimated blood loss was 800 mL and no blood products were given.

Postoperatively, the patient received scheduled acetaminophen and ibuprofen in addition to an epidural infusion. A second dose of 3 mg preservative-free morphine was given on postoperative day 2 prior to removal of the epidural catheter. At the time of maternal discharge from the hospital, the baby remained in the neonatal intensive care unit with a plan for future mandibular distraction.

DISCUSSION

1. What is an EXIT procedure, and what are the indications?

An EXIT procedure is a modification of a cesarean delivery performed with the goal of fetal intervention while the fetus remains on utero-placental support. After uterine incision, the fetus is partially delivered (only the area of the fetus that will be worked on, plus an upper extremity for oxygen monitoring and venous access is exposed). The fetus then undergoes the planned intervention while on "placental bypass." Uterine relaxation is achieved with anesthetic agents, delaying uteroplacental separation and allowing manipulation of the fetus without initiating uterine contractions. The continued uteroplacental perfusion allows the planned intervention to take place while the fetus receives oxygenation from the mother. Once the fetal procedure is complete, the umbilical cord is clamped and uterotonic agents are administered. This procedure is performed at or near term for fetal conditions not compatible with optimal transition to extrauterine life. Historically, isolated anomalies with an otherwise good prognosis have been considered preferable for management via the EXIT procedure.

While the anesthetic principles and considerations are generally the same regardless of indication, the EXIT procedure may be performed for a variety of indications which also modify the nomenclature of the procedure (see Table 52.1). Rapid developments in prenatal diagnosis and surgical advances continue to expand indications for the EXIT procedure, in general. The most common indication is an anticipated difficult airway with severely impaired respiration in a baby immediately following delivery (i.e., EXIT-to-airway), which is discussed here.

All teams involved should extensively educate the mother and her significant other on what this procedure entails, as well as the risks and possible outcomes of the procedure for both the mother and baby prior to obtaining consent. Interdisciplinary communication and planning is critical, and the anesthesiologist should play a key role in determining

TABLE 52.1 INDICATIONS FOR EXIT PROCEDURE

Airway/head and Neck anomalies (EXIT-to-Airway)	Large cervical masses (cervical teratomas, cervical lymphangioma, large goiters) Retromicrognathia/agnathia
Lung or mediastinal masses (EXIT-to-Resection)	Congenital high airway obstruction syndrome Congenital cystic adenomatoid malformation Bronchopulmonary sequestration Compressing mediastinal masses
Cardiopulmonary conditions	Severe congenital diaphragmatic hernia
EXIT to extracorporeal membrane oxygenation (EXIT-to-ECMO)	Certain types of congenital heart disease

Note: EXIT = *ex utero* intrapartum therapy.

whether a patient is an appropriate candidate for an EXIT procedure.

2. What are the key preoperative considerations for the anesthesiologist?

The EXIT procedure involves increased surgical risk for the mother due to the required uterine relaxation which poses a risk for severe peripartum hemorrhage. Therefore, mothers considered for this procedure must be otherwise healthy with very minimal comorbidities.

Typically, two anesthesiologists are assigned to these cases: one dedicated to the care of the mother and the other to the baby. Both anesthesiologists should be knowledgeable about maternal-fetal physiology and the anesthetic implications of the changes occurring in the peripartum/perinatal period.

Anesthesiologist for mother

Preoperative consultation with the mother should involve a discussion of past medical history, past surgical history (particularly any uterine or other abdominal surgeries), and obstetric history. A full history and physical exam with assessment of all imaging and lab work must be done. Blood products for the mother must also be available. A better understanding of the patient's previous deliveries (e.g., vaginal delivery without an epidural versus standard cesarean delivery with neuraxial anesthesia) can help the anesthesiologist to frame the conversation about the differences in anesthetic management of an EXIT procedure. A discussion of the current pregnancy should include any pregnancy-related medical conditions of the mother (e.g., presence of preeclampsia or polyhydramnios), which could have implications for anesthetic management. Procedures performed during this pregnancy (e.g., amnioreductions), as well as any current medications (e.g., for tocolysis), should also be discussed. The anesthetic requirements, if any, for these previous procedures may inform the anesthesiologist about the patient's anxiety level, the need for preoperative anxiolytics, and the degree of uterine irritability. Physical examination should be focused on the airway, cardiopulmonary system, and ease of intravenous access and regional anesthesia placement.

Anesthesiologist for baby

The anesthesiologist assigned to the baby should carefully review the prenatal records including the most recent evaluations of the condition warranting the EXIT procedure. Any other fetal anomalies should be reviewed, considering their possible impact on the anesthetic plan (e.g., limb anomalies affecting intravenous access). A recent estimated fetal weight should be obtained to allow for preparation of medications for the baby. This weight estimate can be obtained from the MFM specialist who will have performed recent ultrasound assessments. The anesthesiologist should also be aware of the current fetal presentation and placental location, as these can alter the surgical plan or approach. While logistics vary amongst institutions, the baby's anesthesiologist has several responsibilities during the EXIT: preparing medications for delivery to the fetus, ensuring adequate pulse oximeter monitoring of the baby, securing intravenous access, and managing the baby's airway after secured by surgical approach, in addition to setting up a second, adjacent operating room in case postnatal surgery becomes necessary. Similar to having blood products for the mother, the anesthesiologist for the baby must ensure the presence of warm type O negative blood in the operating room prior to the start of the surgery (Lin et al., 2013).

Given the nature of these procedures, and logistics in different hospitals, anesthesiologists may find themselves in an unfamiliar environment with a pediatric anesthesiologist providing care in an adult hospital or vice versa. The available medications, equipment, and support may vary, and protocols such as those for massive transfusion may differ between institutions. These issues should be thoughtfully reviewed and explored prior to the day of surgery so delays and complications can be minimized.

Both anesthesiologists should communicate with each other and be well-versed with the operative plan. Depending on the indication for the procedure and specific clinical scenario, the steps may vary significantly and must be discussed among the multidisciplinary team before each surgery. This discussion often occurs in the form of a team meeting, in which members of all medical specialties involved gather to discuss the specifics of the case. Highlights of topics for discussion, include: maternal history and inclusion criteria that qualify her for the procedure, any medical issues with the mother that may have a bearing on surgery or anesthesia, fetal anatomy and review of images such as a fetal MRI, and a step-by-step plan for surgery, including anesthetic preparation and any concerns. Alternate management plans in the face of maternal distress, fetal distress, or failure to complete the fetal intervention should also be discussed at this meeting. All involved team members should be given the opportunity to ask questions before moving forward.

3. What are the main intraoperative anesthetic goals?

Intraoperative goals for the EXIT require special anesthetic considerations (Fig. 52.1). For the mother, these include maintenance of uterine relaxation to allow for adequate fetal manipulation without precipitating uterine contractions, delaying uteroplacental separation, and support of uteroplacental perfusion during fetal intervention. This is followed by the goal of rapid increase in uterine tone once the baby has been delivered. Intraoperative goals for the baby, include: cardiopulmonary monitoring, securing airway and intravenous access, provision of adequate analgesia, and preparation for postdelivery intervention if indicated.

Maternal anesthetic goals:

In contrast to standard cesarean deliveries, EXIT procedures are most commonly performed with general anesthesia for the mother with increased concentration of volatile anesthetic agents to induce uterine relaxation and maintain uteroplacental support. The maintenance of uteroplacental support during fetal intervention precludes the urgency of delivery from time of incision typically associated with cesarean sections. This is inevitably associated with exposure of the fetus to volatile agents for a relatively longer period. After preoperative placement of an epidural (if chosen for postoperative analgesia), and optimizing positioning of the pregnant patient for ease of intubation, rapid-sequence induction and intubation are performed. A primary goal of the maternal anesthetic is optimizing fetal perfusion via two methods: having complete uterine relaxation and sufficient maternal blood pressure (Lin et al., 2016). Maintenance of anesthesia can be achieved using volatile anesthetic alone or in combination with supplemental intravenous anesthesia. Volatile anesthetics at concentrations of 2 to 3 times minimal alveolar concentration (MAC) for a pregnant mother typically help to achieve uterine relaxation, which in turn facilitates surgical exposure and delays uteroplacental separation (Garcia et al., 2011). While any of the different volatile anesthetics can be used to achieve uterine relaxation at the appropriate doses, desflurane has been shown to depress left ventricular function of the fetus at 2 to 3 MAC (Boat et al., 2010). Supplementation of this agent with propofol and remifentanil has been proposed as an alternative to decrease the incidence of this untoward effect on the fetus by desflurane. This method decreases the duration of exposure to the high concentrations of desflurane necessary to provide uterine relaxation. Use of other volatile anesthetic agents (e.g., sevoflurane or isoflurane) at the required concentrations for uterine relaxation have not been reported to be associated with fetal dysrhythmias. There are also reports of this procedure performed under neuraxial anesthesia with a combined spinal-epidural technique using intravenous nitroglycerin infusion for uterine relaxation. However, nitroglycerin has the disadvantage of not being easily titratable, and its use may be associated with pulmonary edema. Nevertheless, the option of a regional technique may be of benefit in patients in whom the use of volatile anesthetics is contraindicated.

Maintenance of uteroplacental perfusion is vital. The patient should be positioned with left uterine displacement to prevent aortocaval compression, and end-tidal carbon dioxide should be maintained at physiological levels for pregnancy, between 30 and 35 mmHg. Beat-to-beat blood pressure monitoring should be facilitated with the aid of an arterial line, and maternal blood pressure maintained within 10% of baseline. This often requires the use of vasopressor infusions (most commonly phenylephrine), due to the required concentrations of volatile agent. The anesthesiologist must carefully monitor blood loss and volume status and remain in constant communication with the surgical team regarding the mother's status. Once the fetal intervention is complete, the cord is clamped and the baby is delivered. Uterotonics are administered after confirming with the surgeon, and the concentration of volatile agent is rapidly weaned to decrease the risk of uterine atony. Discontinuation of the volatile anesthetic and titration of intravenous anesthesia is also an option once the baby has been delivered. If an epidural is in place, it should be loaded with a bolus of local anesthesia and opioid to provide for patient comfort upon emergence.

Fetal anesthetic goals

Once hysterotomy is performed and fetal exposure is achieved, a pulse oximeter probe should be placed on the fetus's hand. This probe is connected to the cable which is passed on to the surgical field by the anesthesiologist covered in a sterile plastic sleeve.

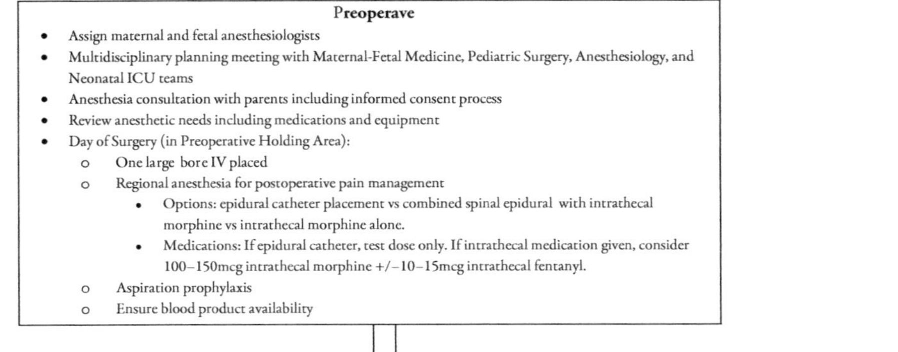

FIGURE 52.1 Sample anesthetic plan for EXIT procedure.

The pulse oximetry waveform is optimized by covering the baby's hand and pulse oximeter with foil to prevent interference by the surgical lights on the field. Expected oxygen saturation while still on uteroplacental support is 50% to 70%. Additional fetal monitoring involves fetal heart rate and contractility monitoring using echocardiography. This is typically performed by a pediatric cardiologist or MFM specialist on the field, but fetal monitoring may also involve other methods, such as, fetal blood sampling or ultrasonography for cerebral blood flow. If abnormal fetal values, such as, decreased oxygen saturation or fetal bradycardia are observed, adequate uteroplacental perfusion should be confirmed by assessing maternal hemodynamics and volume status. Assuming these are acceptable, the umbilical cord should be checked for compression by surgical instruments or positioning of the fetus. The cord can also be palpated on the surgical field to confirm the presence of a good pulse.

The fetus is exposed to both inhaled and intravenous anesthetics administered to the mother but also receives some drugs directly. After the pulse oximeter has been placed on the fetus, an intramuscular combination of an opioid, anticholinergic, and muscle relaxant is administered. This is the most expeditious route of medicine administration to the fetus. Supplemental medications including resuscitation drugs may be administered intravenously after accessing a fetal vein or via the umbilical vein.

Resuscitation

Throughout the fetal intervention, both anesthesiologists must be prepared for resuscitation in the event of maternal or fetal distress (Brusseau & Mizrahi-Arnaud, 2013). For distress of either patient, the maternal anesthesiologist should confirm left uterine displacement, increase inspired oxygen to 100%, and support maternal hemodynamics with vasopressors, blood products, or volume replacement. If the mother continues to decompensate, especially in the setting of uncontrolled hemorrhage, the EXIT may need to be abandoned for cesarean delivery of the baby. In the event of fetal decompensation, the fetal team should confirm umbilical cord perfusion, administer resuscitative drugs and chest compressions as necessary, and prepare for possible abandonment of the EXIT with umbilical cord separation and continued postnatal resuscitation. Given the decreased physiologic reserve of both mother and fetus, these events may happen rapidly and require excellent communication between surgical, anesthetic, and neonatal teams.

4. What are the primary postoperative considerations?

Considerations for the mother

Maternal outcomes after EXIT procedures are comparable to those after standard cesarean deliveries, and the postoperative considerations are relatively similar. Monitoring for postpartum hemorrhage should be performed as with other postpartum patients. While many of these patients will not be able to immediately commence breastfeeding due to the baby's postoperative disposition (most often the baby remains intubated after airway has been secured), rapid return to baseline functioning will facilitate the patient's interaction with her newborn baby. Pain management should be multimodal and include opioids (preferably neuraxial), acetaminophen, non-steroidal inflammatory drugs, and local anesthetics (neuraxial or via regional block; e.g., the transversus abdominis plane or quadratus lumborum block).

Considerations for the baby

Postoperative concerns for the baby vary widely and are related to the indication for fetal intervention. For the EXIT-to-airway, these babies will have an artificial airway in place after the EXIT procedure. Disposition may be directly to the operating room for further surgical intervention or to the neonatal intensive care unit. Anesthetic management should be individualized to the clinical scenario.

SUMMARY

1. As fetal interventions become increasingly common, more anesthesiologists will be tasked with caring for these patients.
2. While more investigation is required to determine the optimal regimen, the anesthetic goals for these procedures have been well defined.
3. Successful anesthesia care for EXIT procedures requires thorough preparation and vigilance, excellent communication skills, and fluency in maternal-fetal physiology.

ANNOTATED REFERENCES

Lin EE, Moldenhauer JS, Tran KM, Cohen DE, Scott Adzick N. Anesthetic management of 65 cases of ex utero intrapartum therapy: a 13-year single-center experience. *Anesth Analg*. 2016;123(2):411–417.

This case series presents data focused on the anesthetic management of 65 EXIT procedures and is the largest case series of its kind to date.

Lin EE, Tran KM. Anesthesia for fetal surgery. *Semin Pediatr Surg*. 2013;22(1):50–55.

This article provides an overview of all 3 types of fetal surgery and reviews key physiologic principles of pregnancy including uteroplacental blood flow and placental transport.

Brusseau R, Mizrahi-Arnaud A. Fetal anesthesia and pain management for intrauterine therapy. *Clin Perinatol*. 2013;40(3):429–442.

This article discusses anesthetic management for the fetus, including specific discussion of fetal access, monitoring, resuscitation, and analgesia.

Garcia P, Olutoye O, Ivey RT, Olutoye OA. Case scenario: anesthesia for maternal-fetal surgery. *Anesthesiology*. 2011;114(6):1446–1452.

This article contrasts the management of an EXIT procedure with a typical cesarean delivery and includes comments from a fetal surgeon.

BIBLIOGRAPHY

Boat A, Mahmoud M, Michelfelder EC, et al. Supplementing desflurane with intravenous anesthesia reduces fetal cardiac dysfunction during open fetal surgery. *Paediatr Anaesth*. 2010;20(8):748–756.

George RB, Melnick AH, Rose EC, Habib AS. Case series: combined spinal epidural anesthesia for Cesarean delivery and ex utero intrapartum treatment procedure. *Can J Anaesth*. 2007;54(3):218–222.

Sviggum HP, Kodali BS. Maternal anesthesia for fetal surgery. *Clin Perinatol*. 2013;40(3):413–427.

PART 12

Challenges in Pediatric Regional Anesthesia and Pain

53

Caudal versus Penile Block

CHERYL MAENPAA, MICHELE HENDRICKSON,
AND KENNETH R. GOLDSCHNEIDER

INTRODUCTION

Circumcision is a commonly performed operation. Although the medical necessity of routine circumcision is debated, common indications for the procedure include: religious beliefs, parental preference, hygienic concerns, phimosis, and paraphimosis. As with any surgical procedure, adequate postoperative pain control is an important consideration. A variety of analgesic options for circumcision exist, each with potential risks and benefits.

LEARNING OBJECTIVES

1. Discuss postcircumcision analgesia.
2. Understand basic anatomy and technique pertaining to caudal and penile blocks.
3. Identify potential risks and benefits of caudal versus penile blockade.

CASE PRESENTATION

*A 2.5-year-old boy presents for circumcision. His parents report that providing adequate hygiene for their son has been difficult due to increasing difficulty with, and pain during, foreskin retraction. He has no allergies, has had no surgeries, and is otherwise healthy. He walks and runs but is not yet toilet-trained. Physical examination reveals **numerous skin bruises** on the shins, knees, and forehead. Exam of the spine reveals a **dimple** that can be probed to an end point. No further dermatologic anomalies are seen. His parents express a desire to "not use strong pain medications" after the operation. During the discussion of **caudal blockade,** they express concern because a neighbor's child was diagnosed with a tethered cord after the pediatrician found a dimple on routine exam. After induction, an ultrasound-guided **penile block** is performed. The child requires acetaminophen and a small dose of fentanyl in the recovery room, and is discharged home with acetaminophen for further analgesia.*

DISCUSSION

1. What is the significance of a sacral dimple?

Physical examination of this patient shows a "sacral **dimple**." Although this variant may occur in up to 4% of normal children, it is a finding that is also associated with tethered cord syndrome (spinal dysraphism). The dimple present in this patient is a simple sacral dimple. These are described in literature as present in the midline within the gluteal cleft, no more than 2.5 cm above the anus, and without additional skin findings. The depth of a dimple does not differentiate a simple sacral dimple from a more complex lesion (Albert, 2016). Additional skin findings in patients with spinal dysraphism include overlying pigmentation changes, hypertrophic growths, lipomas, dermal sinuses, skin appendages, and hemangiomas (Zywicke & Rozzelle, 2011). A review of multiple studies with a total of 5,166 patients with simple sacral dimples found 3.4% of the patients had abnormal spine ultrasounds, which is less than the incidence of 4.8% of abnormal spine ultrasounds found in children without sacral dimples (Albert, 2016).

Significant medical history findings that point to underlying spinal cord and/or vertebral disease, include: progressive motor or sensory deficits, difficulty playing sports due to poor coordination of the lower extremities, frequent falls, and urologic or bowel control problems causing delayed or renewed problems with toilet training. These also include congenital malformations, such as vertebral defects, anal atresia, tracheoesophageal fistula with esophageal atresia, and radial and renal anomalies (VATER); vertebral, anal atresia, cardiac anomalies, tracheoesophageal fistula with esophageal atresia, renal defects, and limb defects (VACTERL); anorectal malformation; or cloacal exstrophy. History or physical examination that is significant for one or more of these issues should lead the anesthesiologist to consider non-neuraxial approaches to postoperative pain. A tethered cord can lead to delayed but progressive neurologic problems. Performing a caudal injection in that context may potentially confound the causality of such changes, thus it is a relative contraindication to performing the block. **Penile blocks** and systemic analgesics provide viable, safe alternatives. If there is a suggestion that the child may have a tethered cord, then further workup, in coordination with the pediatrician, should be discussed with the parents. In this boy, the **dimple** has an easily seen end point and no associated stigmata. Simple sacral dimples such as these are not associated with spinal dysraphism, and reassurance is the only intervention required.

2. What is the innervation of the penis?

The pudendal nerve (S2–S4) and the pelvic plexus give rise to penile innervation. The majority of penile sensation is carried by the pudendal nerve, which divides deep to Buck's fascia, to form the dorsal nerves to the penis. The dorsal nerves travel lateral to the superficial and deep dorsal veins and dorsal arteries on the dorsal aspect of the penis.

3. How are caudal and penile nerve blocks performed?

Caudal blocks are essentially a variant of epidural analgesia. They generally involve a single injection of local anesthetic, with or without additives, into the epidural space. The space is accessed by inserting a needle through the sacrococcygeal ligament, which overlies the sacral hiatus. The landmarks for this block are the posterior superior iliac spines, which form the base of an equilateral triangle projecting downward, with the apex approximating the sacral hiatus. Just prior to the inferior tip of the triangle are the sacral cornua, which can be palpated as two small prominences between 0.3 and 1 cm apart. These form the base of a smaller triangle with the coccyx, which is covered by the sacrococcygeal membrane. To perform a **caudal block**, the child is placed in a lateral decubitus position with knees drawn toward the chest. After confirmation of landmarks and location of the sacral hiatus, the area is prepared with a sterilizing solution such as povidone–iodine or chlorhexidine. As for any neuraxial procedure, strict attention to sterile technique is necessary during this block.

Different practitioners may select different needles for the **caudal block**. Short B-bevel needles are advocated by some for their improved tactile sensation as tissue layers are penetrated. Others prefer intravenous (IV) catheters because they are difficult to advance into the intraosseous space, thereby reducing the potential for intraosseous injection of large volumes of local anesthetic, with subsequent systemic toxicity. One advantage of the catheter technique is that it can be sterilely dressed and left in situ for either continuous infusion or redosing, in a manner similar to traditional epidural catheters.

After the needle pierces the skin just inferiorly to the sacral cornua, the needle is advanced at a 45-degree angle with the bevel facing anteriorly. This orientation of the bevel theoretically reduces the likelihood of puncturing the sacral cortex. Following puncture of the sacrococcygeal membrane, felt as a distinct "pop," the needle's angle is dropped to approximate the angle of the sacral canal. After advancing 1 to 2 mm further, the needle or catheter is advanced. At all points in the procedure, needle and catheter advancement should not meet resistance; otherwise, misplacement of the needle should be suspected, equipment withdrawn, landmarks reconfirmed, and the procedure started again.

A short length of sterile IV extension tubing, connected to and flushed with the syringe containing the caudal block solution, is attached to the needle or catheter hub. It is common practice to connect the syringe directly to the needle; however, the tubing prevents motion in the injecting hand from altering the depth or angle of the needle. Aspiration is performed to check for the presence of blood or cerebrospinal fluid (CSF). Following negative aspiration, the block solution is injected in a slow, fractionated fashion, with repeated checks for blood or CSF. Dosing for caudal blocks has traditionally been cited as up to 1 mL/kg (depending on the concentration of local anesthetic and the size of the child). As the dermatomes involved in circumcision are limited, 0.5 mL/kg will generally suffice and will reduce the potential for toxicity. Epinephrine (adrenaline) can be added to allow for monitoring of electrocardiographic (ECG) changes suggestive of intravascular injection. Some choose to avoid it because ECG changes are not entirely reliable under anesthesia, and the vasoconstrictive effects of larger doses of caudal dosing may affect blood flow to the distal cord. This in theory might cause ischemic damage to the spinal cord or nerve roots. A test dose followed by the balance of the dosing with plain local anesthetic is a reasonable compromise.

A number of different approaches to **penile nerve blocks** have been described. A dorsal penile nerve block (DPNB) is performed by inserting the needle at the inferior edge of the pubic ramus at the midline to a depth (0.5–1 cm, depending on the size of the child) where one feels the needle "pop" through the superficial fascia (Scarpa's fascia). The needle should be angled first to one side of midline, then the other. After negative aspiration, injection of local anesthetic without epinephrine commences. Any resistance to injection should prompt one to reposition the needle to avoid damaging the neurovascular bundle, which is located in the midline. Although this block covers the majority of penile innervation, it may miss lateral and ventral regions of sensation.

Ultrasound seems to have a role in improving the success rate of the **penile block**, and experience with ultrasound is growing. Ultrasound guidance allows one to visualize real-time spread of local anesthetic in the subpubic space. During this approach, local anesthetic is injected deep to Scarpa's fascia in the bilateral subpubic space, contacting Buck's fascia (Sandeman & Diley, 2007). An alternate technique was briefly described in 2015, that involves direct visualization of the neurovascular sheath with perineural administration of local anesthetic within the neurovascular bundle (Qian et al., 2015).

A ring block is performed by subcutaneous infiltration of local anesthetic around the base of the penis. Combining DPNBs with deposition of local anesthetics at different points around the base of the penis has also been described. Whichever penile nerve block is selected, care must be taken to use epinephrine-free solutions to avoid the risk of vasoconstriction-induced penile ischemia.

4. What are the potential risks of caudal versus penile blockade?

Any procedure that involves a needle puncture risks bleeding or infection. All perineural injections carry the risk of injury to nerves, although these appear to be more theoretical than actual. Large retrospective studies suggest that the risks of permanent nerve injury after caudal injection are very small (Giaufré et al., 1996; Llewellyn & Moriarty, 2007). Risks specific to caudal anesthesia include epidural hematoma or abscess, dural puncture with "high" or "complete" spinal anesthesia, postdural puncture headache, and intravascular or intraosseous injection of large volumes of local anesthetic with subsequent systemic toxicity. In addition, the performance of a caudal block requires repositioning, with attendant risk of airway compromise or vascular access dislodgement.

When assessing a patient's risk for bleeding, the physical examination and history must account for the child's developmental stage. In this child, the **numerous bruises** are compatible with an active toddler whose frequent falls will result in bruising that suggests a pattern consistent with forward (if unsteady) motion. Bruising in areas not expected to bear the brunt of falls, such as the buttocks, back, or abdomen, along with bleeding with dental hygiene, would warrant more concern.

Risks of the penile nerve block include hematoma, intravascular injection, penile ischemia (if epinephrine is used), infection, and or block failure. Despite the wide range of variety and severity of complications possible with these techniques, major adverse events are rare.

Due to the rarity of complications and paucity of good data, it is difficult to clearly say which block has higher associated risk. Clinical context should guide one's decision-making when selecting one block versus the other. If there is reason to suspect spinal deformity, then the **penile block** becomes more appealing. A caudal block might be favored if greater coverage is needed for more extensive surgical procedures (e.g., hernia repair) that may accompany the circumcision. Skin infections at the site of intended needle puncture should prompt consideration of alternative regional anesthetic approaches; if they involve the base of the penis or the penis proper, cancellation of the surgery itself may be in order. A medical history significant for bleeding disorders or ongoing use of anticoagulants is a clear contraindication to epidural analgesia.

5. Is there a clear benefit to one regional blockade versus another?

A number of studies have been done comparing different regional anesthetic approaches to postcircumcision analgesia. Most have involved a small number (~50) of patients. The most consistent

TABLE 53.1 PROS AND CONS OF CAUDAL VERSUS PENILE NERVE BLOCKS FOR POSTCIRCUMCISION ANALGESIA

Caudal Block		Penile Nerve Block	
Pros	Cons	Pros	Cons
Decreased intraoperative opioid use Good parent satisfaction Option to perform procedure without general anesthetic Well-known block	Limited duration Increased risk profile vs. penile nerve block Delayed ambulation	Decreased intraoperative opioid use Good parent satisfaction Earlier ambulation Possibly less postanesthesia care unit opioid requirement	Limited duration Increased failure rate vs. caudal

finding of these studies was similar analgesic efficacy (need for additional analgesia in the immediate postoperative period), similar incidences of nausea and vomiting, and comparable parent satisfaction, though motor blockade was seen in patients receiving caudal blocks (Cyna & Middleton, 2009). Ultrasound guidance may improve the success rate of DPNBs compared to traditional landmark techniques (Sandeman et al., 2010) and can facilitate teaching, as it provides direct visualization of local anesthetic spread instead of relying on tactile feedback. For small children, ambulation may not be a practical issue, but for larger children, the need for the parents to carry the child may sway the decision toward a penile block.

Studies comparing DPNB, ring block, and topical local anesthetics in newborns undergoing circumcision suggested more complete blockade of penile sensation with ring blocks (Irwin & Cheng, 1996) and, not surprisingly, that any attempt to provide local anesthesia was more effective than placebo at reducing signs of infant pain (Lander et al., 1997).

One particular advantage of caudal anesthesia is the option to run a continuous infusion of 3% chloroprocaine (Henderson et al., 1993) or provide a dense, single-dose block with ropivacaine or bupivacaine. This technique allows a procedure such as circumcision to be performed without general anesthesia, should that be desired (e.g., in ex-prematures to avoid postoperative apnea related to general anesthesia). A sucrose pacifier along with the continuous block may provide a comfortable experience for a young infant, although it is not effective for older infants and toddlers.

Overall, each block offers benefit to the patient, and choosing between them can be based on need for ambulation postoperatively, operator experience, and availability of appropriate equipment. When available, ultrasound can enhance the efficacy of penile nerve blocks. Table 53.1 summarizes the pros and cons of caudal versus penile nerve blocks for postcircumcision analgesia.

SUMMARY

1. Penile and caudal blocks are effective for circumcision pain, with overall data favoring penile blocks in ambulatory patients.
2. Sacral dimples merit careful examination, but simple sacral dimples are not contraindications to caudal blocks.
3. When circumcision is combined with another procedure, a caudal block poses advantages over a penile block.

ACKNOWLEDGMENTS

The authors wish to thank the first edition authors, Charles B. Eastwood and Kenneth R. Goldschneider.

ANNOTATED REFERENCES

Cyna AM, Middleton P. Caudal epidural block versus other methods of postoperative pain relief for circumcision in boys. *Cochrane Database Syst Rev.* 2009;4:CD003005.

A comprehensive review of the literature comparing caudal blockade to a variety of analgesic approaches for patients undergoing circumcision.

Lander J, Brady-Fryer B, Metcalfe J B, Nazarali S, Muttitt S. Comparison of ring block, dorsal penile nerve block, and topical anesthesia for neonatal circumcision: a randomized controlled trial. *JAMA.* 1997;278(24):2157–2162.

A well-designed study comparing multiple approaches to anesthetizing the penis. An interesting (and controversial) aspect of this study is the inclusion of a placebo control group of patients.

BIBLIOGRAPHY

Albert GW. Spine ultrasounds should not be routinely performed for patients with simple sacral dimples. *Acta Paediatr.* 2016 Aug;105(8):890–894.

Giaufré E, Dalens B, Gombert A. Epidemiology and morbidity of regional anesthesia in children: a one-year prospective survey of the French-Language Society of Pediatric Anesthesiologists. *Anesth Analg.* 1996;83(5):904–12.

Henderson K, Sethna NF, Berde CB. Continuous caudal anesthesia for inguinal hernia repair in former preterm infants. *J Clin Anesth.* 1993 Mar-Apr;5(2):129–133.

Irwin MG, Cheng W. Comparison of subcutaneous ring block of the penis with caudal epidural block for post-circumcision analgesia in children. *Anaesth Intensive Care.* 1996;24:365–367.

Llewellyn N, Moriarty A. The national pediatric epidural audit. *Pediatr Anesth.* 2007;17(6):520–533.

Margetts L, Carr A, McFadyen G, Lambert A. A comparison of caudal bupivacaine and ketamine with penile block for paediatric circumcision. *Eur J Anaesthesiol.* 2008;25:1009–1013.

Qian X, Jin X, Chen L, Pan Y, Wu B, Li J. A new ultrasound-guided dorsal penile nerve block technique for circumcision in children. *Anaesth Intensive Care.* 2015;43(5):662–663.

Sandeman DJ, Diley AV. Ultrasound guided dorsal penile nerve block in children. *Anaesth Intensive Care.* 2007;35:266–269.

Sandeman DJ, Reiner D, Dilley AV, Bennett MH, Kelly KJ. A retrospective audit of three different regional anaesthesia techniques for circumcision in infants. *Anaesth Intensive Care.* 2010;38:519–524.

Weksler N, Atias I, Klein M, Rosenztsveig V, Ovadia L, Gurman GM. Is penile block better than caudal epidural block for postcircumcision analgesia? *J Anesth.* 2005;19:36–39.

Zywicke HA, Rozzelle CJ. Sacral dimples. *Pediatr Rev.* 2011;32:109–114.

54

Neonatal Epidural

DAVID L. MOORE AND KENNETH R. GOLDSCHNEIDER

INTRODUCTION

Over the past decade, the findings surrounding neurotoxicity for the developing brain has cast a pall over the routine usage of various anesthetic drugs. This, coupled with awareness that opioid use for postoperative pain in neonates may not result in the best outcomes for these patients, has resulted in an increased use of regional techniques for postoperative pain in the neonate, particularly epidural anesthesia. The most common location for insertion of epidurals to reach the dermatomal level of the incision in adults and larger children is within a few levels of the target level, often termed "at-level" insertion. Thus local anesthetic (plus adjunct, when used) is delivered centrally covering the dermatomes surrounding the incision. However, many practitioners switch to the caudal or low-lumbar route as the primary means of epidural placement for patients weighing less than 10 kg (about 1 year of age). Caudal and low-lumbar catheters can be used for epidural blocks at any level and theoretically allow for a safer means of placement than the classic at-level loss-of-resistance technique.

LEARNING OBJECTIVES

1. Discuss the risks and benefits of regional techniques versus intravenous (IV) opioids for postoperative pain relief in infants.
2. Understand the technique of placing epidural catheters by caudal and lumbar routes.
3. Describe the methods of confirmation for correct positioning of caudal catheters in babies.

CASE PRESENTATION

A 7-day-old girl, diagnosed antenatally at 20 weeks gestation with a congenital pulmonary adenomatoid malformation, presents to the operating room for excision of the malformation via a right-sided thoracotomy at T6-T7. After smooth induction and intubation, a ***hold point (time out)*** *for epidural placement is observed. The baby is placed in the lateral decubitus position, and her back is prepared in sterile fashion for placement of a thoracic epidural catheter via the caudal space. The distance from the* ***caudal insertion*** *site to desired dermatome (T5-T6) is measured. An* ***18-gauge IV catheter*** *is introduced into the epidural space via the sacrococcygeal ligament using the loss of resistance technique. After negative aspiration for blood and cerebrospinal fluid, a 1-mL bolus of preservative-free 0.9% saline is used to confirm the minimal resistance associated with the epidural space. A styletted 20-gauge catheter is threaded via the IV catheter to the length measured previously. Once placed, the* ***position of the catheter tip is confirmed*** *with* ***ultrasound****. After removing the IV catheter, secure dressing is applied to the insertion site and a 0.5-mL/kg bolus of 0.1% ropivacaine is administered through the catheter. An* ***infusion of 0.2 mg/kg/hr of ropivacaine*** *is initiated and continued into the postoperative period, after an uneventful surgery. The baby is extubated at the end of the procedure and her postoperative course is uneventful and comfortable. The catheter is removed on postoperative day 3 (Tobias et al., 1996).*

DISCUSSION

1. What are the advantages of epidural analgesia in infants?

Patients undergoing thoracic surgery have better pain control, improved postsurgical ventilation including earlier extubation, earlier feeding, and less morbidity with epidural analgesia than with opioid analgesia (Di Pede et al., 2014). As newborns and infants have smaller respiratory reserve than older patients and a decreased ability to metabolize morphine, opioid analgesia carries the risk of sedation and respiratory depression in infants, often requiring postoperative ventilation. Prolonged intubation and mechanical ventilation can lead to iatrogenic disorders such as subglottic stenosis, ventilator-acquired pneumonia, and pulmonary barotrauma. In addition, reducing exposure to opioids reduces the chances for urinary retention, shortens the duration of postoperative ileus, and allows the baby to be awake enough to interact more with the parents after surgery. In an otherwise healthy neonate, epidural analgesia allows extubation shortly after surgery (Tobias et al., 1996). With careful handling, babies with epidurals can be held by their parents, taking full advantage of their wakefulness. In certain surgeries, such as inguinal hernias, some anesthesiologists use regional anesthesia, such as spinals, with little to no supplemental sedation to avoid the neurotoxic effects of general anesthetics (Marhofer et al., 2015). Prior to the rise of concerns regarding anesthetic neurotoxicity, neuraxial anesthesia had been used in ex-premature infants to avoid the risk of postoperative apnea associated with general anesthesia.

2. Are there risks specific to epidurals in infants?

The caudal and low-lumbar approaches to insertion of thoracic catheters are used to minimize the risk of needle trauma to the spinal cord by using an insertion point below the conus medullaris (usually around L3 in newborns). The dural sac terminates around S3 in neonates, so both techniques do have the risk of dural puncture. While there have been no known reports of nerve root injury with this technique, the catheter must still be advanced carefully to avoid injury.

For the first 6 months of life, the clearance of local anesthetics is lower than in older children. Furthermore, infants have lower blood levels of albumin and alpha-1 acid-glycoprotein, the two proteins that account for the majority of local anesthetic binding in the blood. Therefore, total dosing of local anesthetics for patients under 6 months of age must be lower than that for older patients. **Bupivacaine and ropivacaine infusion** rates up to 0.25 mg/kg/hr appear to be safe, although data on exact dosing are lacking. Of note, blood levels of bupivacaine continue to increase 24 hours into infusion, so cardiopulmonary monitoring is crucial, even if the patient looks otherwise stable in the immediate postoperative period. Intravenous administration of intralipid for resuscitation and successful treatment of local anesthetic cardiovascular toxicity in neonates has been noted in the literature (Lin & Aronson, 2010).

2-chloroprocaine is an interesting alternative local anesthetic that may have a role for infants. As an ester, it has a very short half-life, even in fetal blood, and infusion of this drug can be administered for long periods without accumulation (Kuhnert et al., 1986). The tip of the catheter has to be accurately placed at the desired dermatome, as this anesthetic is usually administered alone or in conjunction with clonidine. Intravenous opioids may be administered to supplement this drug, if needed.

The risk of infection is theoretically higher with the caudal approach to neuraxial analgesia because a higher percentage of colonization has been found in caudal catheters compared to lumbar catheters. This is due in part to proximity to the anus but can also potentially be due to the difficulty in maintaining sterile dressings. Contamination of the insertion site by stool is not uncommon and is an indication to remove the catheter. This can be attenuated by tunneling the catheter.

The risk of bleeding during catheter placement may be higher in neonates and young infants who have not received vitamin K supplementation, as this vitamin is critical to the clotting factor pathways but does not cross the placenta. Knowing the vitamin K supplementation status in infants is worthwhile prior to surgery and neuraxial injection.

3. What are the alternative techniques for placing catheters in the thoracic epidural space in infants?

The caudal approach to thoracic catheter placement is presented in this case scenario. It takes advantage of well-known landmarks and is truly just an extension of a very common block (Bösenberg et al., 1988). An **18-gauge IV catheter** is inserted as an introducer for the catheter, although a Crawford or Tuohy needle may also be used. The epidural catheter is then threaded through it, preceded by approximately 1-mL bolus of preservative-free 0.9% saline to open up the epidural space and facilitate threading of the catheter. The disadvantage of this technique is that the insertion site is in close proximity to the intergluteal fold and anus, which limits the ability to maintain sterility postoperatively. The intergluteal fold tends to force the center of the dressing off the skin, allowing urine or feces to get underneath. This logistical problem can limit how long the catheter remains in place. Tunneling of the catheter can reduce rates of bacterial colonization and is worth considering when using the caudal approach (Bubeck et al., 2004).

A second technique is less familiar to many but helps to solve some issues. The modified Taylor technique uses the L5-S1 interspace as the access point (Gunter, 2000). This interspace is the largest in the spinal column and easily allows insertion of an 18-gauge Crawford needle with loss of resistance to preservative-free 0.9% saline or air. The operator should be aware that the depth is usually around 1 cm, and the ligaments are much softer than those of older children, necessitating a careful assessment and detection of loss of resistance. The Crawford needle offers the advantage of being very blunt compared with a Tuohy needle, which enhances the feel of loss of resistance with such soft tissues and theoretically decreases the length of needle in the epidural space when loss of resistance is appreciated. The angle of insertion should be approximately 45 degrees, and angled cephalad, to allow passage of the catheter. Once loss of resistance is appreciated, approximately 1 mL of saline is injected to distend the epidural space, prior to threading the catheter. Advancement of the catheter should be very easy. Any resistance should result in withdrawal of the catheter and re-advancement after repositioning of the catheter or patient. (see later discussion). While less familiar, this technique is easily learned and allows the dressing to be placed above the intergluteal fold and away from the anus.

As with any procedure, a **hold point** (also referred to as a **time out**) should be observed prior to catheter placement, to confirm that the correct procedure is being performed, with the proper equipment and on the correct patient, who is in optimal position. This process is common practice to avoid wrong-site procedures, to ensure that the needed equipment is available and necessary preparations have occurred prior to starting the procedure.

4. If the catheter will not advance, what are techniques to correct this situation?

It is important that the catheter advances easily through the epidural space to avoid traumatic injury to the structures within the spinal canal. Table 54.1 lists approaches to the catheter that is difficult to advance. Of the different techniques that may be used (see later discussion), ultrasound has surpassed fluoroscopy as the primary means for identifying adequate positioning and trajectory of catheters as they are being placed. Withdrawing catheters through a Tuohy needle when malpositionining is identified, is often discouraged due to the risk of shearing off a portion of catheter; however, this risk must be weighed against the risks of reinserting the needle.

5. What are the options for confirming placement of the catheter tip?

Correct positioning of a caudal catheter placed in a blind fashion is not guaranteed (Valairucha et al., 2002). Real-time techniques for assessment include ultrasound, fluoroscopy, and stimulation.

TABLE 54.1 SOLUTIONS FOR INABILITY TO THREAD CATHETER

Lumbar Approach
Immediate resistance
Carefully withdraw catheter; inject ~1 mL saline to recheck loss of resistance and to distend space; lower needle to a more acute angle, and align catheter trajectory with spine.
Delayed resistance
Withdraw catheter ~1 cm and gently twist catheter to change angle slightly while advancing; reduce flexion of spine by repositioning child; consider fluoroscopy to confirm trajectory and rule out coiling of catheter.
Caudal Approach
Immediate resistance
Use a stylet, if not used initially; remove catheter and inject with ~1 mL saline to confirm low resistance and to distend the epidural space; may also detect subcutaneous placement.
Delayed resistance
Use a stylet, if not used initially; withdraw catheter 1 to 2 cm, twirl catheter 90 to 180 degrees, and re-advance; consider fluoroscopic guidance to rule out coiling; gently flex or extend the patient's spine.

Ultrasound is a rapid confirmation technique that does not expose the child to radiation. It is limited to infants under 6 months of age due to the technical difficulty in visualization as the spinous processes begin to ossify (Tsui & Suresh, 2010; Willschke et al., 2007). **Fluoroscopy** can identify the catheter as it is being threaded up, assuming the catheter is radio-paque or has a stylet. Alternatively, a small amount of neurocompatible radiocontrast can be used to confirm placement after the stylet is removed. (usually 0.5 mL will opacify the catheter and extrude enough from the tip to confirm dermatomal level) Patient exposure to radiation and availability of a portable image intensifier are limitations to this approach. Lastly, radiographs can be used, but these lead to delays, especially if placement is incorrect and requires readjustment and repeat confirmation. Certainly, if a catheter is feared to have become dislodged postoperatively, a radiograph taken after a small bolus of neurocompatible contrast can confirm placement and spread of medication. Lastly, **stimulating** catheters can be used to create somatic movement corresponding to the dermatomal level traversed by the catheter as it is threaded (Tsui et al., 2004). Amperage acts as a secondary safety monitor, as extremely low-current requirements suggest intrathecal placement.

SUMMARY

1. Both lumbar (modified Taylor approach) and caudal approaches are viable routes for placing epidural catheters at the thoracic level in babies.
2. Monitoring of epidural infusions in infants differs due to the need to watch for delayed local anesthetic toxicity.
3. Confirmation of catheter placement is best done in real time, using either fluoroscopy, stimulation, or ultrasound.

ANNOTATED REFERENCES

Bösenberg AT, Bland BA, Schulte-Steinberg O, Downing JW. Thoracic epidural anesthesia via caudal route in infants. *Anesthesiology.* 1988;69:265–269.

This is a landmark article in which the authors demonstrate this technique.

Valairucha S, Seefelder C, Houck C. Thoracic epidural catheters placed by the caudal route in infants: the importance of radiographic confirmation. *Pediatr Anesth.* 2002;12:424–428.

This report shows the large error rate in placement of catheters inserted via the caudal route, explaining the need to confirm the position of the catheter.

BIBLIOGRAPHY

Anand K. Pharmacological approaches to the management of pain in the neonatal intensive care unit. *J Perinatol.* 2007;27:S4–S11.

Bösenberg AT. Epidural analgesia for major neonatal surgery. *Pediatr Anesth.* 1998;8:479–483.

Bubeck J, Boos K, Krause H, Thies KC. Subcutaneous tunneling of caudal catheters reduces the rate of bacterial colonization to that of lumbar epidural catheters. *Anesth Analg.* 2004 Sep;99(3):689–693.

Di Pede A, Morini F, Lombardi MH, et al. Comparison of regional anesthesia versus systemic analgesia for post-thoracotomy care of infants. *Pediatr Anesth.* 2014;24(6):569–573.

Flandin-Blety C, Barrier G. Accidents following extradural analgesia in children: the results of a retrospective study. *Pediatr Anesth.* 1995;5(1):41–46.

Gunter JB. Thoracic epidural anesthesia via the modified Taylor approach in infants. *Reg Anesth Pain Med.* 2000;25(6):561–565.

Guruswamy V, Roberts S, Arnold P, Potter F. Anaesthetic management of a neonate with congenital cyst adenoid malformation. *Br J Anaesth.* 2005;95(2):240–242.

Kuhnert BR, Kuhnert PM, Philipson EH, Syracuse CD, Kaine CJ, Yun CH. The half-life of 2-chloroprocaine. *Anesth Analg.* 1986;65 (3):273–278.

Lin EP, Aronson LA. Successful resuscitation of bupivacaine induced cardiotoxicity in a neonate. *Pediatr Anesth.* 2010;20(10):955–957.

Marhofer P, Keplinger M, Klug W, Metzelder ML. Awake caudals and epidurals should be used more frequently in neonates and infants. *Pediatr Anesth.* 2015;25(1):93–99.

Tobias JD, Rasmussen GE, Holcomb GW 3rd, Brock JW 3rd, Morgan WM 3rd. Continuous caudal anaesthesia with chloroprocaine as an adjunct to general anaesthesia in neonates. *Can J Anaesth.* 1996;43(1):69–72.

Tsui BC, Suresh S. Ultrasound imaging for regional anesthesia in infants, children and adolescents: a review of current literature and its application in the practice of neuraxial blocks. *Anesthesiology.* 2010;112(3):719–728.

Tsui BC, Wagner A, Cave D, Kearney R. Thoracic and lumbar epidural analgesia via the caudal approach using electrical stimulation guidance in pediatric patients: a review of 289 patients. *Anesthesiology.* 2004;100(3):683–689.

Willschke H, Bosenberg A, Marhofer P, et al. Epidural catheter placement in neonates: sonoanatomy and feasibility of ultrasonographic guidance in term and preterm neonates. *Reg Anesth Pain Med.* 2007;32(1):34–40.

55

Complex Regional Pain Syndrome for Ambulatory Surgery

CARO MONICO

INTRODUCTION

Complex regional pain syndrome (CRPS) is a disease of the nervous system (abnormal processing by both central and peripheral components) that is characterized by pain out of proportion to the inciting event and is often accompanied by sensory disturbances (allodynia and hyperalgesia), motor/trophic (dystonic reactions, hair and nail growth), vasomotor (swelling, temperature asymmetry between the affected and nonaffected limb), and sudomotor (sweating) signs and symptoms. CRPS is a challenging clinical presentation for many pediatric anesthesiologists due to the heterogeneity of the presentation from one patient to the next, but, even in the same patient, symptoms can and do change through the course of the disease. A biopsychosocial approach is recommended when conducting the initial evaluation of CRPS patients.

LEARNING OBJECTIVES

1. Recognize that chronic pain is a biopsychosocial problem and needs to be managed with an interdisciplinary approach.
2. Identify key features from the history and examination that can help make the diagnosis.
3. Discuss the role of the anesthesiologist and next best steps in managing a patient with CRPS in the ambulatory setting.

CASE PRESENTATION

Samantha is a 12-year-old, 35-kg girl with a history of left foot ***complex regional pain syndrome (CRPS).*** *She presents to the emergency department (ED) with excruciating (9/10) pain in her left foot. Samantha reports hitting her foot on the dining room table this evening, which caused an immediate and intense increase in her left foot pain. Her CRPS began 3 months previously: after a minor twist of her ankle during gymnastic practice, she suddenly developed pain in the heel of her left foot. The pain progressed over 2 days to the point she was unable to bear weight; her foot developed purple mottling and felt cold. No inflammatory, orthopedic, thrombotic, or neurologic etiology was found. The bone scan demonstrated delayed uptake in her left foot, and magnetic resonance imaging showed increased fluid content of the marrow of the left hind foot. Her physician prescribed gabapentin 100 mg twice a day (BID), which was increased over 3 days to 200 mg three times a day (TID). She has used crutches to ambulate since and takes only simple analgesics at home to relieve pain. Samantha has been unable to bear weight, undergo the prescribed physiotherapy, or attend school due to tiredness and pain. Simple analgesics have been ineffective, while codeine and tramadol have caused nausea and retching. Gabapentin improved the pain initially, but this effect diminished over time. She is on no other medication and has no other past medical history.*

The current heel pain is described as a constant burning sensation, associated with shooting pains up to her knee; these sensations are variable in intensity and associated with color and temperature changes. The pain is aggravated with light touch (such as putting on a sock), weight bearing, and leaving the foot in a dependent position. There are no other relieving factors. Her pain is worse at night, and sleep is difficult due to pain from the touch of blankets and the recurrent shooting pains. Samantha's appetite, drive, energy, affect, and eating behavior are normal. On *examination, Samantha is pleasant and interactive. She is afebrile, with normal vital signs. There is no bruising, laceration, or swelling; however, her foot becomes mottled when hanging in a dependent position. Her distal left leg is slightly cooler than her right, and there is intense pain to light touch on the heel of the left foot, which limits examination. When ambulating, she is able to put pressure on the anterior half of her left foot but not her heel. X-ray of her foot is normal. Samantha is given intravenous ketorolac 18 mg, oral acetaminophen (paracetamol) (500 mg), and oral clonidine (40 mcg) with moderate effect after 30 minutes. Following a discussion with the chronic pain management team (***CPMT***), she is given an outpatient pain clinic appointment in 1 week, where she will see an* ***interdisciplinary team*** *comprising a* ***physical therapist****, a* ***psychologist****, and a pain physician and nurse. Her discharge medications are gabapentin 300 mg TID, amitriptyline 10 mg at bedtime, melatonin 3 mg at bedtime, and once-daily topical 5% lidocaine patches.*

DISCUSSION

1. What is CRPS?

CRPS is an unusual condition where pathophysiological changes within the peripheral and central nervous system result in severe pain. The pain is often associated with allodynia (pain from a stimulus that is not normally painful), hyperalgesia (greater-than-normal sensitivity to a painful stimulus or a lowered pain threshold), abnormal sudomotor activity, and changes in the nails, bones, and hair of the affected painful part. A unique feature of CRPS is that pain and the accompanying sensory disturbances are nondermatomal in distribution and vasomotor changes do not obey a vascular territory. However, signs vary between patients, and in individual patients, signs vary with time. Specific diagnostic criteria are now well established (Harden et al., 2007). In children **CRPS** may occur as the result of injury, but often there is no predisposing event. The pain of **CRPS** is of neuropathic nature (shooting/burning character) and often does not respond to medications targeted to nociceptive or inflammatory types of pain.

2. What are the main issues for consideration in the ED?

A thorough history and examination should be performed to *confirm the diagnosis* of CRPS and *exclude an acute remediable cause* for the exacerbation of pain. During this evaluation, it is important to *acknowledge and believe* that the child has pain. Determine the factors, other than pain, that may have significant impact on the child's life, including altered mood or poor sleep, and also to plan appropriate discharge medications. Clarify that the purpose of discharge medications is to provide some analgesia in order to facilitate the initiation and maintenance of physiotherapy and not to provide a completely pain-free state. Medications that are prescribed must be tailored to individual patients. A multimodal approach starting with simple medications is a suitable approach. Follow-up should be organized for the child such that long-term interdisciplinary management can be instituted by a **CPMT**. Wherever possible, avoid "medicalization" and admission. In an extremely busy ED this may not be possible, and a brief admission may be needed to provide analgesia and develop a therapeutic plan.

When faced with a child with CRPS, physicians may struggle with reconciling the pain intensity, psychological distress, and disability experienced by the child with a lack of findings or correspondent mechanism of injury (Logan et al., 2013). A justified concern on the part of physicians of missing occult fractures, cancers, and/or infections can result in unnecessary diagnostic testing and inappropriate medical referrals which may further delay the diagnosis. As a result, a child with CRPS may end up being evaluated by orthopedic surgeons, sports medicine specialists, general pediatricians, neurologists, and rheumatologists before being seen by a pain medicine practitioner in a pediatric chronic pain clinic. In a recent review on the topic, the time to diagnosis varied from 1 to 41 weeks, reflecting the challenge faced by CRPS patients and clinicians alike (Borucki, 2015). Due to the variability in the presenting symptoms of CRPS, there is a lack of an established pediatric diagnostic criteria as well as a poor conceptualization of the pediatric form of the disease.

3. How do we make the diagnosis of CRPS?

Prompt recognition and rehabilitation of the involved extremity are the most important steps in the treatment of CRPS; this begins with obtaining a focused history and physical examination that includes a detailed neurologic exam. During history taking, the clinician should elicit a recount of injuries, travel, recent illnesses, systemic symptoms like fevers, night sweats, unintended weight loss, and so on. A review of systems and a complete medical and surgical history should also be obtained as CRPS is a diagnosis that should be made only after excluding other conditions that could account for the degree of pain and dysfunction. The clinician should listen attentively for neuropathic pain-type descriptors (burning, shooting, stabbing), allodynia (pain caused by an action that is not normally painful like bed sheets, water), and dysesthesia (pins and needles sensation, numbness). Pain-related disturbances in sleep onset and maintenance, school functioning (school attendance, grades), physical activity (sports, physical education), and social functioning should also be assessed. The physical exam begins when the patient enters the room and pain behaviors become manifest. For example, patients with CRPS may adopt protective equipment over a limb to warn others to avoid touch or may avoid weight bearing or wearing socks and shoes in the case of lower extremity CRPS. On physical exam, the clinician should assess passive and active range of motion starting with the most distal joint. Inspection of the affected limb can reveal swelling; red, blue, or mottled skin appearance; hair growth differences; and so on. Motor strength testing and a sensory examination can sometimes be limited by pain but should be performed whenever possible. The clinician should gauge motor strength and sensory deficits to light touch, cold temperature/pinprick, and proprioception deficits. Skin temperature differences between the affected and nonaffected limb should be obtained using an infrared thermometer. Temperature differences between the affected and nonaffected limb are more common in pediatric patients (Stanton-Hicks, 2010). A biopsychosocial approach is recommended when conducting the initial evaluation of CRPS patients; the initial history intake and examination should be done by an interdisciplinary team composed of a pain psychologist, a physical therapist, and a pain physician. CRPS remains a clinical diagnosis as there are no validated pediatric-specific diagnostic criteria. The Budapest Criteria relies on a constellation of signs and symptoms in adult patients with CRPS and has a near 100% (0.99) sensitivity and 70% to 80% specificity. While the Budapest Criteria has not been validated in pediatrics, it is a valuable tool in the clinical setting because it inventories in a uniform fashion, important features of CRPS and encourages the clinician to exclude the diagnosis in the presence of other medical illnesses.

4. Can we predict who will get CRPS?

It is impossible to predict which patients will develop CRPS after surgery, traumatic injuries, or surgically treated traumatic injuries. Like adult CRPS, pediatric CRPS predominately affects females; girls are 6 times more likely than boys to develop CRPS. CRPS is also far more common in the adolescent group (peak age of onset is 12–13). Involvement of a lower extremity is approximately 6 times more common than upper extremity CRPS, and the more common etiology of CRPS in children and adolescents is posttraumatic.

CRPS can develop before and after surgery, particularly in the setting of a prolonged period of immobilization and when restrictions on weight bearing have been placed. Based on an adult data from the Japanese Diagnosis Procedure Combination database, there may be higher risk of developing CRPS after repair of fractures s (open reduction and internal fixation) to the distal end of either the upper or lower limbs. This study also found that longer anesthetics were associated with a higher incidence of CRPS, although it is not known if the longer anesthesia times in this study were due to longer operative time and therefore more complicated surgical repair or if they were associated with longer tourniquet times which have been linked to nerve compression or nerve ischemia. Interestingly, regional anesthesia did not have an impact on the prevalence of CRPS in this study population.

In addition, another adult study found that, in patients with traumatic hand injuries, a CRPS diagnosis was more common in those with a crush injury as well as those with a pain score ≥5 in the first 3 days after surgery (Savas, 2018).

5. How does the pediatric anesthesiologist treat CRPS in the ambulatory setting?

A pediatric anesthesiologist will rarely encounter CRPS in his or her everyday operating room activities. However, they may be involved in the care of

CRPS patients who are admitted to the hospital for pain management or rehabilitation needs and require consultation by the inpatient pain service. Many orthopedic and hand surgeons are familiar with CRPS by virtue of the types of operations they perform. They are unlikely to operate on a child with known CRPS or the unrecognized constellation of CRPS symptoms, particularly if the operation is on the same limb affected by CRPS, unless it is absolutely necessary. Given the complexity of CRPS and the potential for a complicated postoperative pain course, the patient with active CRPS may not be the best candidate for ambulatory surgery but instead may require hospital admission to focus on pain management and rehabilitation after surgery.

If the clinical environment allows for a preoperative identification of patients with CRPS or suspected CRPS, a pain consultation, preferably in conjunction with the chronic pain team, should be obtained. There is no one-size-fits-all for the treatment of patients with CRPS, and there is very little published evidence to support specific pharmacological therapies in children with CRPS. Recommendations are governed by adult studies, pediatric case reports, expert opinion, and the experience and expertise of the pain physician/team dealing with the child (Berde & Lebel, 2005). Simple medications and opioids may be useful if there is an inflammatory or traumatic element to the acute exacerbation of pain but may not be effective for CRPS pain.

6. Should medications or an interventional block be performed in the ambulatory surgical setting?

Medications are used to provide some analgesia to facilitate the initiation and maintenance of physiotherapy. These are tailored to the individual patient and are not intended to provide a completely pain-free state. A multimodal approach using simple medications (gabapentinoids or tricyclic antidepressants) first is a suitable approach. Similarly, interventional blocks should not be used as a "magic wand" to minimize pain but as a means to facilitate paced physical therapy and improve function. The ambulatory surgical setting is not the arena for that purpose. Furthermore, all interventions (medications and invasive intervention) should not be initiated without proper follow-up; they should also be preferentially performed by physician experts in these techniques in children after appropriate psychological screening and preparation of patients and families.

7. What is the long-term management strategy for CRPS?

An interdisciplinary team that includes the child, the family, the family physician, a physiotherapist, psychologist, pain physician, pain nurse, occupational therapist, and a pharmacist, when available, should make up the management team for a child with CRPS. Families may engage in their own research efforts through online community chat rooms and personal websites, so it is important to dispel any misinformation from the outset. Families are often surprised to learn that because of the neuroplasticity of the young brain, pediatric CRPS has excellent outcomes in comparison to adult CRPS. It is extremely important to educate families about the importance of committing to physical therapy and biobehavioral treatment as the majority of pediatric patients do well without additional pharmacologic or interventional interventions. Medications (gabapentinoids, tricyclic antidepressants) can be helpful particularly for those patients with sleep disturbances due to pain. For patients who are unable to participate in physical therapy due to extreme allodynia, continuous neuraxial techniques or peripheral nerve catheters have been used as a bridge to facilitate rehabilitation.

A self-management approach should be promoted from the beginning, allowing children and adolescents to take control of their symptoms and improve day-to-day biopsychosocial functioning (i.e., a functional rehabilitation approach that focuses on sleep, eating, physical activity, mood, and social and school function). The pain and the consequences of pain, such as poor sleep or anxiety, are managed using a combination of concurrent therapies (Fig. 55.1). These include paced and graded physical activity, psychological support, and psychological therapies used in conjunction with medical interventions (medications or interventional blocks). The principal modality that will improve pain and function in children with CRPS is physical therapy. Key to success is early appropriate intervention, education for the child and family, and good communication between team members. The interdisciplinary approach has been shown to be effective for pediatric chronic pain (Eccleston et al., 2003; Logan et al., 2012; Maynard et al., 2010; Sherry et al., 1999; Stanton-Hicks, 2010).

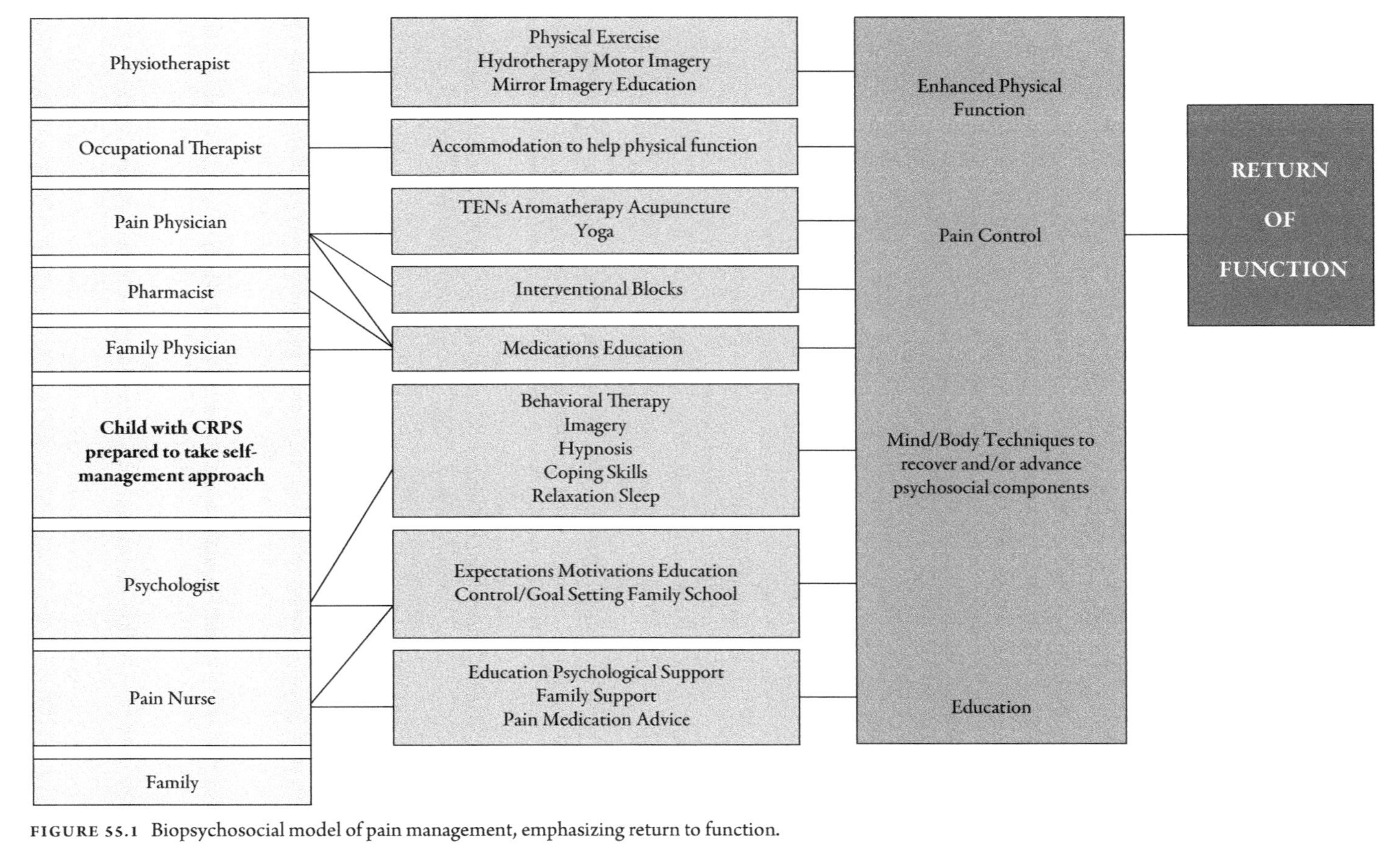

FIGURE 55.1 Biopsychosocial model of pain management, emphasizing return to function.

TABLE 55.1 PHARMACOLOGICAL OPTIONS FOR CHILDREN WITH CRPS

Drug	Characteristics
Gabapentin	***Action***: Binds the alpha-2-delta subunit of the voltage-dependent calcium channel in the central nervous system ***Metabolism:*** None; renal excretion ***Drug interactions***: None; no effect on hepatic microsomal enzymes ***Side effects***: Somnolence, dizziness, peripheral edema, weight gain, and mood swings (including suicidal ideation) ***Comment***: Has a withdrawal syndrome; should be weaned off
Pregabalin	***Action, metabolism, drug interactions, side effects, withdrawal syndrome***: As per gabapentin ***Dosing***: Either once or twice a day ***Comment***: Can be titrated more rapidly than gabapentin
Amitriptyline	***Action***: Prevents the reuptake of serotonin and norepinephrine ***Metabolism***: Hepatic, subject to genetic variance in enzymatic function ***Drug interactions***: Multiple, especially inhibitors of CYP 2D6 (e.g., SSRIs) and those that prolong cardiac QTc interval ***Side effects***: Sedation, dry mouth, blurred vision, weight gain, orthostatic hypotension, and prolonged QTc ***Comment***: An ECG should be strongly considered before starting TCA therapy. Nortriptyline is less sedating, doxepin less anticholinergic. Should be weaned off
Topical lidocaine 5% patch	***Action***: Blockade of upregulated sodium channel receptors in injured nerves ***Metabolism***: N/A, absorption negligible ***Drug interactions***: N/A, absorption negligible ***Side effects***: Mild skin reactions ***Comment***: Useful for very localized CRPS pain
Tramadol	***Action***: Weak μ opioid receptor agonist. Also inhibits spinal cord release of serotonin and reuptake of norepinephrine ***Metabolism***: A pro-drug. Dependent on hepatic microsomal system: hence, interindividual, pharmacogenetic variability ***Drug interactions***: Multiple, especially inhibitors of hepatic P450 systems and SSRIs ***Side effects***: Nausea and vomiting ***Comment***: Serotonin toxicity possible, especially if co-administered with SSRIs, SNRIs, MAOIs, or TCAs. Dose reduction is advised with renal impairment
Opioids	***Action***: Mu-antagonist primarily ***Metabolism***: Hepatic ***Drug interactions***: Additive with sedating medications, alcohol ***Side effects***: Sedation, nausea, constipation, pruritus ***Comment***: Can help to tolerate physiotherapy. Long-term use rarely indicated
Clonidine	***Action***: Selective α2 adrenoceptor agonist with analgesic, sedative, anxiolytic, and cardiovascular effects ***Metabolism***: Hepatic and renal (roughly 50/50) ***Drug interactions***: Beta-blockers, TCAs ***Side effects***: Sedation, dry mouth, hypotension ***Comment***: A useful adjunct; can be used as an opioid-sparing agent

Note: Combined therapy with gabapentin/pregabalin and a TCA seems to be more efficacious than either modality given alone.

CRPS = complex regional pain syndrome; ECG = electrocardiogram; TCA = tricyclic antidepressant; NA = not applicable; SSRI = selective serotonin reuptake inhibitor; SNRI = serotonin–norepinephrine reuptake inhibitor; MAOI = monoamine oxidase inhibitor.

Improvement may take weeks or months. Some children will make a full recovery, others will achieve return to function with ongoing pain, and others may progress to adult life with ongoing complex pain problems.

SUMMARY

1. As for all children with complex needs, appropriate care of CRPS requires a careful history and examination.
2. Emergency care in the ED for these patients requires titration of appropriate medication to provide comfort.
3. Patients should be discharged whenever possible, with a plan for appropriate long-term care, including enough medications to help control their symptoms until they can be seen by a CPMT. Table 55.1 describes different drug modalities for treating CRPS and their mode of action.

ANNOTATED REFERENCES

Berde CB, Lebel A. Complex regional pain syndromes in children and adolescents. *Anesthesiology.* 2005;102(2):252–255.

A good overview on CRPS; includes the differences between the condition in children/adolescents and adults. Also critically appraises the evidence for modalities of treatment, including intravenous regional blockade and continuous nerve blocks.

Harden RN, Bruehl S, Stanton-Hicks M, Wilson PR. Proposed new diagnostic criteria for complex regional pain syndrome. *Pain Med.* 2007;8:326–331.

Clarifies the diagnostic criteria for CRPS.

BIBLIOGRAPHY

Eccleston C, Malleson PN, Clinch J, Connell Sourbut C. Chronic pain in adolescents: evaluation of a program of interdisciplinary cognitive behavior therapy (ICBT). *Arch Dis Child.* 2003;88:881–885.

Gilron I, Bailey JM, Tu D, Holden RR, Jackson AC, Houlden RL. Nortriptyline and gabapentin, alone and in combination for neuropathic pain: a double blind randomized controlled crossover trial. *Lancet.* 2009;374(9697):1252–1261.

Hoebert M, van der Heijden KB, van Geijlswijk IM, Smits MG. Long-term follow-up of melatonin treatment in children with ADHD and chronic sleep onset insomnia. *J Pineal Res.* 2009;47(1):1–7.

Khaliq W, Alam S, Puri N. Topical lidocaine for treatment of post herpetic neuralgia, *Cochrane Database Syst Rev.* 2007;18:CD004846.

Logan DE, Carpino EA, Chiang G, et al. A day-hospital approach to treatment of pediatric complex regional pain syndrome: initial functional outcomes. *Clin J Pain.* 2012;28:766–774.

Logan DF, Williams SE, Carullo VP, et al. Children and adolescents with complex regional pain syndrome: more psychologically distressed than other children in pain? *Pain Res Manag.* 2013;18:87–93.

Perry TL. Neurontin: clinical pharmacologic opinion of Dr. Thomas L. Perry. http://dida.library.ucsf.edu/pdf/oxx18p10

Savaş S, İnal EE, Yavuz DD, Uslusoy F, Altuntaş SH, Aydın MA. Risk factors for complex regional pain syndrome in patients with surgically treated traumatic injuries attending hand therapy. *J Hand Ther.* 2018 Apr–Jun;31(2):250–254.

Sherry DD, Wallace CA, Kelley C, Kidder M, Sapp L. Short- and long-term outcomes of children with CRPS type 1 treated with exercise therapy. *Clin J Pain.* 1999;15:218–223.

Stanton-Hicks M. Plasticity of complex regional pain syndrome (CRPS) in children. *Pain Med.* 2010;11:1216–1223.

56

Perioperative Management of the Child Following an Extremity Amputation

JAMIE W. SINTON

INTRODUCTION

Limb amputations in children are relatively rare and most commonly occur as a result of trauma or malignancy. Traumatic events resulting in limb amputation in children include misadventures with lawnmowers, all-terrain vehicles, and the like. Bone malignancies constitute a large proportion of the indications for limb amputation. The most common appendicular skeletal malignancies in children include osteosarcoma followed by Ewing's sarcoma. These malignancies commonly occur in the distal femoral metaphysis or the proximal tibia.

> **LEARNING OBJECTIVES**
> 1. Explain the types of pain experienced in the perioperative period for children undergoing limb amputation.
> 2. Identify strategies for managing acute postoperative, neuropathic, and phantom limb pain (PLP) for amputation patients.
> 3. Assess the methods available for the prevention of chronic postsurgical pain.

CASE PRESENTATION

Marco is a 12-year-old, 35-kg boy with a history of left distal femur pain. He presents to the operating room with moderate (6/10) pain in his left femur, tenderness of left knee, and obvious deformity due to osteosarcoma. He ambulates with crutches and takes acetaminophen and ibuprofen for analgesia at home.

The current leg pain is a constant burning sensation. The pain is aggravated by long periods of activity. There are no relieving factors. On examination, Marco is pleasant and interactive. He is afebrile, with normal vital signs. There is no bruising or laceration, and his range of motion is restricted for knee flexion and extension.

The surgeon plans to perform an above-the-knee amputation today.

DISCUSSION

1. What is osteosarcoma? How is it treated?

Osteosarcoma is the most common bone malignancy in children. The tumor comprises spindle cells that produce osteoid. Diagnosis involves a plain film with soft tissue mass supported by elevations of alkaline phosphatase and lactate dehydrogenase. Treatment commonly involves 10 weeks of neoadjuvant chemotherapy followed by complete surgical resection with or without amputation. Disease-free survival at 3 years is approximately 65% (Marina et al., 2004).

2. How common is pre-existing preoperative pain in patients with osteosarcoma?

The most common presentation of osteosarcoma is pain and swelling at the tumor site, therefore preoperative pain is almost universal. Trauma or exercise often precipitates the pain and is the impetus for seeking medical attention (Marina et al., 2004).

3. Can Marco's pain be quantified with biologic markers?

Objectively quantifying pain with the use of inflammatory biomarkers such as interleukin-6, tumor necrosis factor-alpha, and so on has been unsuccessful at best. The International Association for the Study of Pain (IASP; 2016) classifies pain as a sensory experience. To date, no definitive way of biologically quantifying pain has been reported. Pain assessment relies on history and physical exam.

4. Does preoperative treatment of preexisting pain improve pain outcomes after surgery?

Yes, Marco's postoperative pain may mirror his preoperative pain (Nikolajsen & Jensen, 2001). A study by Bach et al (1988) randomized adult patients undergoing amputation to receive either preoperative epidurals with morphine and bupivacaine, for 3 days prior to surgery or no pre-operative analgesia (control group). The group randomized to lumbar epidural analgesia remained largely free of PLP at 7 days, 6 months, and 1 year while the control group had more PLP at each time period.

5. What types of postoperative pain can be expected?

Pain sources following surgery are multifactorial. Acute postoperative nociceptive pain can be expected. Following the immediate postoperative period, persistent nociceptive pain can occur with physical therapy. Neuropathic pain is common and results from intraoperative neural trauma. Phantom limb sensations or pain is also a common finding (Anghelescu et al., 2011).

6. What strategies can be used to prevent and treat acute nociceptive postoperative pain? Why is this important?

Many strategies can be employed such as opioids, nonsteroidal anti-inflammatory drugs, opioid-acetaminophen combinations, continuous epidural infusion, tricyclic antidepressants, anticonvulsants, local anesthetic wound infiltration, and continuous peripheral nerve blockade (Anghelescu et al., 2011).

Pain treatment is important primarily for patient comfort but also for return to baseline function, stress, psychologic well-being, and prevention of chronic pain.

7. How common is neuropathic pain following amputation? Does Marco's pain have neuropathic features? What treatments could be recommended?

Neuropathic pain is commonly characterized by tingling, burning, and "pins and needles" sensations. The IASP defines neuropathic pain as pain arising as a direct consequence of a lesion or disease affecting the somatosensory system. It occurs in approximately 83% of pediatric patients following amputation for osteosarcoma (Anghelescu et al., 2017).

The burning sensations in Marco's leg are characteristic of neuropathic pain. Causes of neuropathic pain in this population can be related to chemotherapy or operative neural stretch and injury. Chemotherapeutic agents associated with persistent neuropathic pain include vincristine, cisplatin, and paclitaxel (Friedrichsdorf & Nugent, 2013). Children with osteosarcoma are often prescribed cisplatin, doxorubicin, and/or high-dose methotrexate (Marina et al., 2004).

Nonpharmacologic therapy varies widely, and literature support for any modality is weak at best and only presented in adult literature. Suggested therapies include dietary changes to reduce systemic inflammation, acupuncture, rehabilitation, reiki, and supportive care.

Pharmacologic options include gabapentin, amitriptyline, and methadone. Initiation of gabapentin 3 to 5 days in advance of surgery may reduce neuropathic pain following surgery (Carroll et al., 2013).

8. Is Marco likely to develop phantom limb sensations after surgery?

As many as 100% of patients develop phantom limb sensations and the majority develop PLP following amputation (Krane & Heller, 1995). Children under the age of 4 years are less likely to experience PLP (Pirowska et al., 2014). Children with congenital limb deficiency are less likely to experience PLP than children requiring amputations following surgery or trauma (Wilkins et al., 1998). Unfortunately, there is no universally effective treatment once the pain is established.

9. What is stump pain? Is Marco likely to develop stump pain after surgery?

Stump pain is localized to the stump of the amputated extremity. Commonly, postoperative phantom limb sensations begin with a feeling of a normal-sized limb. Over time, the phantom limb begins to feel smaller and may telescope into the area occupied by the stump. This results in stump pain. Prevention of PLP may reduce stump pain as well (Bach et al., 1988).

10. Could Marco develop chronic postsurgical pain? Could this be prevented?

Yes, approximately 10% of adults develop chronic postsurgical pain and the incidence is unclear in children. Prevention of chronic postsurgical pain depends on several factors. Risk reduction begins with adequate treatment of acute postoperative pain. Untreated acute pain predisposes to the development of chronic pain. Other methods to reduce this phenomenon vary by type of pain, and guidelines have been proposed for adults: gabapentin can be administered 2 hours pre-incision then 3 times per day for 14 days postoperatively. Ketamine 0.5 mg/kg pre-incision can be administered as a bolus dose and then infused at 0.25 mg/kg/hr. Regional anesthesia, if initiated prior to incision can also be used. Ropivacaine 0.75% can be infiltrated into the wound or eutectic mixture of local anesthetic (EMLA) cream can be applied 5 minutes prior to surgery and daily for 4 days following surgery (Carroll et al., 2013).

SUMMARY

1. Patients presenting for amputation usually have pre-existing pain due to tumor burden, trauma or possible exposure to chemotherapeutic agents capable of causing neuropathic pain.
2. Acute postoperative pain control following amputation may prevent the development of chronic pain.
3. Neuropathic pain is very common postoperatively, and preoperative pharmacologic therapy with gabapentin may minimize this.
4. PLP is more common among older children undergoing amputation. The best management of this is preventative care.

ACKNOWLEDGMENT

The author wishes to thank the first edition author, Gillian R. Lauder.

BIBLIOGRAPHY

Anghelescu D, Oakes L, Hankins G. Treatment of pain in children after limb-sparing surgery: an institution's 26-year experience. *Pain Manag Nurs*. 2011;12(2):82–94.

Anghelescu DL, Steen BD, Wu H, et al. Prospective study of neuropathic pain after definitive surgery for extremity osteosarcoma in a pediatric population. *Pediatr Blood Cancer*. 2017;64:e26162.

Bach S, Noreng MF, Tjellden NU. Phantom limb pain in amputees during the first 12 months following limb amputation, after preoperative lumbar epidural blockade. *Pain*. 1988;33:297–301.

Carroll I, Hah J, Mackey S, et al. Perioperative interventions to reduce chronic postsurgical pain. *J Reconstr Microsurg*. 2013;29(4):213–222.

Eccleston C, Malleson PN, Clinch J, Connell Sourbut C. Chronic pain in adolescents: evaluation of a program of interdisciplinary cognitive behavior therapy (ICBT). *Arch Dis Child*. 2003;88:881–885.

Friedrichsdorf SJ, Nugent AP. Management of neuropathic pain in children with cancer. *Curr Opin Support Palliat Care*. 2013;7:131–138.

International Association for the Study of Pain. 2016. http://www.iasppain.org/AM/Template.cfm?Section¼Pain_Definitions

Krane EJ, Heller LB. The prevalence of phantom sensation and pain in pediatric amputees. *J Pain Symptom Manage*. 1995;10:21–29.

Marina N, Gebhardt M, Teot L, Gorlick R. Biology and therapeutic advances for pediatric osteosarcoma. *Oncologist*. 2004;9:422–441.

Nikolajsen L, Jensen TS. Phantom limb pain. *Br J Anaesth*. 2001;87(1):107–116.

Pirowska A, Wloch T, Nowobilski R, Plaszewski M, Hocini A, Menager D. Phantom phenomena and body scheme after limb amputation: A literature review. *Neurol Neurochir Pol*. 2014;48(1):52–59.

Wilkins KL, McGrath PJ, Finley GA, Katz J. Phantom limb sensations and phantom limb pain in child and adolescent amputees. *Pain*. 1998;87:7–12.

PART 13

Challenges in Pediatric Syndromes

57

Down Syndrome

ERICA P. LIN, JAMES P. SPAETH, AND MELANIE HANDLEY

INTRODUCTION

Trisomy 21, or Down syndrome (DS), is the most common human chromosomal syndrome, with an overall incidence of 1 in 691 live births. Its incidence varies greatly with maternal age (e.g., for women age 35–39 years, the incidence increases to 1 in 270; Hobson-Rohrer & Samson-Fang, 2013). Because of its association with other congenital anomalies, children with this syndrome often present for surgical procedures that require general anesthesia. Anesthesiologists caring for these patients must be familiar with the implications of DS on perioperative care.

LEARNING OBJECTIVES

1. Review the clinical presentation of DS.
2. Consider the challenges that are commonly associated with DS, including airway difficulties, cervical spine instability, congenital heart disease (CHD).
3. Identify the implications of general anesthesia for these patients, beginning with preoperative evaluation and extending into postoperative care.

CASE PRESENTATION

A 2-year-old boy with DS presents for bilateral myringotomies with pressure-equalization tube placement and adenotonsillectomy. His medical history is significant for an uncomplicated delivery at term and corrective cardiac surgery in infancy for an ***atrioventricular canal*** *defect. He completed a course of antibiotics 4 days ago for otitis media. Parents note that he is a noisy breather who regularly snores when sleeping and has self-resolving pauses lasting 5 to 10 seconds. The patient has the typical* ***Down's facies****. He breathes with an open mouth and his tongue is slightly protruded. Physical exam is otherwise normal. He has not had any cervical spine x-rays.*

He undergoes inhalational induction with oxygen, nitrous oxide, and sevoflurane. Airway obstruction occurs on induction but resolves with jaw thrust and placement of an oral airway. His heart rate, however, decreases to the 40s. Sevoflurane and nitrous oxide are discontinued. The nurse hastily attempts peripheral intravenous (IV) line placement but is unsuccessful after 2 attempts. At the nadir of 26 beats per minute, his blood pressure is 48/24. Atropine 20 mcg/kg is administered intramuscularly. Shortly thereafter an IV catheter is secured in the right wrist. ***Bradycardia*** *and hypotension persist. Radial pulses remain diminished, despite an additional dose of IV atropine. Epinephrine (adrenaline) (1 mcg/kg) is administered IV with prompt correction of hemodynamics.*

Hyperextension of the neck is carefully avoided during laryngoscopy, and the patient's airway is secured with a 3.5-mm oral Ring-Adair-Elwyn (RAE) endotracheal tube (ETT). Anesthesia is maintained with oxygen, air, and sevoflurane. The otolaryngologist forgoes suspension for the adenotonsillectomy, and the surgery proceeds uneventfully. Fentanyl 2 mcg/kg and dexmedetomidine 0.5 mcg/kg are administered IV for analgesia. The patient is extubated awake, but recovery in the postanesthesia care unit is complicated by ***airway obstruction****,* ***apneic pauses****, and persistent* ***oxygen desaturation****. He is* ***admitted to*** *the* ***intensive care unit (ICU)*** *for continued close monitoring.*

TABLE 57.1 CONSIDERATIONS IN DOWN SYNDROME, BY SYSTEM

System	Pathophysiology	Anesthetic Considerations
Cardiac	Congenital heart disease Pulmonary hypertension	1. Careful preoperative assessment 2. Tailor anesthetic to patient's cardiopulmonary function 3. SBE prophylaxis when indicated
Airway/pulmonary	Narrow nasopharynx, hypoplastic midface, large tongue, micrognathia Hypertrophic tonsils and adenoids Recurrent respiratory infections Subglottic stenosis Sleep apnea	1. Prone to airway obstruction 2. Use an appropriately sized ETT (likely a smaller size); perform a leak test as confirmation. 3. Extubate "awake" when possible 4. Factor airway/respiratory issues into postoperative care plans
Neurologic	Cognitive deficiencies Hypotonia	1. Cooperation and assessment limitations 2. Reduced airway tone with sedation/anesthesia
Musculoskeletal	Atlanto-axial instability Occipito-atlantal instability	1. Careful preoperative assessment 2. Avoid neck extension/flexion/rotation during laryngoscopy, intraoperative positioning.

Note. SBE = subacute endocarditis; ETT = endotracheal tube.

DISCUSSION

1. What are the characteristic physical features of a patient with DS?

Children with DS are easily recognized by their **typical facial features**, which include brachycephaly, flat nasal bridge, epicanthal folds with upslanting palpebral fissures, and Brushfield spots on the iris. Their hands have a single palmar crease (simian crease) and a hypoplastic middle phalanx of the fifth finger, while their feet have a larger-than-normal gap between the large and second toes. The joints are hypermobile, and muscle tone is often decreased. Developmental delays are common, as are short stature and obesity.

Table 57.1 lists anesthesia considerations in DS patients by system.

2. How is the airway altered in these children? How does this affect the ETT size?

In the upper airway, the nasopharynx is often narrow, and the midface is hypoplastic. Micrognathia, large medially displaced tonsils and adenoids, and macroglossia all contribute to airway obstruction and an increased prevalence (as high as 63%–79%) of obstructive sleep apnea (Hamilton et al., 2016). Furthermore, even among those patients whose parents deny sleep problems, a considerable percentage have evidence of obstructive sleep apnea on polysomnography (Marcus et al., 1991).

Airway disorders in children with DS are not restricted to the oropharyngeal and hypopharyngeal regions of the airway. Subglottic stenosis is notably present in all children with DS and can be attributed to decreased tracheal diameter and the predisposition to tracheobronchomalacia (Hamilton et al., 2016). This decrease in tracheal diameter is either congenital or, more commonly, acquired. Children with DS are more likely to require surgery and intubation at a young age. This predisposes them to develop subglottic narrowing from repeated tracheal instrumentation. Additionally, gastroesophageal reflux disease, also common in children with DS, may contribute to the development of subglottic stenosis. Repeated tracheal mucosal injury by gastric acid promotes tracheal scarring and subsequent narrowing of the tracheal diameter.

In general, initial intubation of DS patients should be performed with an ETT 1 to 2 sizes smaller than that predicted for a child of the same age without DS (see Table 57.2). After intubation, it is critical to confirm the fit of the ETT by using a leak test to determine the leak pressure (the inspiratory pressure needed to cause an audible escape of gas around the ETT). A leak between 10 and 30 cm H_2O is desirable (Shott, 2000).

3. Should every patient with DS get cervical spine films preoperatively?

It is widely recognized that children with DS are at risk for craniovertebral joint instability and

TABLE 57.2. ENDOTRACHEAL TUBE SIZES FOR CHILDREN WITH DOWN SYNDROME VERSUS NORMS

Age	Size (ID)	
	Down syndrome	Norms
Premature	2.0 to 2.5	2.5 to 3.0
Full-term newborn to 9 month	2.5 to 3.0	3.5 to 4.0
9 month to 18 month	3.0 to 3.5	4.0 to 4.5
1.5 to 3 years	3.5 to 4.0	4.5 to 5.0
4 to 5 years	4.0 to 4.5	5.0 to 5.5
6 to 7 years	5.0	5.5 to 6.0
8 to 10 years	5.5	6.0 to 6.5
10 to 11 years	5.5	6.5 to 7.0
12 to 13 years	6.0	7.0 to 7.5
≥14 years	6.5	7.5 to 8.0

Reprinted from Shott SR. Down syndrome: analysis of airway size and a guide for appropriate intubation. *Laryngoscope.* 2000;110(4):585–592 Copyright 2000 by Lippincott Williams & Wilkins, Inc.

atlantoaxial subluxation. This instability results from both abnormal joint anatomy and ligamentous laxity. These cervical spine abnormalities can be found in as many as 10% to 30% of patients with DS (Brockmeyer, 1999). The relatively high incidence coupled with the potential for spinal cord damage provoked the question of whether all children with DS should receive routine radiologic evaluation of the cervical spine and, if so, at what age should this occur?

For accurate radiographic evaluation of the cervical spine, the child must have adequate vertebral mineralization, which is typically not achieved until 3 years of age. Additionally, plain radiographs do not predict well which children are at increased risk of developing spine problems. For these reasons, current evidence does not support routine radiologic cervical spine screening in patient with DS, particularly those who are asymptomatic (Bull, 2011).

A thorough history and physical exam are the most important steps to identify patients who may have cervical spine instability. Neurologic manifestations of symptomatic instability include the preference for a sitting position, difficulty walking, abnormal gait, including falling and/or staggering, neck pain, limited neck mobility, torticollis, incoordination and clumsiness, sensory deficits, spasticity, and hyperreflexia. All symptomatic patients should undergo cervical spine radiography followed by prompt referral to a pediatric neurosurgeon or orthopedic surgeon (Bull, 2011).

Certain precautions are advised to reduce the incidence of atlantoaxial subluxation, particularly in patients with unidentified cervical spine instability. With regard to anesthesia, cervical spine precautions should be utilized when performing intubation. This may include the use of video laryngoscopes and flexible fiberoptic bronchoscopes to improve the ease and safety of intubating such patients. Additionally, the cervical spine must be adequately supported and aligned during positioning of the patient for surgery. Avoidance of extreme neck flexion is of great importance in this patient population.

4. How does a history of congenital heart disease (CHD) affect the anesthetic management?

Anesthetic risk in these patients increases in the presence of cardiac disease, particularly when associated with pulmonary hypertension. Approximately 40% to 50% of patients with DS have cardiac malformations (Coté et al., 2013). **Atrioventriculoseptal** defects are the most common, followed by ventricular septal defects, patent ductus arteriosus, and tetralogy of Fallot (Weijerman et al., 2010). Screening affected infants with echocardiography facilitates early identification of CHD and optimal management. Compared to patients without DS, surgical correction in these patients is associated with increased morbidity and mortality secondary to coexisting pulmonary hypertension and an increased susceptibility to recurrent infections, including pneumonia. Postcardiac surgery, patients may have residual defects, including conduction disturbances. Depending on the type of cardiac lesion and the procedure to be performed, antibiotic prophylaxis for subacute bacterial endocarditis may be required. Anesthetic technique should be tailored to each patient's cardiopulmonary function.

5. Does pulmonary hypertension occur in DS patients who do not have CHD?

DS patients are at increased risk of developing pulmonary hypertension. This may be due to several factors other than the presence of CHD with persistent left-to-right shunting. Chronic upper airway obstruction, obstructive sleep apnea, hypoventilation, and chronic hypoxemia from recurrent pulmonary infections can contribute to increased pulmonary vascular resistance. Patients with DS appear to develop pulmonary hypertension at a faster rate and have persistent pulmonary hypertension after corrective cardiac surgery. Although acquired or secondary pulmonary hypertension develops over time, patients with DS also have a higher incidence of idiopathic pulmonary hypertension of the neonate. This finding suggests that these patients may have an intrinsic cause for the development of pulmonary vascular disease (Cua et al., 2007).

6. What anesthesia-related complications should one anticipate?

The most frequent complication is **bradycardia**, specifically **during induction**. A study conducted in 2010 observed the incidence of this phenomenon in children with DS. The authors found that 57% of the patients with DS experienced bradycardia with induction using sevoflurane in comparison to 12% in the control group. Additionally, they confirmed that this clinical finding is not associated with presence of underlying heart disease (Wickham et al., 2011). Since cardiac output is partly dependent on heart rate, especially in younger children, bradycardia can have a profound effect on a patient's hemodynamic stability. Neonates and infants in particular exhibit decreased sympathetic activity and may benefit from vagal blockade with atropine preoperatively. While atropine can help maintain the heart rate, it will not prevent or reverse the negative inotropic effects of volatile anesthetics. Gradually increasing the concentration of inspired sevoflurane during inhalation induction (as opposed to a rapid induction with 8% sevoflurane) will help prevent, but may not completely eliminate, hypotension and bradycardia. Close observation of heart rate and blood pressure during induction is imperative. If bradycardia occurs, immediately decrease the concentration of sevoflurane and administer atropine. Atropine should be administered intramuscularly in the absence of existing venous access. The extreme example in this case is a reminder that if bradycardia does not resolve or if hemodynamic compromise persists, epinephrine (adrenaline) should be given. Other significant anesthesia-related complications include airway obstruction and postintubation stridor (Borland et al., 2004).

7. What are common concerns in the early postoperative period?

Patients with DS are prone to airway complications, specifically **airway obstruction**, **oxygen desaturation**, and postintubation stridor. They have a higher incidence of upper and lower respiratory tract infections, which can contribute to perioperative respiratory compromise as well. Younger patients with a known history of **obstructive sleep apnea** and/or other medical comorbidities may be candidates for **ICU admission** postoperatively, especially following airway procedures. For patients with a known history of airway obstruction, consider placing either an oropharyngeal or nasopharyngeal airway prior to extubation. Patients with DS should generally be extubated awake, not deep, in order to maximize pharyngeal/laryngeal tone. Postintubation stridor can result from subglottic edema due to the use of a larger than necessary ETT. Once identified, stridor can be treated with humidified oxygen, nebulized racemic epinephrine, and IV dexamethasone.

Pain management in the postoperative period can be challenging. While patients with DS clearly experience pain, they may express pain and discomfort more slowly and less precisely due to their developmental delay. Therefore, to accurately assess pain, both behavioral and objective measures of pain, such as heart rate should be observed. Opioids must be administered carefully and incrementally to avoid respiratory compromise in patients who are already at risk for airway complications. When appropriate, regional anesthesia techniques offer excellent long-lasting pain relief without the respiratory depression of opioids.

SUMMARY

1. Patients with DS can have multisystem abnormalities including airway obstruction, sleep apnea, an increased incidence of CHD, cervical spine instability, developmental delay, and obesity.
2. Risks on the induction of anesthesia include airway obstruction, bradycardia, and hypotension.
3. A smaller-than-normal ETT should be utilized with the head maintained in neutral position for intubation.
4. Close postoperative observation for airway obstruction and desaturation is critical.

BIBLIOGRAPHY

Borland LM, Colligan J, Brandom BW. Frequency of anesthesia-related complications in children with Down syndrome under general anesthesia for noncardiac procedures. *Pediatr Anesth.* 2004;14:733–738.

Brockmeyer D. Down syndrome and craniovertebral instability. *Pediatr Neurosurg.* 1999;31:71–77.

Bull M. Clinical report—health supervision for children with down syndrome. *Pediatrics.* 2011;128(2):393.

Coté CJ, Lerman J, Anderson BJ. *A Practice of Anesthesia for Infants and Children.* 5th ed. Philadelphia: Elsevier; 2013.

Cua CL, Blankenship A, North AL, Hayes J, Nelin LD. Increased incidence of idiopathic persistent pulmonary hypertension in Down syndrome neonates. *Pediatr Cardiol.* 2007;28:250–254.

Hamilton J, Yaneza M, Clement W, Kubba H. The prevalence of airway problems in children with Down's syndrome. *Int J Pediatr Otolaryngol.* 2016;81:1–4

Hobson-Rohrer W, Samson-Fang L. Down syndrome. *Pediatr Rev.* 2013;34(12):573.

Marcus CL, Keens TG, Bautista DB, von Pechmann WS, Ward SLD. Obstructive sleep apnea in children with Down syndrome. *Pediatrics.* 1991;88:132–139.

Shott SR. Down syndrome: analysis of airway size and guide for appropriate intubation. *Laryngoscope.* 2000;110:585–592.

Weijerman ME, de Winter JP. Clinical practice. The care of children with Down syndrome. *Eur J Pediatr.* 2010 Dec;169(12):1445–1452.

Wickham K, Stricker P, Gurnaney H, et al. Bradycardia during induction of Anesthesia with Sevoflurane in children with down syndrome. *Surv Anesthesiol.* 2011;55(4):185–186.

58

Muscular Dystrophy

RENEE KREEGER AND JAMES P. SPAETH

INTRODUCTION

Duchenne muscular dystrophy (DMD) is a complex disease which is associated with multiple physiologic perturbations, progressively leading to **cardiomyopathy**, **respiratory failure**, and, eventually, death. Patients with DMD create unique challenges for the anesthesia team, including management of a **difficult airway**, avoidance of **volatile anesthetics** and **succinylcholine**, the need for respiratory support, and discussion of **advance directives**. A thorough and multidisciplinary collaborative approach must be utilized in the care of these patients for the entire perioperative period, including preoperative assessment and optimization, intraoperative support, and postoperative intervention. An abundance of caution guides the anesthesia team, cardiologist, pulmonologist, and intensivist, as all must exercise good judgment, careful monitoring, and thorough evaluation of the patient with DMD to minimize the risk of complications. In addition, all potential interventions must be analyzed to ensure their necessity and contribution to the improvement and/or maintenance of the DMD patient prior to their initiation.

LEARNING OBJECTIVES

1. Identify common comorbidities that may be present in DMD patients who need to undergo surgery.
2. Formulate an anesthetic plan that addresses the DMD patient's cardiopulmonary status and avoids medication that may exacerbate underlying conditions.
3. Review discussion with the patient and use of advanced directives in late-stage DMD.

CASE PRESENTATION

A 17-year-old boy with DMD presents for preoperative anesthesia consultation in anticipation of percutaneous endoscopic gastrostomy tube placement. The patient is wheelchair bound with minimal independent movement. His exam reveals a Mallampati II airway with mildly decreased neck range of motion and mouth opening. His lungs are clear, and heart sounds are normal. The patient reports a significant increase in his respiratory effort and in respiratory illnesses over the past year. His pulmonary function tests from 1 month ago show a significant decrease from previous measurements, with a forced vital capacity of 38% predicted with a peak cough flow of 240 L/min and a maximum expiratory pressure of 55 cmH$_2$O. His room air oxygen saturation is 98%.

Cardiac evaluation from a month ago includes an echocardiogram that demonstrated evidence of stable dilated ***cardiomyopathy*** *with a shortening fraction of 20% and an electrocardiogram (ECG) remarkable for sinus tachycardia with occasional premature ventricular contractions (PVCs). The cardiologist states that the patient is medically optimized, and that she will be available postoperatively to assist with his management as needed. An intensive care unit (ICU) admission is arranged due to the likely need for significant respiratory support postoperatively.*

On the day of the procedure, the patient reports no new issues and his exam and vital signs are unchanged. He is taken to the operating room, where standard American Society of Anesthesiologists monitors are applied. The patient undergoes an intravenous induction with etomidate and fentanyl after preoxygenation. Mask ventilation is somewhat difficult but improves with insertion of an *oropharyngeal airway. Direct laryngoscopy with a Macintosh blade reveals a view of the epiglottis only. With the use of a Miller blade and significant anterior cricoid pressure, the posterior arytenoids are visualized and an endotracheal tube (ETT) is placed. Maintenance of anesthesia is achieved with total intravenous anesthesia consisting of propofol and remifentanil infusions, titrated to effect and hemodynamics. Epinephrine and milrinone infusions are set up for use in the event of the need for cardiovascular support. The surgeon begins the gastrostomy tube insertion, and the patient's oxygen saturation is noted to decrease to 88%. With the reduction of gastric insufflation and adjustments in ventilator settings, including increased positive end-expiratory pressure from 5 to 8 cmH$_2$O and recruitment maneuvers, the oxygen saturation improves to 98%. As the procedure continues, PVCs are noted to increase in frequency; however, the patient's hemodynamics are unaffected. The procedure is completed without further incident, and the patient is transferred to the ICU intubated. The patient is extubated to non-invasive positive pressure ventilation (NPPV) later that afternoon and is weaned to room air with spontaneous ventilation and cough assist by the next day.*

DISCUSSION

1. What is DMD?

DMD is a progressive, X-linked neuromuscular disorder caused by recessive mutations in the dystrophin gene, with a mean age at diagnosis of 4.5 years. Its incidence is approximately 1 in 3,500 male live births, with 8% to 10% of female carriers manifesting symptoms such as mild muscle weakness. The hallmarks of the disease are abnormal motor development, including lack of independent walking by 18 months of age; an inability to run, jump, or climb stairs; and pseudohypertrophy of the calf muscles. The classic Gower's sign, involving the use of a wide-based stance and the aid of hands on the thighs to rise from the floor, is often seen. Approximately 30% of these patients have some degree of developmental delay. These clinical signs are the result of muscular necrosis and replacement with connective or adipose tissue. For two-thirds of children with DMD, no family history of the disease exists. The disease is relentless; patients are wheelchair bound by the age of 12 years and have progressive involvement of respiratory muscles concomitant with the development of a dilated cardiomyopathy. One-third of patients have dilated cardiomyopathy by age 14, with nearly all patients developing cardiomyopathy by age 18. If untreated, the mean age at death is 19 years. With corticosteroid treatment and aggressive pulmonary support and intervention, patients can survive into the third decade (Bushby et al., 2005).

2. What are the cardiovascular concerns for patients with DMD?

Patients with DMD develop a dilated **cardiomyopathy**, which predisposes them to hemodynamic instability and **dysrhythmias,** as well as fulminant cardiac failure. Preoperative assessment of exercise tolerance is limited due to immobility. More subtle signs of cardiac issues may be present, including fatigue and weight loss. ECG abnormalities may include left or right ventricular hypertrophy or other findings such as sinus tachycardia or Q waves (Cripe & Tobias, 2013). Traditional echocardiography may not fully reveal the extent of disease in these patients, as acoustic windows may be poor. Cardiac magnetic resonance imaging is becoming the preferred imaging modality in DMD due to its ability to identify myocardial strain and myocardial fibrosis via late gadolinium enhancement (Brunklaus et al., 2015). The current recommendations include assessment of cardiac function at time of diagnosis or by age 6, with biannual assessment from ages 6 to 10 and annual evaluation starting at age 10 or with symptomatology (Cripe & Tobias, 2013).

Despite an extensive preoperative work-up with reassuring studies, patients with DMD may have significant cardiovascular disease that may not be evident until they are under general anesthesia or sedation. They may also demonstrate dysrhythmias that were not noted preoperatively and may require intervention. As such, anesthesia providers should be prepared for the need for inotropic or other vasoactive support in the form of vasoactive infusions and/or bolus doses. A defibrillator should be immediately available in case cardioversion or defibrillation becomes necessary. In addition, the cardiology and electrophysiology services should be made aware of these patients preoperatively so that they are available to provide assistance in the event of a perioperative issue.

3. What are the pulmonary issues in patients with DMD?

From a respiratory standpoint, these patients are often quite debilitated due to progressive muscular weakness. Many have significant decrements in their pulmonary function that may be acute or chronic. They have a diminished cough reflex, which increases the baseline and postoperative risk of respiratory infection. Many require the use of NPPV, cough assist, or other respiratory intervention at baseline, increasing the likelihood of escalating respiratory support postoperatively. In addition, placement of an ETT is not a trivial matter, as these patients may be difficult to wean from a ventilator once mechanical ventilation it is initiated. Preoperative pulmonary function testing can guide both intraoperative and postoperative respiratory care. Postoperatively, elective admission to the ICU is prudent and allows the patient to receive the level of respiratory support necessary.

4. Are there alternatives to placement of an ETT?

There are reports of the use of alternative airway devices and methods of ventilation such as NPPV with bilevel positive airway pressure, laryngeal mask airways (LMAs), and mouthpieces or nasal masks (Bach et al., 2010; Birnkrant et al., 2006). In addition, alternative anesthetic techniques such as the utilization of dexmedetomidine and ketamine for sedation in a patient with a natural airway have been reported with good success (Kako et al., 2014). These options have been explored for a variety of reasons, including the preference of some patients with end-stage disease not to be intubated. While airway devices have been used successfully, inherent risks are associated with their use. The patient using NPPV may have difficulty breathing with administration of sedatives and spontaneous ventilation may cease. With LMA use, there can be issues with proper fit as well as, in this clinical case, an inability to pass the endoscope to allow for percutaneous endoscopic gastrostomy tube placement. Patients receiving sedation while maintaining a natural airway may suffer hypoventilation and/or apnea, leading to desaturation and the need for escalation of respiratory support. The best approach to DMD patients is one that is individualized to the patient's current medical status and takes into consideration the procedure to be performed and the patient's wishes. No one technique or respiratory device will be applicable in every situation.

5. Are there any formal perioperative guidelines for DMD patients?

The American College of Chest Physicians published a consensus statement in 2007 outlining suggestions for the management of DMD patients undergoing general anesthesia or procedural sedation (Birnkrant et al., 2007). Table 58.1 summarizes their recommendations, providing clinicians with an excellent resource for guiding management of these complex patients.

6. Is there a specific anesthetic technique that is preferred for DMD patients?

Traditional teaching outlines an increased risk of malignant hyperthermia in patients with muscular dystrophies. However, a 2009 review of the anesthesia literature by a group at Children's Hospital of Philadelphia cites an increased risk of a *malignant hyperthermia-like syndrome* with associated rhabdomyolysis in patients with DMD who receive inhaled anesthetics (Gurnaney et al., 2009). Therefore, most anesthesia providers avoid inhalational anesthetics in patients with DMD. A retrospective study at the Hospital for Sick Children in Toronto suggested that anesthesia precautions should be considered for all patients with neuromuscular disease, not just for those with muscular dystrophies (Bamaga et al., 2016).

There is a life-threatening hyperkalemia risk associated with succinylcholine administration in DMD patients which is widely discussed in the literature (Segura et al., 2013). The consensus is that the use of succinylcholine is contraindicated in DMD patients.

Depending on the extent of the cardiomyopathy, a DMD patient may require a high-dose opioid-based anesthetic or ketamine to ensure hemodynamic stability. Induction with etomidate may also be a good option. Medications such as propofol, which may cause significant hypotension when induction doses are administered, should be used judiciously in severely affected patients. The key to management of these patients is thoughtful consideration of the specific patient's physiologic state in choosing an anesthetic technique or particular medication. With close attention to these details, as well as the patient's response to the chosen medications and surgical manipulations, a variety of medications can be used successfully. Careful fluid management and optimization of electrolytes are also important. In more complex procedures, such as spine fusions, blood transfusion should be anticipated, blood products should be ordered preoperatively and be available in the immediate vicinity of the operating room. It is

TABLE 58.1 PERIOPERATIVE CARE OF PATIENTS WITH DUCHENNE MUSCULAR DYSTROPHY

Preoperative
Multidisciplinary approach:
Pulmonary consultation and evaluation: include FVC, MIP, MEP, PCF, and room air oxygen saturation via pulse oximetry
1. FVC: <50 % predicted = increased risk of respiratory complications; <30 % predicted = high risk. Recommend possible preoperative training for NPPV.
2. PCF and MEP: <270 L/min or < 60 cmH_2O respectively = high risk of ineffective cough. Recommend preoperative training in manual and mechanically assisted cough devices.
Cardiology referral: clinical evaluation and optimization
Note: ***normal ECG and echocardiogram results are only modestly reassuring.***
Nutritional assessment with optimization and dysphagia management
Discuss advanced directives, DNR status, anesthesia risks and benefits.
ICU admission planned ahead
Intraoperative
TIVA
Maximize medical personnel available.
Explore options for respiratory support, such as mechanical ventilation with ETT, NPPV, BiPAP, LMA.
Support ventilation via an assisted or controlled mode for patients with FVC <50 %.
Monitoring: standard ASA monitors at minimum
Postoperative
Consider extubating to NPPV in patients with FVC <50 %.
Consider delaying extubation if respiratory secretions are poorly controlled or oxygenation is below baseline.
Use supplemental oxygen with caution while investigating an etiology for decreased oxygen saturation.
Use manual and cough assist devices.
Optimize pain control, delaying extubation if necessary.
Consult cardiology to maximize cardiac function.
Begin a bowel regimen.
If enteral feeding will be delayed >24 to 48 hours, begin parenteral feeding.

Note: MIP = maximum inspiratory pressure, FVC = forced vital capacity, MEP = maximal expiratory pressure, PCF = peak cough flow.

Source: Birnkrant DJ, Panitch HB, Benditt JO, et al. American College of Chest Physicians Consensus statement on the respiratory and related management of patients with Duchenne muscular dystrophy undergoing anesthesia or sedation. *Chest* 2007;132(6):1977–1986.

also prudent to have inotropic and vasoactive support as well as a crash cart, complete with a defibrillator readily available. Due to the multifactorial nature of their disease, as well as their level of deconditioning, DMD patients may require significant resuscitation and intervention, even for "minor" procedures.

7. Can neuromuscular blockade be administered to DMD patients?

Nondepolarizing neuromuscular blockers can be safely used in DMD patients; however, the duration of blockade will be prolonged (Muenster et al., 2006). There is emerging evidence that sugammadex may be utilized for reversal of prolonged blockade in these patients (de Boer et al., 2009). In contrast, depolarizing neuromuscular blocking agents are contraindicated in DMD patients and should not be used.

8. Are advance directives necessary?

Yes. Patients with DMD, particularly as they reach their teenage years and beyond, are keenly aware of their disease, its severity, and their personal wishes for care. It is imperative that clinicians provide DMD patients and their families with the opportunity for initiating advance directives. Consultation with a social worker or other person skilled in these matters will be necessary to ensure that the correct procedures are followed to allow the patient's desires to be honored in the event of a complication or poor outcome. In addition, clinicians must discuss with the patient, specific parameters for resuscitation, intubation, and prolonged dependence on ventilator support. The details of these discussions must then be carefully documented in the medical record.

SUMMARY

1. DMD is an X-linked progressive neuromuscular disease that culminates in cardiomyopathy and respiratory failure. With aggressive treatment and pulmonary support, patients can survive into their third decade of life.
2. While most anesthetic medications can be safely used, the anesthetic plans must be tailored to the individual patient and address the potential need for escalation in care.
3. The use of advanced directives can help guide the medical team on the patient's wishes and desired outcomes in the later stages of disease progression.

ANNOTATED REFERENCES

Birnkrant DJ, Panitch HB, Benditt JO, et al. American College of Chest Physicians Consensus statement on the respiratory and related management of patients with Duchenne muscular dystrophy undergoing anesthesia or sedation. *Chest.* 2007; 132(6): 1977–1986.

This is the best summary of the vital components of the perioperative care of patients with DMD. It provides parameters for assessing risk for complications as well as a proactive multidisciplinary approach to management. It is a must-read for any anesthesiologist who may encounter these patients.

Birnkrant DJ, Ferguson RD, Martin JE, Gordon GJ. Noninvasive ventilation during gastrostomy tube placement in patients with severe Duchenne muscular dystrophy: case reports and review of the literature. *Pediatr Pulmonol.* 2006;41:188–193.

This paper offers alternative methods for airway management in patients with DMD, including LMA and NPPV.

Cripe LH, Tobias, JD. Cardiac considerations in the operative management of the patient with Duchenne or Becker muscular dystrophy. *Pediatr Anesth.* 2013;23:777–784.

This review article provides a look at not only cardiac issues but also general concerns and important considerations associated with the perioperative care of a patient with muscular dystrophy.

BIBLIOGRAPHY

Bamaga AK, Riazi S, Amburgey K, et al. Neuromuscular conditions associated with malignant hyperthermia in paediatric patients: a 25-year retrospective study. *Neuromusc Disord.* 2016;26:201–206.

Brunklaus A, Parish E, Muntoni F, et al. *Eur J Paediatr Neurol.* 2015;19:395–401.

Bushby K, Bourke J, Bullock R, Eagle M, Gibson M, Quinby J. The multidisciplinary management of Duchenne muscular dystrophy. *Curr Pediatr.* 2005;15:292–300.

de Boer HD, van Esmond J, Booij LH, Driessen JJ. Reversal of rocuronium-induced profound neuromuscular block by sugammadex in Duchenne muscular dystrophy. *Pediatr Anesth.* 2009;19:1226–1228.

Gurnaney H, Brown A, Litman RS. Malignant hyperthermia and muscular dystrophies. *Anesth Analg.* 2009;109(4):1043–1048.

Kako H, Corridore M, Kean J, Mendell JR, Flanigan KM, Tobias JD. Dexmedetomidine and ketamine sedation for muscle biopsies in patients with Duchenne muscular dystrophy. *Pediatr Anesth.* 2014;24:851–856.

Muenster T, Schmidt J, Wick, Forst J, Schmitt HJ. Rocuronium 0.3 mg/kg (ED95) induces a normal peak effect but an altered time course of neuromuscular block in patients with Duchenne's muscular dystrophy. *Pediatr Anesth.* 2006;16:840–845.

Segura LG, Lorenz JD, Weingarten TN, et al. Anesthesia and Duchenne or Becker muscular dystrophy: review of 117 anesthetic exposures. *Pediatr Anesth.* 2013;23:855–864.

59

Mucopolysaccharidoses

CATHERINE P. SEIPEL AND TITILOPEMI A. O. AINA

INTRODUCTION

The mucopolysaccharidoses (MPS) are a group of 7 chronic progressive diseases caused by deficiencies of 11 different lysosomal enzymes required for the catabolism of glycosaminoglycans (GAGs). *Hurler syndrome* (MPS IH) is an autosomal recessive storage disorder caused by a deficiency of α-L-iduronidase. *Hunter syndrome* (MPS II) is an X-linked recessive disorder of metabolism involving the enzyme iduronate-2-sulfatase. Many of the MPS clinical manifestations have potential anesthetic implications. Significant airway issues are particularly common due to thickening of the soft tissues, enlarged tongue, short immobile neck, as well as limited mobility of the cervical spine and temporomandibular joints. Spinal deformities, hepatosplenomegaly, airway granulomatous tissue, and recurrent lung infections may inhibit pulmonary function. Odontoid dysplasia and radiographic subluxation of C1 on C2 are common and may cause anterior dislocation of the atlas and spinal cord compression.

LEARNING OBJECTIVES

1. Review the anesthetic issues related to Hurlers syndrome
2. Summarize treatment options for children with MPS.
3. Discuss the management of anticipated difficult intubation in children with MPS.

CASE PRESENTATION

A 14-kg, 4-year-old boy with clinical features suggestive of ***Hurler syndrome (MPS IH)*** *presents with an irreducible umbilical hernia. He was assessed to be unsuitable for* ***bone marrow transplantation*** *as an infant due to neurologic involvement. He has been receiving intravenous* ***enzyme replacement*** *since the age of 3. He has moderate* ***developmental delay****; his general health is good but parents report that he* ***snores*** *a lot at night and sometimes has pauses in his breathing. He is currently being assessed for a* ***nocturnal continuous positive airway pressure (CPAP) device****. His other past history includes a* ***carpal tunnel release*** *12 months ago; at that time the anesthesia record indicates moderate difficulty in visualizing the larynx. On examination, the child is short (height 94 cm). Cardiac auscultation demonstrates a grade III systolic murmur. Echocardiogram shows normal left ventrical function, moderate symmetrical* ***left ventricular hypertrophy****, a thickened tricuspid aortic valve with* ***mild aortic stenosis****, and a thickened,* ***dysplastic mitral valve****. He was not able to comply with a lung function test. Sleep studies demonstrate moderate* ***obstructive sleep apnea*** *with 3 episodes of saturation less than 85% during periods of rapid eye movement sleep. The child is anxious and tearful in the preoperative area, so a midazolam premedication is given.*

Specialized airway devices are prepared for airway instrumentation. After a sevoflurane induction, almost complete ***airway obstruction*** *occurs, the patient's SpO_2 drops to 80%; and attempted mask ventilation is inadequate. Direct laryngoscopy is performed, and no laryngeal structures are recognizable. Rapid desaturation is partially corrected by successful placement of a laryngeal mask airway (LMA). Some resolution of hypoxia is observed, although partial obstruction with rocking chest movements is still present, and only very small tidal volumes are generated. Intubation is attempted using a 2.8-mm fiberoptic bronchoscope. It is passed through the laryngeal* *mask airway and reveals a partial occlusion of the laryngeal inlet by* ***supraglottic tissue*** *and a down-folded epiglottis. Endotracheal intubation is accomplished only after downsizing to size 3.5-mm uncuffed endotracheal tube. Surgery for the hernia is uneventful, but the postoperative period is complicated by repeated failure of extubation and development of postobstructive pulmonary edema. He is reintubated in the same manner as previously and transferred to the pediatric intensive care unit. He receives intravenous dexamethasone and is extubated 24 hours later; he requires mask CPAP for a further 24 hours.*

DISCUSSION

1. What treatment options are available to ameliorate the long-term clinical course of Hurler (MPS IH) and Hunter (MPS II) syndromes?

Treatment options include palliative care, **hematopoietic stem cell transplantation** (HSCT) from bone marrow or umbilical cord blood or recombinant human **enzyme replacement therapy** (ERT). Hurlers syndrome patients receive recombinant human alpha-L-iduronidase (Aldurazyme®, laronidase), whereas MPS II patients with Hunters syndrome receive idursulfase (Elaprase®).

Hurler syndrome: The best clinical outcome of HSCT has been observed in children who receive transplants before they are 2 years old and have a developmental quotient above 70 at the time of transplant (Muenzer et al., 2009). Successful HSCT in patients with Hurlers syndrome modifies disease progression, with increases in life expectancy, resolution of hepatosplenomegaly, stabilization of cardiac disease, and improvement in airway obstruction. The procedure, however, is not curative, and neurologic outcomes are variable. Enzyme replacment therapy (ERT) with alpha-L-iduronidase (laronidase) infusion has been approved by the Food and Drug Administration for patients with the milder or attenuated forms of this disease MPS IH, and for those who have neurologic impairment. The enzyme is not expected to cross the blood–brain barrier or affect central nervous system disease.

Hunters syndrome: As with Hurlers, HSCT is currently not recommended for the severe form of this disease, since neurologic preservation has not been observed. Bone marrow transplantation has been used to treat some symptoms in milder disease forms. Recombinant ERT with idursulfase (Elaprase®) infusion improves exercise tolerance but has produced severe allergic reactions in some patients. ERT also improves obstructive pulmonary function tests in patients with a similar condition, called Hurler Scheie disease (MPS I H/S). There are no data to suggest a reduction in airway complications after HSCT, but the reduction in upper airway soft tissues swelling/thickening following transplant, and to a lesser extent ERT, in children should improve the airway management and the ease of intubation.

2. What are the key features of a preoperative assessment in a patient with Hurlers or Hunters syndrome?

Airway assessment: Ideally, one would review a recent anesthetic record describing the intubation and possible ventilation difficulties (along with techniques used to overcome those difficulties). The case described had these on record from 12 months prior. Before ERT, one could predict this child's airway would become more difficult with time; a careful history of obstructive symptoms gives a surrogate marker as to how the disease has progressed. The alpha-L-iduronidase may have attenuated the disease progression since the last anesthetic. Special investigations could include sleep studies, nasoendoscopy, and cervical spine x-ray (to assess the atlanto-axial joint and odontoid process). Upper airway imaging techniques, such as magnetic resonance imaging and computed tomography (CT), are not routinely used to assess the airway preoperatively but can be performed in cooperative older children (or recreated from previous CT scans of the cervical spine). Clinically significant upper airway obstruction has been reported in 70% of patients with MPS due to enlarged tongue, tonsils and adenoids, narrowed trachea; redundant airway tissue; and thickened vocal cords (Yeung et al., 2009). Patients with very severe Hurlers syndrome, develop obstructive upper airway disease by 2 to 3 years of age.

Respiratory assessment: All MPS patients are at risk of severe respiratory compromise from restrictive lung disease and recurrent infection. Exercise tolerance, compared to their peers, is a useful index of cardiorespiratory function; formal respiratory function testing is difficult in children under 7 years of age and may be impossible with developmental delay.

Cardiology assessment: All patients with a diagnosis of MPS should undergo a cardiology evaluation at time of diagnosis and every 1 to 2 years thereafter (Muenzer et al., 2009). Cardiac manifestations are common and worsen with age. In patients with severe Hurlers, valvular disease, arrhythmia, cardiomyopathy, congestive heart failure, coronary artery disease, and both pulmonary and systemic hypertension may occur. Moderate to severe narrowing of the coronary arteries can occur within the first year of life, and complete coronary occlusion has been reported within the first 5 years of life. In MPS II, valvular heart disease is common (prevalence 50%); cardiomyopathy is less common but can be associated with dysrhythmias.

3. What are clues to a potentially difficult airway in young infants with MPS?

The overall incidence of difficult airway in children with MPS, in the era of HSCT and ERT, is unknown. Before these therapies were available, the incidence of difficult intubation was 25% overall, with much higher rates in Hurler (54%) and Morquio syndrome (50%). Features that would raise suspicion for a difficult intubation are listed in Table 59.1.

4. What airway devices and techniques are appropriate in managing the airway?

Most published series report the need for experienced anesthetists and multiple airway devices. Most authors recommend inhalational induction prior to airway management. In contrast to the steps in an adult difficult airway algorithm, awake fiberoptic intubation is usually not feasible in children with MPS, and emergency tracheostomy is likely to be extremely difficult and prolonged. The most common forms of airway management in patients with MPS involve the use of a supraglottic airway device; these can be used alone or as a conduit for fiberoptic intubation. To maintain the airway and anesthesia during fiberoptic intubation, various devices have been used including LMAs, a modified intubating facemask (VBM Medizintechnik, Sulz, Germany), and a contralateral nasopharyngeal airway. The devices currently available to help with difficult intubation in adults are well described (Niforopolou et al., 2010), and many should be considered for intubating children with MPS.

TABLE 59.1 SOMATIC MANIFESTATIONS OF MPS THAT NECESSITATE DIFFICULT AIRWAY MANAGEMENT

Hurler or Morquio syndrome (higher incidence than Hunter syndrome)
Older children or teenagers not suitable for stem cell transplantation
Previous difficult intubation
Enlarged tongue, adenoids, or tonsils
Obstructive sleep apnea (particularly if the child requires a nocturnal home CPAP machine)
Radiologic evidence of tracheal narrowing or tracheal collapse on neck flexion
Cardiac disease (cardiomyopathy, septal hypertrophy, mitral or tricuspid valve incompetence)
Short or immobile neck
Atlanto-axial subluxation
Obstructive lung disease
Kyphoscoliosis and/or lumbar lordosis

5. What maneuvers can rescue a compromised airway in patients with MPS?

Of all the devices available for anticipated difficult pediatric airway management, only 7 have been reported in MPS patients. Although the successful use of the LMA is well described in these patients (Walker, 2000), it is not universally successful. The other LMA derivatives (including Flexible LMA and LMA ProSeal) have not been described in patients with MPS. The I-Gel LMA has been described in an adult with Hunter syndrome. Emergency tracheostomy in the "can't intubate, can't ventilate" situation is much less of an option for MPS children, due to their having a short neck, impalpable tracheal rings, and pretracheal GAG deposits; in addition, trying to establish this emergenetly may take a prolonged amount of time. In the emergency situation, it may be more prudent to discontinue the anesthetic and wake the patient up, than to struggle with the airway tracheostomy creation for a long period of time. A suggested difficult airway algorithm is presented in Figure 59.1.

6. Is awake regional anesthesia appropriate in this patient?

Neurologic problems due to MPS deposition are recognized in both MPS IH and II, and may represent a relative contraindication to regional anesthesia. There have only been a few successful reports of neuraxial blockade in these children. There is a report of a failed epidural in a 9-year-old boy with Hurlers syndrome; it is thought that the deposition

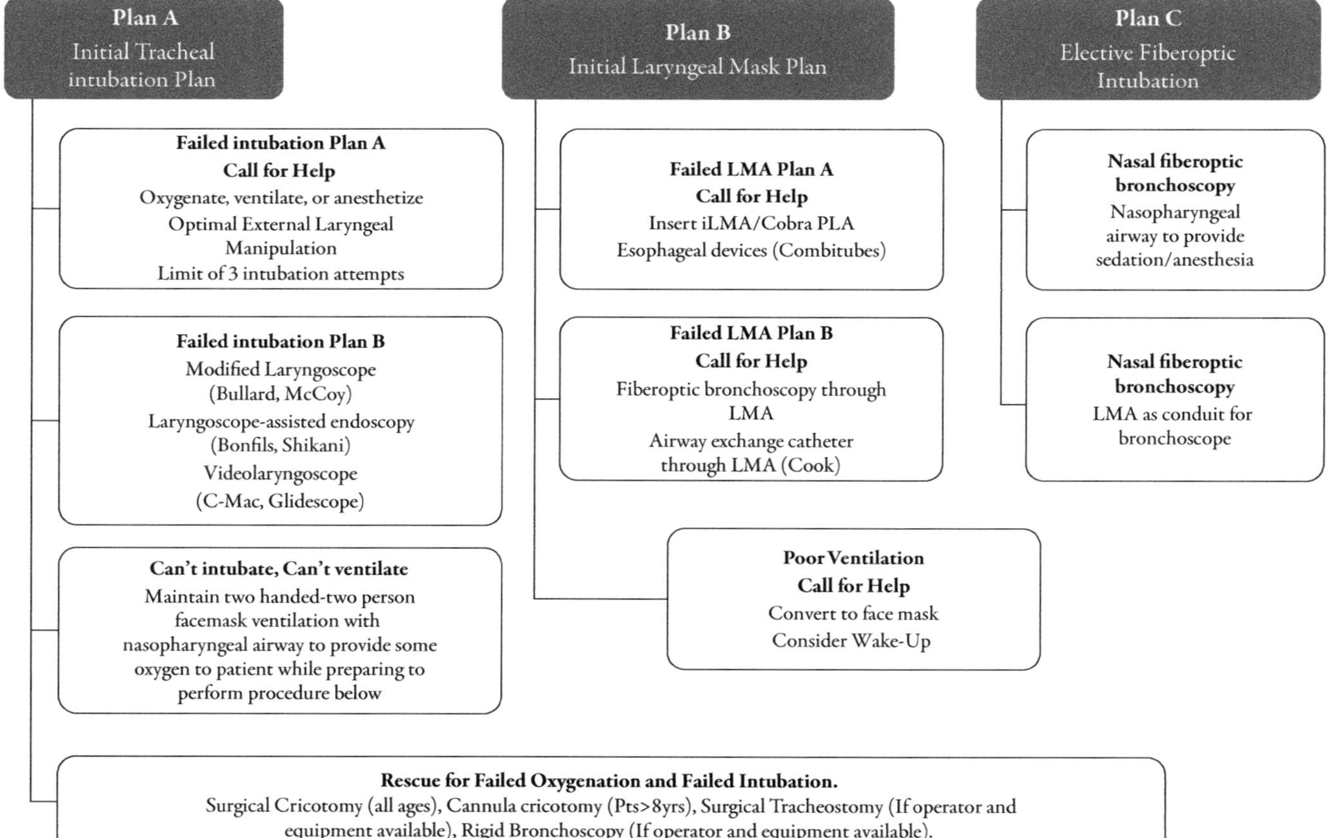

FIGURE 59.1 Suggested difficult airway algorithm for airway management in children with mucopolysaccharidoses.

of GAGs in either the epidural space or the nerve fiber sheath may have prevented the direct access of local anesthetic to the nerve (Vas & Naregal, 2000).

SUMMARY

1. Most children with MPS have significant airway anomalies that predispose to difficult airway management. Undergoing anesthesia requires meticulous assessment, planning and the assistance of an experienced team.
2. Sedation should be avoided if the patient has significant obstructive sleep apnea or upper airway obstruction.
3. Spontaneous respiration should be maintained until the airway is either secured or fully assessed.
4. Ongoing training and regular practice of advanced airway techniques are essential.

ACKNOWLEDGMENT

The authors would like to thank Geoff Frawley for his contributions to the first edition.

ANNOTATED REFERENCES

Muenzer J, Wraith J, Clarke L. Mucopolysaccharidosis 1: management and treatment guidelines. *Pediatrics.* 2009;123:19–29.

This is a consensus paper from a MPS working party that outlines all aspects of disease presentation and management but has minimal anesthetic input.

Walker R, Darowski M, Wraith J. Anaesthesia and mucopolysaccharidoses. *Anaesthesia.* 1994;49: 1078–1084.

A paper from the leading authority on the anesthetic management of MPS details techniques in use prior to the widespread availability of HSCT and ERT.

BIBLIOGRAPHY

Aucoin S, Vlatten A, Hackmann T. Difficult airway management with the Bonfils fiberscope in a child with Hurler syndrome. *Pediatr Anesth.* 2009;19:421–422.

Crocker K, Black A. Assessment and management of the predicted difficult airway in babies and children. *Anaesth Int Care Med.* 2009;10(4):200–205.

Difficult Airway Society. Simple composite chart. 2001. http://www.das.uk.com/guidelines/downloads.html

Mahoney A, Soni N, Vellodi A. Anesthesia and the mucopolysaccharidoses: a review of patients treated by bone marrow transplantation. *Pediatr Anesth.* 1992;2:317–324.

Niforopolou P, Pantazopoulos I, Demestiha T, et al. Video-laryngoscopes in the adult airway management: a topical review of the literature. *Acta Anaesthesiol Scand.* 2010;54:1050–1061.

Sawamoto K, Chen H, Almeciga-Diaz CJ, et al. Gene therapy for mucopolysaccharidoses. *Mol Genet Metab.* 2018;123:59–68.

Vas L, Naregal F. Failed epidural anesthesia in a patient with Hurler's disease. *Pediatr Anesth.* 2000;10(1):95–98.

Walker R. The laryngeal mask airway in the difficult pediatric airway: an assessment of positioning and use in fiberoptic intubation. *Pediatr Anesth* 2000;10:53–58.

Yeung A, Cowan M, Rosbe K. Airway management in children with mucopolysaccharidoses. *Arch Otolaryngol Head Neck Surg.* 2009;135(1):73–79.

60

Epidermolysis Bullosa

KIM-PHUONG NGUYEN

INTRODUCTION

Epidermolysis bullosa (EB) is a genetic skin disorder with multiple modes of inheritance; it is characterized by blister formation due to minimal mechanical shear injury, resulting in extensive scarring. The anesthetic management of children with EB can present an array of unique challenges to the perioperative team. Anticipation and management of a potentially difficult airway as well as the protection of fragile skin and mucous membranes are high priorities during anesthetic planning. Complications can arise with use of even the most routine anesthesia monitors and placement of a simple peripheral intravenous (IV) line. Thorough preoperative planning and meticulous perioperative care will reduce complications ensuring a smooth anesthetic for both patient and clinician.

LEARNING OBJECTIVES

1. Review the pathology and clinical presentation of EB with special focus on anesthetic challenges.
2. Discuss principles of preoperative evaluation and perioperative management of EB patients.
3. Develop an anesthetic plan for EB patients, including induction, monitoring, airway management, and postoperative care.

CASE PRESENTATION

A 10-year-old Caucasian female with a medical history of recessive dystrophic EB, ***esophageal strictures****, and poor nutritional status presents for esophageal dilation and percutaneous endoscopic gastrostomy tube placement. She has had several esophageal dilations for difficulty swallowing due to strictures; however, she continues to lose weight despite oral nutritional supplementation. Her past medical history is otherwise not significant except for dental caries. Parents report* ***difficult intubation*** *with a prior anesthetic performed 2 months ago for dental rehabilitation at an outside hospital. On physical examination, the patient is a cooperative but anxious 22-kg female who has the characteristic features of recessive dystrophic EB: extensive* ***skin blistering*** *in various stages of healing, all extremities wrapped in dressings,* ***pseudosyndactyly*** *of hands and feet, partial alopecia, and flexion contractures of elbows and knees. Her airway exam is significant for* ***microstomia*** *with only 1.4 cm of mouth opening, multiple caps on her teeth,* ***ankyloglossia****, and* ***bullae of the oral mucosal surfaces****.*

After the operating room (OR) is prepared (the difficult airway cart and fiberoptic bronchoscope are available), the patient with one parent is brought to the operating room. Oxygen saturation is measured with a ***clip pulse oximeter probe*** *rather than an adhesive-style probe. The blood pressure cuff is applied over several layers of cotton gauze wrapping the extremity and cycled sparingly. Electrocardiogram leads are placed with the adhesive portion removed and secured to the patient with nonadhesive tape and wraps. A* ***well-lubricated mask*** *is gently applied to the face for inhalational induction with oxygen, nitrous oxide, and sevoflurane. Easy mask ventilation is confirmed. A tourniquet is placed gently over layers of gauze and an IV catheter is placed in the forearm with ultrasound assistance. The IV is then secured with* ***nonadhesive dressing****, wrapped gently with gauze, and then covered with an elastic wrap.*

After the administration of IV muscle relaxant and opioid, laryngoscopy is performed with a lubricated video laryngoscope, and a styletted 5.0 cuffed endotracheal tube (ETT) is placed. The tube is secured loosely behind the neck with cotton ties. The eyes are lubricated with preservative-free eye drops and covered with gauze pads moistened with saline. Using a hydrostatic balloon technique and fluoroscopy, the pediatric surgeon performs esophageal dilation. After the abdomen is prepped with betadine and endoscope appropriately positioned in the stomach, the percutaneous gastrostomy tube is placed. As the surgeon removes the endoscope, the larynx and portions of the oropharynx are inspected for new bullae formation. The patient is ***extubated fully awake*** *and transported to the postanesthesia care unit, where her recovery is uncomplicated with no evidence of airway obstruction. After a period of close observation, she is discharged to the acute care floor for postoperative care. During the follow-up visit the next day, a small bulla was noted on the tongue and several new bullae had formed on her extremity due to accidentally hitting the hospital bed rails while sleeping.*

DISCUSSION

1. What is the basic pathophysiology and clinical presentation of EB?

EB is a group of rare, inherited mechanobullous disorders in which blister formation and subsequent scarring occur with even minor skin trauma. The pathophysiology involves abnormalities in the attachment complexes anchoring the epidermis to the underlying dermis and below. Over 20 clinically different types of EB have been described with 4 main categories of EB notably based on the skin layer in which **blistering** occurs: simplex EB (EBS), junctional EB (JEB), dystrophic EB (DEB), and mixed EB (Kindler syndrome) (Herod et al., 2002). EB simplex (92% prevalence) with autosomal dominant inheritance, is the mildest variant. It results from an abnormality in the basement membrane of the epidermis and causes generalized bullae, but overall the lesions heal without scarring. While rare, EBS may be associated with muscular dystrophy; therefore, questions regarding progressive muscle weakness should be elicited during the history. Junctional EB-JEB (1% prevalence) has an autosomal recessive inheritance pattern and manifests as an abnormality in the basement membrane of the dermis. JEB subtypes have the highest risk of laryngeal stenosis or stricture with airway obstruction. With its extensive mucosal involvement, this variant can result in death from respiratory distress or sepsis before the age of 2 years. Dystrophic EB-DEB (5% prevalence) may be either autosomal recessive or dominant and results from abnormalities below the layer of the basement membrane. Due to its extensive scarring, along with oral and esophageal involvement, this incapacitating, disfiguring variant is the most common type presenting for surgery. Kindler syndrome is a rare autosomal recessive type of EB with only 170 cases reported in the literature. In addition to the skin blistering, it is characterized by photosensitivity and progressive poikiloderma, which is the combination of skin atrophy, telangiectasias, and pigmentary changes. Blistering of the skin occurs in variable locations of the epidermis, dermis, and basement membrane.

Patients with recessive DEB typically have limited mouth opening (**microstomia**) due to scarring and contractures at the corners of the mouth, scarring of the tongue to the floor of the mouth (**ankyloglossia**), and erosions and **bullae of the oral mucosa**. The teeth are often angled inward, and extensive dental caries may be present. Due to eyelid scarring, EB patients often have difficulty closing their eyes and develop recurrent corneal abrasions which may threaten vision in the long term. **Extreme skin fragility** is evidenced by extensive blisters and erosions along with scars from healing wounds. Chronic scarring increases their risk of melanoma and squamous cell carcinoma. Annual or biannual surveillance of skin lesions is highly recommended once patients reach the second decade. **Strictures** may develop in the proximal esophagus due to recurrent injury from swallowing solids. Contractures of the extremities are present, along with fusion of the digits resulting in "mitten" deformities (**pseudosyndactyly**). Osteoporosis and reduced bone densities are attributed to poor nutrition, reduced mobility and weight bearing, delayed puberty, and decreased sun exposure from extensive wound dressings. Growth retardation and failure to thrive due to the high caloric demand of the constant healing process is common and is exacerbated by poor oral intake from dysphagia. Malnutrition and vitamin deficiency can result in impaired immunity and may lead to chronic infection in the face of compromised skin integrity. Anemia due to iron deficiency and chronic disease is often present. Finally, from a cardiorespiratory standpoint, these patients may exhibit aspiration with frequent respiratory infections as well as decreased pulmonary function due to the mechanical restriction created by scarring of the chest wall. Recessive dystrophic patients may develop a dilated cardiomyopathy as a result of severe, chronic anemia and selenium deficiency.

2. Is there a cure for EB?

Currently there is no cure for this rare disease; however, there is promising research that shows potential for stem cell therapy and natural gene therapy. This data will hopefully lead to treatments that will improve the quality of life for patients with EB (Hsu et al., 2014).

3. What issues deserve attention during preoperative evaluation?

A difficult airway may result from a combination of microstomia, ankyloglossia, neck contractures, oropharyngeal bullae, and laryngeal stenosis. A thorough airway exam should be performed with special attention to these physical findings, and management of a **difficult airway** should be anticipated. During childhood, direct laryngoscopy is generally straightforward. As patients approach adolescence and the microstomia becomes more severe, intubation becomes difficult, often requiring **fiberoptic intubation**. Mask ventilation is usually not difficult due to anchoring of the tongue anteriorly from scar formation. Patients may have extensive dental disease as a result of an inability to perform oral hygiene. Careful examination of the patient's dentition to ensure no further dental injury when securing the airway is particularly important. Blistering wounds present before surgery should be well documented so that these may be compared to new bullae formed in the postoperative period.

A complete blood count to assess the degree of anemia and echocardiogram are helpful preoperative tests. Many EB centers have started to obtain annual echocardiograms to screen for cardiomyopathy. Nephrotic syndrome and postinfectious glomeronephritis are rare complications in DEB patients; therefore, laboratory testing to evaluate renal function may be indicated.

A plan for postoperative analgesia can be initiated with the patient and family. DEB patients may have delayed resumption of oral intake after, due to airway swelling or bullae formation. Regional anesthesia can be offered to patients with EB (Herod et al., 2002). In the absence of contraindications, caudal, spinal, or epidural anesthesia for procedures involving the abdomen, pelvis, or lower extremities as well as peripheral nerve blockade for procedures on the extremities are all viable supplements or alternatives to general anesthesia. Care in applying nonadhesive dressings is important, and any indwelling catheters are secured with sutures. Treatment of pruritic side effects from intravenous (IV) or neuraxial opioids are important to reduce further skin blistering from scratching. A multimodal approach with IV acetaminophen, nonsteroidal anti-inflammatory drugs, regional techniques if applicable, and IV opioids (either intermittent or patient-controlled) is typically utilized and effective.

Table 60.1 summarizes perioperative anesthetic care for patients with EB.

4. What procedures are commonly performed in children with EB?

Although patients with EB may present for any type of surgery, certain procedures are commonly performed. These include hand surgery for correction of **pseudosyndactyly**, endoscopy or balloon esophageal dilation with fluoroscopy to diagnose and manage esophageal strictures, percutaneous endoscopic gastrostomy or open gastrostomy for nutritional supplementation, skin biopsies to rule out squamous cell carcinoma, and subsequent excision of squamous cell carcinoma with skin grafting. Dental rehabilitation is often performed to correct extensive decay and to maintain oral hygiene that may otherwise be impossible for the patient due to microstomia and delicate oral mucosa. Finally, anesthesia may be required to provide comfort during wound care such as dressing changes or whirlpool bath treatments for skin debridement.

5. What precautions should be taken in the operating room?

Operating room preparation should include a warm room, a padded operating table, and an egg crate or other soft foam mattress that stays under the patient throughout the perioperative period. Despite the potential for difficult intubation, general endotracheal anesthesia is often the safest and most effective technique for many surgical cases. The airway is protected against aspiration, and optimal surgical conditions are provided for the procedure.

The skin and mucous membranes are very fragile, so minimizing trauma is of the utmost importance.

TABLE 60.1 BASICS OF PERIOPERATIVE ANESTHETIC CARE FOR PATIENTS WITH EPIDERMOLYSIS BULLOSA

General Principles
- Utilize the "no touch or minimal touch" principle.
- Avoid shearing or friction forces to minimize bulla formation.
- Compressive or direct forces to the skin are tolerated.
- Lift the patient during transfer. Avoid rolling or sliding devices.
- Avoid all adhesive tape, electrocardiogram leads, thermometry, and pulse oximeter probes.
- If patient dressings are in place and not in the way, leave them in place.
- Columnar mucosa of nares, larynx, and trachea distal to vocal cords are not affected.
- Tracheal intubation is acceptable.

OR Preparation
- Warm OR to reduce heat loss.
- Use padded OR table with unwrinkled sheet.
- Patient positions self onto bed or gentle transfer of patient.
- Egg crate mattress that stays under patient throughout perioperative period.
- Lubricate eyes with preservative-free, non-lanolin lubricant (Refresh®) and cover eyes with moistened gauze pads or nonadhesive tape (Mepitel® or Mepiform®).
- Assemble all necessary supplies ahead of time.
- Check IV site frequently as IVs tend to become dislodged more easily.

Airway Management
- Mask lubricated with ointment (e.g., Aquaphor®)
- Avoid oropharyngeal or nasopharyngeal airways if possible as it may cause blistering.
- Gentle intubation with well-lubricated laryngoscope and smaller than calculated size ETT
- Anticipate difficult intubation.
- Oral fiberoptic intubation if needed; avoid nasal intubation unless necessary.
- LMA may cause mucosal trauma and pharyngeal bullae.
- Secure ETT with nonadhesive cotton tape or suture to teeth.

Anesthetic Techniques
- General endotracheal anesthesia is advisable for esophageal dilation, dental rehabilitation, or major abdominal procedures.
- Mask anesthesia for brief procedures as appropriate.
- TIVA for whirlpool treatments or peripheral surgery using ketamine, propofol, remifentanil
- Regional anesthesia is acceptable: peripheral blocks, spinal, epidural, caudal (in dwelling catheters should be secured with sutures).
- Muscle relaxants including succinylcholine are acceptable.

Emergence/Postoperative Care
- Smooth emergence to avoid airway and skin trauma.
- Suction gently under direct vision when needed with lubricated suction catheter.
- Awake extubation to minimize airway obstruction and need for mask pressure.
- Appropriate analgesia with avoidance of histamine-releasing medications.
- Care for new skin lesions.
- Preemptively treat postoperative nausea and vomiting.
- Monitor for airway compromise.

Note. OR = operating room; IV = intravenous; ETT = endotracheal tube; LMA = laryngeal mask airway; TIVA = total intravenous anesthesia.

Premedication with oral midazolam helps promote a calm anesthetic induction with minimal anxiety, movement, and restlessness. To minimize patient anxiety, parental presence may be allowed during anesthesia induction. Due to difficulties in establishing venous access, anesthesia is usually induced by mask using inhalational anesthetics. The **anesthesia mask** is **lubricated** with Aquaphor® or

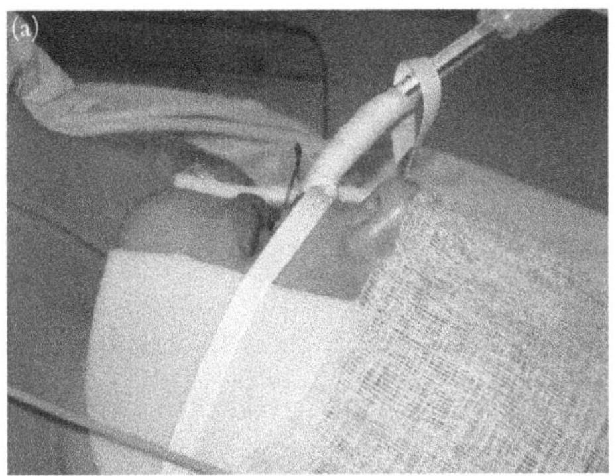

FIGURE 60.1A Airway secured without adhesives, eyes protected with moist gauze.

similar ointment, to minimize skin trauma and must be applied with gentle pressure. Using another approach, nonadhesive dressings (Mepilex®) may be placed on the face where the anesthesia mask and the anesthetist's hands contact the face. There should not be routine oro- or nasopharyngeal airway insertion nor chin lift or jaw thrust unless necessary for ventilation, which can cause damage to the skin. Alternately, venous access may be established in an awake patient for IV induction of anesthesia.

The tourniquet is placed gently over layers of gauze. Once established, venous access is secured with a nonadhesive dressing (Mepitel® or Mepitac®) and then wrapped gently with gauze and Coflex® wrap. For endotracheal intubation, gentle laryngoscopy with a lubricated blade is important to minimize oral trauma. The ETT is secured with cotton ties secured loosely behind the neck. The eyes should be lubricated with eye lubricant containing no lanolin, closed, and covered with saline-moistened gauze pads or nonadhesive tape. *No adhesive tape* of any kind may be used (Figs. 60.1a and 60.1b).

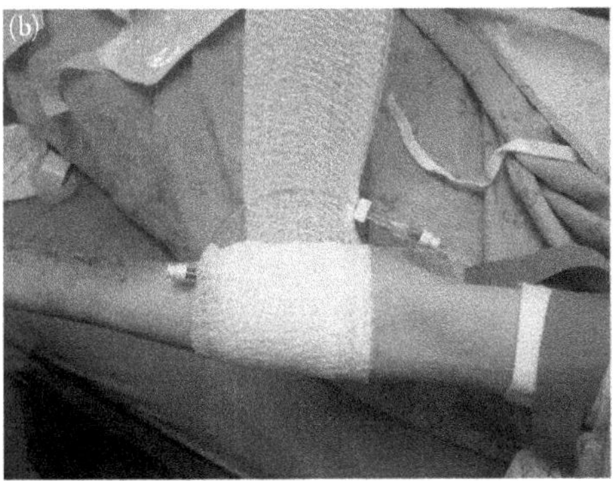

FIGURE 60.1B Peripheral venous catheter, secured without adhesives.

Extreme skin fragility poses challenges to the use of routine anesthesia monitors. A **clip pulse oximeter probe** is preferable to adhesive-style probes. Alternatively, for patients with **pseudosyndactyly**, the adhesive portion of a pulse oximetry probe is removed and the probe wrapped around the radial pulse with nonadhesive wrap. The blood pressure cuff is applied over several layers of cotton gauze wrapped around the extremity. Electrocardiogram pads, if used, must have the adhesive portions removed and secured to the patient with gauze or other nonadhesive wraps. A precordial stethoscope may simply be placed on the chest without adhesive. Prepping the skin for surgery requires gentle tapping of betadine or pouring of the solution onto the skin versus "scrubbing" the skin.

Muscle relaxants may help facilitate intubation after adequate mask ventilation is demonstrated, and antiemetics are given to prevent postoperative nausea and vomiting. Medications that cause histamine release should be avoided to decrease the risk of postoperative pruritus. Suctioning is performed under direct vision as the suction tip vacuum can damage the mucosa. The pharynx and larynx can be inspected prior to extubation to ensure that no glottic or pharyngeal bullosa have formed. Although **awake extubation** at the conclusion of the procedure may be associated with coughing and patient movement, it minimizes the risk of aspiration and the need for continued mask pressure to the face after extubation. While there is a risk of **postoperative airway obstruction from bullae formation**, significant airway obstruction in the recovery period is uncommon. A communication tool or sign placed at the head of the bed reminds staff and personnel about safe monitoring and handling techniques. After a period of close observation, many patients may be discharged home the same day.

6. What supplies are necessary?

- Nonadhesive dressing: for example, Mepitel®, Mepiform®, Mepilex®, Mepitac tape® (Molnlycke Healthcare, Goteburg, Sweden, www.molnlycke.com) or Vaseline gauze/Telfa®
- Nonadhesive wrap: for example, Coflex® (Andover) wrap or Coban® (3M), Kling® (J&J), Webril® (Kendall)

- Methylcellulose eye lubricant
- Cotton ties (umbilical tape) to secure the ETT
- Aquaphor® ointment (or similar) to lubricate anesthesia mask, water-based lubricant (e.g., Surgilube®) to lubricate oral airways, and laryngoscope blade
- Clip pulse oximeter probe
- Silicone-based adhesive remover

SUMMARY

1. EB is a genetically determined, blistering disorder that affects multiple organ systems and can have profound effects on anesthetic care.
2. OR preparation must account for delicate positioning and movement of the patient, as well as difficult airway and IV access.
3. Intraoperative monitoring needs modest adjustments to be performed safely, and postoperative pain management may proceed as for other patients.

ACKNOWLEDGMENTS

The author would like to thank Nancy B. Samol and Eric P. Wittkugel for their contributions to the first edition.

ANNOTATED REFERENCES

Herod J, Denyer J, Goldman A, Howard R. Epidermolysis bullosa in children: pathophysiology, anaesthesia and pain management. *Pediatr Anesth.* 2002;12:388–397.

This comprehensive review article provides a multidisciplinary approach to EB management with an overview of pathophysiology, complications, and practical recommendations for anesthetic care.

Hsu CK, Wang SP, Lee JY, et al. Treatment of epidermolysis bullosa: updates and future prospects. *Am J Clin Dermatol.* 2014;15(1):1–6.

This review article discusses a variety of potential new therapies aimed at curing EB beyond the traditional supportive care for epidermolysis bullosa.

FURTHER READING

Ames WA, Mayou BJ, Williams K. Anaesthetic management of epidermolysis bullosa. *Br J Anaesth.* 1999;82:746–751.

Azizkhan RG, Stehra W, Cohen AP, et al. Esophageal strictures in children with recessive dystrophic epidermolysis bullosa: an 11-year experience with fluoroscopically guided balloon dilation. *J Pediatr Surg.* 2006;41(1):55–60.

Baum VC, O'Flaherty JE. Epidermolysis bullosa. In: Oflaherty JE, ed. *Anesthesia for Genetic, Metabolic and Dysmorphic Syndromes of Childhood.* Philadelphia: Lippincott Williams & Wilkins; 2007:122–124.

Bissonnette B. Epidermolysis bullosa. In: Bissonnette B, ed. *Syndromes: Rapid Recognition and Perioperative Implications.* New York: McGraw-Hill; 2006:272–275.

Goldschneider KR, Lucky AW, Mellerio JE, Palisson F, Vinuela Miranda MDC, Azizkhan RG. Perioperative care of patients with epidermolysis bullosa: proceedings of the 5th International Symposium on Epidermolysis Bullosa, Santiago, Chile, Dec. 4–6, 2008. *Pediatr Anesth.* 2010;20:797–804.

Iohom G, Lyons B. Anaesthesia for children with epidermolysis bullosa: a review of 20 years' experience. *Eur J Anaesthesiol.* 2001;18:745–754.

Mellerio JE, Weiner M, Denyer JE, et al. Medical management of epidermolysis bullosa: proceedings of the IInd International Symposium on Epidermolysis Bullosa, Santiago, Chile, 2005. *Int J Dermatol.* 2007;46(8):795–800.

Spielman F, Mann E. Subarachnoid and epidural anesthesia for patients with epidermolysis bullosa. *Can Anaes Soc J.* 1984;31(5):549–551.

61

Osteogenesis Imperfecta

AIMEE G. KAKASCIK

INTRODUCTION

Osteogenesis imperfect a (OI) is a condition characetrized by weak bones that are prone to fracture. The condition may affect collagen by dominant, recessive, or spontaneous mutations. There are new forms being discovered that affect other genes not associated with collagen. Medical advances have resulted in an increase in survival of patients with OI type II, and more patients with this condition will present for surgery in the future. With careful considerations to the unique features of this condition, affected patients can successfully undergo anesthesia wihout the development of fractures, loss of airway, bleeding, cardiovascular collapse, and hyperthermia which are prone to develop.

LEARNING OBJECTIVES

1. Recognize the common clinical manifestations of OI.
2. Differentiate the types of OI.
3. Review preoperative anesthetic considerations for patients with OI.
4. Develop an anesthetic plan for the patient with OI to lessen complications.

CASE PRESENTATION

A 17-year-old, wheelchair bound male with OI type II and severe scoliosis presents for diagnostic laryngoscopy and bronchoscopy for excision of tracheal granuloma. The tracheal granuloma was diagnosed 1 year ago and recent flexible laryngoscopy through the pediatric 3.5 mm Shiley tracheostomy tube revealed 50% obstruction at the tip of the trachea. He has had this tracheostomy tube for many years and has outgrown this size.

Past medical history:

He was delivered at 36 weeks gestational age via emergency cesarean section secondary to cord prolapse. He spent the first 14 months of life in the neonatal intensive care unit secondary to pneumonia. He has pulmonary hypertension with frequent pneumonias and recently increasing carbon dioxide levels to 50 to 60 mmHg. He suffers from chronic respiratory insufficiency. He uses bilevel positive airway pressure 13 cm H_2O (IPAP) and 9 cm H_2O (EPAP) at night. Despite his developmental delay, he is able to communicate adequately.

Past surgical history:

He has had a tracheostomy, gastrostomy placement with subsequent closure, bilateral inguinal hernia repair, and ventriculo-peritoneal shunt placement.

Physical examination:

- *Tracheostomy dependent, on 0.5–2 L per minute oxygen at home*
- *A 116° curvature to the lower thoracic spine convex to the left with associated kyphosis of 118°*
- *Chest x-ray significant for diffuse skeletal changes, clear lungs, and tracheostomy tube in good position*
- *Existing right wrist fracture present as well as severely contracted extremities*
- *He denies any cough or fever although his temperature routinely averages higher than normal*

Preoperative course:

- *Admission vital signs: Temperature 37°C, pulse 132, respiratory rate 27 per minute, weight 13.7 kg, height 78 cm*
- *Blood pressure not obtained secondary to history of fractures with neonatal settings, automated*

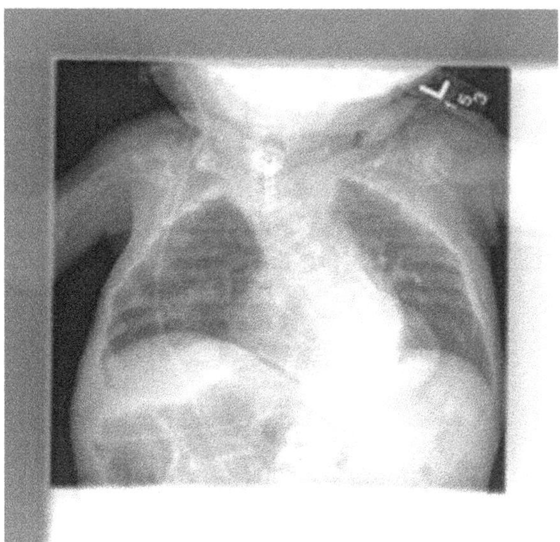

FIGURE 61.1 Chest X-Ray of patient showing clear lung fields and tracheostomy in situ

blood pressure cuffs as well as tourniquets for intravenous (IV) access

- *A 24-gauge peripheral IV is placed in the forehead without the use of a tourniquet*
- *No premedication given*

Intraoperative course:

You obtain assistance with positioning the patient from his personal nurse to prevent fractures. Extensive padding is utilized. A manual sphygmomanometer is utilized to measure blood pressure every 15 minutes by palpation to prevent a fracture from an automated cuff. Standard American Society of Anesthesiologists monitors are also used. The operating room is cooled to 18°C to prevent hyperthermia. An inhalational induction with sevoflurane was performed via the patient's tracheostomy. Spontaneous ventilation is maintained during the procedure. The patient is placed on Heliox shortly after induction to lower the inspired oxygen in order to prevent airway fire and decrease resistance in the occluded tracheostomy. Due to concern for a cervical spine fracture, a 2.8 flexible bronchoscope is used instead of a rigid bronchoscope. A YAG laser is then used to excise the granuloma through the flexible bronchoscope. After the excision, a more flexible 4.0 tracheostomy tube with adjustable length is placed by the surgeon to bypass the site of previous tracheal irritation from the old tracheostomy tube. Dexamethasone 5 mg IV is administered to reduce airway edema along with lidocaine 30 mg IV via the tracheostomy to prevent reactivity. At the end of the surgery, the patient is transported to the recovery room on 100% oxygen via a Jackson-Reese circuit. Normothermia was maintained throughout the surgical procedure and during the postanesthetic recovery period.

Postoperative course:

The postoperative course is uneventful with CO2 level decreasing to 50 mmHg following surgery, and the patient is discharged home the next morning. Figures 61.1 to 61.3 show the granuloma before excision and the trachea following excision.

DISCUSSION

1. What is OI?

OI is a genetic disorder that is characterized by very easily broken bones. The estimate of the number of people affected with OI in the United States is 20,000 to 50,000. OI is caused by genetic defects that affect the body's ability to make strong bones. In dominant (classical) OI, a person is lacking or has poor quality of type I collagen due to a mutation in one of the type I collagen genes. In recessive OI, mutations in other genes interfere with collagen production. Because OI is so rare, it is challenging to have an in-depth understanding of the natural history of the varying disease types. Thus a network of 5 hospitals, the Linked Clinical Research Centers, formed a joint initiative between the Osteogenesis Imperfecta Foundation and the Children's Brittle

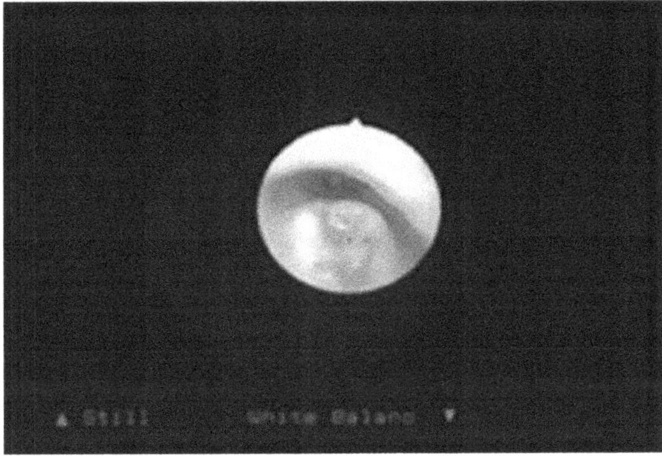

FIGURE 61.2 View via the flexible bronchoscope showing granuloma causing complete occlusion of the airway.

Bone Foundation to increase and improve clinical research as well as patient care of patients with OI (Patel & Nagamani, 2015).

2. What are the different types of OI?

According to the Osteogenesis Imperfecta Foundation, the characteristic features of OI vary greatly even among people with the same type of OI. Types of OI, characteristics and life expectancy of each type are listed in Table 61.1. The majority of cases of OI (85%–90%) are caused by a dominant mutation in a gene coding for type I collagen (types I, II, III, and IV). Types V and VI do not have a type 1 collagen mutation. Types VII and VIII are newly identified forms that are inherited in a recessive manner. The Osteogenesis Imperfecta Foundation (2017) lists the general features of types I to IV as follows:

Type I

- Most common and mildest type of OI.
- Bones fracture easily. Most fractures occur before puberty.
- Normal or near-normal stature.
- Loose joints and muscle weakness.
- Sclera (whites of the eyes) usually have a blue, purple, or gray tint.
- Triangular face.
- Tendency toward spinal curvature.
- Bone deformity absent or minimal.
- Brittle teeth possible.
- Hearing loss possible, often beginning in early 20's or 30's.
- Collagen structure is normal, but the amount is less than normal.

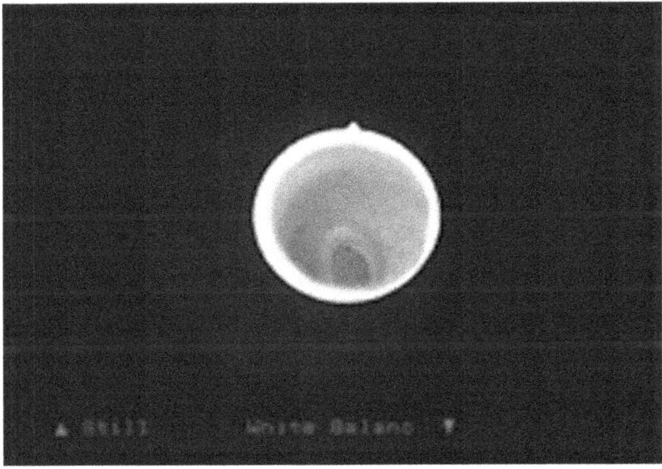

FIGURE 61.3 View via the flexible bronchoscope showing patent airway after excision of the granuloma.

Type II

- Most severe form.
- Frequently lethal at or shortly after birth, often due to respiratory problems.
- Numerous fractures and severe bone deformity.
- Small stature with underdeveloped lungs.
- Tinted sclera.
- Collagen improperly formed.

Type III

- Bones fracture easily. Fractures often present at birth, and x-rays may reveal healed fractures that occurred before birth.
- Short stature.
- Sclera have a blue, purple, or gray tint.
- Loose joints and poor muscle development in arms and legs.
- Barrel-shaped rib cage.
- Triangular face.
- Spinal curvature.
- Respiratory problems possible.
- Bone deformity, often severe.
- Brittle teeth possible.
- Hearing loss possible.
- Collagen improperly formed.

Type IV

- Between type I and type III in severity.
- Bones fracture easily. Most fractures occur before puberty.
- Shorter than average stature.
- Sclera are white or near-white (i.e., normal in color).
- Mild to moderate bone deformity.
- Tendency toward spinal curvature.
- Barrel-shaped rib cage.
- Triangular face.
- Brittle teeth possible.
- Hearing loss possible.
- Collagen improperly formed.

3. How is OI inherited?

Most cases of OI (85%–90%) are caused by a dominant genetic defect. Only 1 copy of the mutation carrying gene is necessary for the child to have OI. Children who have the dominant form of OI have it either as a spontaneous mutation with neither parent having OI or inherited it from a parent. Approximately 10% to 15% of cases of OI are the result of a recessive mutation (Osteogenesis Imperfecta Foundation, 2017).

4. Why is it important to include all caregivers in the preoperative evaluation?

This patient presents a challenging case as most children with OI type II do not survive to the late teenage years. Intraoperative assistance with positioning by a personal caregiver or home nurse who is knowledgeable about the patient's range of motion and other details may help to prevent anxiety, undue discomfort, and the development of fractures. Avoiding pharmacologic premedication minimizes respiratory depression in patients who have chronic respiratory insufficiency and allows for quick emergence from anesthesia.

5. Why did this patient have a tracheostomy tube?

The airway in patients with OI can be extremely difficult to manage. The pressure from applying a facemask can be enough to cause facial fractures. Any neck extension could lead to cervical fracture and paralysis.

6. Why was an inhalation induction used to anesthetize this patient?

Sevoflurane was utilized in order to maintain spontaneous ventilation and to lessen airway reactivity. It will also, prevent further elevations in carbon dioxide.

7. Are patients with OI at risk for malignant hyperthermia?

Temperature elevation in OI patients differs from malignant hyperthermia due to a lack of respiratory acidosis and muscle rigidity (Wilton & Anderson, 2009). Total intravenous anesthesia (TIVA) has been advocated as a way to prevent extreme elevations in temperature that may occur in this group of patients (Ogawa et al., 2009). However, in patients who have received inhalational anesthetics previously with no complications, the use of volatile anesthetics may be a reasonable option. In addition, for this airway procedure, the existing IV access needed to be preserved for rescue drug administration in the event of loss of the airway. Should cardiac compressions be required in the course of this patients care, the ability to administer resuscitation medications via in intravenous access site would be necessary as compressions could result in the development of massive fractures. Pressure as little as that occurring from succinylcholine-induced fasciculations are believed to result in multiple fractures in these patients.

8. What is the risk of using automated blood pressure measurements in patients with OI?

The use of a manual blood pressure cuff decreases the chances of precipitating fractures from excessive pressures which can be generated by an automatic cuff. In this case difficulty was encountered even in finding a place to put the cuff due to extensive existing fractures, and invasive monitoring was also not possible due to extreme contractures. Patients can suffer fractures from the placement of a tourniquet for peripheral IV catheter placement, increased pressures from succinylcholine-induced fasciculations, and certainly from chest compressions. Less severe forms of OI can tolerate automated blood pressures using the neonatal blood pressure cuff.

9. Did this patient have any lung disease?

Yes, he had a chronic elevation of carbon dioxide due to the airway obstruction as well as a restrictive lung disease due to his kyphoscoliosis and chest wall abnormalities. Restrictive lung disease is often seen in patients with OI. After surgery, an improvement was observed in the patient's carbon dioxide level with a decrease to 50 mmHg in the venous blood gas.

10. What cardiovascular conditions may be observed in OI patients?

Type I may have aortic root dilation, aortic insufficiency, or mitral valve prolapse. Type III may have cor pulmonale from severe kyphoscoliosis as present in the patient in this case discussion (Stynowick & Tobias, 2007).

11. Can regional anesthesia be an option in patients with OI?

There have been reports of caudal blocks utilized in pediatric patients with OI (Barros F. 1995). One must be careful as bones can be fractured by the needle and type I patients may have functional platelet abnormality. These platelet abnormalities have led to increased bleeding after cardiac surgery (Stynowick & Tobias, 2007).

12. Is there any risk of hemorrhage in patients with OI?

While the coagulation studies in these patients are usually normal, abnormal bleeding does occur in 10% to 30% of these patients due to defects in the type I collagen which is present in the blood vessels. They may also have problems with platelet adhesion and aggregation as well as blood vessel constriction (Stynowick & Tobias, 2007). Desmopressin and factor VII have been used for excessive bleeding (Keegan et al., 2002).

SUMMARY

1. OI is a collagen deficiency that results in bone weakness.
2. OI can compromise multiple organ systems.
3. Airway management can be difficult, due to inherent airway issues, restricted manipulation of the head and cervical spine, and risk of fracture.
4. Bleeding risk can be elevated and hard to predict.
5. Resuscitation efforts can be difficult due to not being able to use succinylcholine or chest compressions, as these can lead to massive fractures.

TABLE 61.1 MAJOR TYPES OF OSTEOGENESIS IMPERFECTA

Type	Inheritance	Manifestations	Lifespan
I	Autosomal dominant	Fragile bones, blue sclera, hearing impairment, normal stature	Normal
II	Autosomal dominant, sporadic new mutations	Intrauterine fractures, pulmonary function and swallowing compromised from birth	Lethal as neonate
III	Autosomal dominant, sporadic new mutations	Fragile bones, progressive bowing of long bones, short stature, kyphoscoliosis, poor dentition, triangular facies	Decreased
IV	Autosomal dominant	Moderate skeletal fragility, short stature, early blue sclera becoming white with age, dental involvement variable	Normal

ACKNOWLEDGMENTS

The author would like to thank Mario Patino and Anna M. Varughese for their contributions to the first edition.

ANNOTATED REFERENCES

Baum C, O'Flaherty JE. *Anesthesia for Genetic, Metabolic & Dysmorphic Syndromes of Childhood*. 2nd ed. Philadelphia: Lippincott Williams & Wilkins; 2007;283–285.

This text provides an overview of the OI and its effect on each system as well as anesthetic considerations.

Keegan MT, Whatcott BD, Harrison BA. Osteogenesis imperfecta, perioperative bleeding and desmopressin. *Anesthesiology*. 2002;97:1011–1013.

This source provides insight regarding the potential for bleeding as well as the treatment of perioperative bleeding in patients with OI.

Ogawa S, Okutani R, Suehiro K. Anesthetic management using total intravenous anesthesia with remifentanil in a child with osteogenesis imperfecta. *J Anesth*. 2009;23:123–125.

This source provides a case of a patient with OI and discusses the potential for fractures during airway management as well as discusses the use of TIVA.

Osteogenesis Imperfecta Foundation. 2017. http://oif.org.

This website provides information for patients, families, caregivers, and medical professionals regarding OI.

Patel, RM, Nagamani, SM. A cross sectional multicenter study of osteogenesis imperfecta in North America—results from the linked clinical research centers. *Clin Genet*. 2015;87:130–140.

This study combines the data from multiple centers, discusses the very rare condition of OI, and provides a better understanding of the natural history of the disease.

Stynowick GA, Tobias JD. Perioperative care of the patient with osteogenesis imperfect. *Orthopedics*. 2007;30:1043–1049.

This source discusses the delicate management of the patient with OI.

Wilton, N. Anderson, B. Orthopedic and spine surgery. In: Coté CJ, Lerman J, Todres ID, eds. *A Practice of Anesthesia for Infants and Children*. 4th ed. Philadelphia: Elsevier; 2009:652–653.

This text discusses the natural history of OI and orthopedic and anesthetic considerations.

FURTHER READING

Barros F. Caudal block in a child with osteogenesis imperfecta, type II. *Pediatr Anesth*. 1995;5:202–203.

Charnas LR, Marini JC. Communicating hydrocephalus, basilar invagination, and other neurologic features in osteogenesis imperfect. *Neurology*. 1993 Dec;43(12):2603.

Genetics Home Reference. National Institutes of Health. National Library of Medicine. www.ghr.nlm.nih.gov

NORD®. National Organization for Rare Disorders. www.rarediseases.org

62

Cerebral Palsy

MEGHA KANJIA

INTRODUCTION

Cerebral palsy (CP) is a neurologic disorder with an incidence of 2.2 per 1,000 live births, with 80% of cases being acquired prenatally without any obvious insult (Coté et al., 2012). There is a strong association with prematurity and low birth weight, as well as intrauterine growth restriction, intracranial hemorrhage, and trauma (Coté et al., 2012). Eleven percent of babies delivered at 24 to 27 weeks have CP (Brown & Alexis, 2015). Given their comorbidities and complex issues, patients with CP frequently require anesthesia. A thorough understanding of these patients' conditions and comorbidities is imperative to formulate appropriate preoperative, intraoperative, and postoperative anesthetic plans.

LEARNING OBJECTIVES

1. Define cerebral palsy and its clinical manifestations.
2. Recognize anesthetic considerations in a pediatric patient with CP.
3. Formulate an anesthetic plan for patients with CP and existing comorbidities.

CASE PRESENTATION

A 14-year-old male with history of cerebral palsy, epilepsy, grade IV intraventricular hemorrhage, hydrocephalus, and status post ventriculoperitoneal (VP) shunt at birth, presents for surgery. He was born at 25 weeks and had a prolonged stay in the neonatal intensive care unit (NICU), requiring intubation and ventilation as well as a gastrostomy tube for further nutrition. He had a history of a patent ductus arteriosus, which did not require surgical intervention, as well as bronchopulmonary dysplasia. He was eventually discharged from the NICU at 9 months of age and was followed with an Apparent Life-Threatening Event monitor at home for3 months subsequently. He has undergone 4 surgeries related to his VP shunt including replacements and revisions, without major anesthetic issues. While he is developmentally delayed, he has the cognitive capacity of an 11- to 12-year-old child. He presents with acute appendicitis and will be undergoing a laparoscopic appendectomy.

DISCUSSION

1. What causes CP? When does this insult occur? How is the disorder classified?

Birth complications account for only 6% of CP diagnoses, primarily related to asphyxia. Postnatally, infectious causes account for 10% of cases, and may include bacterial meningitis, viral encephalitis, trauma, or metabolic disturbances (Coté et al., 2012). However, during pregnancy, the second trimester can be a period of concern due to several factors that may trigger CP. These factors include insults from teratogenic risks, vascular overgrowth within the lateral ventricles, which may lead to **intraventricular hemorrhage,** and white matter vulnerability. Oligodendrocyte proliferation occurs during the 23rd to 32nd weeks of gestation but this cell proliferation is halted secondary to premature delivery. Hence white matter vulnerability is seen with higher consistency in the premature infant with CP. Since central nervous system maturation and myelination does not occur until the end of the second year of life, perinatal insults that are observed in CP patients can cause a disruption of this neuroproliferative process, resulting in halted or delayed development (Estrada et al., 2013).

2. How is CP classified?

CP is classified by **spasticity**: either spastic or extrapyramidal. Spastic CP patients display increased tone and clonus, while extrapyramidal patients display clonus and rigidity with variable tone. They may also have choreoathetosis, ataxia, or hypotonia. Motor deficits may also be classified as monoparesis (single limb), diparesis, triparesis, or tetraparesis.

CP encompasses a vast spectrum of patients for which the pediatric anesthesiologist may have to take multiple factors into consideration regarding anesthetic management. Though some CP patients may have severely limited physical abilities, others have normal intelligence and can assent for procedures (Coté et al., 2012). It is important to remember that patients may come in for procedures related to their underlying condition of CP but may also come to the operating room for similar procedures as those of healthy children. Common procedures for patients with CP may include surgeries related to VP shunts or other orthopedic procedures to address contractures.

3. What specific comorbidities/other features are commonly seen in patients with CP?

Patients with CP often have a number of concomitant conditions, which may include **gastroesophageal reflux disease (GERD), chronic aspiration, immobility, pulmonary disease, epilepsy, and contractures**. These patients often require additional medications and considerations for their additional comorbidities. Patients with **bulbar and hypothalamic dysfunction** may have ongoing problems with **aspiration, sleep apnea, as well as hypothermia** (Coté et al., 2012).

Chronic or recurrent aspiration may result in poor nutrition as well as poor respiratory reserve, which may require procedures such as fundoplication and a gastrostomy tube for feeding. Additionally, immobility and poor hydration may lead to fecal impaction and electrolyte imbalances that may require ongoing monitoring or treatment.

Pulmonary affectation is the most common cause of death in patients with CP; aspiration, respiratory infections, and **restrictive lung disease** secondary to chronic scoliosis are all contributing factors. Respiratory issues during the perioperative period are the most concerning in this specific group of patients because they are at an increased risk for aspiration and pneumonia and often have very poor residual reserve.

The most common type of procedures that CP patients undergo are orthopedic procedures, which comprise up to 60% of surgeries in this patient population (Darcey, 2010). Common orthopedic procedures include tendon releases for contractures, osteotomies, hip adductor/iliopsoas releases, scoliosis surgery, spinal fusions, and baclofen pump placements. Thirty percent of patients with CP also have epilepsy, so adherence to epilepsy medication schedule should be observed in the peri-operative phase.

4. What are the specific anesthetic considerations for patients with CP?

Pharmacologic considerations

Children with CP may be on any of the following medications: **anticonvulsants, corticosteroids, sedating medications, as well as ketogenic diets**. Anticonvulsants may result in resistance to neuromuscular blockers so the patients may require frequent redosing. Additionally, carbamazepine and valproic acid can cause hepatotoxicity and bone marrow suppression. Use of meperidine promotes accumulation of the metabolite normeperidine, which can precipitate seizures as well (Brown & Alexis, 2015). Additionally, anticonvulsants may affect platelet function, and increase the risk of bleeding in patients with CP (Theroux & Akins, 2005). Pre-operative sedatives should be administered judiciously as many patients with CP also have obstructive sleep apnea (OSA). An increased propensity for aspiration and obstruction may also be observed in CP patients with hypotonia (Thereoux & Akins, 2005).

These patients may also be receiving corticosteroids for treatment of infantile seizures; this may cause adrenal suppression and hypokalemia, therefore electrolytes should be reviewed to rule out any secondary electrolyte disturbances. Other considerations such as ketogenic diet restrictions may be warranted. Appropriate care should be taken to ensure the shortest interval of fasting, adequate glucose monitoring, hydration, and metabolic acidemia suppression. Dextrose-containing fluids and sugar-containing medications/syrups should also be avoided in the perioperative period for patients who are on a ketogenic diet (Brown & Alexis, 2015). It is also crucial to remember that patients with CP will have a normal response to pain and consideration of peripheral nerve blocks, caudal blocks, and epidurals may help reduce overall anesthetic requirements. Lastly, patients with CP may have frank latex allergies and latex precautions may need to be observed in general due to repeated exposure to gloves, Foley catheters, and other medical supplies.

Temperature considerations

Patients with CP often have poorly regulated homeostatic systems and hypothalamic imbalances, which most often lead to hypothermia perioperatively. Hypothermia and temperature dysregulation can lead to poor platelet function, coagulopathy, and decreased metabolism of anesthetic medications. Maintaining the temperature of the patients within normal range in the operating room is a necessity.

Analgesic considerations

Given the frequency of orthopedic surgeries that may be performed in this subset of patients, it is important to consider pain management during the intra- and postoperative periods. Pain is grossly undertreated in patients who are nonverbal or have difficulty in language expression, so they should be closely monitored for other signs of pain and parental input should be encouraged in these instances. While CP patients have an increased risk for opioid-induced respiratory depression, pain should be adequately managed in this patient population as they still have normal analgesic requirements. Mean alveolar concentrations (MAC) of halothane have previously been noted to be decreased by as much as 20% in patients with CP (Darcey, 2010; Theroux & Akins, 2005). Due to differences in anesthetic requirement observed in these patients, some anesthesiologists have argued in favor of the use of the bispectral index monitor in this population (Coté et al., 2012; Frei et al., 1997). The possibility of delayed emergence should be considered particularly in the setting of decreased anesthetic requirements and especially if hypothermia is present as the latter may decrease the metabolism of anesthetic agents in this patient population (Darcey, 2010).

Given the large percentage of patients with CP that have epilepsy, specific questions about the seizures should be asked: What medication regimen is the patient currently on? How well controlled are the seizures? What medications are used as "rescue medications" for ongoing seizures? Patients with significant contractures may have an intrathecal baclofen pump in situ or may be taking baclofen. It is important to continue the baclofen through the perioperative period to avoid precipitating withdrawal or seizures.

Gastrointestinal considerations

Increased activity of the salivary glands can result in copious secretions, which may be difficult to manage, especially with uncoordinated cranial nerve function. Glycopyrrolate and frequent suctioning may be necessary to manage secretions.

Respiratory considerations

Understanding the respiratory needs of the patient, including the use of a home ventilator, bi-level positive airway pressure, or continuous positive airway pressure can help prepare the anesthesiologist for the postoperative course. Anxiolytics, if required, should be administered judiciously as patients may have OSA which will be exacerbated by sedatives. Additionally, these patients may have decreased functional residual capacity and frequent pneumonia may be an issue given difficulty with clearing secretions that is occasionally present.

Developmental considerations

The spectrum of ability and understanding of a child with CP is widespread. It is often helpful to have a solid understanding of the patient's developmental age as this will allow the anesthesiologist to better understand how to approach the patient. It is always important to obtain assent for a procedure if the patient is developmentally appropriate. In addition, child life services are often able to help these patients better understand and cope with the surgery or procedure.

SUMMARY

1. Patients with CP often have developmental delay along with multiple comorbidities including GERD, chronic aspiration, immobility/contractures, pulmonary conditions, and epilepsy.
2. Anesthetic issues commonly seen in patients with CP may include impaired temperature control, challenges with positioning due to contractures, analgesic considerations, respiratory considerations, bleeding, varied developmental ability, and medication dosing variability.
3. Additional postoperative challenges may include evaluation and effective pain management, spasticity, temperature control, and return to respiratory and neurological baseline.

4. Close involvement of the patient's caregiver is in the best interest of the patient, family, as well as the anesthesiologist, as he or she may provide invaluable insight to appropriate anesthetic management in light of the patient's complex medical history.

ACKNOWLEDGMENT

The author wishes to acknowledge the first edition author, George Chalkiadis.

BIBLIOGRAPHY

Brown AK and Alexis RA 2015. Seizure disorder, cerebral palsy, autism. In *Critical Incidents and Essential Topics in Pediatric Anesthesiology*. Cambridge University Press; 2015.

Coté CJ, Lerman J, Todres ID. *A Practice of Anesthesia for Infants and Children*. Philadelphia: Elsevier Health Sciences; 2012.

Darcey M. Anaesthetic management of patients with cerebral palsy. *Anaesthesia Tutorial of the Week*. 2010;196. http://www.frca.co.uk/

Estrada C. Condensed Review of Pediatric Anesthesia by Estrada CR, Stayer SA, Mann DG, Carling NP, Patel NV., Hopkins PW 1st ed. 2013. www.ebookconversion.com

Frei F, Haemmerle M, Brunner R, Kern C. Minimum alveolar concentration for halothane in children with cerebral palsy and severe mental retardation. *Anaesthesia*. 1997;52(11):1056–1060.

Olutoye OA. *Handbook of Critical Incidents and Essential Topics in Pediatric Anesthesiology*. Cambridge, UK: Cambridge University Press; 2014.

Theroux MC, Akins RE. Surgery and anesthesia for children who have cerebral palsy. *Anesthesiol Clin North Am*. 2005;23(4):733–743.

PART 14

Challenges in the Postanesthesia Care Unit

63

Accidental Awareness under General Anesthesia

ERIN S. WILLIAMS

INTRODUCTION

Accidental awareness under general anesthesia (AAGA) is a rare, yet devastating complication. The anesthesiologist has multiple mechanisms in his or her armamentarium to help ensure the patient is adequately anesthetized. There are a variety of factors that can increase or decrease the potential for accidental awareness, such as nature of surgery, type of anesthetic administered, and patient comorbidities. Ultimately it is the sole responsibility of the anesthesiologist to discuss the potential for awareness with the patient during the informed consent process. The anesthesiologist must not only be mindful of the potential risk of awareness but also must be very vigilant in preventing this terrible complication.

LEARNING OBJECTIVES

1. Explain the characteristics of AAGA in children.
2. Review the risk factors for AAGA in children.
3. Understand the principles of preventing AAGA in children.

CASE PRESENTATION

You are in the preoperative holding area preparing to meet your patient and his family. As you enter the room, you notice the 14-year-old boy sitting next to his mother looking quite anxious. He is talking with his mother, stating he is "scared" and that he "does not want to have surgery today." You carefully approach the patient and gently extend your hand for a handshake and introduce yourself as the anesthesiologist who will be taking care of him. He hesitantly shakes your hand and says, "I don't want to do this today. I am afraid I will wake up like last time." The boy's mother reassuringly pats his back and says that he recalls waking up and feeling as though he was constantly choking on something when he had his first esophagogastroduodenoscopy (EGD) 1 year ago.

You ask the mother if she ever talked to the previous anesthesiologist about this, and she says that she thought her son was exaggerating, because he is typically quite dramatic, and she told him that he was fine. They never discussed it again until recently when they discovered he needed to have a repeat EGD for surveillance. Ever since the EGD has been scheduled, he has been quite nervous and constantly stating that he does not want to wake up during the procedure.

You sit next to the patient and ask him to tell you everything he can recall about his last surgery. He again is able to recount feeling as though he was constantly choking on something. He does not recall having frank pain or hearing voices. He even says, "Maybe I was dreaming." You thank your patient for being honest about his experience and you assure him that you will utilize a variety of resources to ensure that he is comfortable during the procedure, and also that he will remain deeply anesthetized until the procedure is completely done. You even show him the different anesthetics and monitors that you will be using during the case. He appears relieved and says, "Thank you for listening to me." You are glad to see his anxiety decrease and the case proceeds.

After a smooth inhalation induction, a peripheral venous catheter is placed and propofol 4 mg/kg, lidocaine 1mg/kg, and fentanyl 1mcg/kg are administered intravenously. The volatile anesthetic is turned off and the patient is successfully intubated.

Correct endotracheal tube (ETT) placement is confirmed with auscultation and end-tidal carbon dioxide. While taping the ETT in place, the alarm on your anesthesia machine goes off informing you that there is no ventilation. You activate the ventilator and turn on sevoflurane with oxygen and air mixture. The EGD is uneventful, and the patient is extubated deep. The patient is transported to the postanesthesia care unit breathing spontaneously and recovers well. Once the patient is awake, you ask the patient about the last thing he remembers, and the patient tells you, "I don't remember anything about the procedure or feeling like I did last time; thank you, I am not scared anymore." You call the patient the next day to determine if there was any recall during the procedure, and the patient's mother reports there was no memory of the intraoperative events. You tell the patient's mother to contact you or your department if any changes occur.

DISCUSSION

1. What is awareness?

Awareness is defined as the explicit recall of an actual event, or events that occurred during the intraoperative period of anesthesia (Tasbihgou et al., 2018). This recollection can be spontaneous and given voluntarily by the patient, or it can be evoked by questioning the patient. As mentioned, the term "awareness" has recently been also called accidental awareness under general anesthesia (AAGA). It is this unintended consciousness during an anesthetic that both patients and anesthesiologists fear.

2. Do children experience awareness?

The incidence of awareness in children is approximately twice as high as the adult population. As children may not be able to verbally express their thoughts, it can be quite challenging for the anesthesiologist to obtain a thorough history of the recalled events, especially from young children.

3. What is the incidence of AAGA?

The literature has suggested that AAGA is higher in the younger population, ranging from 0.2% to 1.2%, which is significantly higher than the adult population in which the incidence of AAGA has been stated to be anywhere from 1:600 patients to 1:17,000 patients (Tasbihgou et al., 2018). One study looked at self-reported occurrences of AAGA and found the incidence to be 1:19,600. Another study found the incidence to be 1:800. The reported incidence of awareness varies based on the type of investigation used to determine the presence of AAGA.

4. What are the risk factors for AAGA?

Factors that can increase the likelihood of AAGA in adults include neuromuscular blockade, cardiovascular instability, trauma, bronchoscopy, obstetric surgery, cardiac surgery, and a family history of awareness.

5. What is the isolated forearm test (IFT)?

There are many studies that have investigated the potential for awareness after induction of anesthesia, by placing a tourniquet on a patient's forearm then checking for the ability to follow commands prior to laryngoscopy and also after laryngoscopy and intubation. These studies showed 72% to 100% of the patients were able to follow commands. However, the patients were overwhelmingly unable to give explicit recall of intraoperative events. Because AAGA that is not associated with explicit recall of events has not been shown to have negative consequences, the IFT method is debatable as to its true confirmation or detection of AAGA.

6. What can be done to prevent AAGA?

There is the rare patient who has a genetic predisposition to metabolize anesthetics differently, thereby increasing the potential of AAGA even at doses that are typically deemed appropriate for rendering a patient unconscious. However, we do not understand the mechanism or cause of awareness in most children. It is therefore difficult to know exactly how to prevent this in children. We do know that children have a higher anesthetic requirement than adults. It may be that children are aware more often because the child did not receive an adequate amount of intravenous or volatile anesthetic, or the anesthesiologist did not wait long enough for the effect site concentration of the volatile anesthetic to be high enough before application of stimulus, such as surgical incision or laryngoscopy. Therefore, the simplest way to prevent awareness in children is to ensure an adequate dose of anesthetic has been administered to the patient and adequate time has been allowed for high enough effect-site levels, prior to any stimulus. A challenge, however, is that the knowledge of the pharmacology of anesthetics in children is still very incomplete. We have a rough idea of how minimal anesthetic concentration (MAC) changes with age, but there are few data on how MAC-awake changes with age. Similarly, we have little idea of the effect-site equilibration times in children.

The processed electroencephalogram (EEG) in the form of the BIS™, monitor is one of the EEG monitoring devices used intraoperatively to guide anesthetic depth. However, there is a paucity of data on the effectiveness of this device in preventing awareness in children. So while these devices may be used, their application does not guarantee absence of awareness. In one randomized trial (Myles et al., 2004), the BIS reduced awareness in high-risk adults. There is substantial evidence that these EEG devices function in older children in a similar way to how they function in adults. The readout numbers go down as the concentration of anesthetic increases, and they have a fair to good discriminative power in differentiating between awake and anesthetized states. As in adults, there are occasions where the performance of these monitors may be compromised, such as when ketamine is used as a sole agent, high-dose opioid anesthesia, or when high concentrations of sevoflurane are administered.

Ultimately, vigilance and meticulous attention is paramount for the pediatric anesthesiologist to prevent this complication.

7. In the event that a patient informs you that AAGA has occurred, what are the appropriate steps to take?

Any time a patient explains that he or she has experienced AAGA, the anesthesiologist must first listen to the patient. It is important to take the patient seriously and address the concern in a nonthreatening, nonjudgmental, nondefensive manner. The ability for a patient to disclose such information takes courage, and we must remember that. Once we are notified of this occurrence, we must seek the necessary interventions for the patient and his or her family. The explicit recall of intraoperative events can lead to significant negative consequences, including posttraumatic stress disorder (PTSD). Thus counseling and psychological interventions must be offered, and follow-up with the patient will be needed. In addition, the anesthesiologist should inform the patient's family of the potential for delayed manifestations of awareness when this is suspected, such as withdrawal, flashbacks, anxiety, or sleep disturbances. The family must also be encouraged to inform all future anesthesiologists of the AAGA occurrence in order to discuss and allay any concerns and also to ensure that this unfortunate incident does not occur again.

SUMMARY

1. Awareness does occur in children.
2. Awareness may occur following different types of anesthesia in children; specific high-risk groups have not been identified.
3. Awareness is usually less distressing in children, though in some children it can lead to severe psychological disturbance.
4. It is unclear why children experience a higher incidence of awareness, but it should be remembered that children have higher anesthetic requirements.
5. In theory, there may be a role for EEG in preventing awareness in children, but it is unproven.
6. Children who describe awareness should be taken seriously.

ACKNOWLEDGMENT

The authors wish to acknowledge the first edition author, Andrew Davidson.

ANNOTATED REFERENCES

Davidson AJ, Huang GH, Czarnecki C, Gibson MA, Stewart SA, Jamsen K, Stargatt R. Awareness during anesthesia in children: a prospective cohort study. *Anesth Analg.* 2005;100:653–661.

The first recent study to show a high incidence of awareness in children.

Davidson AJ, Sheppard SJ, Engwerda AL, et al. Detecting awareness in children by using an auditory intervention. *Anesthesiology.* 2008;109:619–624.

This study found less awareness when a specific measure was used—different noises were played while children were under anesthesia and the children were queried about recall.

Lopez U, Habre W, Laurencon M, Haller G, Van der Linden M, Iselin-Chaves IA. Intraoperative awareness in children: the value of an interview adapted to their cognitive abilities. *Anaesthesia.* 2007;62:778–789.

This study highlights the difficulties in measuring awareness in children.

Osterman JE, Hopper J, Heran WJ, Keane TM, van der Kolk BA. Awareness under anesthesia and the development of post-traumatic stress disorder. *Gen Hosp Psychiatry.* 2001;23:198–204.

A small case series of people with PTSD after awareness. Some were children when the awareness occurred.

BIBLIOGRAPHY

Blusse van Oud-Alblas HJ, van Dijk M, Liu C, Tibboel D, Klein J, Weber F. Intraoperative awareness during paediatric anaesthesia. *Br J Anaesth.* 2009;102:104–110.

Davidson AJ. Measuring anesthesia in children using the EEG. *Pediatr Anesth.* 2006;16:374–387.

Lopez U, Habre W. Evaluation of intraoperative memory and postoperative behavior in children: are we really measuring what we intend to measure? *Pediatr Anesth.* 2009;19:1147–1151.

Lopez U, Habre W, Van der Linden M, Iselin-Chaves IA. Intraoperative awareness in children and post-traumatic stress disorder. *Anesthesia.* 2008;63:474–481.

Malviya S, Galinkin JL, Bannister CF, et al. The incidence of intraoperative awareness in children: childhood awareness and recall evaluation. *Anesth Analg.* 2009;109:1421–1427.

Myles PS, Leslie K, McNeil J, Forbes A, Chan MT. Bispectral index monitoring to prevent awareness during anaesthesia: the B-Aware randomised controlled trial. *Lancet.* 2004;363:1757–1763.

Phelan L, Stargatt R, Davidson AJ. Long-term post-traumatic effects of intraoperative awareness in children. *Pediatr Anesth.* 2009;19:1152–1156.

Tasbihgou SR, Vogels MF, Absalom AR. Accidental awareness during general anesthesia—a narrative review. *Anaesthesia.* 2018;73(1):112–122.

64

Acute Pain Management

NIHAR PATEL

INTRODUCTION

Age-appropriate pain assessment and management is vital in the care of children with acute pain. Assessment should occur regularly with clear documentation; pain should be treated and routinely reassessed. Poor pain management in the acute and postoperative setting can result in both short- and long-term consequences. The most effective plans for analgesia are multimodal. This chapter focuses on the variety of treatment options for pain in the acute setting.

> **LEARNING OBJECTIVES**
> 1. Describe some age-appropriate pain assessment tools for children.
> 2. Discuss the basics of age-appropriate pain management in children.
> 3. Understand the role of opioids, nonsteroidal anti-inflammatory drugs, and patient-controlled analgesia (PCA) in acute and postoperative pain management in children.

CASE PRESENTATION

A healthy 7-year-old boy, weighing 25 kg, fell off the top bunk while wrestling with his brother in the bedroom. He sustained a right-sided tibial fracture. His anxious parents bring the distressed patient to the emergency department, where he complains of severe pain in his leg. His pain is managed acutely in the triage area with 35 μg intranasal fentanyl while local anesthetic cream is applied to the dorsum of his hand for venous access. An x-ray confirms the diagnosis of a comminuted tibial fracture and need for operative treatment. After 10 minutes, his ***pain is assessed*** *again and an additional dose of fentanyl is administered.*

During the open reduction and internal fixation of the fracture in the operating room, the surgeon asks about the postoperative analgesia plan and frowns at the mention of a ***peripheral nerve block*** *or utilization of* patient controlled analgesia *(****PCA****) with opioids postoperatively. He is worried that they will both mask* ***compartment syndrome*** *if one should develop. He also asks that no nonsteroidal anti-inflammatory drugs* ***(NSAIDs)*** *be administered or prescribed.*

DISCUSSION

1. How can one assess the child's pain in the emergency department, postanesthesia care unit, and on the ward?

Good **pain assessment** allows the early recognition of pain and its effective treatment. It should involve the use of an age- and context-appropriate pain intensity measurement tool in the setting of a clinical interview with the child and/or parent/guardian as well as a physical examination. Three fundamental approaches exist in pain assessment in children: self-report, observational/behavioral, and physiological. Verbal self-report is the "gold standard" in pain measurement and should be used whenever possible. Children's understanding of pain and their ability to describe it changes with age and cognitive ability and is also affected by a range of social and cultural factors and other biases. Scales for self-report of pain must therefore be appropriate for the child's age and developmental stage. Assessment should be regularly and uniformly performed by all staff involved in the child's care.

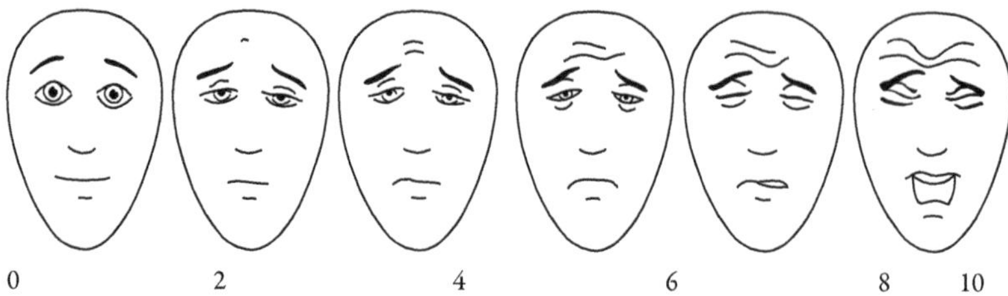

FIGURE 64.1 Faces Pain Scale–Revised (numbers are not shown to the child). From Hicks CL, von Baeyer CL, Spafford P, et al. Faces Pain Scale–Revised: toward a common metric in pediatric pain measurement. *Pain.* 2001;93:173–183. This Faces Pain Scale–Revised has been reproduced with permission of the International Association for the Study of Pain® (IASP®). The figure may not be reproduced for any other purpose without permission.

Self-report of pain is usually possible by the age of 4, and beyond this age children can begin to differentiate "more," "less," or "the same" and can use an image-based, self-report tool such as the OUCHER or Faces Pain Scale (Fig. 64.1). For patients unable to self-report, tools such as the Faces Legs Arms Cry and Consolability (FLACC) scale or Children's Hospital of Eastern Ontario Pain Scale (CHEOPS) can be used. Over 8 years of age, a 0 to 100 visual analog scale or 0 to 10 numeric rating scale may be used.

2. What are the systemic implications of poor pain control in the acute setting?

Pain control is considered one of the core functions of an anesthesiologist—not only because of the desire to relieve suffering as a result of trauma, disease, or surgery itself but also because pain left untreated or poorly controlled, has systemic implications (see Table 64.1).

3. What are the various options for postoperative pain control?

Many options exist to treat pain in the postoperative or acute setting. There is no established method that is considered the gold standard, but it is generally accepted that multimodal analgesia works best. The myriad of options include various pharmacologic agents, which work via different mechanisms of action to treat pain. In addition, peripheral nerve blockade is increasingly performed for isolated extremity surgery.

Acetaminophen (paracetamol) is a well-tolerated and effective analgesic, which should be prescribed routinely and also postoperatively. With an intravenous (IV) formulation readily available, it can be administered via multiple routes. Although there are very few contraindications, namely liver failure, a recent uptick in acetaminophen-related hepatotoxicity has resulted in a regulation of the total daily dose being less than 3250 mg for adults or children older than 12 years of age. The mechanism of action is not completely understood but thought to be via inhibition of cyclooxygenase (COX), especially COX-2

TABLE 64.1 CONSEQUENCES OF POORLY CONTROLLED PAIN BY SYSTEMS

Organ System	Effects
Psychological	Anxiety Fear Depression Poor patient satisfaction
Cardiovascular	Hypertension Tachycardia Increased cardiac workload
Pulmonary	Splinting V/Q mismatch Hypoxia Atelectasis Decreased vital capacity
Gastrointestinal	Postoperative ileus Delayed gastric emptying Nausea
Renal	Urinary retention Oliguria
Musculoskeletal	Weakness Fatigue Limited mobility
Coagulation	Increased risk of thromboembolism
Immunologic	Impaired immune function Poor wound healing
Endocrine	Increased stress hormones Catabolic state Hyperglycemia

in the central nervous system, thereby inhibiting the synthesis of prostaglandins used to relay pain.

Non steroidal anti-inflammatory drugs **NSAIDs** are a separate class of analgesic medications that are often prescribed in combination with acetaminophen as the foundation of a multimodal regimen. Their mechanism of action consists of inhibition of the COX-1 and COX-2 enzymes, thereby preventing the synthesis of prostaglandins and thromboxanes used to mediate pain. While oral formulations of NSAIDs were the dominant forms of administration, IV formulations of ketorolac and ibuprofen have offered alternate routes for patients who are unable to tolerate oral intake. While very safe, side effects of concern include gastric ulceration/bleeding and kidney damage. Caution should be maintained when administering these agents to patients less than 3 months of age and those with a history of gastrointestinal bleed or inflammatory bowel disease. As a component of multimodal analgesia, NSAIDs improve analgesia and decrease opioid consumption, especially when combined with acetaminophen.

Opiates are the analgesic standard by which all other analgesic medications are measured. Their effects are mediated via binding at the opiate receptors to provide potent analgesia in the periphery, spinal cord, and periaqueductal gray of the brain. Opiates typically provide the strongest analgesia in nonregional anesthesia regimens of postoperative pain control. Common side effects include constipation, pruritus, nausea, miosis, sedation, and respiratory depression. Increasing rates of abuse and addiction related to opioids are occurring nationwide so judicious prescription is necessary. Opioids are available in virtually every method of drug delivery possible with IV, oral, and topical patches being the most commonly prescribed routes.

Ketamine has enjoyed a resurgence in the past decade for its potent analgesic effects. The mechanism of action is the antagonism of the *N*-methyl-D-aspartate (NMDA) receptor. As with opiates, it is available in forms suitable for administration by virtually every route. It serves as an IV anesthetic agent at higher doses and provides good sedation at typical doses. It is useful for sedation in the emergency room for painful procedures, as it does not cause respiratory depression. It is particularly useful in the setting of acute on chronic pain as NMDA receptors have been implicated in the central sensitization that is observed in chronic pain states. The greatest benefit to ketamine may be in combination with opioids, where it can reduce the dosages of both drugs considerably when used to relieve pain. It is also particularly helpful in neuropathic pain states and complex regional pain syndrome.

Tramadol is another effective analgesic for postoperative pain. Its side effects are similar to opioids (e.g., nausea and vomiting, sedation, and dizziness) with less constipation and pruritus and a lower risk of respiratory depression.

Lastly, peripheral nerve blockade offers some of the most potent and effective analgesia available. Selective blockade of peripheral or neuraxial nerves with local anesthetics can block transmission of the pain signals to the spinal cord and render the patient pain-free in the immediate postoperative setting. The utility of ultrasound to target specific nerves under direct visualization has led to great resurgence and interest in the technique. Specific local anesthetic agents can deliver targeted therapy commensurate with the desired analgesia and duration. For pain expected to last for longer time periods, peripheral nerve catheters may be placed to infuse local anesthetics to prolong pain relief.

4. What are the various options for opioid administration in acute pain?

IV opioid infusions are safe and effective in the management of postoperative pain in children of all ages. **PCA** can be used in children as young as five but this requires careful patient selection, patient and parent education, and the availability of suitable equipment and trained staff (including monitoring and acute pain service support). Compared with continuous IV opioid infusions, PCA provides similar efficacy and greater dosing flexibility but is associated with higher opioid consumption and a higher incidence of pruritus (but no difference in other opioid-related side effects). Morphine is the PCA opioid of choice. Hydromorphone is an effective alternative when side effects limit the use of morphine, and fentanyl is the alternative opioid of choice in those with renal impairment (or morphine-related side effects). Nausea and vomiting is common (30%–45%) and prophylactic antiemetics (e.g., ondansetron or promethazine) should be prescribed. Pruritus is best treated with low-dose IV naloxone, a change of opioid, or addition of a mixed agonist–antagonist, such as butorphanol or nalbuphine.

5. Does PCA or regional anesthesia mask the diagnosis of the development of compartment syndrome?

There has been sporadic concern that the use of **PCA** or regional anesthesia to treat pain can mask the diagnosis of compartment syndrome. Pain is the most reliable (and earliest) symptom of acute compartment syndrome and should be assessed at rest and with passive movement of the muscles in the affected compartment. The diagnosis can be challenging if the child lacks the cognitive or verbal ability to provide meaningful information or localize symptoms.

Fortunately, the current consensus is that it is very rare for surgical complications to be masked by analgesia. Providing effective analgesia should not increase the risk of a missed diagnosis of compartment syndrome as long as regular monitoring and clinical examination with a high vigilance is carried out to detect the changes in pain scores and analgesic requirements that are early and sensitive indicators of compartment syndrome (Yang & Cooper, 2010). In children at risk of developing compartment syndrome, inadequate analgesia or escalating opioid consumption should immediately trigger orthopedic review to exclude this potentially devastating complication.

6. Do NSAIDs impair bone fusion?

Evidence for an effect on bone fusion is conflicting, and its clinical significance is unknown. There is animal-model evidence of unknown relevance in humans. The evidence comes from retrospective studies looking at high-dose ketorolac following spinal fusion that have reached different conclusions, and, so far, there is no evidence from randomized controlled trials or prospective trials. One retrospective study in children found no effect on postoperative complications after fracture repair (Kay et al., 2010). Ketorolac is often seen as the culprit, but it is hardly representative of **NSAIDs** as a class, especially at the high doses that are administered parenterally. NSAIDs are, however, effective in reducing the complication of postoperative heterotopic bone formation. They do not affect the risk of refracture in any significant way.

SUMMARY

1. Age- and context-appropriate pain assessment and measurement, performed regularly, are important components of pain management in children.
2. Opioids are important analgesics in acute, procedural, and postoperative pain. Multimodal analgesia leads to reduced opioid requirements, better analgesia, and fewer side effects. Nonpharmacological methods should also be incorporated.
3. PCAs provide effective postoperative analgesia. Regular monitoring and clinical examination with a high vigilance for compartment syndrome will allow early identification of this serious complication.
4. There is no good-quality evidence that NSAIDs impair bone fusion in humans, and the analgesic benefits of short-term NSAIDs outweigh this hypothetical risk.

ACKNOWLEDGMENTS

The author would like to thank Jason Chou and George Chalkiadis for their contributions to the first edition.

ANNOTATED REFERENCES

Howard R, Carter B, Curry J, Morton et al. Association of Paediatric Anaesthetists of Great Britain and Ireland. Special Issue: Good Practice in Postoperative and Procedural Pain Management. *Pediatr Anesth.* 2008;18(Suppl):1: 1–81.

Evidence-based article with recommendations on what constitutes good practice. Section 3: Pain Assessment and Section 5: Postoperative Pain are particularly pertinent.

Macintyre PE, Schug SA, Scott DA, et al. *Acute Pain Management: Scientific Evidence.* 3rd ed. Melbourne: Australian and New Zealand College of Anaesthetists and Faculty of Pain Medicine; 2010.

Definitive evidence-based book on acute pain management. Chapter 10 is dedicated to the assessment and management of acute pain in all settings in the pediatric patient.

BIBLIOGRAPHY

Babl FE, Jamison SR, Spicer M, Bernard S. Inhaled methoxyflurane as a prehospital analgesic in children. *Emerg Med Austral.* 2006;18(4):404–410.

Borland M, Jacobs I, King B, O'Brien, D. A randomized controlled trial comparing intranasal fentanyl to intravenous morphine for managing acute pain in children in the emergency department. *Ann Emerg Med.* 2007;49(3):335–340.

Bozkurt P. Use of tramadol in children. *Pediatr Anesth.* 2005;15(12):1041–1047.

Hee HI, Goy RW, Ng AS. Effective reduction of anxiety and pain during venous cannulation in children: a comparison of analgesic efficacy conferred by nitrous oxide, EMLA and combination. *Pediatr Anesth.* 2003;13(3):210–216.

Hicks CL, von Baeyer CL, Spafford PA, van Korlaar I, Goodenough B. The Faces Pain Scale–Revised: toward a common metric in pediatric pain measurement. *Pain.* 2001;93(2):173–183.

Kay RM, Directo MP, Leathers M, Myung K, Skaggs DL. Complications of ketorolac use in children undergoing operative fracture care. *J Pediatr Orthop.* 2010;30(7):655–658.

Lejus C. What does analgesia mask? *Pediatr Anesth.* 2004;14:622–624.

Yang J, Cooper MG. Compartment syndrome and patient-controlled analgesia in children: analgesic complication or early warning system? *Anaesth Intens Care.* 2010;38:359–363.

65

Emergence Delirium

ARVIND CHANDRAKANTAN AND MEHERNOOR WATCHA

INTRODUCTION

Emergence delirium (ED) is a very negative complication that may occur once a child has awakened from an anesthetic. Typically seen in younger patients, this complication is manifested by extreme negative behaviors such as screaming, crying, kicking, and hitting. The patient appears overtly upset. Because ED is transient in nature, it is not always necessary to treat this event unless the patient poses harm to him- or herself or others. Several interventions can potentially minimize and/or prevent ED.

LEARNING OBJECTIVES

1. Define the features of ED and associated risk factors.
2. Describe the different rating scales for measuring ED and the differences between them.
3. Discuss the measures for the prevention and treatment of pediatric ED.

CASE PRESENTATION

A 2-year-old otherwise healthy boy arrives in the recovery room after bilateral inguinal hernia repair performed under general anesthesia via a laryngeal mask airway and supplemented with a caudal block. The anesthesiologist states the intraoperative course was uneventful, and a decrease in the inspired anesthetic gas concentrations during surgery was not associated with cardiovascular responses. Shortly after arrival, the child is thrashing around, incoherent and inconsolable. You and the recovery room nurse are unable to obtain his vital signs.

DISCUSSION

1. What is emergence delirium (ED)?

There is a gradual return of consciousness after discontinuing administration of anesthetic and adjuvant agents at the end of the surgical procedure. In most patients there is a smooth transition from the surgical anesthetic to an awake state, but a variable percentage of both adults and children develop an altered mental state with disorientation, confusion, agitation, disinhibition, hallucinations, and reduced awareness of the environment in the immediate postoperative period. Emergence agitation (EA) or delirium is usually a short self-limiting condition lasting for 15 to 45 minutes. It is more common in children and differs from the longer lasting postoperative cognitive deficits seen in the elderly. The clinical spectrum of pediatric ED ranges from irritability to frank delirium. As it is not possible to evaluate the child's psychological state during emergence, the term "delirium" should be replaced with the terms "agitation" or "excitation." EA has been described as a "dissociated state of consciousness in which the child is irritable, uncompromising, uncooperative, incoherent, and inconsolably crying, moaning, kicking, or thrashing" (Vlajkovic & Sinkjelic, 2007). Although it is short lived and self-limiting, EA is distressing to the patient, parents, and caregivers who are at risk for injuries when the child is thrashing around flailing the arms, and may inadvertently remove intravenous (IV) lines, catheters, drains, and dressings in the process. This disruptive behavior increases the demands on postanesthesia care unit (PACU) nursing staff and leads to dissatisfaction with the postoperative experience for both the parents and nursing personnel. It is therefore important to identify patients at high risk for EA/ED, use validated scales to measure its severity, and determine interventions that reduce the frequency of the condition, along with providing effective treatment when it occurs.

2. What are some proposed mechanisms for EA/ED?

Current theories about the mechanism of anesthesia have focused on the gamma amino butyric acid (GABA) receptor particularly in the amygdala and its connections to the medial prefrontal cortex. This area of the brain is responsible for amnesia during anesthesia. The first sense to return during emergence is hearing, which depends on the synapse between the thalamus and the lateral nucleus of the amygdala. A heightened response to auditory stimuli during emergence similar to that in posttraumatic stress disorder may lead to increased ED, particularly when there is still a diminished cortical regulation from residual anesthetics. In children with ED from sevoflurane, the electroencephalography (EEG) did not pass through sleep and/or drowsy states compared to those without EA/ED. This difference in frontal lobe connectivity during the indeterminate stage of emergence may be observed in subjects with EA/ED.

Animal studies also suggest that excitation of the locus ceruleus neurons by inhalation anesthetics, particularly sevoflurane, may play a role in EA/ED. Another proposed mechanism is an imbalance between inhibition and excitation in the sympathetic nervous system. While the mechanisms for this condition remain to be fully elucidated, more is known about the clinical features including the incidence, risk factors, and interventions for preventing and managing this condition.

3. What are the risk factors for EA/ED?

The incidence of EA/ED in children has been reported to range from as 10% to 80% but varies with the criteria used for the diagnosis. It is important to differentiate pain-related behavior from EA/ED in the PACU. Maladaptive emergence behavior has been reported in children who have been anesthetized for nonpainful procedures such as magnetic resonance imaging scans.

Risk factors for EA depend on the age of the child, anesthetic agents administered, surgical procedure, and use of adjunct drugs (Dahmani et al. 2014). Higher rates (30%–50%) of EA/ED have been repeatedly reported in preschool children aged 2 to 6 years. The association between preoperative anxiety and the probability of developing EA/ED is unclear. A large retrospective study of 800 subjects showed such a relationship, but subsequent smaller prospective studies did not confirm this.

The incidence is lower with propofol-based IV anesthesia compared to inhalation agents (pooled odds ratio 0.25, 95% confidence interval 0.16–0.39) despite a similarity in the speed of emergence. The less soluble inhalation anesthetics sevoflurane, isoflurane, and desflurane are associated with more EA/ED compared to halothane (pooled odds ratio 2.21). This incidence did not change when sevoflurane was gradually decreased in steps to avoid rapid emergence, suggesting that EA/ED with sevoflurane is related to the central nervous system effects of this inhalation agent independent of the speed of emergence. The duration and depth of anesthesia may affect the incidence of EA/ED in adults but not in children. Early studies suggested the EA/ED occurred more often after breast and abdominal surgery in adults and after adenotonsillectomy, urological surgery without neuraxial anesthesia, and strabismus surgery in children. However, this may reflect pain-related behavior rather than EA as the incidence decreases with the adjunctive use of opioids (Martin et al. 2014).

4. How is ED measured?

ED has been measured by multiple scales, namely the Pediatric Anesthesia Emergence Delirium (PAED), the Watcha scale, and the Cravero Emergence Delirium scale (see Tables 65.1–65.3).

The PAED scale is the current standard validated scale for diagnosing ED. It consists of 5 behaviors, each rated on a scale from 0 to 4 with the scores added to give a minimum score of zero and a maximum of 20. A score of 12 or higher has 100% sensitivity and 94.5% specificity for a diagnosis of ED. However, the scale is not a continuous linear scale.

The Watcha and the Cravero scales have not been validated. However, a study comparing these 3 scales revealed all methods had a good correlation with a clinical diagnosis of ED by an experienced practitioner. These authors felt the Watcha scale was simpler to use in clinical practice and may have greater sensitivity and specificity (Bajwa et al., 2010). However, the first 3 factors in the PAED scale (eye contact, purposeful actions, awareness of surroundings) track closely to ED while the restlessness and inconsolability factors are also seen with pain.

5. Can EA/ED be prevented?

Many different pharmacological agents/approaches have been utilized with success in the prevention of ED. The most effective regimen is the elimination of an inhalational agent and utilization of total intravenous anesthesia (TIVA) with propofol (Chandler et al. 2013). It is essential to ensure that adequate analgesia is provided as pain-related behavior is difficult to differentiate from ED. A number of other pharmacological agents have been administered at induction, maintenance, or just before surgery ends to reduce maladaptive emergence when sevoflurane anesthesia is used. These include propofol 1 mg/kg at the end of surgery and intraoperative opioids (intranasal or IV fentanyl, IV remifentanil, sufentanil or alfentanil). Opioids have been shown to reduce the pooled relative risk of EA/ED by 0.49 in a meta-analysis. Midazolam has an inconsistent effect depending on the route and timing of administration. This inconsistency may be the result of postoperative pain and the use of nonvalidated scales for measuring EA/ED. Ketamine 1 mg/kg IV at the start of surgery or a lower dose of 0.25 mg/kg at the end of surgery reduces EA/ED. Dexmedetomidine, at a dose of 0.3 to 1 mcg/kg IV, has generated significant interest not only due to its effects on decreasing ED, but also because of its opioid-sparing effects in addition to possible effects on postoperative nausea and vomiting prevention. However, alpha-2 agonists may prolong the time to hospital discharge. Preoperative gabapentin, dexamethasone, and intraoperative magnesium have all been shown to be effective.

Nonpharmacological approaches which have been tried include preoperative preparation to decrease parental/child anxiety, music therapy, and distraction techniques. The utilization of pharmacological approaches/therapies, including TIVA, should be balanced with the long postprocedural stays associated with their use. Also, the use of opioids, propofol, and dexmedetomidine, with their subsequent hemodynamic/parasympathomimetic effects, requires judicious consideration as well.

The long-term consequences of ED remain unknown, but it is believed to be a self-limiting disorder. There are no unequivocal data that EA/ED leads to postoperative behavioral disturbances beyond the initial 15 to 45 minutes in the PACU or long-term disturbances. However, patients at risk for EA/ED share a number of risk factors that are observed in patients who develop postoperative maladaptive behaviors such as night terrors, enuresis, separation anxiety, temper tantrums, as well as eating and sleep disorders (Banchs & Lerman, 2014). This contrasts strongly with the intensive care unit/perioperative literature in adults, where delirium is a known risk factor for higher morbidity/mortality both on a short- and long-term basis (Abelha et al., 2013).

6. What is the treatment of ED in the PACU?

If a child develops agitation in the PACU, he or she should first be evaluated to rule out potentially dangerous conditions of hypoxemia, hypotension, hypercarbia, and hypoglycemia. Pain, when suspected, must be treated with analgesics. ED is a diagnosis of exclusion and often requires no treatment other than support and prevention of harm. However, some patients will require treatment to prevent disruption of surgical incisions (e.g., plastic surgery). There are no studies available to determine which drug is most effective for treatment of agitation in children in the PACU with the least side effect profile in children. Drugs used for treatment of ED include propofol 1 to 2 mg/kg IV, fentanyl 1 to 2 mcg/kg IV, midazolam 0.05 mg/kg IV, or dexmedetomidine 0.3 mg/kg IV. These drugs all have sedative effects, and it is important to ensure airway patency and hemodynamic stability is maintained following administration. Table 65.4 shows the treatment options for the prevention and management of ED.

SUMMARY

1. ED is a self-limited phenomenon that occurs in up to 80% of pediatric patients and can be distressing to patients, parents, and caregivers.
2. Risks factors for ED depend on age of the patient, use of volatile anesthetic agents, type of surgical procedure, and use of adjunct medications.
3. ED can be graded using the PAED scale.
4. The most effective regimen to prevent ED is the use of total IV anesthesia with adequate analgesia.

TABLE 65.1 PEDIATRIC ANESTHESIA EMERGENCE DELIRIUM SCALE

1. The child makes eye contact with the caregiver.	4 = not at all
	3 = just a little
2. The child's actions are purposeful.	2 = quite a bit
	1 = very much
3. The child is aware of his/her surroundings.	0 = extremely
1. The child is restless.	0 = not at all
2. The child is inconsolable.	1 = just a little
	2 = quite a bit
	3 = very much
	4 = extremely

Maximum total score = 20.

Source. Sikich N & Lerman J. 2004. Development and psychometric evaluation of the pediatric anesthesia emergence delirium scale.

TABLE 65.2 CRAVERO EMERGENCE AGITATION SCALE

Level	Description
1	Obtunded with no response to stimulation
2	Asleep but responsive to movement or stimulation
3	Awake and responsive
4	Crying (for >3 min)
5	Thrashing behavior that requires restraint

Source. Cravero J, Surgenor S, Whalen K. Emergence agitation in paediatric patients after sevoflurane anaesthesia and no surgery: a comparison with halothane. *Anesthesia*. 2000;10:419–424.

TABLE 65.3 WATCHA SCALE FOR EMERGENCE DELIRIUM

Clinical score	Patient characteristic
1	Calm (conversation)
2	Not calm but could be easily calmed
3	Not easily calmed, moderately agitated or restless
4	Combative, excited or disoriented

TABLE 65.4 TREATMENT OPTIONS FOR THE PREVENTION AND MANAGEMENT OF EMERGENCE AGITATION/DELIRIUM

Agent	Emergence Delirium Prevention	Emergence Delirium Treatment
Desflurane	–	NA
Sevoflurane	–	NA
Bolus propofol	+/–	+
Propofol infusion	++	NA
Ondansetron	+/–	+/–
Clonidine or	+	+
Dexmedetomidine	+	+
Fentanyl	+	+
Ketamine	+/–	–
Midazolam	+	+

ACKNOWLEDGMENTS

The authors wish to acknowledge the first edition authors, Charles B. Eastwood and Paul J. Samuels.

ANNOTATED REFERENCES

Bajwa SA, et al. A comparison of emergence delirium scales following general anesthesia in children. *Pediatr Anesth*. 2010;20:704–711.

This article compares the three most common scales for ED in 37 children. It found that the PAED scale was the most sensitive, but the Watcha scale was most easy to use in clinical situations.

Chandler JR, Myers D, Mehta D, et al. Emergence delirium in children: a randomized trial to compare total intravenous anesthesia with propofol and remifentanil to inhalational sevoflurane anesthesia. *Pediatr Anesth*. 2013;23(4):309–315.

This article randomized children to sevoflurane versus TIVA. The sevoflurane group had a far higher incidence of ED.

Dahmani S, Delivet H, Hilly J. Emergence delirium in children: an update. *Current Opin Anaesthesiol*. 2014;27:309–15.

This article discusses the current state of pharmacotherapy for ED including dexmedetomidine.

Martin JC, Liley DT, Harvey AS, et al. Alterations in the functional connectivity of frontal lobe networks preceding emergence delirium in children. *Anesthesiology.* 2014;121:740–752.

This article studies the electroencephalographic patterns (EEG) of children who had ED with those who did not. They were able to describe altered EEG patterns in children with ED.

Vlajkovic GP, Sindjelic RP. Emergence delirium in children: many questions, few answers. *Anesth Analg.* 2007;104:84–91.

This article provides a comprehensive overview of the pathogenesis, risk factors, and background of ED.

BIBLIOGRAPHY

Abelha F, Luís C, Veiga D, et al. Outcome and quality of life in patients with postoperative delirium during an ICU stay following major surgery. *Crit Care.* 2013;17:R257.

Banchs RJ, Lerman J. Preoperative anxiety management, emergence delirium, and postoperative behavior. *Anesthesiol Clin.* 2014;32:1–23.

Sikich N, Lerman J. Development and psychometric evaluation of the pediatric anesthesia emergence delirium scale. *Anesthesiology.* 2004 May;100(5):1138–1145.

66

Stridor after Extubation

CHERYL GORE, JUNZHENG WU, AND C. DEAN KURTH

INTRODUCTION

On occasion, anesthesiologists must manage infants and children who present with postextubation stridor in the recovery room after being intubated and mechanically ventilated during surgery. This stridor may be accompanied by respiratory distress and oxygen desaturation in severe cases. Postextubation stridor can occur anywhere from 3% to 30% of the time after extubation; there is such a variation in the incidence due to the subjective methods surrounding the classification of stridorous sounds and diagnosis. Measures can be taken to help prevent postextubation stridor. If stridor does occur, management of the symptoms and awareness of the objective signs is important.

LEARNING OBJECTIVES

1. Identify risk factors for postextubation stridor.
2. Describe prophylactic measures to ameliorate postextubation stridor.
3. Review management of postextubation stridor to prevent reintubation and subglottic stenosis.

CASE PRESENTATION

A 3-year-old, 16 kg girl presents to your hospital for tonsillectomy and adenoidectomy. Her past medical history is significant for a term delivery with post natal intubation at birth for 2 weeks due to meconium aspiration. She was eventually discharged home without supplemental oxygen or monitors. While she has not had a formal sleep study, her parents state that she does snore with pauses while sleeping at night.

She is taken into the operating room and inhalation induction is performed with standard monitors. An intravenous (IV) line is placed and her trachea is intubated with a cuffed 4.5 endotracheal tube (ETT). Following endotracheal intubation, a negative leak test was performed with no detectable leak at 40 cm of H20. The tube was then exchanged for a 4.0 ETT which had a leak at 30 cm H20. The patient received 0.5 mg of morphine, 1.5 mg of zofran, and 200 cc of lactated Ringer's solution during surgery, was extubated awake with coughing and transferred to the recovery room on blow by oxygen with pulse oximeter monitoring.

After approximately an hour and a half stay in the recovery room, she develops a high-pitched inspiratory sound and is placed on 4 liters of oxygen via nasal cannula. She subsequently develops suprasternal notch retractions; vital signs at this time are as follows: heart rate 150, oxygen saturations 90% on 4L 02, blood pressure 80/60, respiratory rate 40, and temperature 37.5°C. The patient is placed on blow-by cool humidified oxygen mist at 10 L/min. Decadron 8 mg and nebulized racemic epinephrine (adrenaline) are administered but she progresses to further desaturation and respiratory distress requiring intubation with an uncuffed 3.5 ETT. This tube had a leak at 40 cm H20. Propofol 30 mg and rocuronium 15 mg is used to facilitate intubation. The patient is transferred to the pediatric intensive care unit (PICU) and kept intubated for 2 days to allow airway swelling to subside. Fentanyl and midazolam infusions are used to maintain sedation while the patient is on mechanical ventilation. Decadron administration is scheduled every 6 hours and chest x-ray has no evidence of abnormality.

The patient is extubated on day 2 when her tidal volume is 150 ml to 200 ml, saturations are 98% on FiO2 25%, and spontaneous respiratory rate is 30/min with the assistance of pressure support. The air leak around the tube is at 12 cmH20 at this time. Two months later, the patient is diagnosed with subglottic stenosis which is attributed to her previous prolonged intubation as a neonate.

DISCUSSION

1. What are the risk factors of postextubation stridor?

Postextubation croup, also known as postintubation croup, is defined as **inspiratory stridor** developing after extubation. The condition usually presents within 1 hour after extubation, although it may develop as late as the first 24 hours. Postextubation stridor arises from glottic and subglottic edema caused by ischemia of the tracheal mucosa from pressure by the ETT. The symptoms appear after extubation because compression by an in situ ETT prevents narrowing of the tracheal lumen. Upon removal of the endotracheal tube, edema develops to narrow the lumen. Symptoms include **inspiratory stridor, hoarseness,** and **chest retractions**. If the airway obstruction becomes severe, arterial desaturation occurs and reintubation may be required to maintain a patent airway.

Certain factors increase the risk of postextubation stridor, these include the following:

- *ETT* (cuffed or uncuffed): tightly fitting in trachea with a pressure **leak above 25 cmH$_2$O**
- *Age*: children younger than 4 years, due to their disproportionately smaller airway lumen
- *Intubation maneuver:* **multiple** and/or traumatic **attempts**
- *Duration of endotracheal intubation*: risk for trauma or ischemia increases with prolonged intubation. One study showed an increased risk of postextubation stridor with duration of mechanical ventilation greater than 72 hours (Nascimento et al. 2015).
- *Head or neck surgery*: frequent position changes of the head and neck, common with this type of surgery, increase the risk for trauma or ischemia of tracheal mucosa
- *Ongoing upper airway infection*: Mucosal infection results in an inflamed or edematous trachea.
- *Airway trauma or reactivity*: inhalation and burn injury, history of spasmodic croup, or reactive airway disease
- *Extubation*: coughing vigorously with the ETT in situ.
- *Subglottic stenosis*: congenital or acquired lesions or syndromes associated with a disproportionately narrow airway for age, such as Down syndrome (Cohen et al., 2011; Suominen et al., 2006).

2. What are some prophylactic measures to ameliorate postextubation stridor?

To reduce the risk of postextubation stridor, it is necessary to address each risk factor.

Appropriate ETT: An old and common practice was to use an uncuffed ETT in children under 8 years old, and the size was determined by equations such as (age in years + 16)/4. Accumulating data reveal no difference between uncuffed versus cuffed ETTs in the incidence of postextubation stridor. In children, a cuffed ETT with a 0.5 mm outer diameter smaller than determined by the equation, may be used without increasing the risk of postextubation stridor. Cuffed tubes have advantages over uncuffed tubes, including less anesthetic gas contamination, better mechanical ventilation, and decreased risk of aspiration and infection in mechanically ventilated children. Improved mechanical ventilation is especially advantageous when high inflation pressure is required to ventilate the lungs during an acute or chronic lung disease. After intubation, a leak test should be performed. The uncuffed ETT should leak between 20 and 25 cmH$_2$O to permit ventilation and to maintain perfusion of the tracheal mucosa. With a cuffed ETT, the leak should be the same as for the uncuffed ETT when the cuff is fully deflated. If the leak is less than 20 cmH$_2$O, the cuff should be inflated meticulously until the air leak is "just sealed" at 20 cmH$_2$O.

Atraumatic intubation with a high success rate: Multiple and traumatic intubations should be avoided. A skilled anesthetist should perform the intubation if the potential for difficult airway exists, particularly in an infant.

Smooth extubation: Vigorous movement and forceful coughing during extubation increases the risk of subglottic injury and swelling. A good technique during the extubation process minimizes or eliminates these risk factors.

Elective procedure and upper respiratory infection (URI) : Surgery should be postponed if the patient has a recent viral URI and prolonged intubation is required for the procedure.

Dexamethasone: IV administration of dexamethasone prior to extubation helps to reduce airway swelling if the patient is undergoing airway surgery or has experienced multiple and traumatic attempts at intubation.

Air leak test: Infants should remain intubated for as short a time as possible. A negative leak test in a patient who has been intubated for a long period of time may predict the occurrence of postextubation stridor.

3. What is the best way to manage postextubation stridor in order to prevent reintubation and subglottic stenosis?

The incidence of postextubation stridor has decreased significantly during the past 20 years as the pathogenesis has become better understood and preventive measures have been instituted. Although the effectiveness of some treatments for postextubation stridor is still debatable, the following are widely advocated to adequately manage this condition when it occurs:

- Treatment of *postoperative agitation:* Crying and agitation in the postanesthesia care unit (PACU) exacerbates stridor and difficulty breathing. Sedation with dexmedetomidine or other agents and control of pain with opioids have the goal of preventing crying and agitation and promoting smooth respiration.
- *Cool and humidified mist* ameliorates postextubation stridor by reducing mucosal edema and is recommended for use during mild cases when only stridor is present.
- *Racemic epinephrine* is recommended for moderate postextubation stridor, when **retractions** and dyspnea occur. In theory, it reduces mucosal swelling through vasoconstriction. Both in the PACU and in the PICU, the dose is 0.2 to 0.5 mL of 2.25% racemic epinephrine diluted into 3 to 5 mL of normal saline, administered via nebulizer over 5 to 10 minutes. The patient should be observed for 4 hours after administration as there is a potential for a **"rebound effect"**—that is, the stridor could recur as the drug's effect dissipates.
- *Heliox (helium–oxygen mixture):* Heliox, a gas that is less dense than air, increases laminar flow and reduces turbulent flow. A recent study demonstrated its successful use in the PICU for postextubation croup refractory to treatment with racemic epinephrine. Heliox works temporarily to alleviate symptoms of upper airway obstruction and prevents reintubation until other therapies become effective or the disease process naturally resolves
- *Corticosteroids:* Recent data suggest that prophylactic corticosteroids may reduce the incidence of postextubation stridor and the subsequent need for reintubation in patients who have recently undergone prolonged mechanical ventilation or in patients who had an airway operation (Markowitz & Randolph, 2002). Corticosteroids decrease airway swelling putatively by interrupting inflammation resulting from intubation-induced airway injury. **Dexamethasone** may be administered as follows: 0.5 mg/kg every 4 to 6 hours, for a maximum of 40 mg/day, for 2 days in patients at high risk, prior to extubation. Alternatively, aerosolized budesonide may be administered.
- *Reintubation*: In patients with severe stridor and impending ventilatory failure unresponsive to the aforementioned treatments, reintubation should be performed before postobstructive pulmonary edema, hypoxemia, and acidosis ensue. The ETT should be smaller than the one originally placed. An ETT 0.5 sizes smaller than predicted should be used, with appropriate size confirmed by the leak test. The ETT should be left in place for 24 to 48 hours to allow swelling to recede. It is important to provide sedation during this period to avoid further airway trauma. Propofol and a nondepolarizing muscle relaxant are appropriate to facilitate reintubation, followed by an infusion of sedatives, titrated to effect. The patient may be extubated when an appropriate air leak is observed.

Table 66.1 provides an overview of postintubation/post-extubation stridor.

TABLE 66.1 OVERVIEW OF POSTINTUBATION STRIDOR : SUMMARY OF RISK FACTORS AND PREVENTIVE MEASURES FOR POST-INTUBATION STRIDOR

Risk Factors	Preventive Options
Air leak >30 cmH_2O	Maintain air leak around ETT < 30 cmH_2O
Age <4 years	
Multiple attempts at intubation or traumatic intubation	Atraumatic intubation
Prolonged intubation	Shortest possible intubation time
Head/neck surgery	
URI	If child has an URI, delay elective surgery if intubation is required
Airway trauma, inhalation injury (e.g., burn), or spasmodic croup, asthma	
Coughing vigorously prior to extubation	Smooth emergence (avoid coughing)
Subglottic stenosis	Dexamethasone
Signs	**Treatment**
Inspiratory stridor	Manage agitation
Agitation	Cool mist oxygen
Retractions	Inhaled racemic epinephrine
Hoarseness	Dexamethasone IV or inhaled budesonide
Oxygen desaturation	Helium–oxygen mixture
	Reintubation

Note: ETT = endotracheal tube; URI = upper respiratory infection; IV = intravenous.

4. What are the guidelines for discharge in patients who develop postextubation stridor?

In a mild case, defined by inspiratory stridor only with minimal agitation, cool mist, sedation, and pain management are sufficient. Patients still can be discharged after surgery if the situation is improving or has not worsened after an extra hour of observation. The parents should receive appropriate instruction prior to discharge. For a moderate case, defined by stridor, moderate dyspnea, and suprasternal retractions during inspiration, nebulized racemic epinephrine and dexamethasone are added to the treatment. The patient may be discharged home after the symptoms have dramatically improved and the window for potential **"rebound effect"** from racemic epinephrine has passed with no further stridor. The patient should be admitted if symptoms are not improving significantly and additional doses of nebulized racemic epinephrine are administered, especially in infants. Patients who develop severe postextubation stridor presenting with severe difficulty breathing, intercostal retractions, inability to maintain oxygen saturation, and lethargy should be reintubated with a smaller ETT and admitted to the intensive care unit.

SUMMARY

1. Postextubation stridor is most often seen in children under 4 years of age; other risk factors include ongoing URI, history of narrow airway (either congenital or acquired), prolonged intubation, and traumatic intubation.
2. Anticipation and prophylactic treatment of risk factors, followed by prompt recognition and treatment of symptoms, may prevent reintubation.
3. The decision to discharge a patient home depends on the severity of symptoms and their clinical course.

ACKNOLWEDGMENTS

The author wishes to acknowledge the first edition authors, Janzheng Wu and C. Dean Kurth.

ANNOTATED REFERENCES

Markovitz BP, Randolph AG. Corticosteroids for the prevention of reintubation and postextubation stridor in pediatric patients: A meta-analysis. *Pediatr Crit Care Med.* 2002;3(3):223–226.

Data analysis from 6 controlled clinical trials showed convincing evidence that IV steroids reduce the risk of postextubation stridor and reintubation.

Nascimento MS, Prado C, Troster EJ, et al. Risk factors for post-extubation stridor in children: the role of orotracheal cannula. *Einstein.* 2015;13:226–231.

This study is a prospective analysis that looked at intubated patients from June 2008 to August 20011. After reviewing several factors including age, weight, ETT size, cuffed versus uncuffed ETT and duration of mechanical ventilation, the main risk for stridor after extubation was due to prolonged duration of intubation.

Newth CJ, Rachman B, Patel N. The use of cuffed versus uncuffed endotracheal tubes in pediatric intensive care. *J Pediatr.* 2004;144:333–337.

The study results demonstrate the significant advantages using cuffed ETTs in pediatric patients as opposed to the traditional textbook teaching that cuffed tubes should not be used in children younger than 8 years of age.

BIBLIOGRAPHY

Cohen T, Deutsch N, Motoyama EK. Induction, maintenance and recovery. In: Davis PJ, Cladis FP, Motoyama EK, eds. *Anesthesia for Infants and Children*. St. Louis, MO: Mosby-Elsevier; 2011:365–394.

Laryngotracheal stenosis. Wikimedia Foundation; May 27, 2016. https://en.wikipedia.org/wiki/Laryngotracheal_stenosis

Metha R, Hariprakash SP, Cox PN, Wheeler DS. Diseases of the upper respiratory tract. In: Wheeler DS, Wong HR, eds. *Pediatric Critical Care Medicine: Basic Science and Clinical Evidence*. London: Springer; 2007:480–505.

Sinha A, Jayashree M, Singhi S. Aerosolized L-epinephrine vs. budesonide for postextubation stridor: A randomized controlled trial. *Indian Pediatr.* 2010;47:317–322.

Suominen P, Taivainen T, Tuoninen N, et al. Optimally fitted tracheal tubes decrease the probability of postextubation adverse events in children undergoing general anesthesia. *Pediatr Anesth.* 2006;16:641–647.

67

Postoperative Nausea and Vomiting in Patients with Prolonged QTc

ADAM C. ADLER AND MEHERNOOR WATCHA

INTRODUCTION

Postoperative nausea and vomiting (PONV) remains a frequent complication despite the use of various nonpharmacological and pharmacological strategies including drugs with effects on the serotonin, histamine, dopamine, and other receptor sites. However, many of these drugs alter the duration of the QT segment and have the potential to be associated with deleterious life-threatening cardiac arrhythmias including torsades de pointes, particularly in children with congenital or acquired prolonged QT interval. This chapter summarizes the causes of prolonged QT interval, the potential interactions of antiemetics and anesthetics on cardiac rhythm, the choice of approaches in the prophylaxis of PONV in high-risk patients, and an overall anesthetic management plan.

LEARNING OBJECTIVES

1. Understand the basics of cardiac electrophysiology regarding the QT interval and the risks to the patient when it becomes prolonged.
2. Explain the potential effects of first- and second-generation 5-HT_3 receptor antagonists on cardiac repolarization.
3. Review currently used antiemetics and anticipated future developments in this field.
4. Identify an anesthetic strategy that includes PONV management in children with prolonged QT intervals.

CASE PRESENTATION

An 8-year-old, 27-kg boy is scheduled for tonsillectomy for recurrent tonsillitis. His physical examination and past medical history are unremarkable. He just completed a 10-day course of amoxicillin but otherwise takes no medications. Anesthesia is induced with 70% nitrous oxide in oxygen and 8% inspired sevoflurane. After tracheal intubation, anesthesia is maintained with 3% sevoflurane in 70% nitrous oxide supplemented with intravenous (IV) morphine. The child also received dexamethasone 0.1 mg/kg IV and ondansetron 0.1 mg/kg IV. The child was transferred to the postanesthesia care unit (PACU) after tracheal extubation. The arrival electrocardiogram (EKG) revealed ***premature ventricular contractions*** *that deteriorate into sustained* ***ventricular tachycardia****. Sinus rhythm was re-established 20 seconds after the administration of IV* ***lidocaine*** *20 mg. A 12-lead EKG revealed sinus rhythm and a* ***QT interval of 480 msec****.*

DISCUSSION

1. What is the QT interval, which factors affect it, and what are the most common genetic syndromes associated with prolonged QTc?

The electrical activity of the heart is mediated through channels regulating ion flow in and out of cardiomyocytes during the 5 phases of cardiac depolarization and repolarization. These channels consist of a pore-forming component (alpha subunit) with smaller regulatory beta subunits. The normal resting myocyte has a negative potential of 90 mV. During depolarization, there is a large inward current of sodium ions resulting in a rapid reversal of potential to +20mV (phase 0). Repolarization consists of 3 phases. In phase 1, there is a rapid partial repolarization caused by inactivation of inward sodium and the transient efflux of potassium ions. In

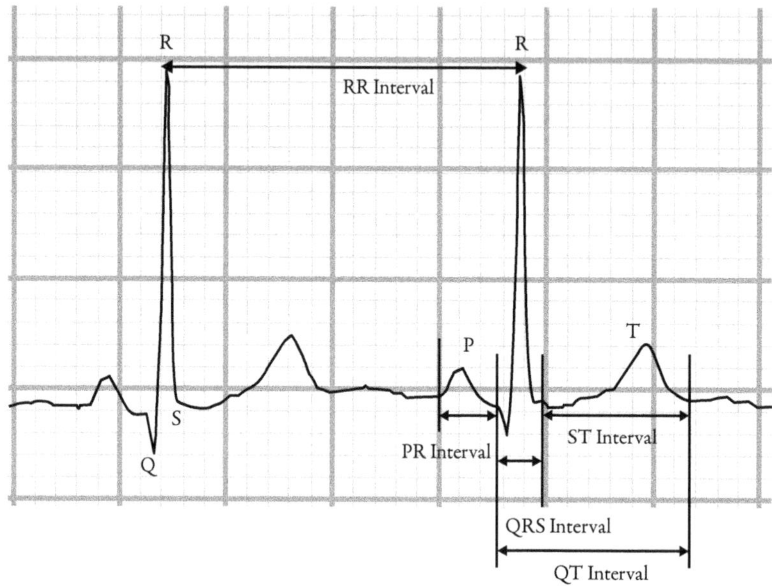

FIGURE 67.1 Normal EKG showing RR interval and QT interval.

phase 2, the action potential reaches a plateau for 0.1 to 0.2 seconds, reflecting a balance between influx of calcium ions through L-type calcium channels and outward repolarizing potassium currents. In phase 3, there is further repolarization from an efflux of potassium ions until the resting potential is achieved and maintained by an inward rectifier current of potassium ions in phase 4. Malfunction of ion channels with inadequate outflow of potassium or excessive inflow of sodium ions may lead to an intracellular excess of positively charged ions with prolonged ventricular repolarization.

The time from the beginning of phase 1 of the action potential to the end of phase 3 is shown in the surface EKG as the period between the start of the QRS complex and the end of the T wave (**QT interval**; see Fig. 67.1). As the QT interval varies with the heart rate, it is necessary to correct the interval for heart rate (**QTc interval**) before a value is considered abnormal. This correction is traditionally calculated by Bazett's formula where the QT interval is divided by the square root of the respiratory rate (RR) interval (QTc = QT interval/$\sqrt{}$(RR interval). In adults, the normal **QTc interval** is less than 450 msec in males and less than 470 msec in females. In children (beyond the neonatal and early infancy period), the normal **QTc interval** is less than 450 msec for both genders. Patients with an uncorrected **QT interval** exceeding 500 msec or the QTc exceeding 470 msec are at risk for unexpected life-threatening arrhythmias such as torsades de point (Fig. 67.2). A preoperative 12-lead EKG should be performed

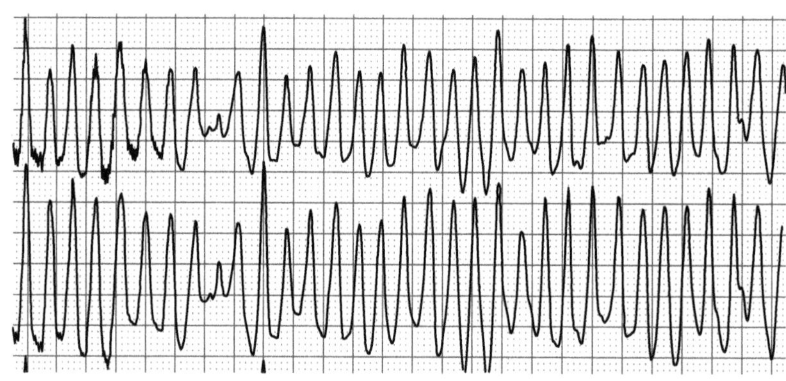

FIGURE 67.2 Torsades de pointes.

in children with undiagnosed syncope or who have a family history of sudden death or unexplained death under anesthesia to determine if an underlying congenital channelopathy with QTc interval prolongation is present.

Factors affecting the duration of the **QT interval** can be divided into congenital channelopathies and those acquired either directly or after the use of pharmacologic agents. The incidence of congenital long QT syndrome (cLQTS) in the population ranges from 1 in 2,500 to 6,500. Five genes (LQT1, 2, 3, 5, 6) code for more than 200 ion channel mutations. Of the cLQTS mutations, 95% involve the K^+ channel (outward flux of potassium during repolarization) as seen in c-LQTS 1 and c-LQTS 2 and only 5% involve the Na^+ channel (slow inward flux of sodium during repolarization) as seen with c-LQTS 3. Romano-Ward syndrome is an autosomal dominant disorder representing 99% of cases, which involves mutations in LQT1 to LQT7. Jervill and Lange-Nielson is an autosomal recessive disorder that occurs in less than 1% of patients with cLQTS and is associated with deafness.

Several acquired conditions such as coronary artery disease, cardiomyopathy, hypertension, bradycardia, hyperthyroidism, female gender, and stroke may result in prolongation of the **QTc interval**. Electrolyte imbalances (hypokalemia, hypomagnesemia, and hypocalcemia) are important precipitating factors for QTc prolongation and may occur in patients with anorexia nervosa, celiac disease, after gastroplasty or following a liquid protein diet.

A large number of commonly used medications have been reported to prolong the QT interval either directly or as a result of associated electrolyte imbalance (e.g., diuretics). Up to 30% of children with cLQTS have a normal phenotype with a normal resting QTc until an initiating event occurs such as stress or drug exposure. Table 67.1 contains a list of the most commonly encountered medications in the perioperative period that may prolong the QTc interval. This effect is usually related to blocking the rapid component of the delayed rectifier potassium channel encoded by the *hERG* gene. Prolonged QT intervals that occur after concomitant administration of drugs during anesthesia may be related to pharmacodynamic or pharmacokinetic interactions. In the former situation, there may be an additive or synergistic effect. Pharmacokinetic interactions occur when both drugs are metabolized by the same pathway (via either CYP3A4 or CYP2D6 enzymes), and plasma concentrations increase. While it may be prudent to avoid these drugs in the immediate perioperative period, it is also important to remember that isolated prolongation of the QTc interval in itself is generally asymptomatic and not always associated with perioperative arrhythmias. Drugs that preferentially lengthen the action potential in epicardial and endocardial cells will increase the QTc interval but reduce transmural dispersion of repolarization and so do not increase the risk of torsades de pointes. In contrast, drugs that increase M cell action potential duration and transmural dispersion of repolarization increase this risk (*vide infra*).

TABLE 67.1 COMMONLY USED PERIOPERATIVE DRUGS THAT MAY PROLONG THE QT INTERVAL

Anti-arrhythmic—Class 1 and Class III (Doftilidine, Procainamide, Sotalol)
Antibiotics—Fluoroquinolones (Lefloxacin, Moxifloxacin, Ciprofloxin)
Antibiotics—Macrolides (Azithromycin, Clarithromycin, Erythromycin)
Antifungal agents—Fluconazole, Ketoconazole, Iitraconazole
Antimicrobial—Other (Quinine, Pentamidine)
Diuretics (Furosemide, hydrochlorothiazide)
Droperidol
Haloperidol
Inhalation Agents (Sevoflurane > Isoflurane)
Opioids (Buprenorphine, Methadone, Oxycodone). Morphine has lower risk
Phenothiazines
Prokinetic Agents—Cisapride

2. What is the main risk in patients with a prolonged QT interval?

Prolongation of the QT interval predisposes susceptible patients to the development of malignant arrhythmias including **premature ventricular contractions**, **ventricular tachycardia**, and **torsades des pointes** (Fig. 67.2). Defects in repolarization requires the presence of two preconditions: a prolonged QTc interval and increased dispersion of repolarization. The dispersion of repolarization is a measure of the variance or heterogeneity of the QT interval across the ventricular cardiac muscle (transmural heterogeneity) or the degree in which the myocardial cells repolarize in unison. As the dispersion of repolarization increases, the risk of malignant arrhythmias increases due to multiple myocardial myocytes acting at varying stages in the "electrical" cycle. In cLQTS 1 patients, beta-adrenergic stimulation increases inward sodium ion current that is relatively unopposed by the smaller increase in outward potassium ion efflux. The consequent prolongation of repolarization during phase 2 and 3 in islands of M cells may increase the susceptibility to arrhythmias. Beta blockade is effective in preventing the generation of arrhythmias in cLQTS 1. Sodium channel blockers (e.g., antihistamines, phenothiazines) can slow intraventricular conduction, thereby establishing a re-entrant circuit, which can result ventricular tachycardia and fibrillation.

3. What are the EKG effects of the 5-HT_3 receptor antagonists?

The current standard of care for PONV prophylaxis in children deemed to be at high risk for vomiting after surgery includes the administration of **5-HT_3 receptor antagonists.** These drugs block the rapid potassium efflux during repolarization in the cardiac myocyte and can prolong the PR, QRS, and **QT interval.** The intensity of this effect is highest with ondansetron, intermediate with granisetron, and lower with dolasetron. However, the active metabolites of dolasetron may block the sodium channels, independent of their effects on 5-HT_3 receptor-blocking activity.

The 5-HT_3 receptor antagonists are routinely administered to asymptomatic children without a preoperative screening EKG. To date, there have been only a handful of reports of polymorphic ventricular arrhythmias including **ventricular tachycardia** and **torsades des pointes** in children after administration of 5-HT_3 receptor antagonists, with the vast majority returning to normal sinus rhythm without incident (McKechnie & Froese, 2010). In healthy children, recent evidence demonstrated that 0.1 mg/kg ondansetron had no clinical effect on the **QT interval**, and in no case did it exceed 500 msec (Mehta et al., 2010).

The second-generation 5-HT_3 receptor antagonist, palonosetron, lacks an indole ring and may bind to the 5-HT_3 receptor at an allosteric site with internalization of the receptor, resulting in a prolonged effect. Palonosetron slightly increases QTc intervals by a mean of 1 to 3 ms compared to 5 to 5.4 ms for the first-generation 5 HT_3 antagonists. Data on its use in pediatric patients is limited, but the relatively minor effect on this drug on QT interval prolongation may make it a viable option in patients with known QT prolongation and either a history of, or current refractory nausea and vomiting. In all cases, the risk of short-term anesthetic-induced PONV must be weighed against the risk for potentially life-threatening drug-induced arrhythmias.

4. Does droperidol affect the QT interval?

Droperidol has been reported to cause prolongation of the QT interval in adults and children with malignant arrhythmias and torsades being reported in several cases. The Food and Drug Administration issued a black-box warning in 2004 recommending continuous EKG monitoring for a minimum of 2 to 3 hours after the administration of droperidol. Studies performed after the black-box warning was introduced showed that a single dose of droperidol 0.02 mg/kg IV significantly increased the **QT interval** in healthy children, although the increase was clinically irrelevant (Mehta et al., 2010). Droperidol is currently not readily available commercially in the United States.

5. What are the alternative strategies to reduce the risk of PONV in children with prolonged QTc?

There are a number of strategies apart from antiemetic therapy, which can be implemented to reduce the baseline risk for PONV in children and adults (Gan et al., 2014). These include (i) avoidance of general anesthesia and the use of regional anesthesia, (ii) preferential use of propofol infusions, (iii) avoidance of nitrous oxide, (iv) avoidance of volatile anesthetics, (v) minimization of perioperative opioids, and (vi) adequate hydration (Gan et al., 2014). Regional anesthesia may reduce opioid requirements and thereby reduce the risks of PONV. However, regional anesthesia is usually performed after induction of general anesthesia in children and is very rarely utilized as the sole mode of anesthesia in children. In older children (pre-adolescents or adolescents), regional anesthesia with supplemental sedation may be a plausible alternative to mitigate the risk of PONV. All inhaled anesthetics increase the risk of PONV and prolong the QT interval (sevoflurane > isoflurane). The preferential use of propofol with the avoidance of nitrous oxide may reduce the risks of both PONV and prolonged QT interval compared to inhaled anesthetics (Booker & Whyte, 2003). However, reports of the effect of propofol on the QT interval are inconsistent with some case reports suggesting it prolongs the QT interval, and others failing to show this. One study demonstrates that propofol rapidly reverses sevoflurane-induced QTc prolongation. Propofol has been successfully used to provide anesthesia in children undergoing procedures for both noncardiac- and cardiac-related procedures such as insertion of pacemakers, implantable cardioverter-defibrillator, and so on (Whyte et al., 2014). Steps to reduce opioid consumption by supplemental regional anesthesia, nonsteroidal anti-inflammatory drugs, and acetaminophen may reduce PONV, but it is important not to allow stress and pain-related release of endogenous epinephrine, which can trigger arrhythmias in these subjects. Midazolam premedication can help calm patients and is associated with reducing PONV. Finally, maintaining adequate hydration by keeping nil per os time to a minimum with liberal IV fluids should be part of a multimodal approach for reducing PONV risks.

In addition, prophylaxis with drugs not affecting the QT interval should be considered in patients at high risk for PONV. Numerous studies have established the antiemetic effect of **dexamethasone** in the perioperative period. Dexamethasone has no effect on the **QT interval and is a useful adjunct in these patients**. The neurokinin antagonist, **aprepitant** has been approved for the prophylaxis of PONV in adults and for managing chemotherapy-induced nausea and vomiting in both adults and children. This drug does not affect the QT interval. However, there is not enough data on its use for managing PONV. The use of palanosetron may be considered in this situation.

Few studies have addressed the efficacy of rescue treatment for established emesis in the PACU after failed prophylactic therapy in children with prolonged **QT intervals**. Metoclopramide is a moderately effective antiemetic, although dystonia has been reported as a side effect. Additionally, metoclopramide may also cause some degree of QT prolongation and should, be used with caution, if its use is required (Ellidokuz & Kaya, 2003). Dimenhydrinate is also moderately effective but produces sedation as a side effect (Vener et al., 1996). Overall, when considering PONV prophylaxis, the risk of emesis must be weighed against the risk for potentially life-threatening drug-induced arrhythmias.

6. Describe an anesthetic plan for managing a child with known prolonged QT syndrome undergoing elective surgery.

A preoperative 12-lead EKG should be performed in children with undiagnosed syncope or who have a family history of sudden death or unexplained death under anesthesia to determine if an underlying congenital channelopathy with QTc interval prolongation is present. The EKG may show broad-based T waves with an indistinct onset and high amplitude in c-LQT 1. Bifid low-amplitude T waves are seen in cLQT2 while peaked T waves with a late onset and long ST segments are noted in cLQT3. Children with c-LQT1 and c-LQT2 may benefit from beta-blockers, which are contraindicated in c-LQT3. Sodium channel blockers are used in c-LQT3.

All patients with cLQT syndromes should be referred to a cardiologist to determine if they will require a pacemaker and/or implanted cardioverter-defibrillator placement before the procedure. The cardiologist should be consulted for specific recommendations about the adequacy of heart rate control (beta-blockers), intraoperative device settings, as well as choice of drugs and their doses for intraoperative emergent therapy of c-LQT-related arrhythmias.

A preoperative review of laboratory tests should ensure normal acid-base and electrolyte balance, particularly for potassium and magnesium levels.

Preoperative sedation with midazolam is helpful, and a defibrillator and transvenous pacer should be ready for prompt use, particularly for children with c-LQT3 disorders. EKG monitoring should include at least two leads. Prevention of intraoperative hypothermia is also important. If extensive surgery with large fluid and electrolyte shifts is anticipated, appropriate invasive vascular monitoring should be placed before the surgical incision. The anesthesiologist should consider the value of cardiac sympathetic denervation via a left stellate ganglion block in patients with c-LQTs who require emergent surgery but do not have pacing devices in place.

The anesthesiologist and surgeon should discuss if surgery may be performed primarily under regional anesthesia, and it may be safer to avoid adding epinephrine to the local anesthetic. If general anesthesia is required, it is important to attenuate perioperative catecholamine release. The time points when this is likely to occur include induction of anesthesia, tracheal intubation, during surgical stimulation, and during emergence from anesthesia. The administration of short acting opioids, esmolol and centrally acting alpha-2 agonists such as dexmedetomidine may attenuate the response during these periods. In addition, application of topical anesthesia spray to the vocal cords can suppress the sympathetic response to tracheal intubation. While rocuronium, vecuronium, atracurium, and cisatracurium have been administered to facilitate tracheal intubation, it is perhaps better to avoid succinylcholine and ketamine. High airway pressures should be avoided, as the Valsalva maneuver is known to lengthen the QTc. Reversal of residual neuromuscular blockade with a combination of anticholinesterase and anticholinergic drugs can prolong the QTc and should be used with caution at the end of the procedure. The choice of prophylactic antiemetics was discussed earlier.

If torsades des pointes develops, magnesium sulphate (bolus 25–50 mg/kg IV; maximum of 2 g over 2–3 mins followed by an infusion of 2–4 mg/min) should be administered. Pacing of the right atrium at 90 to 110 beats/min is recommended if central venous access is available. Ventricular pacing can also be used. Asynchronous defibrillation may be required if ventricular fibrillation occurs.

SUMMARY

1. Children with prolonged QTc intervals are at risk for developing life-threatening arrhythmias including torsades des pointes during anesthesia. Precipitating factors include stress, electrolyte imbalance, and drugs including antiemetics.
2. PONV in children with prolonged QT interval should be managed by reducing baseline risks, prophylactic dexamethasone, and preemptive hydration.
3. In children with prolonged QT interval, exposure to all factors known to prolong the QT interval including sympathetic stimulation must be limited.

ACKNOWLEDGMENTS

The authors wish to acknowledge the first edition authors, Shilpa Rao and Jerrod Lerman.

ANNOTATED REFERENCES

Chiang C-E, Roden DM. The long QT syndromes: genetic basis and clinical implications. *J Am Coll Cardiol.* 2000;36:1–12.

This review introduces the genetics and the clinical presentation of channelopathies of the ventricular muscle for the uninitiated.

McKechnie K, Froese A. Ventricular tachycardia after ondansetron administration in a child with undiagnosed long QT syndrome. *Can J Anesth.* 2010;57:453–457.

An 11-year-old with a recognized long QT interval has ventricular tachycardia after a single dose of ondansetron. After IV lidocaine, the EKG converted to sinus rhythm.

Mehta D, Sanatani S, Whyte SD. The effects of droperidol and ondansetron on dispersion of myocardial repolarization in children. *Pediatr Anesth.* 2010;20:905–912.

This is the first study to measure the QT interval and dispersion of repolarization in children undergoing elective anesthesia after ondansetron, droperidol, both drugs, and neither drug. Although the QT interval increased statistically, the increase was clinically irrelevant, 10 msec. The dispersion of repolarization did not differ before and after the study medications.

Nathan AT, Antzelevitch C, Montenegro LM, Vetter VL: Case scenario: anesthesia-related cardiac arrest in a child with Timothy syndrome. *Anesthesiology.* 2012;117:1117–1126.

This case report provides a good overview of the long QT syndrome and checklist of the guiding principles for the anesthetic management of patients with this condition.

Whyte SD, Nathan A, Myers D, et al: The safety of modern anesthesia for children with long QT syndrome. *Anesth Analg.* 2014;119:932–938.

This multicenter chart review of 103 patients with long QT syndrome (LQTs) undergoing 158 episodes of general anesthesia showed a higher incidence of torsades des pointes in those undergoing LQTs related surgery (pacemaker, cardioverter-defibrillator, etc.) and no episode overtly attributed to the anesthetic regimen. This review suggests that incidental surgery in children with LQTs is safer than previously considered.

Credible Meds. https://crediblemeds.org/index.php/tools/pdfdownload?f=dta_en

This website lists drugs that prolong QT intervals and/or cause torsades des pointes. It classifies them into four groups based on their risks for torsades des pointes: (i) known risk, (ii) possible risk, (iii) conditional risk, or (iv) special risk.

BIBLIOGRAPHY

Apfel CC, Malhotra A, Leslie JB. The role of neurokininin-1 receptor antagonists for the management of postoperative nausea and vomiting. *Curr Opin Anaesthesiol.* 2008; 21: 427–432.

Booker PD, Whyte SD, Ladusans EJ. Long QT syndrome and anaesthesia. *Br J Anaesth.* 2003;90(3):349–366.

Choi EM, Lee MG, Lee SH, Choi KW, Choi SH. Association of ABCB1 polymorphisms with the efficacy of ondansetron for postoperative nausea and vomiting. *Anaesthesia.* 2010;65:996–1000.

Ellidokuz E, Kaya D. The effect of metoclopramide on QT dynamicity: double-blind, placebo-controlled, cross-over study in healthy male volunteers. *Aliment Pharmacol Ther.* 2003;18(1):151–155.

Gan TJ, Diemunsch P, Habib AS, et al. Consensus guidelines for the management of postoperative nausea and vomiting. *Anesth Analg.* 2014;118(1):85–113.

Rojas C, Stathis M, Thomas AG, et al. Palonosetron exhibits unique molecular interactions with the 5-HT3 receptor. *Anesth Analg.* 2008;107:469–478.

Towbin JA, Wang Z, Li H. Genotype and severity of long QT syndrome. *Drug Metab Disp.* 2001;29:574–579.

Van Noord C, Eijgelsheim M, Stricker BHC. Drug and non-drug associated QT interval prolongation. *Br J Clin Pharmacol.* 2010;70:16–23.

Vener DF, Carr AS, Sikich N, Bissonnette B, Lerman J. Dimenhydrinate decreases vomiting after strabismus surgery in children. *Anesth Analg.* 1996;82:728–731.

Vincent GM. The long QT syndrome. *Indian Pacing Electrophysiol J.* 2002;2:127–146.

68

Disclosure after Complication in the Operating Room

DAVID A. YOUNG

INTRODUCTION

It is estimated that approximately 100,000 deaths and 1 million injuries per year occur in the United States due to medical errors. Many of these medical errors occur within the perioperative environment and result in significant morbidity or mortality. In addition, most anesthesiologists have little to no experience or formal training with the disclosure of a poor clinical outcome or medical error. Patients and families overwhelmingly want to be informed regarding matters related to poor outcomes and medical errors. After the occurrence of a medical error, most patients and families highly value an honest and transparent disclosure of the details as well as a sincere apology from those responsible regardless of the amount of apparent harm. Subsequently, they may need, and will greatly appreciate, continued emotional support. Additionally, they anticipate sufficient efforts will be made to identify and prevent similar events from reoccurring in the future. When disclosing a medical error to a parent or patient, an organized approach using a truthful and compassionate discussion as the backbone is the most prudent strategy. Finally, it is imperative that the anesthesiologist notify the appropriate administrative bodies such as quality and safety departments and risk management after the occurrence of a significant medical error including sentinel events.

LEARNING OBJECTIVES

1. Appreciate the differences between medical errors and poor clinical outcomes.
2. Recognize the distinctions between near misses and sentinel events.
3. Characterize the indications for disclosure of medical errors without apparent harm as well as the appropriate use of apology.
4. Develop an approach for the effective disclosure of a pediatric medical error to a parent.

CASE PRESENTATION

An otherwise healthy 12-year-old male presents for emergent exploratory laparotomy. Approximately 1 hour prior to presentation, the patient was playing tackle football and received a direct strike to the abdomen by another player. The patient subsequently complained of severe abdominal pain which resulted in prompt transfer to the local emergency department by ambulance.

In the emergency department, the patient continues to complain of severe abdominal pain. According to the patient's mother, the patient has no past surgical history and the only medical condition reported is a history of well-controlled allergic rhinitis. The patient has no drug allergies and denies use of prescription medications. The patient's vital signs are: temperature 36.7°C, heart rate 114, blood pressure 90/58, respiratory rate 28, room air oxygen saturation 97%. After arrival to the emergency department, the patient has 1 peripheral intravenous line placed; and blood is drawn for laboratory studies to include cell blood count, electrolytes, coagulation studies, and blood cross-matching. The patient has a computed tomography of the abdomen which reveals a significant splenic laceration as well as a large amount of intraabdominal fluid which is strongly suspected to be blood. A general surgeon promptly evaluates the patient and schedules an emergent laparotomy for repair of a splenic laceration versus splenectomy.

The patient is brought emergently to the operating room although the blood products are not initially available. A rapid sequence induction is performed uneventfully, and a second peripheral intravenous line is placed. Vitals signs after induction of anesthesia are similar to preoperative values. After surgical incision and access to the peritoneal cavity, a large amount of intraabdominal bleeding is visualized. The surgeon immediately suctions approximately 700 cc of blood from the abdomen. The blood pressure acutely decreases to 68/46 with a corresponding heart rate of 132. The laboratory results from the emergency department have just been reported and reveal a hemoglobin of 7.9 along with a hematocrit of 22.4%.

Fortunately, a cooler of packed red blood cells arrives from the blood bank. You are very engaged in the management of the acute hypotension which included the preparation of diluted phenylephrine. You quickly check the documents for the blood products with the circulating nurse and administer 2 units of packed red blood cells. The surgical team gains hemostasis and inserts packs into the abdomen. Several minutes later, the patient develops hypotension, diffuse oozing, and red-colored urine. You strongly suspect a transfusion reaction so you discontinue the administration of the second unit of packed red blood cells and institute supportive care. Additional help is summoned, including an emergent consultation with the blood bank pathologist. While providing care to maintain blood pressure and urine output, a blood sample is sent to the blood bank.

The surgeons perform a splenectomy, and the patient is subsequently transferred in critical condition to the intensive care unit. Review of the documents from the blood bank reveal that the paperwork is correct; however, it is noted that the patient's first name on the blood bank papers do not match the name on the blood product. You recall being rushed while checking the blood products due to other simultaneous tasks and only checking the patient's last name. The blood bank pathologist informs you that the patient experienced an acute hemolytic transfusion reaction due to a major blood group incompatibility. You give the intensive care unit staff a detailed handoff and you prepare to go to the surgical waiting room to speak with the patients parents.

DISCUSSION

1. How would you define a medical error? How do medical errors compare with poor clinical outcomes? What type of event(s) do you think occurred in this case?

An injury or complication attributable to the medical management of a patient is considered an adverse event. An adverse event specifically is any harm caused by the medical care rather than by the patient's underlying disease process (Lipira & Gallagher, 2014) A medical error can be defined as a failure of the planned action to be completed as intended. Another definition of a medical error is the delivery of an inappropriate method of care or the use of a wrong plan to achieve a goal (Richardson WC et al., 2000). Examples of medical errors include administration of wrong medication, wrong medication dose, or wrong site surgery, wrong patient, misdiagnosis, and retained foreign bodies. This is in contrast to a poor clinical outcome, which is an unfavorable result (i.e., death) but not necessarily related to a medical error. Poor clinical outcomes typically are related to an underlying disease process (i.e., acute heart failure). An adverse event (i.e., cardiac arrest) can be caused by a medical error and/or due to the underlying disease process. If a medical error has occurred, families want to know what went wrong, why it happened, and what measures will be instituted to prevent it from happening again (Brandom et al., 2011).

In this case, the failure to recognize that the packed red blood cells were for another patient with the same last name, is the most likely cause for the development of the acute hemolytic transfusion reaction. According to The Joint Commission, a nonprofit organization responsible for the accreditation and certification of approximately 21,000 health care organizations and programs in the United States, development of an acute hemolytic transfusion reaction due to a major blood group incompatibility is a type of sentinel event (see Question 3). In summary, a medical error occurred in this patient that was a sentinel event which also resulted in a poor clinical outcome.

2. Hypothetically, if the event resulted in no detectable morbidity or harm, would it change your decision to disclose a medical error?

A medical error may or may not result in a poor clinical outcome. Likewise, a poor clinical outcome may or may not be due to a medical error. Typically, a poor clinical outcome is foreseeable and associated with an identified preoperative morbidity and/or high-risk surgical procedure. Medical errors are encouraged to be disclosed regardless of the severity and association with a poor clinical outcome. Many experts would argue it is easier to disclose a medical error if no detectable morbidity has occurred. From, a legal perspective, disclosure of a medical error after no detectable harm has occurred, would be expected to have minimal to zero associated liability since no measurable damage has occurred. From a medical perspective, disclosure of a medical error which did not result in any detectable harm, may have favorable clinical consequences. For example, the unintentional administration of a medication thought to be associated with an allergic reaction (i.e., antibiotic) that resulted in no apparent reaction may warrant allergy testing as well as provide additional options for the future administration of antibiotics.

3. What is a sentinel event? What are some examples of sentinel events? How does a sentinel event differ from a near miss? What actions are required by the institution after a sentinel event occurs?

According to The Joint Commission, sentinel events are serious adverse events that require an immediate institutional response. These events are unanticipated, not related to the patient's illness or underlying condition, and may result in serious physical and/or psychological injury. These events are called "sentinel" because they indicate the need for immediate investigation and response. Each accredited organization is strongly encouraged, but not required, to report sentinel events to The Joint Commission. Examples of sentinel events that are plausible to occur within the perioperative environment include death; permanent harm; severe temporary harm; hemolytic transfusion reaction resulting from the administration of blood or blood products having major blood group incompatibilities; invasive procedures on the wrong patient or the wrong site; the wrong procedure; fire, unanticipated smoke, or heat occurring during patient care; and unintended retention of a foreign object in a patient.

A near miss is an event that could have resulted in patient harm but the event did not occur due to multiple factors including timely intervention by health care providers, the patient and family or due to chance. Near misses have also be referred to as "close calls" or "good catches." A near miss under different circumstances could have easily resulted in patient harm and the development of a sentinel event.

All sentinel events must be investigated by the institution and are subject to review by The Joint Commission. Accredited hospitals are expected to have policies in force that identify and respond appropriately to all sentinel events. An appropriate institutional response to a sentinel event would include a formalized response that stabilizes the patient, discloses the event to the patient and family, and provides support for the family as well as the staff involved in the event. After appropriate patient care has occurred, the institutional response begins with notification of the hospital clinical and administrative leadership. Additionally, any medications, devices, and documents that are relevant to the event should be obtained for analysis.

The institutional investigation of a sentinel event includes completion of a comprehensive systematic analysis for identifying the causal and contributory circumstances of the event. This analysis should include strong corrective actions developed from the identified factors that eliminate or control system hazards or vulnerabilities, results in sustained improvement over time, and contains a time line for implementation of the identified corrective actions. A root cause analysis (RCA) is the most common form of a comprehensive systematic analysis used for identifying the factors related to a sentinel event. This utilizes a retrospective process that must be performed within 45 days of the sentinel event; the RCA focus is to prevent recurrence rather than assign blame (Tung, 2014).

4. Will your disclosure of this medical error to the family, including the use of an apology, impact the risk for future legal liability?

The Joint Commission requires institutions to disclose unanticipated outcomes to patients and families if related to a sentinel event. Avoiding confessions of fault in cases of medical error has been a previously well-accepted strategy used to potentially reduce legal liability. There is a commonly held belief that acknowledgement of error can later be used during legal proceedings against doctors and hospitals. Thirty-six states have "apology laws" which prohibit certain statements, expressions, or other evidence related to disclosure, from being admissible in a lawsuit. Most states simply include expressions of empathy or sympathy, while a few states protect admissions of fault. In addition, acts of empathy have been viewed very favorably by many families, and it has been proposed that a comprehensive disclosure, including the use of disclosure, apology, and offer (DA&O) has reduced the frequency of medical malpractice lawsuits as well as the monetary amounts awarded (Kachalia et al., 2010).

Some institutions and health systems have adopted an open disclosure policy and have demonstrated that effective disclosure practices can reduce legal liability. Health systems that have implemented an open disclosure policy have reduced the number of medical malpractice lawsuits, the amount of judgments paid, and the cost of attorneys' fees. For example, the University of Michigan adopted an open disclosure policy in which doctors admit mistakes and apologize in cases of medical error. Since the commencement of this policy, the university has reduced the time to resolve complaints, attorneys' fees have been reduced by approximately two-thirds, and the number of medical malpractice lawsuits has decreased (Kachalia et al., 2010). As health care compensation becomes more influenced by measured quality and safety outcomes, providers and institutions may be driven to pursue aggressive performance improvement programs which focus on system-wide error identification and prevention initiatives.

5. What is your strategy for the effective disclosure of this medical error to the parents? What preparations should you make prior to speaking with the parents? In general, what do you think should be discussed with the parents?

After the occurrence of this medical error, a discussion should ideally take place with the parents, attending surgeon, and attending anesthesiologist. Timing of the response should be prompt, typically soon after completion of patient care. The first discussion with the patient and/or family should focus on what happened, how it will affect the patient, and the prognosis. Make every effort to have all involved parties at a single meeting for the initial disclosure. This will avoid the family hearing multiple and possibly different explanations which can result in the family having decreased trust in all involved parties. If there is an obvious medical error, an acknowledgement is made and an expression of regret and an apology are offered. Patients do not only desire information after an adverse event or medical error but also want emotional support, including an empathic apology (Lipira & Gallagher, 2014). However, if the mechanisms for injury are unclear, disclosure of possible causes should be initially mentioned and then possibly modified after more information is available. Medical providers who have a primary relationship with the family should also be updated on the circumstances related to the medical error including ongoing medical conditions and the current medical therapies being administered.

Regardless of whether the medical error is immediately identified, the discussion should occur in a quiet and private location. A discussion with the involved patient care team should occur prior to speaking with the parents in order to review the intraoperative events, prevent conflicting stories, and promote a thoughtful discussion. Social workers, clergy, and language interpreters should all be offered to the parents if deemed appropriate. Plan what to say to the parents in advance. Discussion with parents should be objective, compassionate, and at an appropriate educational level for the parents. Be prepared to repeat all previous discussions with the parents. Many parents may only recall portions of your discussions due to the severe emotional stress from the event. Disclosures for an unanticipated medical error are complex; these discussions should be tailored to the nature of the event, the clinical context, and the patient–provider relationship.

Several factors should be considered to make this experience as effective as possible. Disclose only the facts. Tell the parents what you know and what you do not know. Take as much time as needed. Attempt to explain the medical conditions that occurred by using the most appropriate descriptions as possible. Explain what has been done and what future care plans are anticipated. Be compassionate; it is appropriate to say, "I'm sorry" regarding the medical error. Ask the parents if they understand and if they have any questions. Sometimes parents may request to hear limited information only; this may especially occur soon after an unexpected adverse event. Respect the parents' wishes as much as possible.

Follow-up visits should continue to coordinate care, answer questions, and maintain a good rapport with the parents. Place only objective findings in the medical record, and avoid corrections to the medical record. Document all discussions with the parents including follow-up visits and future care plans. New information may become available as time passes, an

TABLE 68.1 KEY COMPONENTS FOR THE EFFECTIVE DISCLOSURE OF A PEDIATRIC MEDICAL ERROR TO THE PARENTS

Plan discussion of disclosure promptly after completion of patient care
Review the main events with the involved providers and hospital administration prior to disclosure to families
Determine the attending physician who will speak to the family
Plan the suggested topics for discussion prior to the disclosure
Obtain social workers, language interpreters, and/or clergy to be present
Speak with parents in a private location
Discuss only the facts and avoid speculation
Communicate what you know and what you do not know
Provide an objective and compassionate discussion on an appropriate level
Offer an apology if a known medical error has occurred
Ask the parents if they understand and if they have any questions
Be available for future questions from parents
Expect to repeat previous discussions due to emotional distress
Plan for ongoing follow-up and coordination with primary medical providers

investigation is completed, and the condition of the patient changes. Update the parents as new information becomes available. Continue to provide postoperative visits and offer your expertise to the primary team caring for the patient. There are a number of resources that help physicians deliver bad or negative news systematically (Minichiello et al., 2007). Table 68.1 lists the key components for the effective disclosure of a pediatric medical error to the parents.

SUMMARY

1. Families expect and deserve a transparent as well as honest communication after a medical error regardless of whether harm has occurred and also after a poor clinical outcome which is not associated with a medical error.
2. Open disclosure, including the use of apology, has numerous benefits including maintaining trust and reducing moral anguish.
3. A demonstration of empathy along with a commitment to investigate and make future improvements is crucial to convey during disclosure of medical errors.
4. Future improvements in safety and quality are dependent upon accurate disclosure and reporting of medical errors including sentinel events.
5. The use of an organized disclosure process after a medical error will maximize the effectiveness of communication during a time of significant stresses to the family and the physician.

ACKNOWLEDGMENTS

The author wishes to acknowledge the first edition authors, Mark J. Meyer and Norbert J. Weidner, for their contribution.

ANNOTATED REFERENCES

Brandom BW, Callahan P, Micalizzi DA. What happens when things go wrong? *Pediatr Anesth.* 2011 Jul;21(7):730–736.

This review article describes the responses from parents and health care providers after a significant medical adverse event or death.

Kachalia A, Kaufman SR, Boothman R, et al. Liability claims and costs before and after implementation of a medical error disclosure program. *Ann Intern Med.* 2010;153(4):213–221.

This article discusses the University of Michigan Health System implementation of a full disclosure program with offer of apology that shows no increase in the total claims or liability costs.

Lipira LE, Gallagher TH. Disclosure of adverse events and errors in surgical care: challenges and strategies for improvement. *World J Surg.* 2014 Jul;38(7):1614–1621.

This article discusses several strategies to promote a culture of effective and complete disclosure of surgical adverse events.

Minichiello TA, Ling D, Ucci DK. Breaking bad news: a practical approach for the hospitalist. *J Hosp Med.* 2007 Nov;2(6):415–421.

This article describes a step-wise, practical approach for breaking bad news using case examples.

Richardson WC, Berwick DM, Bisgard JC. The Institute of Medicine report on medical errors. *N Engl J Med.* 2000 Aug 31;343(9):663–4; author reply 665

Tung A. Sentinel events and how to learn from them. *Int Anesthesiol Clin.* 2014;52(1):53–68.

This review article describes near misses, sentinel events, and the RCA process.

FURTHER READING

Bell SK, Moorman DW, Delbanco T. Improving the patient, family, and clinician experience after harmful events: the "When Things Go Wrong" curriculum. *Acad Med.* 2010;85:1010–1017.

Eaves-Leanos A, Dunn EJ. Open disclosure of adverse events: transparency and safety in health care. *Surg Clin North Am.* 2012 Feb;92(1):163–177.

Etchegaray JM, Ottosen MJ, Burress L, et al. Structuring patient and family involvement in medical error event disclosure and analysis. *Health Aff.* 2014 Jan;33(1):46–52.

Gallagher TH, Waterman AD, Ebers AG. Patients' and physicians' attitudes regarding disclosure of medical errors. *JAMA.* 2003;289(8):1001–1007.

Gazoni FM, Amato PE, Malik ZM, et al. The impact of perioperative catastrophes on anesthesiologists: results of a national survey. *Anesth Analg.* 2012 Mar;114(3):596–603.

Heard GC, Sanderson PM, Thomas RD. Barriers to adverse event and error reporting in anesthesia. *Anesth Analg.* 2012 Mar;114(3):604–614.

Hickson GB, Federspiel CF, Pichert JW, Miller CS, Gauld-Jaeger J, Bost P. Patient complaints and malpractice risk. *JAMA.* 2002;287:2951–2957.

Hobgood C, Peck CR, Gilbert B, Chappell K, Zou B. Medical errors—what and when: what do patients want to know? *Acad Emerg Med.* 2002;9:1156–1161.

Matlow AG, Moody L, Laxer R, Stevens P, Goia C, Friedman JN. Disclosure of medical error to parents and pediatric patients: assessment of parent's attitudes and influencing factors. *Arch Dis Child.* 2010;95:286–290.

McDonnell WM, Guenther E. Do state laws make it easier to say "I'm sorry?" *Ann Intern Med.* 2008;149:811–815.

McLennan SR, Engel-Glatter S, Meyer AH, et al. Disclosing and reporting medical errors: cross-sectional survey of Swiss anaesthesiologists. *Eur J Anaesthesiol.* 2015 Jul;32(7):471–476.

Sage WM, Gallagher TH, Armstrong S, et al. How policy makers can smooth the way for communication-and- resolution programs. *Health Aff.* 2014 Jan;33(1):11–19.

Sage WM, Jablonski JS, Thomas EJ. Use of nondisclosure agreements in medical malpractice settlements by a large academic health care system. *JAMA Intern Med.* 2015 Jul;175(7):1130–1135.

Wu AW, Boyle DJ, Wallace G, et al. Disclosure of adverse events in the United States and Canada: an update, and a proposed framework for improvement. *J Public Health Res.* 2013 Dec 1;2(3):e32.

PART 15

Challenges in Ethics

69

Managing Blood Loss in a Jehovah's Witness Patient

MICHELLE DALTON

INTRODUCTION

Approximately 8 million individuals worldwide and 2.1 million in the United States practice the Jehovah's Witness (JW) faith. One of the tenets of this religion that is most familiar to the medical community is the refusal of blood transfusion even if it may result in death (Woolley, 2005). Specifically, JW patients do not accept what they consider the primary components of blood: red cells, white cells, plasma, and platelets (Frank et al., 2014). Transfusion of minor fractions, such as albumin and cryoprecipitate, as well as salvaged blood kept in continuity with the vascular system, is acceptable to some (Resar et al., 2016). The acceptability of these components is a matter of personal conscience, according to church leaders. In caring for pediatric JW patients, refusal of transfusion by the parents and/or legal guardians can be overridden based on ethical grounds and legal precedent. Nevertheless, efforts can and should be made to respect parental and patient wishes through careful preoperative planning and discussion. Bloodless medicine centers have emerged that specialize in the management of patients who refuse or cannot receive blood transfusions. Results from these centers suggest that "bloodless" patients not only do as well as, but may also have better outcomes than, traditionally managed patients who receive transfusion.

LEARNING OBJECTIVES

1. Appreciate acceptable versus nonacceptable blood loss management strategies in accordance with JW beliefs.
2. Develop a strategy for preoperative optimization in advance of elective surgery and intraoperative blood loss reduction.
3. Review transfusion thresholds in healthy pediatric patients.
4. Understand legal and ethical ramifications of transfusion refusal by the pediatric patient.

CASE PRESENTATION

A 14-year-old girl with neuromuscular scoliosis presents to the anesthesia preoperative clinic in preparation for elective spinal instrumentation to take place in 6 weeks. Her parents accompany her and inform you that they are Jehovah's Witnesses and therefore will not accept blood transfusion. The patient, who is mentally age-appropriate, confirms in an interview separate from her parents that she refuses transfusion. Discussion with the surgeon indicates he is familiar and comfortable with caring for JW patients. Both the patient and family history do not suggest anemia or a bleeding disorder, although the patient does report heavy menstrual periods. She is not taking any medications or supplements. She sees a pulmonologist for management of mild-moderate restrictive lung disease. She weighs 48 kg and is 5′5″tall.

You ask the parents what, if any, transfused products they are comfortable with their daughter receiving. They tell you that albumin and other fractions are okay. You clarify which fractions are acceptable to them, including clotting factors and cryoprecipitate. They do not want blood salvage to be used as it is their understanding that the blood administered under this technique, is separated from the body to be cleaned prior to transfusion. Similarly, they do not want their daughter to donate her own blood unless it can be done in a way that keeps the blood in continuity with her circulatory system. They ask you about artificial blood, and you discuss the potential risks and benefits of blood substitutes, informing them that at present none are Food and Drug Administration (FDA) approved. They also ask about medications that can help their daughter make more blood. You explain that although erythropoietin-stimulating agents (ESAs) can be helpful for some patients, they are probably not indicated in this case. During this interview, you counsel the parents and patient that, although every effort will be made to respect their wishes and avoid transfusion, if in your judgment the risk for death is high due to the degree of blood loss, you will proceed with transfusion. They accept this and wish to proceed with surgery.

The patient's pulmonologist is consulted. She recommends postoperative extubation to bilevel positive airway pressure (BiPAP) as tolerated. Using low-volume tubes for phlebotomy, a complete blood count is ordered which reveals hemoglobin (Hgb) 10.5 g/dL and hematocrit (Hct) 32.0%. Testing for von Willebrand disease is negative. Oral iron, B12, and folate supplements are ordered.

On the morning of surgery, a wearable convection blanket is placed on the patient while she waits in the holding area. Her Hgb and Hct are 12.2 g/dL and 36%. A current type and crossmatch are available in the blood bank. You have discussed the case with the perioperative team who are all aware that the patient is a Jehovah's Witness and the plan is to avoid transfusion if safely possible. You and the surgeon agree on a minimum acceptable Hgb of 9 g/dL and permissive hypotension to no lower than 30% of baseline systolic or mean arterial pressure (MAP). After induction of general anesthesia, an arterial line with in-line reinfusion device is placed. The patient is positioned prone with special care to avoid pressure on the abdomen. Normocapnia is maintained with mechanical ventilation, and high intrathoracic pressures are avoided. You administer a loading dose of tranexamic acid followed by infusion. Euvolemia is maintained with crystalloids. Somatosensory evoked potentials (SSEPs) are used to monitor for potential spinal cord ischemia. Blood loss as expected is steady despite meticulous surgical technique. Though no change is noted in the SSEPs, the MAP is steadily declining even after discontinuation of hypotensive agents. The surgeon notes that bleeding seems to be increasing and a bedside ROTEM suggests hypofibrinogenemia so you administer cryoprecipitate. You check a Hgb and find that it is 7.9 g/dL. You inform the surgeon who decides the surgery should be stopped in view of likely ongoing bleeding intra- and postoperatively.

You extubate the patient awake. In recovery, she has an oxygen requirement in addition to a need for BiPAP but she tolerates it well. She is able to follow commands and move all extremities. Initial postoperative Hgb is 7.0 g/dL, and she is admitted to the intensive care unit (ICU). You and the surgeon meet with the parents to discuss the intraoperative course and decision to stage surgery. You also reiterate that although she did not require transfusion during surgery, their daughter could still require transfusion during hospitalization. They express understanding and their appreciation for your efforts. During the ICU admission, daily labs are not drawn per routine but rather as clinically indicated using microtainer tubes when possible. After an uneventful hospitalization, the patient is discharged home with an Hgb of 8.1 g/dL. Six weeks later she returns for completion of surgery.

DISCUSSION

1. What is the threshold for transfusion in a pediatric patient?

The goals of blood and blood product transfusion are to prevent end-organ ischemia and reduce bleeding in at-risk patients. Transfusion recommendations exist for stable pediatric ICU patients but not for their surgical counterparts. Hgb levels are frequently used as an indicator for when to transfuse. However, a poll of pediatric intensivists in the United States and Canada revealed that in addition to absolute Hgb values, indicators such as respiratory or cardiovascular insufficiency prompted transfusion. Furthermore, complicating factors such as the presence or absence of cardiac disease or sepsis tend to bias practitioners toward more liberal transfusion practice. Data suggest that in the absence of cardiac disease, stable pediatric ICU patients who do not receive transfusion, do not have an increased risk of morbidity or mortality if Hgb exceeds 7 g/dL. Below 5 g/dL, there appears to be an increased risk of death, and transfusion is indicated. No clear evidence exists currently to recommend transfusion thresholds for stable children with Hgb between these values. This data comes from stable ICU patients without active bleeding or other complicating factors (e.g., cancer, congenital heart disease) who may have higher requirements.

2. What is the significance of the patient's preoperative anemia?

The World Health Organization defines anemia as Hgb <12g/dL in women and <13 g/dL in men. More refined definitions of anemia based on age range can be found in *Nathan and Oski's Hematology of Infancy and Childhood.* Anemia is present in anywhere from 5% to 75% of all patients, depending on the patient population and definition of anemia. Anemia is more common in hospitalized patients and due to its prevalence may often be overlooked or ignored. Preoperative anemia in pediatric surgical patients may be an independent risk factor for in-hospital mortality and as such probably warrants preoperative correction when feasible.

3. What can be done preoperatively to reduce the risk for transfusion?

Strategies to reduce transfusion can be applied not only to those who refuse blood based on religious grounds. Evidence suggests that conservative management that reduces or eliminates transfusion results in comparable, and possibly better, patient outcomes. The Bloodless Medicine and Surgery Program at Johns Hopkins reported in a retrospective case-control study that hospitalized patients who did not receive transfusion were at no greater risk for adverse outcomes than controls and had an overall lower mortality, though the latter was not significant ($p = 0.46$). However, they also noted that the study was limited by the fact that patients who refused transfusion may not have been offered surgical options. Bloodless medicine programs are multidisciplinary collaboratives designed to reduce risk to surgical patients who refuse blood transfusion. Although children and adolescents may not legally be able to refuse transfusion (see later discussion), a coordinated plan to reduce need for transfusion should still be considered in this population. Planning begins with scheduling elective surgery at least 4 to 8 weeks after preoperative evaluation. This allows time for a thorough history and physical; diagnosis and treatment of anemia; elimination or replacement of medications and supplements that increase bleeding risk; consultation with the patient's primary and/or specialty care physicians; and discussion between the surgeon, anesthesiologist, and perioperative staff regarding expectations and endpoints such as expected blood loss and minimum acceptable Hgb. Preparing weeks ahead of surgery also allows the family time to discuss transfusion with their religious leaders and ask clinicians for clarification regarding techniques such as blood salvage and acute normovolemic hemodilution. Not all JW patients refuse or accept the same blood components, so it is worthwhile to have a detailed discussion regarding what they find acceptable. The ban on accepting blood transfusion is rooted in a number of Biblical passages that refer to the condemnation of eating blood. The consequence of violating this prohibition is loss of eternal life. However, in 1990 the JW Watchtower Society published a reader's argument that because certain blood components naturally pass freely between a mother and fetus, it followed that minor blood fractions might also reasonably be transfused without being disloyal to the faith. Thus human albumin (and albumin-containing products such as Epogen) may be acceptable to some. Cryoprecipitate, fibrinogen, and factor concentrates may also be considered minor fractions. Further, if blood remains in a continuous circuit with a patient, it may not be considered a transfusion. This may allow for normovolemic hemodilution as long as the tubing to the blood withdrawn from the patient is clamped but not disconnected.

Previously undiagnosed anemia, as noted, is relatively common and workup may include evaluation for common conditions such as von Willebrand's disease, iron studies, and consideration of occult bleeding. Patients found to have von Willebrand's disease should be evaluated for response to desmopressin. Menorrhagia can be medically controlled with progesterone. Iron deficiency can be treated with oral iron, folate, and B12 supplements. Anemia of chronic disease (anemia of inflammation) in which iron stores are adequate but inaccessible may need to be treated with intravenous iron in combination with ESAs. ESAs are somewhat controversial and do carry a black-box warning from the FDA due to the possible risk of increased tumor growth in cancer patients and the risk of thrombotic events. While their use in pediatric craniofacial surgery patients appears to decrease transfusion requirements, at least one study of pediatric orthopedic patients reflected no benefit to its use. Finally, any comorbidities present should be optimized, as should the patient's nutritional state.

4. What intraoperative strategies can further reduce transfusion risk?

In managing a JW patient, it is ideal to have a perioperative team that is familiar and comfortable with techniques to reduce blood loss. The surgical facility should have an appropriate level of care available for recovery (e.g., an ICU bed). From the surgical side, judicious use of tourniquets, endoscopy, or laparoscopy in lieu of open procedures; use of cautery and fibrin glues to promote hemostasis; and consideration for staging surgery can all reduce blood loss. Blood salvage has been used in JW patients, but one should be clear when describing the type of device used. Some devices involve processing of blood in batches and unequivocally separates the final product from the patient. However, some continuously processing devices do stay in-line with the patient, and this may be acceptable. Blood salvage should not be used in any situation in which it would be otherwise contraindicated (e.g., blood bacterial contamination with pus, cancer patients in whom dissemination of malignant cells might occur).

Intraoperative administration of lysine analogs such as tranexamic acid and aminocaproic acid reduces blood loss. These agents bind to fibrin clots and inhibit plasminogen activation thus preventing clot breakdown by plasmin. They are typically administered as a loading dose followed by an infusion which is discontinued at the conclusion of surgery. As much as possible, low-volume microtainer tubes should be used for lab draws, and blood should be drawn for lab work only when clinically indicated. Use of an in-line reinfusion device for arterial blood draws eliminates waste that is frequently thrown out when sampling the line. Controlled hypotension appropriate to the patient's underlying medical condition is frequently used even in non-JW patients undergoing major orthopedic procedures such as posterior spinal fusion. Hypercapnia promotes bleeding and should be avoided. Mechanical pressures that reduce venous return to the heart may increase venous bleeding, so increased intrathoracic or abdominal pressure should be avoided. Hypothermia is a known cause of platelet and coagulation factor dysfunction and should be prevented or treated as necessary; preoperative application of a wearable warm air device is useful in patients at risk for intraoperative hypothermia. As mentioned earlier, acute normovolemic hemodilution is a technique that might be acceptable to some JW patients as long as blood stays in continuity with the patient's vascular system: phlebotomy is performed, the tubing is clamped, and the volume of blood removed is replaced with crystalloid. Blood is then returned to the patient after the period of greatest surgical blood loss is over or when it is clinically indicated. Neuraxial analgesia, often implemented after induction of general anesthesia in pediatric patients, might be associated with less postoperative bleeding and transfusion and should be considered in the absence of any contraindications.

In addition to traditional coagulation panels, point-of-care thromboelastography (TEG) or thromboelastometry (ROTEM) devices are used in some institutions for a more rapid assessment of coagulopathy. Volume replacement only without replacing factors or other blood components, may lead to a dilutional coagulopathy, and information from these tests may be used to guide transfusion of plasma, cryoprecipitate, fibrinogen concentrate, and platelets. Of these, only the cryoprecipitate and fibrinogen are likely to be acceptable to a JW patient. Familiarity with the device used and an understanding of how to interpret the results is required. A Cochrane review of randomized controlled trials comparing use of TEG or ROTEM versus traditional coagulation panels and/or clinical judgment to guide transfusion observed no difference in the need for surgical reintervention, significant bleeding, or massive transfusion, but the quality of evidence was low.

Blood substitutes can primarily be divided into 2 categories: Hgb-based oxygen carriers and perfluorocarbons. The former is derived from human or bovine hemoglobin and may or may not be acceptable to a JW patient. Significant vasoconstriction and an association with myocardial infarction and death are among the concerns with these products. The perfluorocarbons are completely artificial and thus do not conflict with JW beliefs. Immunosuppression, pulmonary reactions, and risk of stroke have been noted with these agents. Currently no blood substitutes are approved by the FDA for routine administration. However, 2 products (Sanguinate and Hemopure, both Hgb-based) are available for compassionate use with emergency FDA approval.

5. What are the parents' rights in deciding whether or not their child can receive a blood transfusion? How does the mature minor doctrine affect the decision to transfuse against the patient's wishes?

The JW faith was founded in 1881 by Charles Taze Russel. However, it was not until 1944–1945 that blood transfusions were banned by the faith (Lason & Ralph, 2015). The first US court case of parental transfusion refusal occurred in 1951. Custody of the child was granted to the probation service, which approved the transfusion. The Illinois Supreme Court subsequently heard the parents' appeal but upheld the ruling. The decision to permit state intervention upheld an earlier decision made by the US Supreme Court in 1944, *Prince vs Massachusetts*, which was a case of violation of child labor law. A minor had accompanied her aunt, who was her legal guardian, to distribute JW literature on a public street while soliciting donations. Though this case did not involve the medical welfare of the child, the conclusion included language that addressed this issue: "The right to practice religion freely does not include liberty to expose the community or the child to communicable disease or the latter to ill health or death/. . . Parents may be free to become martyrs themselves. But it does not follow that they are free . . . to make martyrs of their children before they have reached the age of full and legal discretion when they can make that choice for themselves." This ruling has generally been used in the United States as the basis for cases of JW parents refusing transfusion for their children. In these cases, the basic principles have been that the welfare of the child and state outweigh parental rights; parental rights do not grant life and death authority; and, specifically, religious beliefs do not give parents an absolute right to refuse medical treatment.

In the case of an adolescent patient, the authority to transfuse against the patient's wishes is less clear. In the United States, special cases exist for minors where they can legally make decisions regarding their own health care. These fall into 3 categories: patients seeking care related to specific diagnoses and treatment (e.g., sexually transmitted disease, contraception), patients who are legally emancipated (e.g., married patients), and mature minors. The last category listed is the least well defined. There is no absolute age above which one automatically has the maturity to understand informed consent, and data suggest that even up to 50% of adults do not fully comprehend what they agree to in the informed consent process. The American Academy of Pediatrics (AAP) recommends approaching medical decision-making in adolescents in a way that incorporates respect for the patient's experience and the family's concerns as well as current data regarding adolescent neurodevelopment and decision-making. Not surprisingly, the science of adolescent decision-making capacity is complex. Essentially, it appears that adolescents, even those with apparently good impulse-control versus reward-seeking behavior, make decisions differently than adults do.

If an adolescent who seems reasonably mature refuses transfusion, the clinician is tasked with making a judgment on whether that individual is mature enough to make a decision, based on religious conviction, which could put his or her life in jeopardy. Further, one must consider the degree to which family and community pressure influence the patient's decision. Conversely, medical caregivers should not unduly coerce the patient into acceptance of transfusion against his or her inclination. Further complicating this issue is that not all states recognize the mature minor doctrine. Precedents do exist in which JW minors have been granted the right to refuse transfusion. The Illinois Supreme court ruled in *Illinois vs E.G.* (1989) that E.G., a 17-year-old Jehovah's Witness with leukemia, had the maturity to refuse transfusion. Among those testifying to her maturity was a psychiatrist who specialized in determining maturity and competence in minors. In a 2007 county court case in Mt. Vernon, Washington, a 14-year-old Jehovah's Witness with leukemia was allowed to refuse transfusion; he died shortly after the ruling. This ruling was against his biological parents' wishes but in compliance with his and his legal guardian's.

The concept of informed refusal by mature minors can be applied to non-JW patients as well. The AAP endorses the consideration of refusal while taking into account such factors as the patient's cognitive level, social situation, and presence of chronic disease; all these experiences can impart a greater degree of capacity to make these decisions. When family conflict arises, consultation with services such as palliative care (when appropriate), ethics, and psychiatry is encouraged. Regardless of the decisions made, respect for the patient and family should be communicated.

SUMMARY

1. JW patients generally refuse blood, plasma, and platelets but may accept certain products. All Jehovah's Witnesses do not accept the same products; thus a detailed conversation is warranted in cases where significant blood loss is possible.
2. Children of JW parents can legally be transfused against parental wishes, and this should be communicated clearly and respectfully in advance of elective surgery. Efforts to accomplish surgery and recovery without transfusion should be made.
3. A multidisciplinary approach to perioperative management of the JW pediatric patient can reduce the risk and possibly eliminate the need for transfusion without adversely affecting patient outcome.
4. Tenets of transfusion risk reduction include diagnosis and treatment of anemia and also minimization of blood loss. Preparation should begin 4 to 8 weeks in advance of surgery.
5. Mature JW adolescents who do not wish to receive blood may legally be able to make this decision, although this may vary from state to state. Factors to consider are family and community pressures, cognitive ability, and apparent neurodevelopmental maturity.

REFERENCES

Lacroix J, Tucci M, DuPont-Thibodeau G. Red blood cell transfusion decision making in critically ill children. *Curr Opin Pediatr.* 2015;(27):286–291.

This article discusses whether transfusion status has any impact on length of stay or mortality.

Lason T, Ralph C. Perioperative Jehovah's Witnesses: a review. *Br J Anaesth.* 2015;115(5):676–687.

This article provides a thorough review of the perioperative management of the JW patient.

Resar LMS, Wick EC, Almasri TN, Dackiw EA, Ness PM, Frank SM. Bloodless medicine: current strategies and emerging treatment paradigms. *Transfusion.* 2016;56:2637–2647.

This article discusses a variety of bloodless medicine strategies.

Woolley S. Children of Jehovah's Witnesses and adolescent Jehovah's Witnesses: what are their rights? *Arch Dis Child.* 2005;90:715–719.

This article provides insight into the JW patient's desires for bloodless surgery as well as the ethical and legal ramifications.

BIBLIOGRAPHY

Faraoni D, DiNardo JA, Goobie SM. Relationship between preoperative anemia and in-hospital mortality in children undergoing noncardiac surgery. *Anesth Analg.* 2016;123:1582–1587.

Frank, SM, Wick EC, Dezern AE, et al. Risk adjusted clinical outcomes in patients enrolled in a bloodless program. *Transfusion.* 2014;54:2668–2677.

Katz AL, Webb SA. Informed consent in decision-making in pediatric practice. *Pediatrics.* 2016;138: e20161485.

Ruchika G, Cushing MM, Tobian AAR. Pediatric patient blood management programs: not just transfusing little adults. *Transf Med Rev.* 2016;30:235–241.

Secher EL, Stensballe J, Afshari A. Transfusion in critically ill children: an ongoing dilemma. *Acta Anaesthesiol Scand.* 2013;57:684–691.

Wikkelso A, Wetterslev J, Moller AM, Afshari A. Thromboelastography (TEG) or thromboelastometry (ROTEM) to monitor haemostatic treatment versus usual care in adults or children with bleeding. *Cochrane Database Syst Rev.* 2016;8:CD007871.

70

Organ Donation after Cardiac Death in the Pediatric Patient

CAITLIN D. SUTTON AND DAVID G. MANN

INTRODUCTION

Based on the US Organ Procurement and Transplantation Network Data in 2015, the number of organ transplants performed in the United States exceeded 30,000, representing a 5% increase from the prior year. Despite this, the number of individuals who are actively listed and waiting for an organ transplant remains above 75,000. In 2017 there were over 34,000 organ transplants. This number is ever growing. The need for organ transplantation is great as there are tens of thousands of people awaiting a life-saving organ.

Acceptable organ donation methods in the United States currently include living donation, donation after brain death (DBD), and donation after cardiac death (DCD). While DCD represents approximately 10% of total donors in the United States (8.9% in 2015), the number is expected to continue rising. DCD has been suggested as a possible means of closing the supply to demand gap for transplantable organs.

However, a number of ethical concerns exist surrounding organ procurement through DCD, particularly for pediatric donors. The process of DCD, as well as the various ethical controversies surrounding the practice, are described in this chapter.

LEARNING OBJECTIVES

1. Identify whether a potential donor is eligible for DBD or DCD.
2. Explain the steps that occur in the DCD process, from the decision to withdraw life support to the procurement of organs.
3. Discuss the various ethical controversies surrounding DCD.

CASE PRESENTATION

Annie, a 7-year-old female who was involved in a motor vehicle accident 6 weeks ago, has been in the pediatric intensive care unit (PICU) at your hospital for over a month after being transferred from an outside hospital. She has been intubated and has required full ventilator support since she was admitted. Despite undergoing emergent craniotomy for decompression immediately after the accident, she has unfortunately showed no signs of neurologic improvement. Over the last several days, she has required increasing hemodynamic support with vasopressors; however, the exam for brainstem death has remained unchanged, and Annie has not been declared "brain dead."

The neurosurgery, neurology, and pediatric critical care teams have had weekly meetings with Annie's family to ensure open, ongoing communication. Last week, the critical care team suggested that the palliative care team be involved for ongoing support, and the family accepted this recommendation gratefully. This consultation led to a frank but compassionate conversation about Annie's poor prognosis. Annie's family explained that they understood the prognosis, but they needed a few more days to process all the information. After ongoing discussion and meetings, Annie's doctors and family establish that she will not have a meaningful recovery.

At the end of the following family meeting during which the discontinuation of life support is discussed openly by the team and family, Annie's mother asks if she can bring up a question. She tearfully states how grateful she has been for the support of the PICU team and how helpful the palliative care consultation has been. She then explains that she has also gained a significant amount of support from the other parents she has met in the PICU waiting room and that she has been particularly impacted by a mother whose daughter has just woken up after receiving a liver transplant. She states, "As hard as it is for me to bear if Annie isn't going to make it, I wondered if would she be able to be an organ donor, to help save other children who may still have a chance to recover?"

The critical care and palliative care teams offer emotional support for this difficult decision and contact the local organ procurement organization to discuss the next steps. Over the next few days, arrangements are made. Following the institutional protocol, Annie is taken to the operating room with her family, who is given time to say goodbye. The PICU physician withdraws ventilation support, and, within 3 minutes, Annie is pulseless and the doctor declares cardiopulmonary death. After 5 minutes of pulselessness, a transplant team begins organ procurement. Annie's lungs, liver, pancreas, and kidneys are all successfully recovered and each organ is subsequently transplanted in for 5 separate children.

DISCUSSION

1. What is organ DCD? How does it differ from organ DBD?

Deceased-donor organs come from patients declared legally dead by either neurologic (brain death) or cardiopulmonary (cardiorespiratory death) criteria. Under DCD, critically ill patients who do not meet the neurologic criteria for death are declared dead using the cardiopulmonary criteria. DCD donors are commonly divided into 5 categories, based on the Maastricht classification (Table 70.1). In the ideal, controlled situation, the declaration of death by cardiopulmonary criteria occurs only after life-sustaining support is withdrawn. In the United States, both controlled and uncontrolled DCD occur, but controlled DCD is more common and therefore is the type of DCD discussed in this chapter.

TABLE 70.1. MODIFIED MAASTRICHT CLASSIFICATION OF NON-HEART-BEATING DONORS

Category I	Dead on arrival
Category II	Unsuccessful resuscitation
Category III	Awaiting cardiac arrest*
Category IV	Cardiac arrest in a brainstem dead donor
Category V	Unsuspected cardiac arrest in a critically ill patient

*Category III is considered "controlled" donation after cardiac death.

One key difference between controlled DCD and DBD is the timing of the patient's death relative to the legal decision by the surrogate to pursue organ donation. In DBD, a patient is declared dead by neurologic criteria before the surrogate is offered the opportunity to pursue organ donation. Because these bodies continue to have cardiac function, organs remain perfused while preparations are made for organ donation, including matching organs to recipients and coordinating transplant teams. In DCD, cessation of cardiac function at the time of death leads imminently to organ ischemia. For this reason, controlled DCD requires that the decision for organ donation be made before support is withdrawn and organ ischemia ensures.

2. Who is a potential DCD donor?

DCD is used when surrogates recognize that their loved one will never recover consciousness, even though the patient cannot be declared dead by neurologic criteria. In addition, the family (or surrogate) wishes to achieve a positive outcome through organ donation despite losing their loved one. For controlled DCD, the patient must be on life-sustaining support and should have a high probability of dying shortly after withdrawal of the support. Examples of patients eligible for DCD include those with end-stage musculoskeletal disease or irreversible brain injury which do not meet brain death criteria. In general, a clear definition of death should exist in order for the public to maintain trust in the medical doctor.

3. What does a DCD protocol look like?

See Figure 70.1.

4. What institutional variations exist?

Depending on the existing institutional protocol, support may be withdrawn in the ICU or in operating room. Some centers use extracorporeal membrane oxygenation (ECMO) to decrease warm ischemic time, with large vascular cannulation occurring before withdrawal of support, although ethical controversy surrounds this practice. In these cases, aortic or carotid occlusion balloons are used with ECMO to

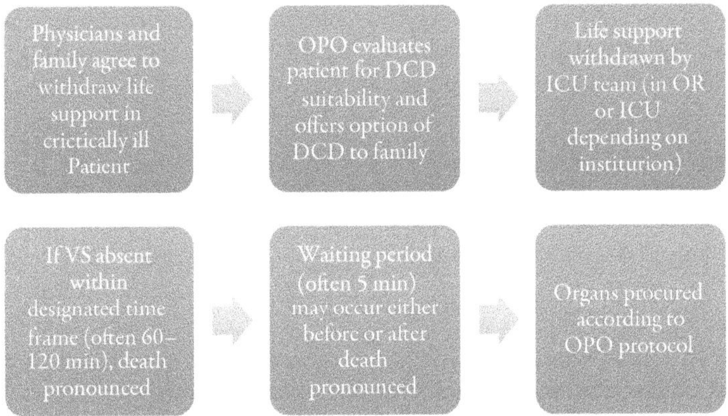

FIGURE 70.1: Sample organ procurement protocol.
OPO, organ procurement organization; DCD, donation after cardiac death; VS, vital signs.

prevent "reanimation" from return of cerebral perfusion. The role of the anesthesiologist here is variable as well and ranges from no involvement to assisting with logistics or, in rare instances, assisting with withdrawal of care. In instances in which the anesthesiologist is involved in withdrawal of care, he or she may not be involved in organ procurement or transplant procedures in order to prevent a conflict of interest.

5. What are the outcomes?

The number of organs recovered per donor is less with DCD donors (mean 2.7 organs per donor) versus standard criteria donors (mean 3.9 organs per donor) and the functional outcomes also vary by organ. Data has shown similar graft survival rates between DCD and DBD donors for kidney and lung transplants, although the incidence of delayed graft function is increased in DCD kidneys. In contrast, there is a higher risk of graft failure in DCD liver transplants, and this is primarily related to increased rates of biliary stricture.

6. What is the anesthesiologists' role in DCD?

The role of the anesthesiologist in DCD is highly variable between institutions. In fact, many transplant center protocols omit any mention of anesthesiologists for DCD. This can lead to confusion and discomfort on the part of the providers, who are less familiar with the operating room environment and equipment. Despite this, anesthesiologists are often asked to participate in some aspect of DCD because of their role as leaders in the operating room environment. This can range from simply assisting with logistics of assigning an operating room to being present to assist with the withdrawal of life-sustaining support. As anesthesiologists are generally not trained in end-of-life care and generally do not have a long-standing relationship with the patient or family members, questions have been raised regarding the appropriateness of their involvement in the withdrawal of support.

To avoid serious conflicts of interest, it is important to ensure that no care provider is involved in both the procurement and transplantation process for a given organ.

7. What are the ethical controversies surrounding DCD?

Current legal standards in the United States require that organ donation adheres to the "dead donor rule." This rule states that any determination of death (whether by neurologic or cardiopulmonary criteria) requires both *cessation of function* and *irreversibility.* The National Conference on Donation after Cardiac Death affirmed DCD as an "ethically acceptable practice of end-of-life care," stating that it does not violate the dead donor rule. Despite this, DCD remains the subject of ethical controversy.

While the principles of beneficence and nonmaleficence are universally agreed to be the foundation of the ethical care of patients, their application in DCD have been argued both to favor the prolongation of life and in support of a patient's wish to donate his or her organs. In addition, many other DCD-related issues have been discussed in the ethics literature. These include the timing of death relative to initiation of organ donation process, adequacy of informed consent for donor family and recipient, and conflict of interest between donor and recipient care. Additionally, some institutional protocols call for specific interventions that remain controversial, such as premortem intervention and the use of ECMO. In particular, the placement of aortic or carotid occlusion balloons to prevent reanimation when ECMO is used calls into question the dead donor rule's requirement that death be irreversible.

8. Do special considerations exist when the donor is a pediatric patient?

Organ donation can offer some solace to families dealing with the death of a child. However, the timing of the decision for organ donation in DCD has caused some to voice concern over the protection of critically ill children. Compared with adults, there is more controversy surrounding pediatric DCD for several reasons (Harrison et al., 2008).

First, there is more uncertainty regarding the neurological prognosis for neurologically devastated children. This is an important consideration, because physicians have less data to help inform families regarding expectations for their child's recovery. Theoretically, the desire to donate an organ could potentially lead to premature withdrawal of life-sustaining support in a pediatric patient who could have otherwise recovered some meaningful brain function.

These concerns are further complicated by the greater difficulty surrounding the informed consent process for DCD in children than in adults. As in other aspects of the care of pediatric patients, a child's ability to voice his or her own preferences varies with development and maturity. Because many children are unable to choose or consent for organ donation on their own behalf, special consideration must be given to organ donation in this vulnerable population.

As discussed in question 7, the application of the principles of beneficence and nonmaleficence could imply either providing life-sustaining support or fulfilling the patient's (or family's) wish to donate his or her organs. In the case of a child, both of these are more complicated: with the prolongation of life, neurological prognosis is uncertain, and the child may not have ever reached a developmental stage in which he or she could express the desire to donate his or her organs. Thus the "substituted judgment" standard is inappropriate, and choices are made using the "best interests" standard; exactly what constitutes the best interests of a child in this setting remains controversial. For these reasons, some advocate only adopting DCD for competent adults and mature or emancipated minors.

SUMMARY

1. As the number of DCD donors continues to rise, pediatric anesthesiologists working in transplant centers may be asked to participate in DCD procurements or transplants.
2. A thorough understanding of the DCD process and anticipation of ethical issues that may arise will be helpful to the pediatric anesthesiologist presented with this situation.

ANNOTATED REFERENCES

Harrison CH, Laussen PC. Controversy and consensus on pediatric donation after cardiac death: ethical issues and institutional processes. *Transplant Proc.* 2008;40(4):1044–1047.

A paper written summarizing the multidisciplinary approach undertaken to resolve controversy surrounding the DCD policy at Boston Children's Hospital.

Statement on Controlled Organ Donation After Circulatory Death Committees of Origin: Critical Care Medicine, Ethics and Transplant Anesthesia (Approved by the ASA House of Delegates on October 25, 2017). http://www.asahq.org/~/media/sites/asahq/files/public/ resources/standards-guidelines/statement-on-controlled-organ-donation-after-circulatory-death.pdf

A statement by the American Society of Anesthesiologists that is intended to serve as a guide for institutions implementing DCD organ procurement and transplantation policies.

Steinbrook R. Organ donation after cardiac death. *N Engl J Med.* 2007;357:209–213.

A concise but clear explanation of DCD, supplemented by historical context of the implementation of DCD in the United States.

Van Norman GA. Another matter of life and death: what every anesthesiologist should know about the ethical, legal, and policy implications of the non-heart-beating cadaver organ donor. *Anesthesiology.* 2003;98:763–773.

A discussion of DCD written for the anesthesiologist.

71

Do-Not-Resuscitate Orders in the Operating Room

CAITLIN D. SUTTON AND DAVID G. MANN

INTRODUCTION

End-of-life care for pediatric patients is complex and presents many challenges. The pediatric anesthesiologist must thoroughly discuss the patient's wishes, concerns and the relevance to the perioperative period. Such an extensive communication requires time but most importantly requires a commitment to executing to the best of one's ability, the desires of the patient. Depending on the nature of the surgery and the patient's condition, various aspects of the do-not-resuscitate (DNR) order may need to be rescinded, continued, or modified for the perioperative period. Adequate communication with the patient and patient's family, the pediatric anesthesiologist and surgeon is necessary to develop an appropriate plan for the patient with DNR orders in the perioperative setting.

LEARNING OBJECTIVES

1. Outline the special implications in the perioperative period, for pediatric patients with standing DNR orders.
2. Discuss the ethical principles relevant to perioperative DNR orders for pediatric patients.
3. Explain the various options for patients with a standing DNR who are scheduled to undergo surgery, highlighting the benefits and challenges of each option.
4. Outline the components of an ideal consent discussion regarding perioperative DNR orders.

CASE PRESENTATION

A 15-year-old boy named Billy has a diagnosis of terminal lymphoma. He is scheduled semi-emergently for the surgical creation of a pericardial window to relieve increasing tamponade physiology. In the preoperative holding area, you find him sitting upright in bed looking uncomfortable, and you note that his SpO_2 is 95% on 10 L non-rebreathing face mask and that his breathing is labored. After introducing yourself to Billy, his father tearfully states, "Before we start I need to tell you, we have signed the form designating him as DNR. He's been through so much and we don't want him to suffer any more, so we don't want him to be intubated or resuscitated."

During the preoperative assessment, you encourage Billy and his dad to talk about why they've elected the DNR designation. His father is adamant "that Billy doesn't want to suffer any more." In fact, he admits, Billy hadn't wanted the last bout of chemotherapy; however, the cancer doctors offered a new and promising drug that was only available under their research protocol. This prompted his father to essentially force Billy to accept the new drug. After starting the treatment, Billy developed supraventricular tachycardia and was "shocked" out of it. Later, as a small fluid collection around his heart continued to grow, he became ineligible to continue treatment under the study protocol. After that whole experience, his father feels tremendous guilt that he now needs a surgically placed drain to remove the fluid from around his heart in order to breathe better during his final days. All of them accept that the end is near.

As you review the DNR order, you note that "no resuscitative drugs may be administered, and aggressive interventions or therapies, including intubation, mechanical ventilation, and CPR are not to be performed."

DISCUSSION

1. Why does a perioperative DNR require special consideration?

There are several compelling reasons that a DNR order in the perioperative period requires special consideration. First, many components of an anesthetic would be considered "resuscitation" in a nonoperative setting. Patients are often unaware of the routine use of intubation and pharmacologic intervention in the operating room (OR). If a strict, procedure-oriented DNR were to be held in place, a standard anesthetic may be either impossible or unsafe to perform (Truog et al., 1999).

Also, DNR orders are typically understood to be related to cardiorespiratory insufficiency or collapse related directly to a patient's disease process. In the perioperative period, events related specifically to anesthesia or surgery can lead to cardiorespiratory derangements that are more readily reversible in most patients. This means that rates of success for resuscitation in the OR are significantly higher, calling into question the "futility" of resuscitation attempts. A systematic review of perioperative cardiopulmonary resuscitation (CPR) revealed a rate of 32.0% to 55.7% survival (approximately 25% survival with favorable neurologic outcome), compared to a less than 15% success rate for out-of-hospital CPR (Kalkman et al., 2016).

Finally, the OR environment is less conducive to some end-of-life preferences, such as family presence and the involvement of critical care or palliative care physicians who are more experienced in end-of-life care and support.

TABLE 71.1. OPTIONS FOR REQUIRED RECONSIDERATION

Principle	Impact on Perioperative DNR Decision-Making
Beneficence	Choosing treatment strategies that are expected to reliably produce an overall balance of goods over harms
Nonmaleficence	Providing care that considers the medical, social, financial, and other possible harms that may result from intervention (or nonintervention)
Autonomy	Selecting care plans that are aligned with the patient's perspectives and preferences, including medical and nonmedical concerns
Surrogacy	Using an alternative decision-maker when the patient does not have capacity due to age, medical condition, etc. Surrogates are generally expected to choose based on substituted judgment (e.g., what the patient would have wanted) in instances where the patient has previously had the ability to determine his or her own preferences.
Assent	Making decisions supported by the patient who is unable to legally give consent (e.g., a 16-year-old patient who can express preferences)

2. What ethical foundational principles are relevant to perioperative DNR orders for the pediatric patient?

In the ethical system of principlism, various principles are used to support the decision-making process. For perioperative DNR discussions, the key principles are beneficence, nonmaleficence, autonomy, and surrogacy/assent. We have listed these principles and their relevance to perioperative DNR orders in Table 71.1.

3. What are the options for patients with DNR when they come to the OR?

Though some hospitals and anesthesiologists incorrectly believe that automatically rescinding DNRs for surgical patients is standard, this is no longer accepted. The American Society of Anesthesiologists, American College of Surgeons, and Association of Operating Room Nurses all have guidelines to support "required reconsideration" of DNR orders in the perioperative period. Only after reconsideration, which involves thorough communication and documentation, would DNR orders be rescinded, continued, or (most commonly) modified. A full DNR is only continued throughout the perioperative period after appropriate, thorough education with the subsequent patient/family choice to maintain the DNR as ordered.

More commonly, the DNR is modified in one of two ways: goal-directed or procedure-directed (Truog et al., 1999). Goal-directed modification of a DNR emphasizes outcomes rather than specific interventions. In goal-directed modifications, patients and family members are less concerned about technical details and more concerned about overall values and preferences. This requires immediate availability of physicians who are intimately aware of the patient's goals. Trust between the patient and team is essential, which requires a relationship and thorough communication. As surgery is a specific, timed event, the perioperative period is often conducive to this sort of communication and relationship-building, but it requires deliberate and thoughtful planning on the part of the providers. Caregivers are often called upon to be flexible in their care plans as the clinical situation changes. Documentation is often performed using narratives, and simple checklists typically would not suffice.

Procedure-directed modification may seem simpler, in that it is amenable to a checklist and interventions are predetermined and specifically defined. However, in the dynamic clinical environment of surgery, procedure-directed modification is often difficult and confusing (e.g., requesting drugs can be administered but declining the chest compressions necessary to circulate those drugs). This type of alteration also places more responsibility on the patients/family to make specific decisions that can be very complex.

Whether goal or procedure directed, any modification to a DNR order requires a specific time frame for when the original DNR comes back into effect. Whether based on a date/time or an event (e.g., 2 hours postoperatively or after transfer from the postanesthesia care unit), this must be specifically determined, communicated, and enacted.

All health care providers including the surgeon, anesthesiologist, and all intraoperative personnel must be aware of decision and have the opportunity to recuse themselves from the care of the patient (with appropriate provider substitution).

4. How should we approach the discussion about perioperative DNR orders?

The involved parties should include the patient, family, surgeon, anesthesiologist, and primary team. Ideally, a discussion should be held between health care providers first, followed by a meeting with the team and patient/family as well as any supportive personnel such as a chaplain.

The meetings should allow ample time for questions, consideration, and discussion. Therefore, it should not occur in the preoperative holding area or on the way to the OR. Ideally, a policy should be enacted whereby the surgeon booking a case for a patient with a DNR triggers a protocol in which the anesthesiologist is notified and a meeting with the stakeholders is scheduled prior to surgery.

In the meeting, the following items should be discussed:

- Patient conditions, prognosis, and expectations separate from the procedure
- Goals of the procedure, including expected and possible outcomes
- Options for care with and without modification of the DNR
- Likelihood of successful resuscitation

The health care provider leading the discussion should emphasize that the primary goal will be to prevent the need for resuscitation and that the discussion is being held so that everyone clearly understands the next steps should resuscitation be required. Once the patient and family have heard this information and have had the opportunity to ask questions, open-ended questions soliciting their goals and preferences should be asked (See Table 71.2).

A discussion of the time frame for the modification should follow the decisions. This must include a discussion of withdrawal of interventions made during the DNR modification (e.g., extubation of a patient who was intubated for surgery but was unable to be extubated due to unforeseen complications). In these cases, the health care team should emphasize that withdrawal is ethically (but rarely emotionally) equivalent to not initiating an intervention.

The team should then summarize the plan to confirm with the family, which will then be documented in the chart. Prior to proceeding to the OR, all perioperative team members must be informed and given the opportunity to recuse themselves from the care of the patient if they so desire, provided that a suitable replacement is found.

CASE RESOLUTION

During your preoperative discussion of anesthetic management, you explain that during the normal course of anesthesia, "resuscitative" drugs are routinely administered to manipulate a patient's heart rate and blood pressure. In essence, it's difficult to safely administer anesthesia without using these drugs when necessary. Billy's father asks him if it would be ok for you to treat him with these drugs, just like any other patient

TABLE 71.2. OBJECTIVES AND DISCUSSION PROMPTS FOR THE ANESTHESIOLOGIST ON PERIOPERATIVE DNR WITH PATIENT AND FAMILIES

Goal: Clarify patient's goals for care.
Example:
"How did you decide to have a DNR?"
"When you made this decision with your pediatrician; what was
important to you?
What are your goals for medical care? What are your goals for this procedure?"
Goal: Discuss the risks of the present anesthetic specific to the patient and the procedure.
Example:
"The anesthetic for this procedure causes breathing to stop. A ventilator and breathing tube are needed. I am concerned that your son will need the ventilator for several hours after the procedure until he can breathe on his own. What are your thoughts about that? Is that consistent with your goals?"
Goal: Consider contingency planning for the unexpected or unlikely.
Example:
"If his heart were to stop in the operating room during the procedure, we could start CPR with chest compressions and give medications to restart the heart. In my judgment, it is unlikely that his heart would restart. We should talk about how we should handle that if it occurs."

under anesthesia. He nods in agreement and says, "The drugs are okay, but no CPR." Acknowledging his concern, you explain that a drug administered through the intravenous line in Billy's wrist can't work unless it gets to his heart, which requires blood circulation, and sometimes the only way to circulate the blood is to perform chest compressions. His father looks surprised and says that "nobody's ever explained it like that before." Looking at Billy, you ask if CPR for this purpose would be okay with him. Billy again nods his assent but adamantly states that he does not want any "shocks." After a clear discussion of the risk and implications of this, you all mutually agree that given the trauma Billy experienced during his previous cardioversion and his strong stance against receiving another shock even if he is anesthetized, you will not "shock" Billy under any circumstance, even if not doing so means allowing him to die.

Noting the "no intubation or mechanical ventilation" provision of the DNR, you tell Billy and his dad that for this procedure you do not plan to place a breathing tube; however, if the drug that he needs is oxygen, an efficient way to deliver it is through a breathing tube. His father replies that they don't want Billy to spend his final days on a breathing machine. You point out that placing a breathing tube does not have to be permanent. If treatment with the breathing tube is not achieving the therapeutic goal, it can be removed. His father says that a nurse told them "it's better not to start a treatment because once it's started, it can't be stopped." Based on this information, they don't want to put him on a breathing machine because she told them that "he'd never get off it." You agree that there is a lot of "folklore" about how it's illegal or unethical to stop a treatment once it's been started; however, the "folklore" is just that, "folklore," and you explain that it's neither illegal nor unethical to stop a treatment that is inconsistent with the therapeutic goal. You suggest an alternative to them: if intubating Billy is appropriate, they could agree to permit it for a predetermined "trial period," perhaps 24 hours. In other words, the breathing tube would be removed after 24 hours because at that point it would be inconsistent with the therapeutic goals for Billy. Appearing to trust you, they agree to allow Billy to be intubated in the OR with a 24 hour "therapeutic trial."

In the OR, Billy receives ketamine, and remains spontaneously breathing with a natural airway, while the surgeon creates a pericardial window. As the dressing is being placed, Billy's heart rate acutely increases from 88 bpm to 190 bpm, and you note a narrow-complex QRS on the electrocardiogram monitor. You check a noninvasive blood pressure (NIBP) which is 118/58; it had previously been stable at 145/90. You direct the anesthesia fellow to perform carotid massage while you reach for adenosine. Following the carotid massage maneuver, the NIBP is 78/42. Following the adenosine, a sinus rhythm is re-established at a rate of 79 bpm and the NIBP reads 128/68. However, almost immediately the heart rate returns to the 190s, again with a narrow-complex QRS, and the next NIBP is not measurable. Despite your best efforts (without administering electrical cardioversion), a perfusing rhythm is never re-established and Billy dies.

After informing Billy's father of his death, and the events leading up to it, you sit quietly with him as he cries. A few minutes later, he shakes your hand and thanks you for respecting Billy's humanity and acting according to his wishes.

SUMMARY

1. Patients with a standing DNR order who are to undergo surgery may present many challenges to the anesthesiologist.
2. Using ethical principles as a foundation, the DNR should ideally be modified in a goal-oriented manner with a clearly defined timeline, and all team members must be aware of the modification.
3. Providing the patient and family with information and allowing the parents to play an active role in the decision-making process is preferred (de Vos et al., 2015). Proactive, thoughtful communication on the part of the anesthesiologist facilitates optimal care of the patient with a standing DNR.

ACKNOLWEDGMENTS

The authors wish to acknowledge the first edition authors, Mark J. Meyer and Norbert J. Weidner.

ANNOTATED REFERENCES

de Vos MA, Bos AP, Plotz FB, et al. Talking with parents about end-of-life decisions for their children. *Pediatrics*. 2015;135(2):e465–e476.

This article uses information obtained from a Dutch survey to show that parents may be able to have a more active role in end-of-life decision-making than they are often given. It provides insight from the parents' perspective that can be useful in these difficult situations.

Kalkman S, Hooft L, Meirjerman JM, et al. Survival after perioperative cardiopulmonary resuscitation: providing an evidence base for ethical management of do-not-resuscitate orders. *Anesthesiology*. 2016;124:723–729.

This article discusses the fact that the survival rate after perioperative CPR is twice as high compared to other settings; thus such a difference warrants reconsideration of DNR orders in this setting.

Truog R, Waisel D, Burns J. DNR in the OR: a goal-directed approach. *Anesthesiology*. 1999;90(1):289–295.

This article provides a thorough discussion of goal-directed modifications of DNR orders.

FURTHER READING

Campise-Luther RJ, Diaz CD. Pediatric patients: do not resuscitate decisions. In: Jericho B, ed. *Ethical Issues in Anesthesiology and Surgery*. Cham, Switzerland: Springer; 2015:59–66.

Fallat ME, Deshpande JK. Do-not-resuscitate orders for pediatric patients who require anesthesia and surgery. *Pediatrics*. 2004;114(6):1686–1692.

Michelson KN, Frader JE. Do not resuscitate decisions in pediatric patients. In: *Clinical Ethics in Anesthesiology: A Case-Based Textbook*. Cambridge, UK: Cambridge University Press; 2011:39–43.

Sumrall WD, Mahanna E, Sabharwal V, Marshall T. Do not resuscitate, anesthesia, and perioperative care: a not so clear order. *Oschner J*. 2016;16:176–179.

INDEX

Page numbers followed by *f* and *t* indicate figures and tables, respectively. Numbers followed by b indicate boxes.

www.ingramcontent.com/pod-product-compliance
Ingram Content Group UK Ltd.
Pitfield, Milton Keynes, MK11 3LW, UK
UKHW051131260726
13967UKWH00010B/2984

9 780190 678333